Transfusion Microbiology

Transfusion Microbiology

Edited by

Professor John A. J. Barbara, MA (Cantab), MSc, PhD, FIBiol, FRCPath

Formerly Head of National Transfusion Microbiology Laboratories, National Blood Service, UK
Emeritus Consultant in Microbiology to NHS Blood and Transplant
Visiting Professor in Transfusion Microbiology, University of the West of England, Bristol, UK

Dr Fiona A. M. Regan

NHSBT and Hammersmith Hospitals NHS Trust, London, UK

Professor Dame Marcela Contreras, MD, FRCPath, FRCP, FMedSci, DBE

Royal Free and University College Hospitals Medical School, London, UK
Formerly Director of Diagnostics, Development and Research, National Blood Service, UK

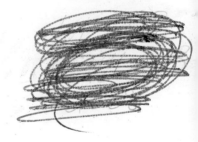

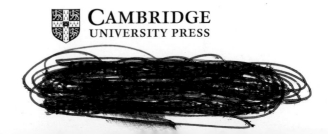

CAMBRIDGE
UNIVERSITY PRESS

CAMBRIDGE UNIVERSITY PRESS
Cambridge, New York, Melbourne, Madrid, Cape Town, Singapore, São Paulo, Delhi

Cambridge University Press
The Edinburgh Building, Cambridge CB2 8RU, UK

Published in the United States of America by Cambridge University Press, New York

www.cambridge.org
Information on this title: www. cambridge.org/9780521453936

First published 2008

Printed in the United Kingdom at the University Press, Cambridge

A catalogue record for this publication is available from the British Library

Library of Congress Cataloguing in Publication Data

Transfusion microbiology / edited by John A. Barbara, Fiona A. M. Regan, Dame Marcela C. Contreras.
   p. ; cm.
Includes bibliographical references and index.
ISBN 978-0-521-45393-6 (hardback)
1. Bloodborne infections.   2. Blood–Transfusion–Complications.
I. Barbara, John A. J.   II. Regan, Fiona A. M.   III. Contreras, Marcela.
[DNLM: 1. Blood Transfusion–adverse effects.   2. Blood-Borne Pathogens.
3. Disease Transmission–prevention & control.   4. Infection Control–methods. WB 356 T77291 2008]
RA642.B56T73 2008
615'.39–dc22

                                                                                     2008006740

ISBN 978-0-521-45393-6 hardback

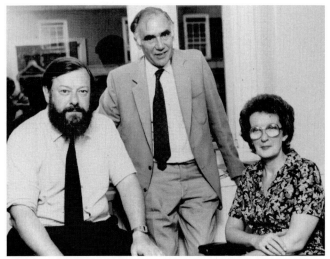

Dr Colin Cameron
Dr David Dane
Moya Briggs

This book is dedicated to the memory of Dr David Dane and Dr Colin Cameron who, together with Moya Briggs, in 1970, identified the infectious agent of hepatitis B and who for the next two decades worked to advance all aspects of transfusion microbiology.

CONTENTS

Contents

CONTRIBUTORS

Jean-Pierre Allain, MD, PhD, FRCPath, AcMedSc
Department of Haematology
The Division of Transfusion Medicine
Cambridge Blood Centre
Cambridge, UK

David J. Anstee, PhD, FRCPath, FMedSci
Bristol Institute for Transfusion Sciences
NHS Blood and Transplant
Bristol, UK

Yasmin Ayob, MD
National Blood Centre
Kuala Lumpur, Malaysia

John A. J. Barbara, MA, MSc, PhD, FIBiol, FRCPath
Emeritus Consultant in Microbiology to NHS Blood and
Transplant and Visiting Professor in Transfusion Microbiology
University of the West of England
Bristol, UK

Carol Bienek, BSc, PhD
Protein Fractionation Centre
Scottish National Blood Transfusion Service
Edinburgh, UK

M. A. Blajchman, MD, FRCP(c)
Canadian Blood Services and McMaster University
Hamilton, Ontario, Canada

Kevin E. Brown, MD
Consultant Medical Virologist
Unit Head, Immunisation and Diagnosis
Virus Reference Department
Centre for Infections
Health Protection Agency
London, UK

Moira Bruce, PhD
Institute for Animal Health
Neuropathogenesis Unit
Edinburgh, UK

Michael P. Busch, MD, PhD
Director, Blood Systems Research Institute
Vice President Research and Scientific Programs
Blood Systems, Inc. and Professor of Laboratory Medicine
University of California, USA

Rebecca Cardigan, PhD
Head of Components Development
NHS Blood and Transplant Cambridge
Cambridge, UK

Katy Davison, MSc
Scientist (Epidemiology)
Immunization Department
Health Protection Agency
Centre for Infections
Colindale, London, UK

Roger Y. Dodd, PhD
Vice President, Research and Development
American Red Cross
Holland Laboratory
Rockville, MD, USA

Brian C. Dow, BSc, PhD, CSci, FIBMS
Consultant Clinical Microbiologist
Head, Scottish National Blood Transfusion Service
National Microbiology Reference Unit
West of Scotland Transfusion Centre
Glasgow, UK

Denis M. Dwyre, MD
Assistant Professor, Department of Pathology
University of California Davis Medical Center
Sacramento, CA, USA

Roger Eglin, BSc, MSc, PhD
Head, National Transfusion Laboratories
NHS Blood and Transplant
Colindale, London, UK

Eberhard W. Fiebig, MD
Associate Professor/Vice Chair
UCSF Department of Laboratory Medicine
Chief, Laboratory Medicine Service
San Francisco General Hospital
San Francisco, California, USA

Peter R. Foster, BSc, MSc, PhD, CS, CSci, CEng, FIChemE
Protein Fractionation Centre
Scottish National Blood Transfusion Service
Edinburgh, UK

Paul R. Grant, PhD
Head of Molecular Diagnostics
Department of Virology
University College London Hospitals
London, UK

Helen Harris, BSc, PhD
Clinical Scientist, Epidemiology Research Associate
Immunization Department
Health Protection Agency, Centre for Infections
Colindale, London, UK

Patricia E. Hewitt, FRCP, FRCPath
Consultant Specialist in Transfusion Microbiology
NHS Blood and Transplant,
Colindale, London, UK

Paul V. Holland, MD
Clinical Professor of Medicine and Pathology
University of California,
Davis Medical Center Sacramento, CA, USA
and Scientific Director, Delta Blood Bank
Stockton, CA, USA

James W. Ironside, CBE, FRCPath, FRCPEdin, FMedSci, FRSA
Professor of Clinical Neuropathology
National CJD Surveillance Unit
University of Edinburgh
Western General Hospital
Edinburgh, UK

Virge James, BM, BCh, MA, DM, FRCPath
NHS Blood and Transplant
Sheffield, UK

Alan D. Kitchen, PhD
Head, National Transfusion Microbiology
Reference Laboratory
NHS Blood and Transplant
Colindale, London, UK

David A. Leiby, PhD
Chief of Parasitology
American Red Cross Holland Laboratory
Rockville, MD, USA

Elizabeth M. Love, MB, ChB, FRCP, FRCPath
Consultant Haematologist (Transfusion Medicine)
Lead Clinician for Blood and Tissues Safety Assurance
NHS Blood and Transplant
Manchester Blood Centre and Central Manchester and
Manchester Children's Hospitals University NHS Trust
Manchester, UK

Carl P. McDonald, BSc, MSc, PhD
Head of Bacteriology
NHS Blood and Transplant
Colindale, London, UK

Gary Mallinson, BSc, PhD
Bristol Institute for Transfusion Sciences
NHS Blood and Transplant
Bristol, UK

Chris Moore, BSc, MBBS
Associate Specialist in Transfusion Microbiology
c/o NHS Blood and Transplant Colindale
Colindale, London, UK

Joan O'Riordan, MCRP, FRCPath
Consultant Haematologist
Irish Blood Transfusion Service
National Blood Centre
Dublin, Ireland

Arturo Pereira, MD, PhD
Service of Hemotherapy and Haemostasis
Hospital Clinic
Barcelona, Spain

Juraj Petrik, PhD
Head, Microbiology Research and Development
Scottish National Blood Transfusion Service
TTI Department
Royal (Dick) Veterinary College
Edinburgh, UK

Chris Prowse, MA, DPhil, FRCPath
Research Director
National Science Laboratory
Scottish National Blood Transfusion Service
Edinburgh, UK

Peter D. Rogan, MPhil, BA FIBMS
NHS Blood and Transplant
Manchester, UK

W. Kurt Roth, MD
Professor of Medicine, CEO
GFE Blut mbH,
Altenhoeferallee 3,
Frankfurt am Main, Germany

Kate Soldan, BA, MSc, PhD
Epidemiologist, HIV/STI Department
Health Protection Agency
Centre for Infections
Colindale, London, UK

Susan L. Stramer, PhD
Executive Scientific Officer
American Red Cross
Gaithersburg, MD, USA

Richard S. Tedder, MA, MB, BChir, FRCP, FRCPath
Professor of Medical Virology
Centre for Virology
University College London Hospitals NHS Trust
London, UK

Gary E. Tegtmeier, PhD
Community Blood Center of Greater Kansas City
Kansas City
Missouri, USA

Marc L. Turner, MB, ChB, MBA, PhD, FRCP, FRCPath
Professor of Cellular Therapy
University of Edinburgh
Clinical Director/Consultant Haematologist
Edinburgh and S.E. Scotland Blood Transfusion Centre
Royal Infirmary of Edinburgh
Edinburgh, Scotland

Eleftherios C. Vamvakas, MD, PhD
University of Ottowa Faculty of Medicine
Department of Pathology and Laboratory Medicine
Ottawa, ON, Canada

Elizabeth Vinelli, MD
Programa Nacional de Sangre
Comayaguela, Honduras

Silvano Wendel, MD, PhD
Medical Director, Blood Bank
Hospital Sírio Libanês
São Paulo, Brazil

Lorna M. Williamson, BSc, MD, FRCP, FRCPath
Reader in Transfusion Medicine, University of Cambridge
Medical Director
NHS Blood and Transplant
Cambridge, UK

FOREWORD

Microbiology has been intertwined with transfusion medicine from the outset. It was not long after the development of transfusion as we know it, that viral hepatitis was recognized as an inevitable and largely intractable complication of transfusion. More than fifty years later, we are almost in control of this, and other transfusion-transmissible viruses, but we are, in common with others, facing the unexpected problems of emerging infections. Human immunodeficiency virus, the first of these, was, and still is, an enormous human tragedy. As such, it taught us that blood safety must be managed by action, not words. Further unpredictable challenges have appeared and will continue to beset us. In 1950, who could have dreamed that artificial changes in the way that cattle are fed would result in a crisis in the perception of transfusion safety? Even in 2001, we did not predict the impact of West Nile virus on blood safety – in part because experience had told us that acute infections were rarely transmitted by transfusion.

John Barbara, one of the editors of this book, coined the term 'transfusion microbiology', which turns out to be a discipline much greater than the sum of its parts. Managing the risk of transfusion-transmitted infection involves knowledge of a wide range of pathogens, of their pathology and epidemiology, and of the strange interface between human infection, risk behaviour, truthfulness and motivation. Furthermore, the practitioner of transfusion microbiology must have a grip on the finer points of laboratory detection of infection and infectivity, and of the unfamiliar disciplines of quality systems and regulatory scrutiny. Also, a working knowledge of transfusion medicine and of the immune status of transfused patients are needed. Constant surveillance of information about seemingly unconnected infectious diseases is also required.

Undoubtedly, these and other fields of science contribute to transfusion microbiology, but it is not a one-way street. The need to maintain transfusion safety has stimulated excellence in the development of sensitive and accurate screening assays, but it has also directly provoked extraordinary achievements, such as the collaboration of transfusion scientists and molecular biologists that led to the characterization of hepatitis C virus. This was the very first virus to be fully characterized solely from its genomic sequence. It does not take much thought to recognize many such examples of the contributions of transfusion-based studies to our understanding of pathogens.

This wonderful book covers all of these issues, and many more, in extraordinary detail, from the familiar agents of the past, such as hepatitis B virus, to the bizarre world of prions. Means to control the safety and quality of blood are fully covered, from donor selection and testing to haemovigilance. Quality, regulation and risk assessment are equally well managed. The careful reader of this book may, or may not, become a fully-fledged transfusion microbiologist, but will certainly gain a full appreciation of the field and will have learned from the best of experts.

I have reserved my final comment for the final chapter. I suspect that most readers of this book will live and work in a developed country where disproportionate resources are directed towards reducing transfusion risks to immeasurably low levels. We must also stop and consider the toll on human life that is exacted by the inadequate levels of blood safety that are available to the inhabitants of the developing world. Let us all work to ameliorate this, the biggest of blood safety problems.

Roger Y. Dodd

PREFACE

Prior to the early 1970s infections transmitted by transfusion were relatively common. In developed countries the introduction of routine screening for hepatitis B virus infection marked the beginning of the recognition, and implementation of systematic measures to reduce the risk from transmission, of viruses by blood transfusion. Currently, extensive measures are taken in many countries to ensure that blood transfusion poses a minimal microbiological hazard to recipients. Continual refinements to donor selection criteria, microbiological testing, technologies, processes such as leucodepletion, viral inactivation and associated quality management systems seek to improve the safety even further, yet there is a diminishing safety yield for ever escalating costs with each new intervention. In less affluent countries, the level of risk from transfusion-transmitted infections is often undetermined and there is a chronic insufficiency of blood donors. The few donors available may well be non-voluntary and this adds to the potential risk from transfusion infections. Fortunately, progress is being made in several regions in establishing voluntary, non-remunerated, blood donor panels. So what does the future hold in the field of transfusion microbiology?

Inevitably, 'new' infectious agents will emerge that are potentially pathogenic, which will have to be assessed in terms of the degree of risk to recipients of blood. The way in which these risks are addressed will continue to evolve. Available options for prevention of transmission will have to be assessed not only in terms of efficacy but also in terms of cost-effectiveness and, in many countries, prioritized against other demands for health care resources. Expectations from the public and the media of infectious risks of blood transfusion will always play a part in decision making and these perceptions of risk themselves may also have to be addressed. Ultimately, decisions regarding the introduction of new 'safety' measures for the blood supply will be taken by the political powers who will be governed by the precautionary principle and the fear of litigation.

John A. J. Barbara
Fiona A. M. Regan
Marcela Contreras

ACKNOWLEDGEMENTS

The editors would like to express their gratitude for the tremendous secretarial support over the duration of this endeavour, particularly to Tahera Lakha, Carmel McGinn, Marina Mobed and Faye Fisher; without their help this book would have never been completed.

We would also like to thank many of our colleagues for their input in a reviewing capacity, with particular thanks to Dr Alan Kitchen, Dr Roger Eglin and Dr Brian Dow for their extensive support with this project.

In addition to our very patient and hardworking contributors to the chapters, we would also like to thank Dr Cees L. van der Poel and Dr David Howell for their advice.

Professor John A. J. Barbara, Dr Fiona Regan and
Professor Marcela Contreras

GLOSSARY

Abbreviations for major viruses are included in this glossary. Other viruses will be covered in individual chapters.

AIDS	Acquired immunodeficiency syndrome	IBCT	Incorrect blood component transfused
ALT	Alanine aminotransferase	IHA	Indirect haemagglutination assay
Anti-HBc	Antibody to hepatitis B core antigen	IVIg	Intravenous immunoglobulin
Anti-HBe	Antibody to hepatitis e antigen	IVDU	Intravenous drug user
Anti-HBs	Antibody to hepatitis B surface antigen	LCR	Ligase chain reaction
AST	Aspartate aminotranferase	LD	Leucodepletion
ATL	Adult T-cell leukaemia and lymphoma	LDH	Lactate dehydrogenase
ATR	Acute transfusion reaction (within 24 hours)	MCD	Multicentre Castleman's disease
BCBL	Body cavity based lymphoma	MHRA	Medicines and Healthcare Products Regulatory Agency
B19V	Parvovirus B19		
bDNA	Branched DNA signal amplification assay	NANBH	Non-A, non-B hepatitis
CARD	Catalyzed reporter deposition	NASBA	Nucleic acid sequence based amplification
CIE	Counter immune electropheresis	NAT	Nucleic acid testing
CCD	Charge coupled device camera	NBS	National Blood Service, England and N. Wales
CHIKV	Chikungunya fever virus	NIBSC	National Institute for Biological Standards and Control
CJD	Creutzfeld-Jakob disease		
CMV	Cytomegalovirus	PBMC	Peripheral blood monocyte cells
CPMP	Committee for Proprietary Medicinal Products	PCC	Prothrombin complex concentrate
		PCR	Polymerase chain reaction
DALy	Disability adjusted life year	PI/PR	Pathogen inactivation/pathogen reduction
DID	Double immune diffusion	POEMS	Polyneuropathy, organomegaly, endocrinopathy, M protein and skin changes
DTR	Delayed transfusion reaction (beyond 24 hours)		
EC	European Commission	PrP	Prion protein
EIA	Enzyme linked immunosorbent assay	PTP	Post-transfusion purpura
EMEA	European Medicines (evaluation) Agency	PRCA	Pure red cell aplasia
EQAS	External quality assurance system	QA	Quality assurance
EU	European Union	QC	Quality control
FDA	Food and Drugs Agency	QALY	Quality adjusted life year
FFP	Fresh frozen plasma	RCA	Rolling circle amplification
GBV-C/HGV	GB virus-C/Hepatitis G virus	RPHA	Reverse passive haemagglutination assay
GMP	Good manufacturing practice	RIBA	Recombinant immunoblot assay
HAM	HTLV-I associated myelopathy	RLS	Resonance light scatter
HAV	Hepatitis A virus	RPR	Rapid plasma reagin test
HBeAg	Hepatitis B e antigen	SACTTI	Standing Advisory Committee on Transfusion Transmitted Infection
HBsAg	Hepatitis B surface antigen		
HBV	Hepatitis B virus	SARS	Severe acute respiratory syndrome
HCC	Hepatocellular carcinoma	SD	Solvent detergent
HCV	Hepatitis C virus	SEN-V	SEN virus
HDV	Hepatitis D virus	SFV	Simian foamy virus
HEV	Hepatitis E virus	SHOT	Serious hazards of transfusion
HHV8	Human herpes virus 8	SNP	Single nucleic acid polymorphisms
HIV	Human immunodeficiency virus	SNBTS	Scottish National Blood Transfusion Service
HPA	Health Protection Agency	SPC	Statistical process control
HRP	Horseradish peroxidase	SPM	Statistical process monitoring
HSV	Herpes simplex virus	SPR	Surface plasmon resonance
HTLV	Human T-cell lymphotropic virus	TAC	Transient aplastic crisis

TACO	Transfusion-associated circulatory overload		TSA	Tyramide signal amplification
TA-GVHD	Transfusion-associated graft versus host disease		TSP	Tropical spastic paraparesis
			TTI	Transfusion transmitted infection
			TTV	TT virus
TMA	Transcription mediated amplification		vCJD	Variant Creutzfeld-Jakob disease
TPHA	*Treponema pallidum* haemagglutination assay		VDRL	Venereal diseases research laboratory
			VZV	(Herpes) varicella-zoster virus
TPPA	*Treponema pallidum* particle agglutination assay		WHO	World Health Organization
			WNV	West Nile virus
TRALI	Transfusion related acute lung injury		WP	Window period (of an infection)

INTRODUCTION: TRANSFUSION-TRANSMITTED INFECTIONS, THEN AND NOW

John A. J. Barbara and Roger Eglin

In 1983, a small textbook was published entitled *Microbiology in Blood Transfusion* (Barbara, 1983).

At the beginning of this book the characteristics of microbial agents that might predispose them to the potential for transmission by transfusion were explored. Some of the characteristics identified included:

- Presence of the agent in one or more of the constituent components of blood
- Propensity for causing asymptomatic (sub-acute) infections
- Protracted incubation period to the development of symptoms
- A long-term carrier state of expressed microbial components (e.g. HBsAg in the case of hepatitis B virus)
- A long-term latency of the agent via incorporation of the microbial nucleic acid into the white cells of the infected host. The microbial nucleic acid could reactivate to initiate infection in the recipient of a transfusion from an infected donor.

In any table of transfusion-transmissible infections (TTIs) summarizing the situation at that time, the predominant microbial agents featured would typically be persistent rather than acute. More recently, the risk (actual or potential) from acute infections, especially in situations of high incidence and attack rates in a population, has also become a significant issue. The epidemic of West Nile fever virus (WNV, see Chapters 6 and 15) is a very good example of this. A summary of the currently clinically significant TTIs is shown in Table 1. These agents will all be covered in detail throughout the ensuing chapters. Chapter 6 also considers the potential risks from 'new' or newly recognized agents.

In the 1983 book, the newly recognized acquired immune deficiency syndrome featured in a small paragraph, with the observation that the associated level of risk to transfusion recipients remained to be determined. Subsequently, as the tragic outcome of transfusion-transmitted HIV infections gradually became all too clear, the scope of transfusion microbiology changed irrevocably. Risk analysis (see Chapter 26), quality aspects (see Chapter 17) and regulatory control (see Chapter 27) became increasingly prominent. The transfusion risks from WNV in North America and vCJD in the UK clearly demonstrate that the potential risks of transfusion infection demand careful and continuing monitoring and surveillance.

As a result of the above, increasingly sophisticated analyses and assessments of potential microbial threats to the safety of transfused blood have been developed. The following is an approach used by the UK Standing Advisory Committee on Transfusion Transmitted Infection (SACTTI) to assess the risk of potentially transfusion-transmissible agents (see Table 2). It was developed by Dr Roger Eglin, together with Professor Peter Simmonds, based on an original analysis by Dr Brian McClelland. It is summarized with the permission of Dr P Hewitt, chair UK SACTTI. The analysis is considered in several sections. In many instances, several questions may not have clear answers, or estimates (for example the duration of viraemia following certain infections) may have to be used. Gathering of data and extensive review of the literature is a crucial requirement. Even then, the analysis is more qualitative than quantitative: but even if it only generates a comprehensive checklist of the available data relevant to transfusion risk for a given agent, the often difficult decisions for managing possible risk will at least be better informed.

The development of risk analysis methodology (Chapter 26) together with improvements in standardization, enhanced quality measures (see Chapter 17) and increasing regulatory control (see Chapter 27) has led to the consistency of both current microbiology testing and assessment of new and emerging agents within a standardized framework. Evidence of the latter is seen in the Blood Services' reaction to the transfusion risks presented by the emergence of WNV in North America and vCJD in the UK. In addition, the continuing requirement for careful and continuing monitoring and surveillance of the potential risks of infection by transfusion is clearly demonstrated.

The information is collated in individual templates and then used to complete Table 3 'Characteristics of New/Emerging Infectious Agents'. This Appendix also includes estimates of risk and cost effectiveness. Key entries into Table 3 automatically transfer into Table 4, which comprises levels 0 to 4, with level 0 equating to 'no action required for donors but continue surveillance' to level 4 equating to 'priority action required', for example HIV. The level is determined by the extent to which the entry 'yes' extends towards the bottom of this table.

This sort of analysis can be applied to any newly recognized potential risk to the blood supply. Risk levels and a detailed checklist of possible interventions will then be readily available as a basis for informed decision making by blood services. Typical recent examples of agents that are being monitored by blood services as potential TTIs are simian foamy virus (SFV) and Chikungunya fever virus (CHIKV). Because cases of SFV transmission from infected chimpanzees to humans in contact with them have been reported (see Khan and Kumar, 2006, for detailed references), blood transfusion experiments from infected to uninfected macaques have shown that SFV can be transmitted by transfusion of blood (see Khan and Kumar, 2006). With CHIKV, the concern is that because infections have reached epidemic levels in parts of India and islands in the Indian Ocean since 2005, and viraemia can be demonstrated in symptomatic cases, there may be a potential transfusion risk from pre-symptomatic

Transfusion Microbiology, eds John A. J. Barbara, Fiona A. M. Regan and Marcela C. Contreras. Published by Cambridge University Press. © Cambridge University Press 2008.

Table 1 Clinically significant transfusion transmissible infections.

Parasitic protozoa

  Malaria (*Plasmodium falciparum, P. vivax, P. malariae, P. ovale*)

  Chagas' disease (*Trypanosoma cruzi*)

  Nantucket fever (North America, *Babesia microti*)

  Toxoplasmosis (rare, *Toxoplasma gondii*)

  Leishmaniasis (rare, *Leishmania donovani*)

Bacteria (and endotoxins): no fungal transmissions reported

  Endogenous ('infection')

  Exogenous ('contamination')

Viruses

  Hepatitis viruses A[a], B, C, D and E

  Herpes viruses (EBV, CMV, HHV8)

  Retroviruses: HIV1, HIV2

             HTLV I, HTLV II

  Parvovirus B19 (human erythrovirus)[a]

  West Nile fever virus (WNV)[a]

  Colorado tick fever virus (rare, transmitted as a 'passenger' in red cells)

Prions

  Variant Creutzfelt-Jakob disease (vCJD)

[a] Agents that transmit only in the acute (non-persistent) phase of infections.

Several 'novel' viruses cloned from recipients suffering from post-transfusion hepatitis (GB-virus C – sometimes inaccurately referred to as hepatitis G virus, TT-virus (TTV) and SEN virus) have fortunately proven to be non-pathogenic, that is, not the causes of post-transfusion hepatitis in the recipients.

Table 2 Information on agent epidemiology, pathogenicity and transmissibility by transfusion

(1) Agent category
   (a) Emerging (increasing prevalence in donors).
   (b) Pre-existing (already present in donors).
   (c) Potentially present (frequency of infection in donors unknown).
   (d) Newly discovered.
(2) Pathogenicity of infectious agent
   (a) Known disease associations in humans.
   (b) Availability of disease prevention and/or treatment.
   (c) Influence of transfusion route of infection on disease outcome.
(3) Frequency and dynamics of infection in blood donors
   (a) Frequency of infection, seasonal variation.
   (b) Existence of identifiable risk factors in donors.
   (c) Duration of infectious stage.
   (d) Relationship between viraemia/bacteraemia and identifiable symptoms or signs that may lead to donor deferral.
   (e) Prevalence and incidence in donors.
   (f) Frequency of persistence or re-occurrence of infection in donors.
(4) Identifiable risk groups (recipients)
   (a) Frequency of individuals with generalized increased risk of infection and/or disease (e.g. immunosuppressed individuals).
   (b) Their representation amongst blood recipients.
   (c) Availability of methods to identify individuals specifically susceptible or resistant to infection (tests for detection of past exposure and/or immunity).
   (d) Identification of individuals specifically at risk of development of disease.
(5) Transfusion-transmissibility
   (a) Presence and concentration of infectious agent in each blood component (plasma, buffy coat, red cells and platelets).
   (b) Evidence that disease has been transmitted by transfusion.
   (c) Availability of information on relationship between the concentration of the agent in the blood and transmissibility.
   (d) Frequency of susceptibility to infection in recipients (e.g. immunity arising from past infection).
   (e) Occurrence of reinfection in already infected individuals; impact on existing disease occurrence.
   (f) Possibility of secondary spread of transfused agent to contacts of infected recipient. If yes, is this a common or a rare event (i.e. how many times, over what time period, in what at risk population, has disease transmission by transfusion been reliably reported)?

Existence of preventive, inactivation or removal steps for the infectious agent

(1) Exclusion of infected donors
   (a) Existence of specific risk factors for infection in donors.
   (b) Existence of serological or NAT-based assays that could be used to identify infected donors before donation processing or release for transfusion.
   (c) Compatibility of candidate assays with existing screening methods.
   (d) Availability of information on the effectiveness of proposed donor screening test.
   (e) Sensitivity and specificity of assays for detection of infection.
   (f) Impact of testing in the reduction or elimination of transfusion-transmitted infections and occurrence of disease.
(2) Modification of blood collection and storage
   (a) Methods for prevention of skin contamination of blood (e.g. enhanced skin cleansing, discarding of initial few ml of blood collected).
   (b) Prevention of bacterial growth during red cell and platelet storage.
   (c) Monitoring of bacterial contamination during storage.
   (d) Interception of bacterially contaminated units before transfusion.
(3) Infectious agent removal during blood product processing
   (a) Availability of information on susceptibility of infectious agent to inactivation procedure.
   (b) Previously collected evidence for the specific agent.
   (c) Data for closely related agents with similar predicted physicochemical properties.
   (d) Likely effectiveness of inactivation in 'worst case' scenario, where agent properties are unknown and/or unpredictable.
   (e) Existence of evidence for the effectiveness of conventional blood product inactivation procedures to remove infectivity in fractionated blood products (e.g. dry heat).
   (f) Information on agent size and likelihood of removal by nanofiltration.

Table 2 (cont.)

(g) Scope for modification of blood product/component inactivation procedures to specifically inactivate infectious agent.

(h) Impact of the introduction of modified inactivation procedures on the manufacturing process and quality/activity of blood products.

(4) Infectious agent removal during blood component processing

(a) Information on cell types infected by the infectious agent.

(b) Effectiveness of agent removal by leucodepletion.

(c) Proportion of agent removed.

(d) Reduction in infectivity of blood component.

(e) Residual infectivity in washed red cells.

(f) Demonstrated or predicted efficacy of inactivation methods proposed for platelets and red cells.

(g) Impact of the above processes on the quality, activity and effectiveness of blood components, for example the loss of red cells during leucodepletion or the reduction in activity of platelets after certain pathogen inactivation procedures.

(5) Recipient assessment

(a) Scope for introduction of additional donation screening for identified susceptible recipients (e.g. as with current anti-CMV screening).

(b) Introduction of methods to assess recipient susceptibility (e.g. antibody tests for measurement of past infection/immunity).

(c) Enhanced surveillance of blood recipients to enable early detection of transfusion-associated infections.

(d) Effectiveness and availability of immunization in multi-transfused individuals (e.g. HAV and HBV vaccines for haemophilia and thalassaemia patients).

(e) Scope for prophylaxis or treatment of identified transfusion-associated infections.

Impact of the infectious agent and methods to prevent transmission on blood supply and cost

(1) Blood donors

(a) Impact of screening on blood collection and blood donors.

(b) Assessment of the possible effect of modified donor interviews on the blood collection process.

(c) Staff resource issues associated with extended donor interviews.

(d) Willingness of donors to donate blood (voluntarily).

(e) Quality of information on prognosis and treatment options available for donors identified as being infected.

(2) Impact on public perception of blood safety

(a) Adverse publicity associated with identified new transfusion-transmitted infectious agent (TTIA).

(b) Potential positive and negative changes in the perception of the safety of blood transfusion associated with the introduction of new screening measures.

(3) Investigation of previous donations from identified infected donors

(a) Options for look-back studies among recipients of blood components and the identification of previously infected blood recipients.

(b) Scope for monitoring and potential treatment of potentially infected recipients.

(c) Likelihood of successful compensation claims.

(d) Identification and potential disposal of blood products manufactured from infected donations; product recall where appropriate.

(e) Assessment of likelihood of virus inactivation and potential residual infectivity in different blood products.

(f) Establishment of specific screening programmes for multiply treated individuals (e.g. haemophiliacs)

(4) Blood component supply

(a) Frequency of donations reactive in assays for the infectious agent, proportion of donations lost through additional screening.

(b) Availability of methods to confirm infection.

(c) Assessment of transfusion risk for donations reactive in assays for infectious agent.

(d) Impact of donation disposal and donor deferral on blood supply.

(e) Re-admission criteria for donors with false-positive results or with transient infections (e.g. parvovirus B19, HAV).

(f) Potential for matching infection status of positive donations with identified recipients (e.g. limiting transfusion of positive units to previously infected individuals).

(5) Blood product supply and quality

(a) Potential reduction in supply of plasma for fractionation.

(b) Impact of modified inactivation procedures on product quality and economic cost.

(c) Lower yield of active constituents, reduced clinical efficacy and/or increased dose requirements.

(d) Greater toxicity.

Assessment of efficacy of donation screening

(1) Frequency of transmission

(a) Frequency of infectious blood donations in blood supply.

(b) Duration of viraemia in donor.

(c) Distribution of infectious agent in different blood components.

(d) Frequency of blood recipient susceptibility to infection.

(e) Frequency of development of post-transfusion disease induced by the infectious agent.

(2) Effectiveness of intervention

(a) Availability, feasibility and effectiveness of donor or donation screening measures for identifying active infection or contaminated blood components.

(b) Screening test sensitivity and specificity.

(c) Predicted reduction in donor pool size after exclusion of infected donors.

(d) Reduction in blood supply after discard of blood components, including plasma, reactive in screening assays.

(e) Predicted reduction in incidence of post-transfusion infection.

(f) Predicted reduction in incidence of post-transfusion disease.

For a given agent, what information is missing?

(1) Contributory to risk assessment

Section A: Properties of the infectious agent

Section B: Prevention of transmission through transfusion

Section C: Impact of possible preventive measures

Section D: Effectiveness of preventive measures

Table 3 Characteristics of new/emerging infectious agents.

Class		WNV	Simian FV	Cox B	CMV
Infection characteristics					
IC1	Evidence of pathogenicity in immunocompetent humans	Y	N	Y	Y
IC2	Evidence of disease in exposed humans and/or general population	Y	N (may enhance other infections)	Y	Y
IC3	Evidence of antibody response in specifically exposed humans	Y	Y	Y	Y
IC4	Evidence of acute/persistent/chronic/latent (=/− reactivation) infection in humans	acute	latent	acute	latent/per.
IC5	Natural mode of transmission (droplet, faecal/oral, contact, percutaneous, vector, blood vertical)	v	percut.	dr, f/o	contact
IC6	Epidemic periodicity (years)	annual	not applicable	annual	constant
IC7	Seasonality (months)	6	not applicable	summer?	not applicable
IC8	Severity of infection (morbidity and mortality as a proportion of infections)	<1%	0%	5%	0%
IC9	Incubation period	7d	no disease	7d	3–12 wks
IC10	Incidence and prevalence of infection	rv	monkey handlers	high	rv
IC11	How long has agent been known	endemic in EU	since 1942	years	years
IC12	Other related organisms	JEV	retros	enteros	HHVs
Transmission					
T1	Transmissible to human	Y	Y	Y	Y
T2	Present in blood during infection	Y	Y	Y	Y
T3	Duration of blood detection (days)	14	lifelong	10	constant
T4	Plasma or cells infectious	p	cells	p	cells
T5	Transmissible through blood	Y	Y (animal model only)	Y	Y
T6	TTI evidence	Y	N (0/3)	N	Y
T7	Frequency of TTI	low	0	0.024%	low
Donors					
D1	Exclusion at pre-donation level feasible	Y	Y	Y	N
D2	Effectiveness of pre-donation exclusion	high	high	moderate	low
D3	Screening test available	Y	N	Y	Y
D4	Effectiveness of screening assay	high	n/a	high	high
D5	Risk reduction by leucodepletion	N	N	N	Y?
D6	Pathogen inactivation/removal step feasible	Y/N	N	N	Y/N
D7	Effectiveness of inactivation/removal	high/−	high	high	high
D8	Vaccine available	N	N	N	N
D9	Treatment available	N	?N	N	Y

Table 3 (cont.)

Risk assessment of the threat of an agent to blood safety to include

R1	Risk of infective donation entering the blood supply, without a given intervention
R2	Yield: infective donations kept out of the blood supply each year
R3	Impact: patients protected from infection in a year
R4	Impact: number and type of donors deferred in a year
R5	Impact: donations lost to the supply chain

Cost effectiveness

C1	(For > level 2 action) QALY gained per year
C2	Cost of preventing one potentially infective unit entering the blood supply
C3	Cost of preventing one recipient becoming infected
C4	Cost of preventing one recipient becoming ill as a result of TTIA
C5	Cost per QALY gained

GLOSSARY

CMV	Cytomegalovirus
Cox B	Coxsackie B
d	days
dr	droplet
enteros	enteroviruses
EU	European Union
f/o	faecal/oral
HHV's	human herpes viruses
JEV	Japanese Encephilitis Virus
N	no
per	persistent
percut	percutaneous
prev	prevalence
QALY	Quality adjusted life year
retros	retroviruses
rv	regional variation
Simian FV	Simian foamy virus
TTI	Transfusion-transmissible infections
v	vector
wk	weeks
WNV	West Nile virus
Y	yes

Table 4 Suggested risk levels

	Infection characteristics	WNV	Sim. foamy v.	Cox B	CMV
Level 0 **No action required for donors but continue surveillance**					
(1) Evidence of pathogenicity in immunocompetent	IC1	Y	N	Y	Y
(2) Evidence of disease in exposed humans and/or the general population	IC2	Y	N (may enhance other)	Y	Y
(3) Evidence of antibody response in specifically exposed humans	IC3	Y	0	Y	Y
(4) Evidence of persistent/chronic/latent (+ or reactivation) infection in humans	IC4	acute	latent	acute	latent/per
(5) Evidence of TTI	T6	Y	N (0/3)	N	Y
Level 1 **Consider precautionary measures and continued surveillance**					
(1) Evidence of pathology in immunocompetent humans	IC1	Y	N	Y	Y
(2) Evidence of disease in exposed humans and/or the general population	IC2	Y	N (may enhance other)	Y	Y
(3) Evidence from other related organisms	IC12	JEV	retros	enteros	HHVs
(4) Exposure has occurred, cases would be recognized and reported but no cases reported yet	IC2	Y	N (may enhance other)	Y	Y
(5) Evidence of TTI	T6	Y	N (0/3)	N	Y
(6) Evidence of resolved infections (serological response)	IC3	Y	0	Y	Y
Level 2 **Consider precautionary measures and continue enhanced surveillance**					
(1) Serological evidence of infection in humans	IC3	Y	0	Y	Y
(2) Incidence and prevalence of infection	IC10	0	monkey handlers	0	prev 30%
(3) Humans exposed and cases would be recognized and reported	IC2	Y	N (may enhance other)	Y	Y
(4) Evidence of TTI	T6	Y	N (0/3)	N	Y
Level 3 **Action required**					
(1) Human cases recognized and reported	IC2	Y	N (may enhance other)	Y	Y
(2) Evidence of person to person spread	IC5, T1	Y	Y	Y	Y
(3) Evidence of TTI	T6	Y	N (0/3)	N	Y
(4) Persistence of infection established at the present time	IC4	acute	latent	acute	latent/per
Level 4 **Priority action required**					
(1) Human cases recognized and reported	IC2	Y	N (may enhance other)	Y	Y
(2) Person to person spread reported	IC5, T1	v	per cut	d, f/o	contact
(3) Evidence of TTI	T6	Y	N (0/3)	N	Y
(4) Persistence of infection established at present time	IC4	acute	latent	acute	latent/per
(5) Proportion of symptomatic cases may be high/low or not yet established	IC10	0	monkey handlers	0	prev 30%?
(6) Proportion of cases with severe/fatal outcome or not yet established	IC8	0	0%	5%	0%
SUGGESTED LEVEL:		**4**	**0**	**1**	**4**

GLOSSARY (see Table 3)

or asymptomatic infections. Several countries are therefore applying appropriate donor exclusion criteria.

However, a balance needs to be achieved. As governments and transfusion practitioners become increasingly sensitized to potential microbial risks to transfusion saftety there is a danger of over-reacting. On the one hand one might apply the 'precautionary principle' where, even if the level of a possible risk is not known, preventative measures which might reduce the risk are implemented. The pressure to employ this 'better safe than sorry' approach is heightened by legislation such as the European Consumer Protection Act (see Chapter 26) which leads to the concepts of 'product liability' and 'fitness for purpose'. In this Act, blood (for transfusion) is considered as a product and so,

regardless of whatever blood safety measures are in place, producers are liable for any adverse events that might occur as a consequence of the transfusion of blood or blood derivatives.

On the other hand, this approach may well conflict with the actuarial opinion that a risk equal to, or less than, one in a million can be considered as virtually nil.

REFERENCES

Barbara, J. A. J. (1983) *Microbiology in Blood Transfusion*. Bristol, John Wright.

Khan, A. S. and Kumar, D. (2006) Simian foamy virus infection by whole-blood transfer in rhesus macaques: potential for transfusion-transmission in humans. *Transfusion*, **46**, 1352–9.

SECTION 1: AGENTS

1 HEPATITIS VIRUSES

Denis M. Dwyre and Paul V. Holland

Introduction

Transmission of hepatitis through blood transfusion was first reported in 1943 (Beeson, 1943; Morgan and Williamson, 1943). Hepatitis transmitted through faecal-oral mechanisms was termed hepatitis A ('epidemic hepatitis'), while hepatitis transmitted through blood and its derivatives ('serum hepatitis') was termed hepatitis B. These terms were formally adopted by the World Health Organization in the 1970s (Dienstag, 2002).

Prevention of the transmission of hepatitis by blood transfusions began with donor screening through the use of a donor questionnaire, primarily for a history of hepatitis, commonly referred to as 'yellow jaundice'. Laboratory screening for hepatitis B virus began in 1969, with the testing of blood donors for what eventually became known as the hepatitis B surface antigen (HBsAg). Soon after regular testing of donor blood for HBsAg was initiated and tests for antibody to the hepatitis A virus became available, it became apparent that the majority of cases of transfusion-transmitted viral hepatitis were not related to hepatitis A or hepatitis B. The then undefined virus, named non-A, non-B (NANB) hepatitis virus, was believed to be the cause of a large number of transfusion-related infections. In an effort to reduce the number of transfusion-transmitted NANB viral hepatitis infections, 'surrogate' or substitute testing of donor blood was evaluated in the 1970s, initially in the USA.

In 1981, an association between elevated serum levels of alanine aminotransferase (ALT) in blood donors and transfusion-transmitted NANB hepatitis in recipients was reported (Aach et al., 1981; Alter et al., 1981). But implementation of testing donor serum for ALT as a surrogate marker was not adopted in most countries while the need for a randomized study was debated and additional studies for the agent (or agents) of NANB hepatitis were initiated. Antibody to the hepatitis B core antigen (anti-HBc) in blood donors was also found to be associated with an increased risk of transfusion-transmitted NANB hepatitis in recipients (Koziol et al., 1986; Stevens et al., 1984). Without an assay for non-A, non-B hepatitis forthcoming and with a wider appreciation of the morbidity and chronicity of the disease caused by this agent(s), implementation of surrogate marker testing of blood donations using ALT and anti-HBc was instituted in the USA in 1986. Screening specifically for anti-HCV was not available until 1990, when assays based on cloned HCV antigen became available.

Data evaluating surrogate testing in the USA, from part of a large, historically controlled study, concluded that implementation of surrogate testing of blood donations reduced the hepatitis C virus (anti-HCV version 1.0) seroconversion rate from 3.84% to 1.54% in multi-transfused patients (Donahue et al., 1992). This same group subsequently evaluated all the patients in their study using a second-generation anti-HCV assay (anti-HCV version 2.0) on the patients and found a negligible effect of surrogate testing in those receiving multiple transfusions from 4.49% before, to 4.43% after implementation (Nelson et al., 1993). On the other hand, anti-HCV screening of donors using the 1.0 version had a dramatic effect, lowering the seroconversion rate in recipients to 1.08%.

Data on transfusion-transmitted hepatitis also have to be interpreted in light of the source of the blood. Paid individuals, as opposed to those who are unpaid volunteers, are associated with a higher risk of transfusion-associated hepatitis, in all prospective studies conducted to date (Aach et al., 1978; Alter et al., 1981; Walsh et al., 1970), and have higher rates of positive surrogate markers (Aach et al., 1978; Walsh et al., 1970). Also important is the linear increase in transfusion-transmitted infection with the number of transfused units received (see Figure 1.1). It is important to note that patient-directed blood donations (often from family members) have a transfusion-transmitted hepatitis rate between that of volunteer donors and paid individuals (Aach et al., 1978). There is also a background rate of hepatitis in all hospitalized groups not receiving transfusions, ranging from 1–3% (Aach et al., 1978; Alter et al., 1981). Thus, only with prospective serological or nucleotide marker data on implicated donors and infected patients can a viral hepatitis be considered transfusion-transmitted, rather than acquired by more usual routes before or after a blood transfusion, and simply be 'associated' with the blood transfusion.

With the implementation of anti-HCV testing, ALT testing became irrelevant, especially with the introduction of nucleic acid amplification testing (NAT) for HCV RNA. However, despite the presence of a high false-positive rate in blood donors, anti-HBc testing is still being used in a number of countries. It is not being used as a surrogate marker for HCV infection, but as another marker for hepatitis B virus carriers where hepatitis B surface antigen is absent.

Hepatitis A virus

Definition and characteristics

Hepatitis A virus (HAV) infection is the most common cause of acute viral hepatitis in the world (see Figure 1.2). The virus is transmitted primarily via the faecal-oral route. Hepatitis A virus is endemic throughout many parts of the less developed world, including most of Africa, South and Central America, Southern/

Transfusion Microbiology, eds John A. J. Barbara, Fiona A. M. Regan and Marcela C. Contreras. Published by Cambridge University Press. © Cambridge University Press 2008.

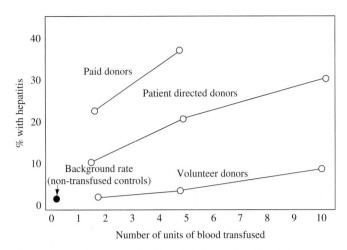

Figure 1.1 Transfusion-transmitted hepatitis virus study – effect of donor status and number.

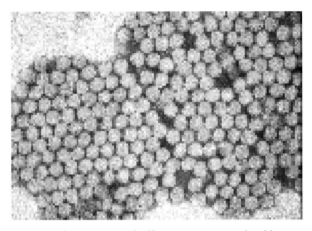

Figure 1.2 Electron micrograph of hepatitis A virus, reproduced from CDC (http://www.cdc.gov).

South-east Asia and Eastern Europe. The seroprevalence in many of these areas approaches 100%. Endemic transmissions predominantly occur via person-to-person contact, and primarily in children under the age of five years (Koff, 1998). Sporadic local epidemics occur worldwide, primarily through contaminated food and water. In low prevalence areas with only local outbreaks, the seroprevalence is low, with Scandinavian countries having some of the lowest rates, near 13% (Catton and Locarnini, 2005; Melnick, 1995). There are an estimated 1.4 million new infections of HAV annually worldwide (Previsani *et al.*, 2004).

First identified in 1973, HAV is a non-enveloped (no lipid coat) single-stranded RNA virus (Feinstone *et al.*, 1973). Along with human poliovirus and human Coxsackie viruses, HAV is classified in the picornavirus family. Four human strains of HAV have been identified, but all appear antigenically similar. In fact, only one serotype has been identified. The virus is resistant to extremes in temperature (−20 to 70°C), acid, and detergents (Previsani *et al.*, 2004). The lack of a lipid coat on HAV is of importance to transfusion medicine in that, while the presence of a lipid coat allows destruction of a virus by solvent/detergent processing, the lack of a lipid envelope confers resistance to destruction by this processing. The plasma from one donor

incubating HAV can thus contaminate the large plasma pool (of 100 to more than 2500 donations) and resist solvent/detergent inactivation whilst processing for fresh frozen plasma or plasma derivatives, like factor VIII (Chudy *et al.*, 1999).

Upon infection, following ingestion of faecally contaminated food or water, HAV crosses the intestinal epithelium, travels via the bloodstream, and infects only the hepatocyte. In the hepatocyte cytoplasm, the viral RNA acts as messenger RNA, initiating the translation of viral proteins in the host cell. After cell lysis, the virus then travels to the biliary system (where it is resistant to the detergent-like bile), and is subsequently secreted back into the intestine. From the intestine, HAV re-enters the environment via the faeces, thus completing its life cycle.

Clinical features

When infected, a patient with HAV infection generally goes through four phases of illness. The first phase is the asymptomatic incubation period, lasting from 10–50 days. Due to the lack of symptoms, it is this first stage where the risk of transmission (either via contaminated food/water or transfusion) is greatest. During this asymptomatic phase, people infected with HAV do not know they are infected and infectious since they feel well and continue their normal activities. The second phase of the infection, the prodromal phase, may last for up to a week. In this pre-jaundice period, a wide range of symptoms may occur, including nausea, vomiting, diarrhoea, fever, weakness, anorexia, headache and other systemic symptoms. Dark urine and pale stools may develop at this stage.

In the third phase, the icteric phase, clinical jaundice occurs, where total serum bilirubin levels exceeding 340–680 μmol/L (20–40 mg/dL) can occur. The symptoms that occurred in the prodromal phase usually persist. Hepatomegaly, with or without right upper quadrant pain and tenderness, can also be present. Laboratory findings include marked elevation of the aminotransferases, aspartate amino transferase (AST) and alanine aminotransferase (ALT)), often reaching 5000 IU/L. Elevation of lactate dehydrogenase (LDH) can also occur. Jaundice often peaks in 1–2 weeks. During the fourth or convalescent phase, resolution of the signs and symptoms occur over the course of 4–15 weeks. Only rarely are other organs affected by HAV infection. Many infections are completely asymptomatic, especially in those under five years of age.

Infectivity, as measured by stool viral shedding, begins during the asymptomatic period and persists until the icteric phase in immunocompetent individuals. However, in some immunoincompetent patients (e.g. neonates), stool viral shedding can persist for months (Rosenblum *et al.*, 1991). Viraemia can precede stool viral shedding, and persists also until the icteric phase. One recent study noted prolonged viraemia for a median period of 42 days after infection, detected by polymerase chain reaction (PCR) (Tjon *et al.*, 2006).

Complete recovery within months with only symptomatic treatment is the norm for an acute HAV infection. However, rarely liver necrosis with acute liver failure can occur in a small minority of patients. The incidence of acute liver failure is more common

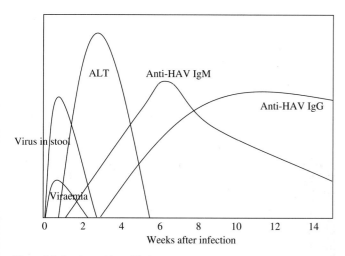

Figure 1.3 Serology of hepatitis A.

in developing countries (Shah *et al.*, 2000), and increases with age (Brown and Persley, 2002; Kyrlagkitsis *et al.*, 2002; Purcell and Emerson, 2005). A prolonged cholestatic hepatitis condition can occur with this complication. However, typically, prognosis is still excellent, with complete recovery. A relapsing HAV course has also been well documented (Raimondo *et al.*, 1986; Sagnelli *et al.*, 2003), but recovery and prognosis are usually excellent (Koff, 1998).

With HAV infection and recovery, lifelong immunity develops. There is no known chronic HAV infectious condition and, thus, no chronic carrier state.

Diagnostic testing

All viral hepatidities can look alike clinically. Similarly, all viral hepatidities can produce similar biochemical results (elevated bilirubin and aminotransferases, plus other abnormal 'liver function' tests). Serological testing is required to make a definitive diagnosis of HAV infection. The diagnosis of acute hepatitis A infection requires identification of anti-HAV IgM in the acute-phase serum (see Figure 1.3). The presence of anti-HAV IgG connotes past infection. In general, the IgG persists indefinitely and correlates with immune protection. As only one serotype exists, false-negatives secondary to multiple serotypes do not occur (or have not been reported). Alternatively, detecting HAV RNA from blood or stool via a nucleic acid amplification technology (NAT), such as PCR, would be diagnostic of an acute infection.

Total and IgM anti-HAV can be measured by radioimmunoassay, enzyme linked immunoassays (EIA), or competitive solid phase assays (Lemon, 1997). Commercial kits to detect anti-HAV are available. The administration of IVIg usually does not affect testing for IgM anti-HAV, but will provide passive transfer of IgG anti-HAV (Lemon, 1997). Tracing and proving transfusion-transmitted HAV infections can be accomplished by identifying seroconversion in an implicated donor or by detecting HAV RNA in a sample from the transfused component using PCR (Gowland *et al.*, 2004).

Although generally not performed for diagnosis, HAV can be grown in cell culture. The process is too time consuming for clinical use, and HAV produces little to no cytopathic effect on cultured cells.

Window period

As HAV is only rarely transmitted by transfusion of blood components and products (Gresens *et al.*, 2003; Lee *et al.*, 1992), and as most adult blood donors with an acute HAV infection are symptomatic, testing for HAV in donors is not performed. Establishing the 'window period' (WP), defined as the period between potential for infectivity and the presence of symptoms or positive test results, for a blood donor infected with HAV is difficult. Conceivably, the entire incubation period could potentially be the WP. In reality, this is not the case. More likely, the short period (days) between viraemia and symptoms is the effective WP. If serological testing were to be instituted for anti-HAV IgM, few infectious donors would be identified, as HAV disappears rapidly from the blood when anti-HAV appears. To identify asymptomatic donors with HAV in their blood would require NAT. Pathogen inactivation technology would be a better way, however, to prevent transfusion-transmission of HAV. Solvent/detergent (SD) treatment alone, however, is insufficient for elimination of HAV transmission as there have been confirmed cases of transfusion-associated HAV from SD treated factor VIII concentrates (Chudy *et al.*, 1999). Additonal heat treatment is effective for the treatment of plasma derivatives.

Risk factors for infection

Groups of people at risk of infection include international travellers to areas where HAV is endemic or people who reside in such areas. Additionally, people who live with infected people or spend extended time in crowded or poor sanitary conditions (for example institutionalized people, daycare children and caretakers, military, refugee camps) are at risk of acquiring HAV infection. Homosexually active men and IV drug users are also considered at higher risk. Additionally, medical personnel and food handlers are considered higher risk groups. All of these groups should receive the HAV vaccine. Nevertheless, many would not qualify as blood donors due to other risk factors.

Fortunately, the current blood donor questions should eliminate most people at higher risk for transmitting HAV through transfusion. In general, those travellers from HAV endemic areas would be deferred due to the fact that these are, in general, the same areas where malaria is common. Donors in the WP could still potentially transmit HAV through their donated blood, but transfusion-transmitted HAV is quite rare, estimated at 1:1 000 000 (Goodnough *et al.*, 1999).

Estimated risk of transmission by transfusion

Transmission of HAV by pooled plasma derivatives and blood component transfusion is a rare, but well documented event (Azimi *et al.*, 1986; Barbara *et al.*, 1982; Giacoia and Kasprisin,

1989; Gresens *et al.*, 2003; Hollinger *et al.*, 1983; Ishikawa *et al.*, 1984; Nigro and Del Grosso, 1990; Noble *et al.*, 1984; Seeberg *et al.*, 1981; Sheretz *et al.*, 1984; Skidmore *et al.*, 1982). Outbreaks of HAV have occurred from infected factor VIII in Europe, before the use of recombinant factor VIII (Gerritzen *et al.*, 1992; Mannucci, 1992; Mannucci *et al.*, 1993; Peerlinch and Vermylen, 1993; Temperley *et al.*, 1992). Such events point out the increased risk of HAV transmission (and all transfusion-transmitted infectious diseases) with the use of pooled plasma and pooled plasma-derived products. Due to its rarity, it is difficult to determine accurately the risk of transfusion-transmitted HAV. A recent study of Portuguese blood donors did not identify any HAV viraemic donors in a group of 5025 donors. The authors estimated a maximum risk of 0.06% risk/unit based upon this study (Henriques *et al.*, 2005). Another recent abstract estimated the risk to be 1 in 1 million (Gresens *et al.*, 2003).

As a non-enveloped virus, solvent/detergent treated plasma would not be expected to affect the infectivity of an HAV infected unit in the pool. This mode of infectivity came to light in the 1980s and 1990s with reports of multiple HAV transmissions in haemophilia patients receiving factor VIII concentrates in the USA (Chudy *et al.*, 1999; Soucie *et al.*, 1998). This was in part due to the low prevalence of anti-HAV in plasma donors, combined with the single step solvent/detergent step used for viral inactivation. The risk of pooled, solvent/detergent plasma transmitting HAV is dependent on the number of units of plasma in the pool (often from 2500 to 5000). However, further processing, including the combination of antibody-mediated neutralization, partitioning with freezing/lyophilization and anion-exchange chromatography resulted in significant reduction of HAV infectivity in pooled plasma (Henriques *et al.*, 2005). Heat treatment would also be expected to inactivate HAV.

Other important information

Although not routinely implemented in all developed countries, HAV vaccine provides immunity against the disease. Furthermore, as there is only one serotype, vaccination against one antigen strain will provide protection against all HAV infections. As the rate of infection, and especially transfusion-transmitted infection, is low in developed countries, widespread vaccination may not be economically feasible. For those exposed to HAV, either parenterally or non-parenterally, the clinical signs and symptoms, but not the infection, can be modified by passive immunization with immune serum globulin. Hepatitis A virus vaccination may also be of benefit, but it takes up to 30 days to develop an immune response, which may not be detectable at the beginning by commercial tests for anti-HAV (Betlach *et al.*, 2000).

Hepatitis B virus and hepatitis D virus (delta virus)

Definition and characteristics

Discovered in 1963 by Blumberg, hepatitis B virus (HBV) was the first human hepatitis virus identified (see Figure 1.4). Initially

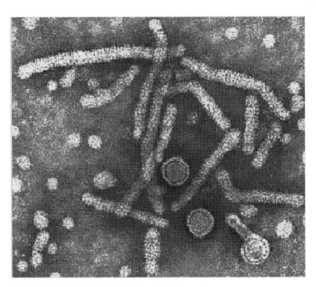

Figure 1.4 Electron micrograph of hepatitis B virus, reproduced from CDC (http://www.cdc.gov).

termed the Australia antigen, due to its original description in an Australian aborigine, and linked to leukaemia, HBV was eventually noted to have a high prevalence in multiply transfused patients (Blumberg *et al.*, 1965). Hepatitis B virus infection is now known to be a very common infection, with over 300 million carriers worldwide, which is approximately 5% of the world's population (Zarski *et al.*, 2002). There is a wide range of prevalence of HBV infection, as measured by hepatitis B surface antigen positivity (HBsAg), ranging from 8–15% in the Far East, Middle East, Africa, and parts of South America to less than 2% in most of the United States, Canada, Northern Europe, and parts of South America (Andre, 2000; Zarski *et al.*, 2002). Other regions (e.g. some Mediterranean areas) are intermediate in prevalence (2–8%). There are over 4 million new cases of acute clinical hepatitis yearly. One million of those infected die annually from chronic hepatitis B infection or one of its complications – cirrhosis and hepatocellular carcinoma (Previsani *et al.*, 2004).

Hepatitis B virus is a member of the virus family *Hepadnaviridae*. Multiple other animal species, including woodchucks, ground squirrels, other primates, herons and ducks, are known to be susceptible to infection with related hepatitis viruses from the same family (Mason and Jilbert, 2003). Hepatitis B virus is a partially double stranded circular DNA, enveloped (lipid coated) virus (see Figure 1.5). The presence of a lipid coat is important in transfusion medicine in that treatment of plasma with solvent/detergent destroys HBV.

Hepatitis B virus is primarily transmitted by blood. Perinatal transmission from mother to newborn is an important mode of transmission in areas where the disease has a higher prevalence, together with infection within the first year of life. Sexual contact and the sharing of needles in intravenous drug users are the most important modes of transmission of HBV, especially since HBsAg screening is in widespread use to test blood components intended for transfusion. Viraemia can reach 10^8 to 10^{10} viral particles per millilitre of serum or copy numbers of 10^5 to 10^7 per millilitre of serum (Kann and Gerlich, 2005). From the blood, HBV

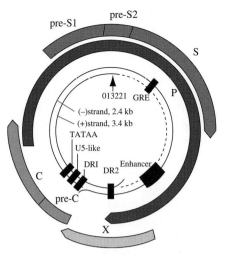

pre-S1
pre-S2
S
P
013221 GRE
(−)strand, 2.4 kb
(+)strand, 3.4 kb
TATAA
U5-like
DRI Enhancer
DR2
C
pre-C
X

Figure 1.5 Genome of hepatitis B virus, reproduced with permission from Dr Alan J. Cann (http://www-micro.msb.le.ac.uk/3035/HBV.html).

binds to a receptor on the hepatocyte. In the hepatocyte, HBV enters the nucleus, and becomes a circular supercoiled DNA molecule that is used for transcription of viral RNA (Previsani *et al.*, 2004). Hepatitis B virus RNA is then transcribed into viral DNA via a reverse transcriptase. Viral particles are shed in the blood after replication. Persistent viraemia is important in the chronic infectious state and the continual potential for infectivity; approximately 5–10% of infections (especially in neonates and the immunosuppressed) evolve into a persistent carrier state.

Hepatitis B virus is composed of an outer shell containing lipid. Serologically, the outer shell is named the hepatitis B surface antigen (HBsAg); excess viral coat protein devoid of DNA is produced with HBV infection, especially in the chronic carrier state. The inner core contains the infectious DNA. In the laboratory, core is determined serologically by the presence of hepatitis B core antigen (HBcAg). This assay may be useful for monitoring anti-viral therapy (Kimura *et al.*, 2003); the assay is not available clinically, however. Both HBsAg and HBcAg are highly immunogenic. It is the purified HBsAg from the plasma of carriers which was the first HBV vaccine, now largely replaced by recombinant HBsAg. A third moeity, hepatitis B e antigen (HBeAg), is an antigen associated with the nucleocapsid of the HBV, and correlates with infectivity.

Hepatitis D virus (HDV), also known as the delta agent, is an RNA virus that can infect the liver only in association with HBV. In 1980, it was discovered that HDV was a distinct virus that relied on HBV for its transmission, as it uses HBsAg as its own viral coat (Previsani *et al.*, 2004). It is transmitted by blood, via routes similar to HBV. Inoculation of HDV viral particles without HBV will not result in infection, as HBV is required for its infectivity. The presence of HDV viraemia signifies active liver disease.

Hepatitis D virus has the same worldwide distribution as HBV. Some countries with high HBV prevalence, such as China, however, have low HDV prevalence (Previsani *et al.*, 2004). There are more than 10 million HDV infected people globally. The number of new infections has been decreasing, however, with the increased use of HBV vaccination.

Clinical features

The clinical presentation of HBV infection is variable and depends upon the age at infection and immunological competency (Previsani *et al.*, 2004). The acute infection may be asymptomatic, especially in neonates and children. When symptomatic, patients generally have non-specific constitutional symptoms, including nausea, vomiting, anorexia, headaches and diarrhoea. Mild splenomegaly and/or hepatomegaly with vague abdominal pain can also occur. Symptoms tend to be less severe in children. The incubation period lasts from 1–6 months. Jaundice can sometimes develop during this time period although the majority of infections are anicteric. When jaundice occurs, serum levels of bilirubin are only increased modestly. Almost uniformly, however, marked increases in serum aminotransferase levels occur during this period of infection, sometimes reaching up to 100 times normal levels; remarkably, the levels of aminotransferases do not correlate with prognosis (Previsani *et al.*, 2004).

The acute hepatitis generally resolves with only symptomatic treatment over the course of 4–8 weeks. The clearance of the virus (serum viral DNA and HBsAg) results in protective immunity with the formation of antibody to HBsAg (anti-HBs) in 95% of infected patients (Hyams, 1995; Previsani *et al.*, 2004; Zarski *et al.*, 2002). About 5% of patients fail to clear the viral DNA and become chronic carriers, at risk of progressive liver damage, continued infectivity and potential transmission to others. Failure to clear the virus with a resultant lifelong, chronic infection/carrier state is highly age dependent; over 90% of those infected as neonates become chronic carriers, while this reduces to approximately 5% in adults. A well-known complication of chronic HBV infection is the risk of developing hepatocellular carcinoma (HCC) after persistent carriage, with resultant cirrhosis (Beasley, 1988; Previsani *et al.*, 2004; Zarski *et al.*, 2002). The prevalence of HCC geographically mirrors the endemic areas of chronic HBV infection (Previsani *et al.*, 2004). Hepatocellular carcinoma, with underlying HBV cirrhosis, is one of the most common causes of cancer-related deaths in parts of Asia and Africa.

The most grave result of acute HBV infection is fulminant liver failure, usually occurring within eight weeks of primary infection. Although rare (less than 1% of infections), the mortality is high with virtually no chance of recovery once encephalopathy occurs. Patients with this course present with liver synthesis dysfunction, elevated liver enzymes and serology consistent with acute HBV infection.

Extrahepatic complications of HBV infection are not uncommon, seen in 10–25% of patients (Previsani *et al.*, 2004; Zarski *et al.*, 2002). Arthralgias and dermatoses are the most frequent extrahepatic symptoms. Polyarteritis nodosa can occur in acute or chronic HBV infection. Immune complex formation with a serum sickness-like illness can also occur. Membranous glomerulonephritis has also been associated with immune complex deposition in the basement membrane of the kidneys. Other autoimmune phenomena, including mixed cryoglobulinaemia, polyneuropathy and Reynaud's syndrome, are also associated with HBV infection. Rarely, other cancers, such as cholangiocarcinoma, have been linked to HBV infection (Patel, 2006).

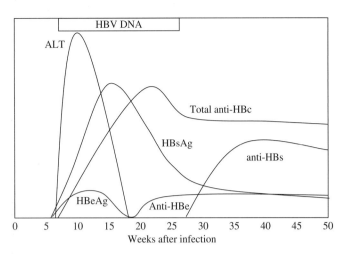

Figure 1.6 Serology of hepatitis B. Laboratory serology studies after infection with hepatitis B. Note, anti-HBe generally develops only if HBe antigen is cleared. HBV DNA can be detected by nucleic acid amplification testing.

Epididymitis has recently been reported in association with acute HBV infection (Tasar *et al.*, 2005). Asymptomatic autoantibody formation can also be found in HBV infected patients (Cacoub *et al.*, 2005).

Hepatitis D virus coinfection with HBV usually results in an acute hepatitis clinically. The chronic form of HDV is seen in approximately 5% of those infected, similar to HBV alone (Macnaughton, 2003; Previsani *et al.*, 2004). Coinfection can be associated with fatigue persisting for a longer period of time. Superinfection with HDV (infection with HDV in a patient with pre-existing HBV) can result in a more severe acute hepatitis, with a higher incidence of chronic HDV infection and higher incidence of cirrhosis (Previsani *et al.*, 2004).

Diagnostic testing

As with other viral hepatitis infections, elevations in serum levels of aminotransferases, up to 100 times normal (Previsani *et al.*, 2004), generally occur. Bilirubin elevations are usually mild to moderate, generally reaching 85–170 µmol/L (5–10 mg/dL).

Hepatitis B surface antigen is present in the serum of HBV infected patients some weeks after HBV DNA is detectable but before symptoms appear (see Figure 1.6). As HBsAg is also often present in chronic HBV infections, the presence of anti-HBc IgM, along with HBsAg, is usually also required for the diagnosis of an acute infection. The presence of HBsAg also indicates the potential for infectivity. Some patients never test positive for HBsAg, even with clinical symptoms of hepatitis. These patients, however, will usually have an antibody response: antibody to the hepatitis B core antigen (anti-HBc), both IgM and IgG. The presence of the hepatitis B e antigen (HBeAg) is significant not only for active disease, but is also a marker of high infectivity. With clearance of HBsAg, anti-HBs appears; similarly, with disappearance of HBeAg, anti-HBe appears.

Chronic HBV carriers maintain HBsAg in their sera, but not always at levels detectable by serologic tests. Cases of chronic carriers with no evidence of HBsAg in their sera (false-negatives)

but who have HBV DNA, do occur. The HBV in the livers of these patients may have undergone mutations, affecting their detection by standard serologic assays. Chronic carriers usually fail to develop protective immunity in the form of anti-HBs. In some patients who are unable to eliminate the virus, low levels of anti-HBs may co-exist with HBsAg. The presence of anti-HBs, either produced in response to an infection or by vaccination, generally indicates immunity. The presence of anti-HBc without the presence of HBsAg or anti-HBs is often indicative of a false-positive test, especially in low risk individuals, such as blood donors; however, infections which occurred long ago can also show a similar pattern. Anti-HBc persists after HBV infection for longer than anti-HBs. Where anti-HBc is used to screen blood donations, detection of this antibody on two separate occasions usually results in indefinite donor deferral, whether the anti-HBc is a true or a false-positive result. (Please refer to Chapter 2.)

In blood donation screening, testing for HBsAg is standard, with permanent deferral of donors with a confirmed, reactive test. Testing for anti-HBc was first implemented in the USA as a surrogate test for carriers of NANB viral hepatitis. After the discovery of the hepatitis C virus (HCV) and implementation of anti-HCV testing, the testing of anti-HBc was continued in some countries, as it was shown to detect some HBV infected, HBsAg-negative donors (though anti-HBc testing is associated with numerous false-positives).

Testing for HBsAg is usually performed using EIA, radioimmunoassay or other immunological based assays. The latest, most sensitive HBsAg detection method uses chemiluminescence; this method is widely used in Canada, Europe, and parts of Asia (Biswas *et al.*, 2003). Since the inception of HBsAg testing in 1971, the sensitivity has increased by two orders of magnitude ($2 \log_{10}$) (Stramer, 2005). The choice of the method used to detect HBsAg is not standardized. The only requirement for HBsAg testing is the licensing or accreditation of the test in the country where the test is used; tests may be licensed for diagnostic use and/or screening of blood donors. Approaches to test selection vary in different countries.

Numerous commercial kits are available for HBsAg testing. Positive tests are often confirmed by retesting the sample after incubation with anti-HBs, to see if the HBsAg result can be neutralized. True positive tests for HBsAg will have the antigen neutralized by the specific antisera. In countries where blood donor centres have limited resources, rapid and less expensive immunofiltration, latex based, or immunochromatographic methods are used, often without confirmatory or neutralization testing (WHO, 2001). Testing for anti-HBc, anti-HBs and anti-HBe is usually performed by radioimmunoassay or enzyme-based immunoassays. Sometimes, when 'in-house' reagents are used in countries without formal kit licensing requirements, simultaneous presence of anti-HBc and/or anti-HBe strengthens the validity of an HBsAg positive result.

Alternatively, the presence of HBV DNA, determined by nucleic acid testing (NAT), is evidence of infection and infectivity. Nucleic acid testing has been able to reduce the WP significantly for infectivity with human immunodeficiency virus (HIV) and hepatitis C virus (HCV); however, a similar dramatic reduction in the WP has not been shown with testing for HBV DNA (Biswas *et al.*, 2003; Brojer, 2005; Roth and Seifried, 2002; Stramer *et al.*, 2004; Stramer, 2005). Thus, routine blood donation screening using NAT for HBV DNA is currently only used in a few countries, in addition to research studies at some blood centres.

Since HDV is only present as a coinfection with HBV, it is not routinely tested for in blood services. When superinfection is a clinical suspicion, testing for HDV antigen or anti-HDV can be performed using methods similar to those used for HBV. Testing for anti-HDV markers is unnecessary in blood services; donors found positive would have been permanently deferred from donation because of the presence of HBsAg.

Window period (WP)

For HBV testing, the WP is defined as the period between infection and emergence of HBsAg in the serum. The WP using earlier versions of HBsAg tests has been estimated at 59 days, ranging from 37–87 days (Kleinman *et al.*, 2005; Mimms *et al.*, 1993; Schreiber *et al.*, 1996). In order to increase detection of the number of infectious units donated during the window period, consideration of the implementation of NAT for HBV versus the current sensitive HBsAg tests and/or anti-HBc screening has been debated recently (Biswas *et al.*, 2003; Kleinman and Busch, 2001; Kleinman *et al.*, 2005; Stramer, 2005). Window-period HBV infections have been detected by NAT, even in a mini-pool format of 16 to 96 donor samples and with anti-HBc in place; the yield, however, would be improved by pools of less than eight, or NAT of individual samples.

In areas with low prevalence, such as North America, much of Europe, and Australia, there is no consensus on the significance of the number of WP units detected by NAT for HBV DNA and the reduction in the WP. It has been estimated that the WP would be reduced by ten days with the introduction of mini-pool NAT (Biswas *et al.*, 2003; Kleinman *et al.*, 2005). With single donor unit testing, the reduction in WP is estimated to be an additional 13 days (Biswas *et al.*, 2003). The question of single donor unit testing, with the inherent higher expense and the need for automation, will require further evaluation. In countries with higher prevalence of HBV infections and the ability to afford NAT, such as Japan, WP reduction will result in more HBV infectious blood donations eliminated (Comanor and Holland, 2006). A comparison of the detection rates of HBV mini-pool NAT with HBsAg serology from a recent study by the Japanese Red Cross is shown in Figure 1.7 (Comanor and Holland, 2006, reprinted with permission).

Risk factors for infection

Risk factors for both HBV and HDV are similar. As HBV is an infection transmitted by blood and body fluids, risk factors include those conditions and behaviours that put people into contact with infectious blood or body fluids. Hepatitis B surface antigen has been found in virtually all body fluids; however, in humans, only blood, semen and vaginal/menstrual fluid have been shown to be infectious (Previsani *et al.*, 2004). Sexual,

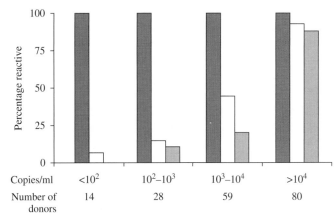

Copies/ml: <10^2, 10^2–10^3, 10^3–10^4, >10^4

Number of donors: 14, 28, 59, 80

NAT = nucleic acid amplification technology
CLIA = chemiluminescent immunoassay, PRISM, Abbott Laboratories
EIA = enzyme immunoassay, Auszyme II, Abbott Laboratories

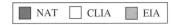

■ NAT   □ CLIA   ▨ EIA

Figure 1.7 Comparison of detection rates of HBV mini-pool NAT testing with HBsAg serology in 181 HBV NAT yield cases (Comanor and Holland, 2006). Reprinted with permission from authors.

mother to infant transmission, iatrogenic, sharing intravenous drug needles, syringes and transfusions are all important and likely, in this order. Thus, a person with sexual or close household contact with an HBV infected person is at higher risk of contracting HBV. Men who have sex with men are noted to be especially at risk. Intravenous drug users and people who have had tattoos or body piercings using unsterile needles are also at higher risk.

In the past, haemodialysis patients have long been known to be at higher risk, as well as recipients of blood components and products, including pooled plasma (Barker *et al.*, 1970; Barker and Murray, 1972). Children in day care settings or residential settings, prisoners, and heath care workers are also at higher risk. Perinatal transmission is also an important mode of transmission, especially in endemic areas (see earlier). Additionally, people living in or travelling to endemic areas are at higher risk due to increased potential for exposure. Over one-third of people infected with HBV report no known risk factor (CDC, 1991; Previsani *et al.*, 2004).

Estimated risk of transmission by transfusion

Prior to HBsAg screening of the blood supply in 1971, it was estimated that the risk of transfusion-transmitted HBV infection was 6% of all multiply transfused patients (Alter and Houghton, 2000). After the introduction of HBsAg screening, the risk of transfusion acquired HBV was reduced to approximately 0.3%–1.7% (Hoofnagle, 1990). Introduction of anti-HBc screening in the mid-1980s, which was initially developed for detecting NANBH carriers, allowed for detection of remote, HBsAg negative HBV infections. After utilization of this test in the USA, the risk of transfusion-transmitted HBV was reduced to a level where mathematical estimates had to be used to determine the risk as approximately 1 in 63 000 (Schreiber *et al.*, 1996). It is difficult to measure the impact of anti-HBc testing of donors on reducing

HBV transmission, especially since these units from chronic, low-level HBV carriers without detectable HBsAg are much less likely to transmit HBV than units collected in the window period (Satake, 2005). However, the low specificity of anti-HBc testing has led to many permanent donor deferrals, 23–75% of whom may be false-positives, and no answers on how to re-enter those false-positive donors into the donor pool (Stramer, 2005). (Please refer to Chapter 2.)

The impact on prevention of transfusion-transmitted HBV infection using NAT methodology to screen donations is difficult to estimate due to limited data and multiple variables (e.g. size of donor sample pools, prevalence in the population, using NAT alone or in combination with traditional testing, etc.). Two recent studies in the USA have studied the effects of NAT for HBV. Kleinman *et al.* concluded that, using NAT on pools of 24 donations, 39 additional units could be interdicted, preventing 56 cases of HBV transmission annually in the USA (Kleinman *et al.*, 2005). Biswas *et al.* concluded that NAT would detect 15–21 HBV positive units per 10^7 units (Biswas *et al.*, 2003). It should be noted that single donor unit testing (vs. mini-pooling) will increase yield as well accounting for 13–15 additional units detected for 10^7 units tested (Biswas *et al.*, 2003). The very high levels of infectious virions of HBV in samples was first demonstrated in 1972 when the inoculation dose (or viral load) of the infected blood (or pooled plasma product) was demonstrated to be related to potential for infectivity (Barker and Murray, 1972). Dilutions of 1 ml of HBV infectious plasma 10 million fold were still infectious, probably beyond detection even by sensitive NAT assays for HBV DNA.

Other important information

Hepatitis B virus infection has a worldwide prevalence noteworthy for its infectivity, chronicity and ability to cause substantial morbidity and mortality, in the form of cirrhosis and HCC. However, the development of a vaccine in the 1980s and the progressive implementation of vaccine programmes around the world may affect the way that HBV testing is looked upon in the future.

Presently, advances in NAT technology will enable more sensitive testing of the blood supply, but at a high cost. Due to the now rarer presence of HBsAg negative, anti-HBc positive infections

with low levels of viraemia, elimination of traditional testing methods is unlikely to occur in the near future (Busch, 2004; Kleinman *et al.*, 2005; Stramer, 2005). For countries with a moderate to high prevalence of HBsAg, testing for HBsAg and HBV DNA by NAT would appear optimal; for low prevalence countries, HBV DNA by NAT and anti-HBc testing may be superior to HBV DNA by NAT and HBsAg testing.

Pathogen inactivation will possibly have a role in increasing the safety of blood products in the future, including reducing the risk of transfusion-transmitted HBV (Klein, 2005; Lin *et al.*, 1997; Snyder and Dodd, 2001). Processes, such as the use of psoralen-based chemicals and ultraviolet light, have been shown to inactivate HBV-like viruses in blood products (Lin *et al.*, 1997). Additionally, solvent/detergent treatment of pooled plasma is known to destroy lipid-coated viruses, such as HBV; this treatment assists in the reduction of transfusion-transmitted HBV in plasma and plasma products. However, such treatment is not appropriate for red blood cells or platelets.

Hepatitis C virus

Definition and characteristics

After the discovery of HAV and HBV, and after the introduction of tests for these viruses, a large residuum of patients with clinical (presumed viral) hepatitis were diagnosed with what was termed non-A, non-B (NANB) hepatitis. It was known that NANB hepatitis was associated with intravenous drug use, treatment with pooled plasma derivatives before viral inactivation processes were implemented and transfusions prior to 1990. After the cloning of its genome in 1989 (Choo *et al.*, 1989), NANB hepatitis, now termed hepatitis C virus (HCV), was determined to be a major aetiological agent of chronic viral hepatitis worldwide. Over 2 million people are infected with HCV annually. The prevalence varies between less than 2% in North America, Europe, and Australia to greater than 5% in Africa (Quer and Mur, 2005).

Hepatitis C virus is a single-stranded, RNA, enveloped (lipid coated) virus in the viral family *Flaviviridae* (see Figure 1.8). This lipid coat can be destroyed by solvent/detergent, leading to HCV inactivation. Hepatitis C virus is transmitted primarily through contact with blood. Intravenous drug use is the major risk behaviour. Before anti-HCV testing was available, blood transfusion

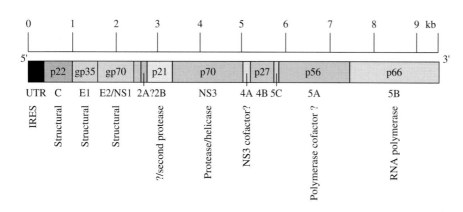

Figure 1.8 Genome of hepatitis C virus. Reproduced with permission from Dr Alan J. Cann (http://www-micro.msb.le.ac.uk/3035/HCV.html).

recipients were at high risk for HCV infection. Historically, testing for elevated transaminases during blood donation was a surrogate test for NANB hepatitis in donor blood, but as shown retrospectively, along with anti-HBc testing in the USA, surrogate testing had little impact on HCV transmission (Nelson *et al.*, 1993), despite initially appearing to be of benefit (Donahue *et al.*, 1992). The virus is also known to be transmitted through sexual contact, albeit inefficiently, and from mother to infant perinatally.

In HCV infection, the virus travels via the blood to the primary target cell, the hepatocyte. Once in the liver, the virus attaches to the receptor, CD81 (Pileri *et al.*, 1998), and enters the hepatocyte cytoplasm. In the cytoplasm, the viral RNA is translated into proteins using host rough endoplasmic reticulum. Nascent RNA is then made from negative strand viral RNA (unlike HBV, which uses DNA and a reverse transcriptase). Also, unlike HBV, only primates are known to have been infected with HCV or HCV-like viruses (Farci *et al.*, 1992; Garnier *et al.*, 2002).

There is significant genetic heterogeneity with hepatitis C, which is generally classified into six major genotypes. Initially, the genotypes were separated based upon molecular methods; however, the genotypes have been shown to have a distinct geographical distribution, predilection for modes of infection (for example intravenous drug use), and, most importantly, can be predictive of response to treatment (Muerhoff and Dawson, 2004). Despite the differences in genotype, no distinct serotypes have been discovered yet.

Clinical features

Hepatitis C virus is predominantly transmitted parenterally via blood exposure. Before blood donation testing in 1990, blood transfusion was a major mode of transmission. Intravenous drug use was, and continues to be, known as the most important risk factor for HCV transmission. The symptoms of acute HCV infection are insidious or not reported at all. When acute HCV infection is documented, patients generally report mild non-specific symptoms of nausea, anorexia, abdominal pain, malaise and occasional jaundice. The symptoms of this mild acute hepatitis, when present, usually occur within 7–8 weeks of exposure, with a range of 2–26 weeks (Lauer and Walker, 2001). The acute illness, when present, persists for 3–12 weeks, with quick resolution of jaundice (when present) and other symptoms, despite the infection usually persisting. Only mild to modest elevations of aminotransferases and serum bilirubin levels are noted when acute HCV infection is diagnosed. Anti-HCV is present in 70% of patients at the time of symptoms and in virtually all patients by six months after exposure (Garnier *et al.*, 2002). Fulminant hepatitis can occur rarely after acute HCV infection (Farci *et al.*, 1996).

In general, HCV infection results in a chronic disease, regardless of the presence of acute signs and symptoms. Chronic hepatitis develops in the vast majority of patients. As the acute symptoms are often absent, the length of chronicity is often unknown. The development of cirrhosis has been known to occur up to 30 years after initial infection (Lauer and Walker, 2001), and there are believed to be many undiagnosed asymptomatic carriers without overt evidence of liver disease. Most

chronic infections will lead to 'hepatitis' at some time, and most have some hepatic fibrosis (Lauer and Walker, 2001). Occasionally, the infection clears on its own, but the exact percentage of infections that do this is unclear (Lauer and Walker, 2001; Takaki *et al.*, 2000). Severe complications, including cirrhosis, hepatic failure and death, are estimated to develop eventually in 15–20% of those infected (Lauer and Walker, 2001). Factors which predispose to progression are male gender, infection after the age of 40, and concomitant use of alcohol.

Chronic HCV patients can also have thrombocytopaenia, increased serum gamma globulins, or increased serum ferritin levels, all of which connote a worse prognosis (Garnier *et al.*, 2002). The presence of HCV RNA and/or anti-HCV is indicative of infection, and thus persistent infectivity of the patient. Coinfection with HBV or HIV is not uncommon with HCV, and can lead to faster progression of the disease. Coinfection with HAV, with resultant acute hepatitis, has a high mortality; for this reason, patients with HCV should be vaccinated against HAV (Garnier *et al.*, 2002; Lauer and Walker, 2001).

Those infected with HCV can have a variety of extrahepatic manifestations; in fact, these conditions may lead to the diagnosis of underlying HCV infection. Most of these conditions are related to autoimmune or lymphoproliferative phenomena that are believed to be an interaction between genetic factors and the infection (Lauer and Walker, 2001; Zignego and Brechot, 1999). Mixed cryoglobulinaemia, membranoproliferative glomerulonephritis, porphyria cutanea tarda, Sjögren's syndrome, and lymphoproliferative disorders are associated with HCV infection.

Diagnostic testing

Because many HCV infections are asymptomatic in the acute setting, the diagnosis is often made during the chronic phase. Only mild to moderate elevations of aminotransferases and serum bilirubin occur acutely. Aminotransferases can remain elevated throughout the chronic disease or be elevated at times and within the 'normal range' at other times. Testing for aminotransferase levels is often used in assessing response to treatment, but levels of HCV RNA are more predictive.

Definitive diagnosis of HCV requires serological or molecular based (NAT) assays. Hepatitis C antigen (HCVAg) is present initially, then anti-HCV develops in the weeks following infection, during the acute phase of the disease (see Figure 1.9). In rare instances, anti-HCV may not develop. Hepatitis C virus antigen is present in the serum until anti-HCV appears, which can often be detected indefinitely (Lauer and Walker, 2001; Takaki *et al.*, 2000). However, disappearance of antibody can occur over time in a minority of infections. An alternative non-nucleotide based assay has been studied (Aoyagi *et al.*, 1999; Bouvier-Alias *et al.*, 2002; Courcouce *et al.*, 2000; Icardi *et al.*, 2001; Laperche *et al.*, 2003; Lee *et al.*, 2001; Letowska *et al.*, 2004; Peterson *et al.*, 2000; Piccoli *et al.*, 2001; Tanaka *et al.*, 2000; Tobler *et al.*, 2005) and recently developed commercially (Tobler *et al.*, 2005), for the detection of HCV core antigen (HCVAg). The investigators of the commercial assay concluded that the antigen-based test approaches the sensitivity of NAT, and that the test might be

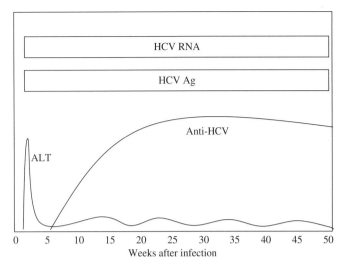

Figure 1.9 Serology of hepatitis C. Laboratory serology studies after infection with hepatitis C. HCV RNA can be detected by RNA amplification testing.

useful in areas where NAT is not available. (Biorad combined HCV Ag/Ab is now available.) The presence of antibodies to HCV does not denote protective immunity. Antigen and antibody testing used to test blood donors for HCV is similar to other antiviral antibody testing. Enzyme immunoassays (EIA) are most often used, with supplementary immunoblot assays.

Nucleic acid testing of plasma intended for fractionation and of blood donations for HCV RNA began in the late 1990s when methodologies became available. Nucleic acid for HCV is now required in many countries, using either 'home-brew' or commercial technology. Nucleic acid testing for HCV involves primers specific for the HCV RNA; testing for HCV RNA is usually performed using mini-pools (16 to 96 donor samples per pool). Hepatitis C virus can be grown in (hepatic) cell culture, but this method is not used clinically or diagnostically in blood banking. Furthermore, the 'gold standard' for diagnosing hepatitis is a biopsy with histological examination. With the development of molecular studies, the role of invasive studies, such as liver biopsy, is now limited.

Window period

With the introduction of NAT on blood donations, the WP for HCV has been affected more than any other transfusion-transmitted infectious disease. Before NAT, using anti-HCV testing only, the WP for HCV was approximately 70 days. After NAT, which became mandatory in the USA and many European countries in the late 1990s/early 2000s, the WP for HCV has been reduced to 12 days (Gonzalez et al., 2005; International Task Force on Nucleic Acid Amplification Testing of Blood Donors, 2000). Window-period reduction is also achieved by testing for HCVcAg on individual donor samples, but detection is delayed by 4–5 days compared with NAT for HCV RNA (Tobler et al., 2005).

The 95% detection limit of sensitivity for HCV NAT ranges between 6.2 – 280 IU/ml, depending on the nucleic acid technology used (Brojer, 2005; Hourfar et al., 2005; Jarvis et al., 2005; Koppelman et al., 2005). A study comparing NAT with HCVcAg

antigen testing showed a detection level of 8 000–32 000 copies/ ml for the antigen EIA test (Tobler et al., 2005) This finding is consistent with the delayed WP for HCVcAg testing.

Risk factors for infection

Hepatitis C virus is transmitted predominantly by blood exposure, and secondarily by sexual contact. As such, intravenous drug users are one of the higher risk groups. Recipients of blood products were a high-risk group prior to anti-HCV testing of donations in 1990. The risk is much lower today, with mandatory anti-HCV screening for blood donations, and the subsequent addition of NAT. Health care workers, with potential exposure to needlestick injuries, are at increased risk. Hepatitis C has been known to be transmitted by organs, transplanted tissues (Pereira et al., 1991; 1992), colonoscopy (Bronowicki et al., 1997), dialysis (Katsoulidou et al., 1999) and during surgery (Esteban et al., 1996; Ross et al., 2000).

Although less efficient, HCV is known to be transmitted by the sexual route. Mother to infant transmission occurs variably, but may occur up to 6% of the time (Ohto et al., 1994; Zanetti et al., 1995). The transmission appears to be higher in mothers also infected with HIV (Zanetti et al., 1995).

Estimated risk of transmission by transfusion

Prior to anti-HCV screening, the risk of HCV transmission via blood transfusion was substantial. As the seroprevalence in low-prevalence countries was up to 2% (1.8% in the USA) (Lauer and Walker, 2001), and approximately 75% of these had viraemia, the risk of HCV transmission from transfusion was substantial: about 1% per unit transfused (0.1% per unit in the UK). With the introduction of anti-HCV screening in the early 1990s and improvement in the anti-HCV testing over time, the risk was reduced to approximately 1 in 100 000 transfused units (Schreiber et al., 1996).

With the introduction of NAT, because the low level of residual risk precludes simple and effective data collection from prospective trials, mathematical modelling has had to be used to estimate the risk of transfusion-transmitted HCV. Today, it is estimated that such risk in the USA is approximately 0.03 to 0.5 in 1 000 000 units using mini-pool donor testing (Busch et al., 2005; Dodd et al., 2002; Jarvis et al., 2005; Seed et al., 2005; Soldan et al., 2005; Stramer et al., 2004). Potential further reduction of transmission to 0.25 in 1 000 000 is achievable with single-donor unit NAT (Soldan et al., 2005). It is believed that the vast majority of these NAT positive, anti-HCV negative units are WP donations. Three cases of immunologically silent chronic HCV infections were documented, however, in one study (Stramer et al., 2004). Of note, first-time donors are twice as likely to be infected with HCV than repeat donors (Dodd et al., 2002). This has also been noted by epidemiological analysis in England (J. Barbara and K. Soldan, personal communication).

From the calculated risks noted above, the impact of HCV NAT depends upon prevalence. In very low prevalence countries, such as Scotland, it was determined that only one WP HCV positive donation was interdicted in five years (Jarvis *et al.*, 2005). In the USA and other countries with similar seroprevalence, it is estimated that two to three additional HCV positive units per 1 000 000 will be detected annually (Busch *et al.*, 2005). In countries with higher endemnicity and the ability to institute NAT, such as Italy, the impact is expected to be much greater (Gonzalez *et al.*, 2005). Although predicted yields of extra positives detected have been borne out in actual practice in some countries, this has not been the case in all countries.

Other important information

As with other enveloped viruses, HCV would be expected to be destroyed by solvent/detergent treatment during pooled plasma processing. Pathogen inactivation (PI) of individual units of plasma and platelets may be a method in the future to further reduce transfusion-transmitted HCV (Klein, 2005; Lin *et al.*, 1997; Snyder and Dodd, 2001). One method of PI using a psoralen-based product and ultraviolet light has been shown to eliminate a HCV-like virus from blood components (Lin *et al.*, 1997). Until PI methods are in widespread use, the use of NAT will be the best protection from transfusion-transmitted HCV. In the future, there is hope of a vaccine which will be protective against HCV. Thus far, no vaccine is available, but progress has been made using animal models for HCV vaccination (Houghton and Abrignani, 2005).

Hepatitis E virus

Definition and characteristics

Hepatitis E virus (HEV) is a single stranded, non-enveloped RNA virus, classified in the genus *Hepevirus*. Like HAV, HEV is enterically transmitted and is a major source of morbidity in developing countries. Unlike HAV, HEV is less hardy, and is sensitive to harsh conditions, such as freezing. Generally, HEV infection is a self-limiting disease affecting primarily only the liver. Two features that make HEV unique to the viral hepatidities are the high mortality rate with infection during pregnancy, and the potential for HEV to be a zoonosis, most notably between humans and swine (Anderson and Shrestha, 2002). Transmission between humans and non-human primates can also occur.

Hepatitis E virus is primarily transmitted through faecally contaminated water. As such, this viral infection is endemic in developing countries, with the highest endemic rate being in India, Egypt and parts of China (Anderson and Shrestha, 2002). Due to the zoonotic nature of the infection, areas where humans and pigs live in close proximity are areas where endemic rates are higher. There is a seasonal variation, and relationship to flooding in developing countries has been known to play a role in epidemics (Balayan, 1997). Direct human-to-human transmission is not believed to be an efficient mode of transmission. In more developed countries, recent travellers to endemic areas are the most commonly affected. The seroprevalence rate of the infection in developed countries is low. A 1–2% rate of anti-HEV has been reported in studies from the USA and Europe (Balayan, 1997;

Jameel, 1999; Mast *et al.*, 1996; Mast *et al.*, 1997; Zanetti and Dawson, 1994). One study from the USA showed disparate results; it demonstrated a much higher rate of anti-HEV of 21.3% in blood donors (Thomas *et al.*, 1997). The authors of this study could not rule out cross-reactivity with an antigenically related virus. Higher rates are seen in endemic areas, and in populations exposed to swine.

Like HAV, HEV enters the host via the enteric endothelium. From there, it almost exclusively targets the hepatocyte. In the hepatocyte, the RNA behaves like the host mRNA, directing translation of viral proteins. Four major genotypes of HEV are recognized, with important antigenic variation; antigenic cross-reactivity does exist, however. Serotyping of the strains has been more problematic, but only one serotype is believed to exist (Jameel, 1999).

Clinical features

The course of clinical disease caused by HEV is similar to HAV. Many infections are sub-clinical and asymptomatic, especially in children. For symptomatic patients, after exposure, there is an asymptomatic incubation period of approximately 30 days (Chauhan *et al.*, 1993). Viruses can generally be found in the stool for only one to two weeks following clinical symptoms, but similar to HAV, protracted stool virus shedding can occur (Nanda *et al.*, 1995). Viraemia is transient, and generally disappears prior to the onset of symptoms (Chauhan *et al.*, 1993; Nanda *et al.*, 1995). Prolonged viraemia can occur in patients where protective antibody development is delayed (Nanda *et al.*, 1995). These persistently viraemic individuals are believed to be human reservoirs for the disease.

Following viraemia, constitutional symptoms of nausea, vomiting, fatigue, malaise and a low-grade fever generally occur as the first symptoms. The icteric phase follows, with clinical jaundice and pale stools. Abdominal pain can occur with splenomegaly (10–15% of patients) (Anderson and Shrestha, 2002). Recovery generally occurs over 4–6 weeks.

Laboratory findings during HEV infection generally mimic those of HAV. Serum levels of aminotransferases and serum bilirubin increase moderately. In severe infections, where liver synthesis function is affected, elevation of the prothrombin time and a decrease in serum albumin may be seen. Anti-HEV IgM levels increase as viraemia resolves, at about the time of symptomatology. Immunoglobulin G production follows soon after IgM appears, and seems to persist for years, if not for life.

Diagnostic testing

Identification of HEV viral antigens, RNA, or antibodies to the virus is required for diagnosis. Similar to HAV, antigen detection using stool samples was initially the mainstay of diagnosis, but due to poor sensitivity, the method has been abandoned. Detection of viral RNA, until recently, has only been a research tool. A new, real-time PCR assay has been developed for the detection of the virus (Jothikumar *et al.*, 2006).

Antibody detection for anti-HEV is the most common method for determination of infection. Many commercial EIAs are available. Identification of anti-HEV IgM is an indication of recent or acute infection. Absence of IgM with the presence of anti-HEV IgG is indicative of a past infection. Routine evaluation of HEV antibodies is not performed in blood donor centres; this would only serve to identify donors with immunity to HEV, not those in the viraemic phase of the window period.

Window period

Hepatitis E virus transmission via blood transfusion is a rare event, even in areas where the infectious agent is endemic and of moderate prevalence. As such, defining a window period (the period between potential for infectivity and the presence of symptoms or positive testing results), is not possible. The unknown factor is the potential for infectivity. It is known that protracted viraemia can occur (Nanda et al., 1995) and asymptomatic cases are common; therefore, the window period could potentially be months. In reality, as transfusion-transmitted HEV is rare, the potential WP is likely to be short, but unpredictable. Of importance is the fact that, in industrialized countries, most potentially HEV infected donors would be deferred during the WP due to potential malarial exposure during overseas travel.

In order to identify HEV infected donors in the WP, serologic testing for anti-HEV IgM or NAT (or other nucleotide-based molecular technology) would have to be instituted. Anti-HEV testing would identify few potentially infectious donors as the virus is generally cleared rapidly with antibody formation. Hepatitis E virus NAT technology is generally not considered a practical option in industrialized countries (Matsubayashi et al., 2004). Hepatitis E virus screening of blood is being debated in endemic areas, however (Aggarwal, 2004; Khuroo et al., 2004). Although solvent/detergent would not be expected to be effective in killing this non-lipid coated virus, pathogen inactivation could be an effective method of reducing HEV infection.

Risk factors for infection

The major risk factor for HEV infection is exposure to faecally contaminated food or water. In blood donors in developed areas of the world, this exposure most often occurs during travel to an endemic area, especially during a rainy season. Although quite rare, several reports of potential transfusion-transmitted HEV exist (Aggarwal, 2004; Khuroo et al., 2004; Lee and Shih et al., 2005; Matsubayashi et al., 2004; Mitsui et al., 2004; Wang et al., 1993; 1994), but few conclusively documented (PCR proven) cases have been reported (Boxall et al., 2006, Matsubayashi et al., 2004). Cases of vertical (Khuroo et al., 1995) and sexual (Montella et al., 1994) transmission have also been reported. There have also been multiple reports of acquisition of HEV from the consumption of wild deer or boar meat (Hsieh et al., 1998; Masuda et al., 2005; Tei et al., 2003). Therefore, there is a theoretical, but highly unlikely, potential of transmission of HEV from a donor who recently consumed certain (poorly cooked or raw) wild animal meat.

Estimated risk of transmission by transfusion

Hepatitis E virus is generally not suspected in cases of acute hepatitis and not tested for routinely in blood donor centres. Therefore, the risk of transfusion-transmitted HEV exists. In reality, only a few case reports have suspected HEV transmission via blood components (see above). A potential HEV transfusion-transmitted infection was averted recently by the donor choosing to self-exclude due to post-donation symptoms (Lee and Chau et al., 2005). To date, the actual risk of HEV is exceeded by the risk of transfusion-transmitted HAV, which is itself estimated to be about 1 in 1 million (Gresens et al., 2003).

Viral inactivation processes, other than solvent/detergent, render HEV non-infectious in plasma derivatives. One would need pathogen inactivation processes for blood components to (essentially) eliminate the risk of HEV infection.

Other important information

As there is only one known serotype for HEV (with at least four genotypes), the prospects for an effective HEV vaccine are good (Koff, 2003; Wang and Zhuang, 2004; Worm and Wirnsberger, 2004). The inability to grow HEV effectively in cell culture has been a hindrance. Vaccines developed from recombinant proteins and RNA based vaccines are under investigation; methods include expression of HEV in prokaryotes, tomatoes, insect and yeast cells (Koff, 2003; Wang and Zhuang, 2004; Worm and Wirnsberger, 2004). Many vaccines have been developed, but only one has reached a phase 1 trial in the USA. Further investigation continues. The role of a vaccine would be, in addition to the prevention of epidemics in the developing world, useful for travellers from more developed countries.

Other viruses that can cause hepatitis

Other newly discovered viruses, such as HHV-8, and TTV, can cause a viral hepatitis condition. The implication of these hepatitis-associated viruses will be discussed in Chapter 6. Retroviruses, most notably HIV, can also cause a clinical hepatitis. This infection will be discussed in detail in Chapter 6. Epstein-Barr virus (EBV) and CMV have also been associated with hepatitis. These agents are discussed in Chapter 6, along with the other herpes viruses. In addition, parvovirus B19 has been reported to cause a viral hepatitis (see Chapter 6).

REFERENCES

Aach, R. D., Lander, J. J., Sherman, L. A., et al. (1978) Transfusion-transmitted viruses: interim analysis of hepatitis among transfused and non-transfused patients. In Viral Hepatitis: a Contemporary Assessment of Etiology, Epidemiology, Pathogenesis and Prevention, eds G. N. Vyas, S. N. Cohen and R. Schmid, pp. 383–96. Philadelphia, Franklin Institute Press.

Aach, R. D., Szmuness, W., Mosley, J. W., et al. (1981) Serum alanine aminotransferase of donors in relation to the risk of non-A, non-B hepatitis in recipients: the transfusion-transmitted viruses study. New Engl J Med, 304, 989–94.

Aggarwal, R. (2004) Hepatitis E: is it a blood-borne pathogen? J Gastroenterol Hepatol, 19, 729–31.

Alter, H. J. and Houghton, M. (2000) Hepatitis C virus and eliminating post-transfusion hepatitis. *Nature Medicine*, **6**, 1082–6.

Alter, H. J., Purcell, R. H., Holland, P. V., *et al.* (1981) Donor transaminase and recipient hepatitis. Impact on blood transfusion services. *JAMA*, **246**, 630–4.

Anderson, D. A. and Shrestha, I. L. (2002) Hepatitis E virus. In *Clinical Virology*, eds D. D. Richman, R. J. Whitley and F. G. Hayden, pp. 1061–74. Washington DC, ASM Press.

Andre, F. (2000) Hepatitis B epidemiology in Asia, the Middle East, and Africa. *Vaccine*, **18**, S20–S22.

Aoyagi, K., Ohue, C., Iida, K., *et al.* (1999) Development of a simple and highly sensitive enzyme immunoassay for hepatitic C virus core antigen. *J Clin Microbiol*, **37**, 1802–8.

Azimi, P. H., Roberto, P. R., Guralnik, J., *et al.* (1986) Transfusion acquired hepatitis A in a premature infant with secondary nosocomial spread in an intensive care nursery. *Am J Dis Child*, **140**, 23–7.

Balayan, M. S. (1997) Epidemiology of hepatitis E virus infection. *J Viral Hepat*, **4**, 155–65.

Barbara, J. A., Howell, D. R., Briggs, M., *et al.* (1982) Post-transfusion hepatitis A. *Lancet*, **1**, 738 (letter).

Barker, L. F. and Murray, R. (1972) Relationship of virus dose to incubation time of clinical hepatitis and time of appearance of hepatitis-associated antigen. *Am J Med Sci*, **263**, 27–33.

Barker, L. F., Shulman, N. R., Murray, R., *et al.* (1970) Transmission of serum hepatitis. *JAMA*, **211**, 1509–12.

Beasley, R. P. (1988) Hepatitis B virus. The major etiology of hepatocellular carcinoma. *Cancer*, **61**, 1942–56.

Beeson, P. B. (1943) Jaundice occurring one to four months after transfusion of blood or plasma: report of seven cases. *JAMA*, **121**, 1332–4.

Betlach, B., Paglieroni, T. and Holland, P. V. (2000) Delayed anti-HAV response to hepatitis A vaccine. *Antivir Ther*, **5**(S1), A13.

Biswas, R., Tabor, E., Hsia, C. C., *et al.* (2003) Comparative sensitivity of HBV nucleic acid tests and HBsAg assays for detection of acute HBV infections. *Transfusion*, **43**, 788–98.

Blumberg, B. S., Alter, H. J., Visnich, S. (1965) A 'new' antigen in leukemia sera. *JAMA*, **191**, 541–6.

Bouvier-Alias, M., Patel, K., Dahari, H., *et al.* (2002) Clinical utility of total HCV core antigen quantification: a new indirect marker of HCV replication. *Hepatology*, **36**, 211–8.

Boxall, E., Herborn, A., Kochethu, G., *et al.* (2006) Transfusion-transmitted hepatitis E in a 'nonhyperendemic' country. *Transfus Med*, **16**, 79–83.

Brojer, E. (2005) Implementation of donor screening for infectious agents transmitted by blood by nucleic acid technology in Poland. *Vox Sang*, **89**, 267–8.

Bronowicki, J. P., Venard, V., Botte, C., *et al.* (1997) Patient-to-patient transmission of hepatitis C virus during colonoscopy. *N Engl J Med*, **337**, 237–40.

Brown, G. R. and Persley, K. (2002) Hepatitis A epidemic in the elderly. *South Med J*, **95**, 826–33.

Busch, M. P. (2004) Should HBV DNA NAT replace HBsAg and/or anti-HBc screening of blood donors? *Transfus Clin Biol*, **11**, 26–32.

Busch, M. P., Glynn, S. A., Stramer, S. L., *et al.* (2005) A new strategy for estimating risks of transfusion-transmitted viral infections based on rates of detection of recently infected donors. *Transfusion*, **45**, 254–64.

Cacoub, P., Saadoun, D., Bourliere, M., *et al.* (2005) Hepatitis B virus genotypes and extrahepatic manifestations. *J Hepatol*, **43**, 764–70.

Catton, M. G. and Locarnini, S. A. (2005) Epidemiology (Hepatitis A). In *Viral Hepatitis*, eds H. C. Thomas, S. Lemon, A. J. Zuckerman, pp. 92–108. Malden, MA, Blackwell.

Centers for Disease Control (1991) Hepatitis B virus: a comprehensive strategy for eliminating transmission in the United States through Universal childhood vaccination: recommendations of the Immunization Practices Advisory Committee (ACIP). *MMWR*, **40**, 1–19.

Chauhan, A., Jameel, S., Dilawari, J. B., *et al.* (1993) Hepatitis E virus transmission to a volunteer. *Lancet*, **341**, 149–50.

Choo, Q. L., Kuo, G., Weiner, A. J., *et al.* (1989) Isolation of a cDNA clone derived from a blood-borne non-A, non-B viral hepatitis genome. *Science*, **244**, 359–62.

Chudy, M., Budek, I., Keller-Stanislawski, B., *et al.* (1999) A new cluster of hepatitis A infection in hemophiliacs traced to a contaminated plasma pool. *J Med Virol*, **57**, 91–9.

Comanor, L. and Holland, P. (2006) Hepatitis B virus blood testing: unfinished agendas. *Vox Sang*, **91**, 1–12.

Courcouce, A. M., Le Marrec, N., Bouchardeau, F., *et al.* (2000) Efficacy of HCV core antigen detection during the preseroconversion period. *Transfusion*, **40**, 1198–202.

Dienstag, J. L. (2002) Transfusion-transmitted hepatitis B, A and D. In *Rossi's Principles of Transfusion Medicine*, eds T. L. Simon, W. H. Dzik, E. L. Snyder, C. P. Stowell and R. G. Strauss, pp. 733–41. Philadelphia, PA, US, Lippincott Williams & Wilkins.

Dodd, R. Y., Notari, E. P. and Stramer, S. L. (2002) Current prevalence and incidence of infectious disease markers and estimated window-period risk in the American Red Cross blood donor population. *Transfusion*, **442**, 975–9.

Donahue, J. G., Munoz, A., Ness, P. M., *et al.* (1992) The declining risk of post-transfusion hepatitis C virus infection. *New Engl J Med*, **327**, 369–373.

Esteban, J. I., Gomez, J., Martell, M., *et al.* (1996) Transmission of hepatitis C virus by a cardiac surgeon. *N Engl J Med*, **334**, 555–60.

Farci, P., Alter, H. J., Shimoda, A., *et al.* (1996) Hepatitis C virus-associated fulminant hepatic failure. *N Engl J Med*, **335**, 631–4.

Farci, P., London, W. T., Wong, D. C., *et al.* (1992) The natural history of infection with hepatitis C virus (HCV) in chimpanzees: comparison of serologic responses measured with first- and second-generation assays and relationship to HCV viremia. *J Infect Dis*, **165**, 1006–11.

Feinstone, S. M., Kapikian, A. Z. and Purcell, R. H. (1973) Hepatitis A: detection by immune electron microscopy of a virus like antigen associated with acute illness. *Science*, **182**, 1026–8.

Garnier, L., Inchauspe, G. and Trepo, C. (2002) Hepatitis C virus. In *Clinical Virology*, eds D. D. Richman, R. J. Whitley, F. G. Hayden, pp. 1153–76. Washington DC, ASM Press.

Gerritzen, A., Schneweis, K. E., Brackmann, H. H., *et al.* (1992) Acute hepatitis A in haemophiliacs. *Lancet*, **340**, 1231–2.

Giacoia, G. P. and Kasprisin, D. O. (1989) Transfusion-acquired hepatitis A. *South Med J*, **82**, 1357–60.

Gonzalez, M., Regine, V., Piccinini, V., *et al.* (2005) Residual risk of transfusion-transmitted human immunodeficiency virus, hepatitis C virus, and hepatitis B virus infections in Italy. *Transfusion*, **45**, 1670–5.

Goodnough, L. T., Brecher, M. E., Kanter, M. H., *et al.* (1999) Transfusion medicine: first of two parts, blood transfusion. *New Engl J Med*, **340**, 438–47.

Gowland, P., Fontana, S., Niederhauser, C., *et al.* (2004) Molecular and serologic tracing of a transfusion-transmitted hepatitis A virus. *Transfusion*, **44**, 1555–61.

Gresens, C. J., Flynn, N. M., Simon, N. F., *et al.* (2003) Transfusion (and related secondary) transmission of hepatitis A virus. Proceedings of the 11th International Symposium on Viral Hepatitis and Liver Disease, Sydney, eds A. R. Jilbert, E. V. L. Grgacic and K. Vickery, pp. 471–2.

Henriques, I., Monteiro, F., Meireles, E., *et al.* (2005) Prevalence of parvovirus B19 and hepatitis A virus in Portuguese blood donors. *Transfus Apher Sci*, **33**, 305–9.

Hollinger, F. B., Khan, N. C., Oefinger, P. E., *et al.* (1983) Post-transfusion hepatitis type A. *JAMA*, **250**, 2313–7.

Hoofnagle, J. H. (1990) Post-transfusion hepatitis B. *Transfusion*, **30**, 384–6.

Houghton, M. and Abrignani, S. (2005) Prospects for a vaccine against the hepatitis C virus. *Nature*, **436**, 961–6.

Hourfar, M. K., Schmidt, M., Seifried, E., *et al.* (2005) Evaluation of an automated high-volume extraction method for viral nucleic acids in comparison to a manual procedure with preceding enrichment. *Vox Sang*, **89**, 71–6.

Hsieh, S. Y., Yang, P. Y., Ho, Y. P., *et al.* (1998) Identification of a novel strain of hepatitis E virus responsible for sporadic acute hepatitis in Taiwan. *J Med Virol*, **55**, 300–4.

Hyams, K. C. (1995) Risks of chronicity following acute hepatitis B infection: a review. *Clin Infect Dis*, **20**, 992–1000.

Icardi, G., Ansaldi, F., Bruzzone, B. M., *et al.* (2001) Novel approach to reduce the hepatitis C virus (HCV) window period: clinical evaluation of a new enzyme-linked immunosorbent assay for HCV core antigen. *J Clin Microbiol*, **39**, 3110–4.

International Task Force on Nucleic Acid Amplification Testing of Blood Donors (2000) Nucleic acid amplification testing of blood donors for transfusion-transmitted infectious diseases. *Transfusion*, **40**, 143–59.

Ishikawa, K., Sato, S., Sugai, S., *et al.* (1984) A case of post-transfusion hepatitis A. *Gastroenterol Jpn*, **19**, 247–50.

Jameel, S. (1999) Molecular biology and pathogenesis of hepatitis E virus. *Expert Rev Mol Med*, 6 Dec., 1–16.

Jarvis, L. M., Dow, B. C., Cleland, A., *et al.* (2005) Detection of HCV and HIV-1 antibody negative infections in Scottish and Northern Ireland blood donations by nucleic acid amplification testing. *Vox Sang*, **89**, 128–34.

Jothikumar, N., Cromeans, T. L., Robertson, B. H., *et al.* (2006) A broadly reactive one-step real-time PCR assay for rapid and sensitive detection of hepatitis E virus. *J Virol Methods*, **131**, 65–71.

Kann, M. and Gerlich, W. H. (2005) Hepatitis B virus: structure and molecular virology. In *Viral Hepatitis*, eds H. C. Thomas, S. Lemon and A. J. Zuckerman, pp. 149–180. Malden, MA, Blackwell.

Katsoulidou, A., Paraskevis, D., Kalapothaki, V., *et al.* (1999) Molecular epidemiology of a hepatitis C virus outbreak in a haemodialysis unit. Multicentre haemodialysis cohort study on viral hepatitis. *Nephrol Dial Transplant*, **14**, 1188–94.

Khuroo, M. S., Kamili, S. and Jameel, S. (1995) Vertical transmission of hepatitis E virus. *Lancet*, **345**, 1025–6.

Khuroo, M. S., Kamili, S. and Yatoo, G. N. (2004) Hepatitis E virus infection may be transmitted through blood transfusions in an endemic area. *J Gastroenterol Hepatol*, **19**, 778–84.

Kimura, T., Rokuhara, A., Matsumoto, A., *et al.* (2003) New enzyme immunoassay for detection of hepatitis B virus core antigen (HBcAg) and relation between levels of HBcAg and HBV DNA. *J Clin Microbiol*, **41**, 1901–6.

Klein, H. G. (2005) Pathogen inactivation technology: cleansing the blood supply. *J Intern Med*, **257**, 224–37.

Kleinman, S. H. and Busch, M. P. (2001) HBV: amplified and back in the blood safety spotlight. *Transfusion*, **41**, 1081–5.

Kleinman, S. H., Strong, D. M., Tegtmeier, G. G., (2005) Hepatitis B virus (HBV) DNA screening of blood donations in mini-pools with the COBAS AmpliScreen HBV test. *Transfusion*, **45**, 1247–57.

Koff, R. S. (1998) Hepatitis A. *Lancet*, **351**, 1643–9.

Koff, R. S. (2003) Hepatitis vaccines: recent advances. *Int J Parasitol*, **33**, 517–23.

Koppelman, M. H., Sjerps, M. C., Reesink, H. W., *et al.* (2005) Evaluation of COBAS AmpliPrep nucleic acid extraction in conjunction with COBAS AmpliScreen HBV DNA, HCV RNA and HIV-1 RNA amplification and detection. *Vox Sang*, **89**, 193–200.

Koziol, D. E., Holland, P. V., Alling, D. W., *et al.* (1986) Antibody to hepatitis B core antigen as a paradoxical marker for non-A, non-B hepatitis agents in donated blood. *Ann Intern Med*, **104**, 488–95.

Kyrlagkitsis, I., Cramp, M. E., Smith, H., *et al.* (2002) Acute hepatitis A virus infection: a review of prognostic factors from 25 years' experience in a tertiary referral center. *Hepatogastroenterology*, **49**, 524–8.

Laperche, S., Le Marrec, N., Simon, N., *et al.* (2003) A new HCV core antigen assay based on disassociation of immune complexes: an alternative to molecular biology in the diagnosis of early HCV infection. *Transfusion*, **43**, 958–62.

Lauer, G. M. and Walker, B. D. (2001) Hepatitis C virus infection. *N Engl J Med*, **345**, 41–52.

Lee, C. C., Shih, Y. L., Laio, C. S., *et al.* (2005) Prevalence of antibody to hepatitis E virus among haemodialysis patients in Taiwan: possible infection by blood transfusion. *Nephron Clin Pract*, **99**, 122–7.

Lee, C. K., Chau, T. N., Lim, W., *et al.* (2005) Prevention of transfusion-transmitted hepatitis E by donor-initiated exclusion. *Transfus Med*, **15**, 133–5.

Lee, K. K., Vargo, L. R., Le, C. T., *et al.* (1992) Tranfusion-acquired hepatitis A outbreak from fresh frozen plasma in a neonatal intensive care unit. *Pediatr Infect Dis J*, **11**, 122–3.

Lee, S. R., Peterson, J., Niven, P., *et al.* (2001) Efficacy of a hepatitis C virus core antigen enzyme-linked immunosorbent assay for the identification of 'window-phase' blood donations. *Vox Sang*, **80**, 19–23.

Lemon, S. M. (1997) Type A viral hepatitis: epidemiology, diagnosis and prevention. *Clin Chem*, **43B**, 1494–9.

Letowska, M., Brojer, E., Mikulska, M., *et al.* (2004) Hepatitis C core antigen in Polish blood donors. *Transfusion*, **44**, 1067–71.

Lin, L., Cook, D. N., Wiesehahn, G. P., *et al.* (1997) Photochemical inactivation of virus and bacteria in platelet concentrates by use of a novel psoralen and long-wavelength ultraviolet light. *Transfusion*, **37**, 423–35.

Macnaughton, T. B. (2003) New directions and predictions for the future – hepatitis D. Proceedings of the 11th International Symposium on Viral Hepatitis and Liver Disease, Sydney, eds A. R. Jilbert, E. V. L. Grgacic and K. Vickery, pp. 237–40.

Mannucci, P. M. (1992) Outbreak of hepatitis A among Italian patients with haemophilia. *Lancet*, **339**, 819 (letter).

Mannucci, P. M., Gdovin, S., Gringeri, A., *et al.* (1993) Transmission of hepatitis A to patients with hemophilia by factor VIII concentrates treated with organic solvent and detergent to inactivate viruses. The Italian Collaborative Group. *Ann Intern Med*, **120**, 1–7.

Mason, W. S. and Jilbert, A. R. (2003) Hepatitis B virus: an unresolved problem. Proceedings of the 11th International Symposium on Viral Hepatitis and Liver Disease, Sydney, eds A. R. Jilbert, E. V. L. Grgacic and K. Vickery, pp. 254–62.

Mast, E. E., Favorov, M. O., Shapiro, C. N., *et al.* (1996) Hepatitis E virus infection in the Americas. In *Enterically-transmitted Hepatitis Viruses*, eds Y. Buisson, P. Coursaget and M. Kane, pp. 282–93. Tours, France, La Simarre.

Mast, E. E., Kuramoto, I. K., Favorov, M. O., *et al.* (1997) Prevalence of and risk factors for antibody to hepatitis E virus seroreactivity among blood donors in northern California. *J Infect Dis*, **176**, 34–40.

Masuda, J. I., Yano, K., Tamada, Y., *et al.* (2005) Acute hepatitis E of a man who consumed wild boar meat prior to the onset of illness in Nagasaki, Japan. *Hepatol Res*, **31**, 178–83.

Matsubayashi, K., Nagaoka, Y., Sakata, H., *et al.* (2004) Transfusion-transmitted hepatitis E caused by apparently indigenous hepatitis E virus strain in Hokkaido, Japan. *Transfusion*, **44**, 934–40.

Melnick, J. L. (1995) History and epidemiology of hepatitis A virus. *J Infect Dis*, **171**(Suppl. 1), S2–S8.

Mimms, L. T., Mosley, J. W., Hollinger, F. B., *et al.* (1993) Effect of concurrent acute infection with hepatitis C virus on acute hepatitis B virus infection. *Br Med J*, **307**, 1095–7.

Mitsui, T., Tsukamoto, Y., Yamazaki, C., *et al.* (2004) Prevalence of hepatitis E virus infection among hemodialysis patients in Japan: evidence for infection with a genotype 3 HEV by blood transfusion. *J Med Virol*, **74**, 563–72.

Montella, F., Rezza, G., Di Sora, F., *et al.* (1994) Association between hepatitis E virus and HIV infection in homosexual men. *Lancet*, **344**, 1433 (letter).

Morgan, H. W. and Williamson, D. A. (1943) Jaundice following administration of human blood products. *BMJ*, **1**, 750–3.

Muerhoff, A. S. and Dawson, G. J. (2004) Hepatitis C virus. In *Viral Hepatitis: Molecular Biology, Diagnosis, Epidemiology and Control (Perspectives in Medical Virology, volume 10)*, ed. I. K. Mushahwar, pp. 127–71. Amsterdam, Elsevier.

Nanda, S. K., Ansari, I. H., Acharya, S. K., *et al.* (1995) Protracted viremia during acute sporadic hepatitis E virus infection. *Gastroenterology*, **108**, 225–30.

Nelson, K., Ahmed, A., Ness, P. M., *et al.* (1993) Efficacy of donor screening methods on reducing the risk of transfusion-transmission of hepatitis C virus. *Fourth International Symposium on HCV*, Tokyo, **40** (abstract).

Nigro, G. and Del Grosso, B. (1990) Transfusion acquired hepatitis A in a patient with β-thal major. *J Infect*, **20**, 175–6.

Noble, R. C., Kane, M. A., Reeves, S. A., *et al.* (1984) Post-transfusion hepatitis A in a neonatal intensive care unit. *JAMA*, **252**, 2711–5.

Ohto, H. S., Terazawa, S., Sasaki, N., *et al.* (1994) Transmission of hepatitis C virus from mothers to infants. *N Engl J Med*, **330**, 744–50.

Patel, T. (2006) Cholangiocarcinoma. *Nat Clin Pract Gastroenterol Hepatol*, **3**, 33–42.

Peerlinch, K. and Vermylen, J. (1993) Acute hepatitis A in patients with haemophilia A. *Lancet*, **341**, 179 (letter).

Pereira, B. J., Milford, E. L., Kirkman, R. L., *et al.* (1991) Transmission of hepatitis C virus by organ transplantation. *N Engl J Med*, **325**, 454–60.

Pereira, B. J., Milford, E. L., Kirkman, R. L., *et al.* (1992) Prevalence of hepatitis C virus RNA in organ donors positive for hepatitis C antibody and in the recipients of their organs. *N Engl J Med*, **327**, 910–5.

Peterson, J., Green, G., Iida, K., *et al.* (2000) Detection of hepatitis C core antigen in the antibody negative 'window' phase of hepatitis C infection. *Vox Sang*, **78**, 80–5.

Piccoli, P. L., Franchini, M., Gandini, G., *et al.* (2001) HCV core antigen assay. *Transfusion*, **41**, 1172 (letter).

Pileri, P., Uematsu, Y., Campagnoli, S., *et al.* (1998) Binding of hepatitis C virus to CD81. *Science*, **282**, 938–41.

Previsani, N., Lavanchy, D. and Siegl, G. (2004) Hepatitis A. In *Viral Hepatitis: Molecular Biology, Diagnosis, Epidemiology and Control (Perspectives in Medical Virology, volume 10)*, ed. I. K. Mushahwar, pp. 1–98. Amsterdam, Elsevier.

Purcell, R. H., and Emerson, S. U. (2005) In *Viral Hepatitis*, eds H. C. Thomas, S. Lemon and A. J. Zuckerman, pp. 109–25. Malden, MA, Blackwell.

Quer, J. and Mur, J. I. E. (2005) Hepatitis C virus: epidemiology. In *Viral Hepatitis*, eds H. C. Thomas, S. Lemon and A. J. Zuckerman, pp. 407–25. Malden, MA, Blackwell.

Raimondo, G., Longo, G. and Caredda, F. (1986) Prolonged, polyphasic infection with hepatitis A. *J Infect Dis*, **153**, 172–3.

Rosenblum, L. S., Villarino, M. E., Nainan, O. V., *et al.* (1991) Margolis HS. Hepatitis A outbreak in a neonatal intensive care unit: risk factors for transmission and evidence of prolonged viral excretion among preterm infants. *J Infect Dis*, **164**, 476–82.

Ross, R. S., Viazov, S., Gross, T., *et al.* (2000) Transmission of hepatitis C virus from a patient to an anesthesiology assistant to five patients. *N Engl J Med*, **343**, 1851–4.

Roth, W. K. and Seifried, E. (2002) The German experience with NAT. *Transfus Med*, **12**, 255–8.

Sagnelli, E., Coppola, N., Marrocco, C., *et al.* (2003) HAV replication in acute hepatitis with typical and atypical clinical course. *J Med Virol*, **71**, 1–6.

Satake, M. (2005) Lookback study for transfusion-related HBV infection in Japan. *Transfusion*, **45**, 9A–10A (abstract).

Schreiber, G. B., Busch, M. P., Kleinman, S. H., *et al.* (1996) The risk of transfusion-transmitted viral infections. *N Eng J Med*, **334**, 1685–90.

Seeberg, S., Brandberg, A., Hermodsson, S., *et al.* (1981) Hospital outbreak of hepatitis A secondary to blood exchange in a baby. *Lancet*, **1**, 1155–6.

Seed, C. R., Kiely, P. and Keller, A. J. (2005) Residual risk of transfusion transmitted human immunodeficiency virus, hepatitis B virus, hepatitis C virus and human T lymphotropic virus. *Intern Med J*, **35**, 592–8.

Shah, U., Habib, Z. and Kleinman, R. E. (2000) Liver failure attributable to hepatitis A virus infection in a developing country. *Pediatrics*, **105**, 436–8.

Sheretz, R. J., Russell, B. A. and Reuman, P. D. (1984) Transmission of hepatitis A by transfusion of blood products. *Arch Intern Med*, **144**, 1579–80.

Skidmore, S. J., Boxall, E. H. and Ala, F. (1982) A case of post-transfusion hepatitis A. *J Med Virol*, **10**, 223.

Snyder, E. L. and Dodd, R. Y. (2001) Reducing the risk of blood transfusion. *Hematology* (Am Soc Hematol Educ Program), 433–42.

Soldan, K., Davison, K. and Dow, B. (2005) Estimates of the frequency of HBV, HCV and HIV infectious donations entering the blood supply in the United Kingdom, 1996 to 2003. *Euro Surveill*, **110**, 17–9.

Soucie, J. M., Robertson, B. H., Bell, B. P., *et al.* (1998) Hepatitis A virus infections associated with clotting factor concentrate in the United States. *Transfusion*, **38**, 573–9.

Stevens, C. E., Aach, R. D., Hollinger, F. B., *et al.* (1984) Hepatitis B virus antibody in blood donors and the occurrence of non-A, non-B hepatitis in transfusion recipients. An analysis of the Transfusion-transmitted Viruses Study. *Ann Intern Med*, **101**, 733–8.

Stramer, S. L. (2005) Pooled HBV DNA testing by nucleic acid amplification: implementation or not. *Transfusion*, **45**, 1242–6.

Stramer, S. L., Glynn, S. A., Kleinman, S. H., *et al.* (2004) Detection of HIV-1 and HCV infections among antibody-negative blood donors by nucleic acid-amplification testing. *N Eng J Med*, **351**, 760–8.

Takaki, A., Wiese, M., Maertens, G., *et al.* (2000) Cellular immune responses persist and humoral responses decrease two decades after recovery from a single-source outbreak of hepatitis C. *Nat Med*, **6**, 578–82.

Tanaka, E., Ohue, C., Aoyagi, K., *et al.* (2000) Evaluation of a new enzyme immunoassay for hepatitis C virus (HCV) core antigen with clinical sensitivity approximating that of genomic amplification of HCV RNA. *Hepatology*, **32**, 388–93.

Tasar, M. A., Bostanci, I., Karabulut, B., *et al.* (2005) A rare extrahepatic syndrome related to acute hepatitis type B: epididymitis in an adolescent. *Acta Gastroenterol Belg*, **68**, 270–1.

Tei, S., Kitajima, N., Takahashi, K., *et al.* (2003) Zoonotic transmission of hepatitis E virus from deer to human beings. *Lancet*, **362**, 371–3.

Temperley, I. J., Cotter, K. P., Walsh, T. J., *et al.* (1992) Clotting factors and hepatitis A. *Lancet*, **340**, 1466 (letter).

Thomas, D. L., Yarbough, P. O., Vlahov, D., *et al.* (1997) Seroreactivity to hepatitis E virus in areas where the disease is not endemic. *J Clin Microbiol*, **35**, 1244–7.

Tjon, G. M. S., Coutinho, R. A., van den Hoek, A., *et al.* (2006) High and persistent excretion of hepatitis A virus in immunocompetent patients. *J Med Virol*, **78**, 1398–405.

Tobler, L. H., Stramer, S. L., Lee, S. F., *et al.* (2005) Performance of ORTHO HCV core antigen and trak-C assays for detection of viraemia in pre-seroconversion plasma and whole blood donors. *Vox Sang*, **89**, 201–7.

Walsh, J. H., Purcell, R. H., Morrow, A. G., *et al.* (1970) Post-transfusion hepatitis after open-heart operations. *JAMA*, **211**, 261–5.

Wang, C. H., Flehmig, B. and Moeckli, R. (1993) Transmission of hepatitis E virus by transfusion? *Lancet*, **341**, 285–6.

Wang, J. T., Lin, J. T., Sheu, J. C., *et al.* (1994) Hepatitis E virus and post-transfusion hepatitis. *J Infect Dis*, **169**, 229–36.

Wang, L. and Zhuang, H. (2004) Hepatitis E: an overview and recent advances in vaccine research. *World J Gastroenterol*, **10**, 2157–62.

World Health Organization (2001) Hepatitis B surface antigen assays: operational characteristics (May), Geneva, World Health Organization.

Worm, H. C. and Wirnsberger, G. (2004) Hepatitis E vaccines: progress and prospects. *Drugs*, **64**, 1517–31.

Zanetti, A. R. and Dawson, G. J. (1994) Hepatitis E in Italy: a seroepidemiological survey. Study group of hepatitis E. *J Med Virol*, **42**, 318–20.

Zanetti, A. R., Tanzi, E., Paccagnini, S., *et al.* (1995) Mother-to-infant transmission of hepatitis C virus. *Lancet*, **345**, 289–90.

Zarski, J. P., Ganem, D. and Wright, T. L. (2002) Hepatitis B virus. In *Clinical Virology*, eds D. D. Richman, R. J. Whitley and F. G. Hayden, pp. 623–57. Washington DC, ASM Press.

Zignego, A. L. and Brechot, C. (1999) Extrahepatic manifestations of HCV infection: facts and controversies. *J Hepatol*, **31**, 369–76.

ANTIBODY TO HEPATITIS B CORE ANTIGEN

Joan O'Riordan

Introduction

In the mid-1980s some countries introduced blood donor screening for antibody to hepatitis B core antigen (anti-HBc) as a surrogate test for non-A, non-B hepatitis (Aymard *et al.*, 1986; Koziol *et al.*, 1986). Once anti-hepatitis C virus (HCV) antibody screening was implemented, anti-HBc testing was retained to reduce the risk of hepatitis B transmission and to detect populations at high risk of HIV infection. With data documenting the declining efficacy of anti-HBc as a surrogate marker for the prevention of HIV infection (Busch *et al.*, 1997), anti-HBc screening has been retained to detect the rare hepatitis B virus (HBV) infectious, HBsAg negative donation (Busch, 1998). On a global level the frequency of anti-HBc is proportional to the prevalence of HBV in the population, with the highest prevalence rates in Asia and Africa, moderate rates in South and Central America and Southern Europe and lowest rates in Northern Europe and North America (Busch, 1998).

With the advent of nucleic acid amplification testing (NAT) of blood donations for HCV and HIV in North America and in many European countries, the role of anti-HBc screening and of mini-pool HBV DNA NAT is being investigated (Kleinman and Busch, 2001).

Hepatitis B virus serology

Please refer back to Chapter 1.

In general, in the immune response to hepatitis B infection, antibodies to the core of hepatitis B virus (IgM class followed by IgG) are the first antibodies produced and may be detected a few days after the appearance of HBsAg. HBsAg declines over a period of several weeks and is replaced by detectable levels of antibody to HBsAg (anti-HBs), the presence of which was thought to predict immunity and lack of infectivity. Acute HBV is asymptomatic in 50–70% of adults and spontaneously resolves in 95% of adults with apparently no long-term sequelae. About 5% of HBV infections become chronic in immunocompetent subjects and a smaller proportion generate a severe HBV-related disease. After the resolution of an acute HBV infection, anti-HBc typically persists for the lifetime of the individual, while anti-HBs levels may decline and become undetectable.

Anti-HBc testing of donations helps to reduce the risk of HBV transmission by detecting individuals with low-level chronic HBV infection in whom HBsAg is not detectable. In addition, during the early convalescent period of acute HBV, when neither HBsAg nor its homologous antibody are detectable (core window period), anti-HBc persists and may be the only detectable serological

marker of HBV infection (Busch, 1998). Anti-HBc may also identify HBV 'escape mutants', not detected by HBsAg tests (Jongerius *et al.*, 1998; Zuckerman and Zuckerman, 2000).

Anti-HBc positive donors who are HBsAg negative but are unequivocally positive for anti-HBs are thought to have resolved HBV infection and to be non-infectious (Mosley *et al.*, 1995; NIH, 1995). This serological definition of immunity is imperfect. There have been numerous reports of transmission of HBV via liver allografts from donors after complete serological recovery from HBV (Dickson *et al.*, 1997; Dodson *et al.*, 1997; Douglas *et al.*, 1997). This reactivation may be especially problematical in liver transplantation, in which a substantial viral load is transplanted (Wachs *et al.*, 1995). Recrudescence of apparently cured HBV infection has also been described after renal and bone marrow transplantation, and 'reverse seroconversion' from anti-HBs to HBsAg positivity has been observed (Dhedin *et al.*, 1998; Marcellin *et al.*, 1991). Traces of HBV DNA are often detectable in the blood for many years after clinical recovery of acute hepatitis despite the presence of antibodies and HBV-specific cytotoxic T-lymphocytes (CTLs) (Rehermann *et al.*, 1996). Sterilizing immunity to HBV frequently fails to occur and traces of virus can maintain the CTL response for decades, apparently keeping the virus under control, perhaps for life (Hennig *et al.*, 2002; Rehermann *et al.*, 1996).

Residual risk of transfusion-transmitted (TT) – hepatitis B virus infection

At present, estimation of the residual risks of transfusion-transmissible viral infections (TTIs) is mainly based on mathematical risk modelling (Korelitz *et al.*, 1997; Schreiber *et al.*, 1996). (Please refer to Chapter 25.) The residual risks of TT-HIV and HCV, which are already very low, have been reduced to extremely low levels after implementation of mini-pool (MP) NAT (Dodd *et al.*, 2002). The yield of donors found positive by NAT but not by serology for HIV-1 and HCV RNA in the USA was consistent with that predicted from the mathematical models (Stramer *et al.*, 2004). Although HBV risk estimates need to be evaluated with some caution, because of limited data on the window period and because incidence rates for HBsAg are adjusted to account for the transient presence of HBsAg, HBV remains the most likely of the major viral agents to be transmissible by transfusion. For HIV and HCV the pre-seroconversion window period accounts for 90% of the total residual risk of transmission by transfusion. This is also the case for HBV in countries performing anti-HBc screening, whereas HBsAg negative, anti-HBc reactive chronic carriers probably contribute a level of risk equal to or greater

Transfusion Microbiology, eds John A. J. Barbara, Fiona A. M. Regan and Marcela C. Contreras. Published by Cambridge University Press. © Cambridge University Press 2008.

than that from early seroconversion window-period risk in the absence of anti-HBc screening (Glynn *et al.*, 2002; Roth *et al.*, 2002). Residual risk estimates for HBV (with large confidence intervals), are similarly low for France (1 in 470 000) (Pillonel *et al.*, 2002) and Australia (1 in 483 000) (Seed *et al.*, 2002), intermediate for the USA (1 in 205 000 for repeat donors) (Dodd *et al.*, 2002) and Germany (1 in 230 000 without and 1 in 620 000 with MP-NAT) (Offergeld *et al.*, 2005) and highest in Spain (1 in 100 000) (Alvarez do Barrio *et al.*, 2005) and Switzerland (1 in 115 000) (Niederhauser *et al.*, 2005). The UK have adapted the Schreiber incidence/window-period model (Schreiber *et al.*, 1996) to take account of the risk due to test or process errors, the incidence rate in new donors and a longer infectious window period for HBV (52 days for early acute +30 days for late acute window-period infections). This gave a point estimate of 1 in 260 000 for the time period 1993–2001 (Soldan *et al.*, 2003) declining to 1 in 450 000 for the time period 2002–2003 (Soldan *et al.*, 2003). There appears to have been a decline in risk in repeat donors over the last decade in France, the USA, UK and Spain. In France, the most recent estimate for the period 2001–2003 is 1 in 640 000 donations which represents an almost six-fold decline when compared to the period 1992–1994 (Pillonel *et al.*, 2005). An important factor contributing to this decline has been attributed to improved rates of vaccination of the French population (Pillonel *et al.*, 2002; Pillonel *et al.*, 2005).

There is a disparity between predicted cases of TT-HBV and observed cases in countries of low endemicity for HBV. In the USA, there have been few well documented cases of TT-HBV in the recent past (Stramer *et al.*, 2005). Of 7381 cases of acute hepatitis B reported to the US Centres for Disease Control and Prevention (CDC) in 2003, ten were confirmed by the CDC as acute cases of HBV corresponding to the time of transfusion (i.e., transfusion within the past six months), of whom only one case could be associated with an identified single infected unit (Stramer, 2005). This disparity may be due to the large percentage of asymptomatic HBV infections leading to under-reporting both in the general population and probably in the transfused population, but in addition, the entire window period may not be infectious, whereas this is assumed in the risk estimate models (Stramer, 2005).

Since the enhanced surveillance of TTIs commenced in the UK in 1995, only ten documented cases of TT-HBV were reported up until 2004 (Serious Hazards Transfusion Annual Report, 2005). Soldan *et al.* reported that all six cases of TT-HBV identified between 1998 and 2001 were the result of infectious donations collected from donors with acute HBV infection. This is in contrast to the series reported during 1991–1997, when only 3 of 14 similar cases were caused by acute infections in donors; the majority of incidents were due to chronic infection in donors. The authors postulate that the change over a decade may reflect improvements in the sensitivity of HBsAg assays and/or a decrease in prevalence of chronic HBV infection in the UK (Soldan *et al.*, 2002).

Between 1995 and 2003, the Paul-Ehrlich-Institut (PEI) in Germany received a total of 36 reports of probable or confirmed cases of HBV transmission by cellular blood products and fresh

frozen plasma. In at least 7 of the 18 cases, in which it was possible to prove the causal relationship of the blood components by genomic comparison, anti-HBc testing would have prevented the transmissions (Burger, 2005).

In Japan, which implemented anti-HBc screening in 1989 because of high endemic rates of HBV infection, 103 cases of suspected TT-HBV infections between 1997 and 1999 (before the implementation of HBV mini-pool NAT), have been reported to the Japanese surveillance programme (Matsumoto *et al.*, 2001). Sixteen were confirmed to be due to transfusion. According to the results of anti-HBc in implicated donations and the results of follow-up testing of the donors, it was estimated that at least ten were due to window-period donations. Five of these ten would have been detected by a more sensitive HBsAg assay (Auszyme II EIA) (Matsumoto *et al.*, 2001); of the five donors who were negative by more sensitive assays, four were HBV DNA positive, HBV genome was estimated to be 3300, 3000, 800 and 500 geq/ml respectively, but even individual donor (ID) NAT with a sensitivity of 50 copies/ml would have missed detecting HBV in one donation. A further 2 of the 16 transmissions were from units that were anti-HBc positive but at titres (32 and 16) that were permissible for transfusion. The causes for the remaining four cases of HBV transmission were difficult to characterize (Matsumoto *et al.*, 2001).

What is the evidence that a proportion of donors with antibody to hepatitis B core antigen in the absence of hepatitis B surface antigen are infectious for hepatitis B virus?

(1) Quantitative analysis of serological data from the Transfusion-Transmitted Viruses Study conducted in the 1970s and re-evaluated in the 1990s indicated five possible transmissions of HBV by anti-HBc positive donations (Mosley *et al.*, 1995). Only high level anti-HBc reactivity in the presence of borderline or no anti-HBs reactivity was associated with HBV transmission; no HBV transmission was observed when anti-HBs sample-to-negative control values were ≥ 10 (Mosley *et al.*, 1995). By contrast, a post-transfusion study by the National Institutes of Health found no association between anti-core positivity in donors and HBV infection in recipients (Busch, 1998; Koziol *et al.*, 1986) and the Canadian Post-transfusion Hepatitis Prevention Study failed to detect HBV in 138 recipients of anti-HBc reactive, HBsAg negative blood (Blajchman *et al.*, 1995), but a larger study is probably required to achieve significance.

(2) A decline in reported cases of HBV has occurred in countries coincident with the implementation of anti-core screening (Busch, 1998; Chambers and Popovsky, 1991, Japanese Red Cross non-A, non-B Hepatitis Research Group, 1991; Mosley *et al.*, 1995). To avoid excessive donor deferrals, the Japanese Red Cross implemented anti-HBc testing in 1989 and restricted the transfusion of some, but not all anti-HBc-positive units. Anti-HBc detection was by an in-house haemagglutination inhibition technique. Units were transfused if the anti-HBc titre was $<2^4$; if the anti-HBc titre was $>2^5$, units

were still eligible for transfusion if the anti-HBs titre was $>2^4$ (approx $\geq$200 mIU/ml) (Yoshikawa et al., 2005). However, as noted above, two cases of TT-HBV have been reported from units that were anti-HBc positive but at titres that were permissible for transfusion (one had a titre of 32 and the other, 16); the one sample that could be quantitated had 400 copies/ml of HBV DNA (Matsumoto et al., 2001). Since June 1997 the criteria for anti-HBc screening were changed such that the level of acceptable anti-core titre was reduced from 64 to 32 (Matsumoto et al., 2001). Since the implementation of MP-NAT HBV in Japan in 1999, the above anti-HBc screening policy has been maintained except that now all units are tested by NAT apart from those donors who are HBsAg positive or who have high titre anti-HBc without detectable anti-HBs who are already excluded and therefore not tested by NAT (Yoshikawa et al., 2005).

(3) In a look-back study in the UK of persons who had received units of blood from donors who subsequently tested positive for anti-HBc, two cases of probable HBV transmission were found; it was estimated that the transmission of HBV from HBsAg negative, anti HBc positive donors occurred in one per 52 000 donations (95% CIs, 1 in 12,821–1 in 333,333) (Allain et al., 1999).

(4) Hepatitis B virus DNA concentrations during the later stages of HBV infection are extremely low, as are detection rates but they vary depending on the sensitivity of tests used and also according to the prevalence of HBV infection. Detection rates for HBV DNA generally are <5% in low prevalence areas but have been found in 4–24% of anti-HBc positive individuals in high-prevalence areas (Allain, 2004).

The Retrovirus Epidemiology Donor Study (REDS) investigators in the USA have reported a detection rate of HBV DNA in 4 out of 395 (1%) anti-HBc positive specimens (107 of whom were anti-HBs neg and 288 were anti-HBs pos at 3–100 IU/L) from a repository of allogeneic donations collected between 1991–1995 (Kleinman et al., 2003). The 4 PCR positive specimens were anti-HBs negative; estimated levels of HBV DNA were 10–30 copies/ml in two and 50–100 copies/ml in the other two. The HBV DNA detection rate in anti HBs-negative samples was 3.7% and the projected rate among all anti-HBc reactive samples was 0.24%, leading to an estimate that about one HBV DNA-containing unit in 49 000 allogeneic donations (95% CI, 1 in 16 600–1 in 152 600) would have been released for transfusion, if anti-HBc testing had not been performed. Only one of the four with an estimated copy number of HBV DNA of 50 to 100 copies/ml was confirmed positive for HBsAg by the Abbott PRISM HBsAg. This study concluded that MP-NAT will not detect most potentially infectious units from anti-HBc positive donors because of the low viral load (Kleinman et al., 2003).

An American Red Cross study of HBV DNA prevalence in anti-HBc positive, HBsAg negative specimens, (not tested for anti-HBs), showed that only 17 of 3000 (0.57%) were detected in a very sensitive ID NAT assay; the majority had viral loads below 100 geq/ml (Busch, 2004).

Kleinman et al., recently reported the results of the US clinical trial of the Roche COBAS AmpliScreen HBV assay (Kleinman

et al., 2005). The 95% limit of detection of the assay on an individual donor sample was 5 IU/ml (20 copies/ml) and was 120 IU (480 copies)/ml in a pool of 24. Of a total of 2900 anti-HBc-positive, HBsAg negative specimens, that were evaluable by MP and ID-NAT, 12 were HBV DNA positive; only one was detected by MP and 11 by ID NAT, giving a detection rate of 0.41% (95% CI 0.21–0.72%). Overall, 1 in 48 942 donations were HBV DNA-positive, HBsAg negative, anti-HBc positive. Only three of the twelve HBV DNA positives were positive by alternative DNA assays (900–1200 copies/ml). Six of these donors had consistently negative ID AmpliScreen HBV DNA results on follow-up, three of whom were positive for anti-HBs. Lack of detection could have been due to fluctuating low level viraemia or a false-positive ID NAT result (Kleinman et al., 2005).

A Japanese study reported HBV NAT data for 1103 samples which tested negative by Abbott PRISM HBsAg chemiluminescent immunoassay (CLIA) and positive by anti-HBc testing (titre $\geq$32). Twelve (1.1%) of these contained HBV DNA, all at very low copy numbers (projected at 10–100 copies/ml) and in addition all 12 samples had anti-HBe reactivity (Sato et al., 2001). Seven out of twelve of these low-level chronic infections could also be detected by PRISM CLIA-HBsAg if a 30% reduction in the assay cut-off was applied (S: CO, 0.7) (Sato et al., 2001).

Another Japanese study showed a 38% HBV DNA positive rate in donors who were HBsAg (EIA, sensitivity 1.0 ng/ml) negative and anti-HBc positive at high titres (Yotsuyanagi et al., 2001). These results were markedly discrepant from the low detection rates in previously reported studies, but Iizuka et al., also from Japan, had previously shown an apparent correlation between HBV DNA and titres of anti-HBc: HBV DNA was detected in 12 (6.9%) of 175 blood units with anti-HBc HI titres $\geq$2^6$, which is significantly more than detecting HBV DNA in none of 119 units with anti-HBc titres $\leq$2^5$ (p <0.01) (Iizuka et al., 1992).

In a further recent study among isolated anti-HBc positive donors from Japan, plasma viraemia was also more frequently observed in groups with a high anti-HBc titre (Yugi et al., 2006). In the group of donors with high anti-HBc titres who were anti-HBs negative and who are not normally subjected to the Japanese Red Cross HBV MP-NAT screening system, the proportion of HBV-NAT positives was very high and ranged from 25% to 100%, with increasing anti-HBc HI titres from 2^6 to 2^{12}. Perhaps some of the donors in these studies (Iizuka et al., 1992; Yotsuyanagi et al., 2001; Yugi et al., 2006) would have had detectable HBsAg if more sensitive assays had been used. This group also reported that when a large volume of sample (e.g. 2ml) was used for extraction, HBV DNA was detected in 8 of 500 of donors with isolated low titre anti-HBc reactivity (2^4 or less by HI), four of whom had HBV DNA levels of ten copies or less (Yugi et al., 2006).

In a study on the frequency and load of HBV DNA in first-time blood donors in Germany, 216 (1.5%) of 14 251 donors tested positive for anti-HBc in two different assays and 205 of them (16 HBsAg pos, 189 HBsAg neg) were tested for HBV DNA by PCR (95% detection limit of assay 27.8 IU/ml) (Hennig et al., 2002).

Hepatitis B virus DNA was repeatedly found in 14 (87.5%) of the HBsAg positive blood donors and in three (1.59%) of the HBsAg-negative donors, representing 0.02% of the core reactive HBsAg negative donors. Hepatitis B virus DNA was seen at a low level, <1000 IU/ml; even 6 of the 14 HBsAg and HBV DNA positive samples were quantified to be <100 IU/ml. In the three HBV DNA positive, HBsAg negative cases, anti-HBe and anti-HBs (>100 IU/l) were also detectable.

In a study on the value of anti-HBc screening of blood donors in north-western Greece, anti-HBc reactivity was found in 998 of 6696 (14.9%) donors screened; 716 (71.7%) had protective anti-HBs titres (>20 mIU/ml), whereas the remaining 282 donors (28.3%) had either anti-HBc reactivity alone or in combination with either or both anti-HBe and low titre anti-HBs <20 mIU/ml. None of the 282 donors tested HBV DNA positive by a combination assay based on PCR and a DNA EIA (lower detection limit between 100 and 1000 copies/ml). No transfusion-associated HBV infections were recorded in the recipients of the blood donated by these 282 donors (Zervou et al., 2001).

Anti-HBc was found to be a surrogate marker for previous risk behaviour in the Danish blood donor population. The prevalence of confirmed positive HBc antibodies was 0.70% (76 in 10 862). None were HBV DNA positive (detection limit of PCR assay was <100 geq/ml) (Christensen et al., 2001).

The German experience with MP-HBV NAT identified six HBV PCR positive, HBsAg negative donations after screening of 3.6 million donations in Central Europe (Germany, Austria, Luxembourg) (Roth et al., 2002). Two were from infected donors in the pre-seroconversion window period and four were from chronic anti-HBc positive, anti-HBs negative, low-level HBV carriers. The detection limit for the mini-pool HBV NAT was 1000 geq/ml for each individual donation. In addition, the investigators reported that a recipient-directed look-back revealed two anti-HBc positive recipients of HBsAg negative, mini-pool PCR-negative, anti-HBc positive and single-sample PCR positive blood components. After testing 729 randomly selected HBsAg negative, mini-pool PCR negative, anti-HBc positive donors, by single-sample enrichment PCR, seven were identified with ≤10 HBV DNA geq/ml of donor plasma. Six of the seven were positive for anti-HBs, three of whom had an antibody titre higher than 100 IU/ml. The authors concluded that MP-PCR and even single sample PCR would not be sensitive enough to provide a risk reduction factor with respect to chronic low-level carriers similar to that of anti-HBc screening. More extensive results of the voluntary (non-mandatory) NAT testing in Germany were reported in a recent review which showed that 47 HBV NAT-only positives were detected from testing 21 733 529 donations in MP-NAT, (mini-pool size of 96) giving a yield rate of 1: 462 416; of the first 42 cases, two-thirds (28) were anti-HBc positive (Comanor and Holland, 2006).

In an evaluation of anti-HBc screening of blood donations in New Zealand, a strongly reactive anti-HBc donation with anti-HBs of <10 IU/l, was found to be HBV DNA positive when tested by the Chiron Ultrio assay. Hepatitis B virus DNA positivity was confirmed in an additional assay. One stored aliquot from the most recent 12 donations of this regular donor was Ultrio

reactive, but none of four recipients of these donations had markers suggestive of HBV infection. Overall, 682 of 10 000 donations were anti-HBc reactive (6.8%) and the authors concluded that the high level of anti-HBc reactivity in their study suggested that anti-HBc screening would not be an appropriate test to reduce the risk of HBV in New Zealand (Flanagan et al., 2005).

Anti-HBs levels of >100 IU/l in the presence of anti-HBc reactivity are thought to be protective against transmission as the anti-HBs might neutralize any HBV that is present. There is clear evidence that latent virus in the liver is infectious when such donors are used for liver transplantation. Whether this holds true for concurrent HBV DNA positivity in blood is uncertain. In Japan, the transfusion of anti-HBc reactive units with a titre of anti-HBs >1 in 16 (approx 200 IU/l) is permitted and has not been linked to post-transfusion HBV transmission (Matsumoto et al., 2001). In the TTVS study, only high level anti-HBc reactivity in the presence of borderline or no anti-HBs reactivity was associated with HBV transmissibility (Mosley et al., 1995). A case report from Germany showed that transfusion of units from a donor with anti-HBc, anti-HBs and intermittently detectable HBV DNA (concentration ranging from 8 to 260 IU/ml) did not result in transmission of HBV to any of the nine patients who received RBC or plasma from these anti-HBc and anti-HBs positive donations (Dreier et al., 2004). In the UK anti-HBc look-back study, the two probable HBV transmissions resulted from the transfusion of components from anti-HBc positive, anti-HBs negative donors (Allain et al., 1999).

The inoculation of small amounts of serum and lymphocytes from three patients who were HBsAg negative, anti-HBs positive, anti-HBc positive, and with low-level HBV DNA positivity (ranging from 265 to 2023 DNA copies/ml) into three chimpanzees did not lead to infections in any of the animals (Prince et al., 2001). Further studies with larger volumes of inoculum (e.g. a unit of blood) should be conducted. However, it can be concluded that sera and PBMNCs in this study were one-tenth to one-hundredth as infective as were materials derived from HBsAg positive blood from subjects with acute HBV infection (Prince et al., 2001). Further look-back investigations and animal transmission studies are required.

Even in the absence of anti-HBs, it is not known to what extent units with low concentrations of HBV DNA will transmit infection. Yugi et al., recently reported on HBV (genotype A) transmission experiments in chimpanzees which showed that the minimum infective dose of HBV was equivalent to ten copies of HBV DNA when acute phase plasma was used as the inoculum (Yugi et al., 2006).

The implementation of MP-NAT for HBV in Japan sheds further light on TT-HBV. Repository samples from previous donations were investigated for HBV by means of ID-NAT when repeat donors seroconverted for viral markers or first tested positive by 50-pool-screening NAT and a look-back was performed (Satake et al., 2005). Only 11 of 71 evaluable patients in whom the transfused donation was ID-NAT positive but negative for MP-NAT showed evidence of HBV transmission. Ten out of eleven implicated components were derived from window-period donations, that is, were HBcAb negative; the remaining one component was HBcAb weakly positive. Ten of thirty-one recipients (32%) of window-period derived donations versus 1 of 40 (2.5%) recipients of chronic carrier derived ID-NAT positive components showed evidence of transmission.

A prospective study of transfusion recipients from Taiwan, a hyperendemic country for HBV, identified 39 HBV-naive recipients who had been transfused with blood from 147 donations (Wang et al., 2002). Eleven samples from these HBsAg (EIA) negative donations tested anti-HBc positive and HBV DNA positive by PCR at a low concentration, (50–500 copies/ml). Only 1 of 11 recipients of these 11 HBV DNA positive donations developed acute, mild, transient HBV infection. Another recipient appeared to have either an abortive infection or HBV carry-over.

While the limited data in these two studies suggest that units donated by chronic carriers may be less infectious than units donated during the window period, the immune status of recipients is likely to be an important factor, as illustrated by HBV transmissions in four immunocompromised patients with haematological malignancies in Japan from a single apheresis platelet donor whose retrospective infectious donations tested ID-HBV NAT positive ($<10^2$ copies/ml) on only one occasion (Inaba et al., 2005). The authors conclude that the implementation of more sensitive anti-HBc tests than the HI assay used in Japan, such as enzyme immunoassay, would not be possible because of high donor loss. However it is not known whether more sensitive HBsAg assays now in use might have been positive and therefore detected HBV.

Comparative sensitivity of hepatitis B surface antigen and hepatitis B virus nucleic acid testing

Pre-hepatitis B surface antigen window period

Anti-HBc testing will not detect HBsAg negative donors in the pre-seroconversion window phase. Hepatitis B virus infection is endemic in Japan, and therefore the risk of transmission by blood transfusion in the pre-HBsAg-infectious window period is expected to be high. Because the doubling time in the period of exponential increase in HBV DNA – the 'burst' so-called 'ramp-up' phase of acute HBV infection is slow, estimated at approximately 2.6 days (Biswas et al., 2003; Yoshikawa et al., 2005), a highly sensitive NAT would be required to detect donors in the pre-HBsAg infectious WP. Unlike the situation with HCV and HIV, HBV NAT has only been mandated in Japan, and since January 2005 in Poland, a country of medium endemicity for HBV (Brojer, 2005). In addition, the majority of donations in Germany undergo voluntary MP-NAT for HBV DNA. The low uptake of HBV NAT reflects the fact that assays such as the Abbott PRISM HBsAg CLIA have equal sensitivity to prototype and commercial HBV NAT assays using pool sizes of 16–24 donations (Biswas et al., 2003; Koppelman et al., 2005; Stramer et al., 2001). It has been estimated from a US study on HBV seroconversion panels that HBsAg concentration at cut-off for new unlicensed (in the USA) tests ranged from 0.07 to 0.12 ng/ml with a median estimated viral load at cut-off of 720 HBV DNA copies/ml for the most sensitive HBsAg assay (US version) (Biswas et al., 2003). Mini-pool NAT

would reduce the 59-day seroconversion window period for HBV by 9 to 11 days, the most sensitive unlicensed (in the USA) HBsAg assay by 9 days and a sensitive single-sample NAT by approximately 18 days compared to the most sensitive HBsAg assay (Biswas et al., 2003). The authors concluded that sensitivity, WP closure, and yield projections for newer HBsAg assays and pooled-sample-NAT are comparable.

A Japanese study showed that for a mini-pool NAT system (95% detection rate 100 copies/ml) to be more efficacious than the PRISM HBsAg assay, NAT mini-pools needed to be no larger than 25 donations (Sato et al., 2001). They further demonstrated, by analysing 95 seroconversion samples, that HBsAg detection by PRISM CLIA (S/C ratio of 1.0) corresponded to 1644 HBV DNA copies/ml.

An American Red Cross study compared the sensitivities of HBV NAT and HBsAg assays by testing serial samples from 17 seroconversion plasma donor panels (Stramer et al., 2001). Hepatitis B virus DNA (no pooling) was detected for a mean of 21 days prior to HBsAg by the most sensitive assay; however, the median HBV DNA titres in HBsAg negative samples was 100–500 copies/ml. Hepatitis B surface antigen detection by PRISM corresponded to approximately 1400 copies/ml.

Recently, a European multicentre study demonstrated that the Procleix Ultrio™ (Chiron/Gen-Probe) NAT assay (which simultaneously detects HIV-1, HCV RNA and HBV DNA by transcription-mediated amplification) had a 95% detection limit of 11 IU/ml (WHO International Standard) for HBV DNA (Koppelman et al., 2005). By testing 15 seroconversion panels, the Ultrio assay demonstrated an advantage over the PRISM HBsAg assay with a window-period reduction by an average of three days (range, 0–5 days) with pools of 16, 6 days (range, 3–8 days) with pools of 8 and 14 days (range, 11–18 days) with ID NAT. No window-period reduction was observed in a pool of 24, with PRISM being more sensitive in about half the panels tested.

Results of a large multicentre clinical trial of the COBAS AmpliScreen HBV test (Roche Molecular Systems) on screening 1.2 million units in the USA, in mini-pools of 24, yielded four HBV DNA positives, HBV serology negative donations (Kleinman et al., 2005). Viral loads of the four samples reported were: 200 copies in a previously HBV vaccinated donor who had high-titre anti-HBs and never produced HBsAg, and 2000, 2300 and 61 000 copies/ml respectively for three samples from donors who developed HBsAg 7 to 17 days after the index donation. The index donation with a HBV DNA concentration of 61 000 copies/ml, which tested negative for HBsAg, was positive in an alternative HBsAg assay. It is not known how many of the remaining 3 samples would have detectable HBsAg if more sensitive assays, including the US version of PRISM, had been used (Stramer, 2005).

Since October 1999, the Japanese Red Cross (JRC) has implemented NAT nationwide for HBV, HCV and HIV, initially utilizing a pool size of 500, moving to a 50-pool size in 2000 and since August 2004 mini-pool size has been 20 (Yugi et al., 2005). Samples with HBsAg positivity by the relatively insensitive reverse passive haemagglutination (RPHA) assay (sensitivity approx 2 ng/ml) and with high-titre anti-HBc, but without detectable anti-HBs are excluded from testing by NAT and the pertinent units are discarded (Yoshikawa *et al.*, 2005). It has been previously shown from parallel testing 540 161 Japanese donors, that of 1 153 CLIA-HBsAg confirmed reactive samples only 837 (72.6%) were also positive by the RPHA-HBsAg (Sato *et al.*, 2001). From 2000 to end of 2002, the JRC screened 16 012 175 units with their multiplex in-house PCR (mini-pool size 50), demonstrating an HBV DNA yield of 308 cases (1 in 51 987), representing 86% of their total NAT yield (Mine *et al.*, 2003).

Mineghishi *et al.*, reported on 181 HBV DNA positive donations which were detected during testing of over 11 million donations by the JRC between February 2000 and October 2001, giving a yield of 1 in 61 000 (Mineghishi *et al.*, 2003). Out of 181 HBV-DNA positive donations, 105 (58%) were positive when tested by PRISM CLIA-HBsAg, giving an adjusted yield of 1 in 145 000. Reactivity on CLIA correlated with HBV DNA concentration: a total of 99 (74%) of the 133 samples with HBV DNA copies of >1400 were CLIA reactive compared with only six (12.5%) of the 48 samples with HBV DNA copies of <1400/ml (Mineghishi *et al.*, 2003). The estimated viral load corresponding to the positive cut-off for PRISM HBsAg testing was 2100 copies/ml. The 95% limit of detection (LOD) of the ID-HBV NAT was 22–60 copies/ml for HBV or 1100–3000 copies/ml in a 50-sample NAT pool. The authors suggested that the effect of the Poisson distribution in PCR test systems explains the ability of the system to detect the 42 HBV DNA positive samples with HBV DNA of <1000 copies/ml, even though this is less than the 95% LOD (Mineghishi *et al.*, 2003).

Yoshikawa *et al.*, in a further report, have shown that the 50 mini-pool, HBV NAT screening in use by the JRC detected HBV DNA in both the early (so-called serological window period) and late stages of acute HBV infection (Yoshikawa *et al.*, 2005). Out of 170 evaluable HBV NAT positive samples, 125 (45%) were found to have an increasing viral load and 45 (16%) a decreasing viral load. Sixty per cent of HBV NAT positive samples with an increasing viral load, and 77% of those with a decreasing viral load, were positive when tested by CLIA for HBsAg. The authors comment that their 50 mini-pool, 0.2 ml input volume, multiplex HBV NAT system shows greater sensitivity relative to the effectiveness of CLIA than previous estimates, which may be related to the use of donor samples in their studies, whilst previous studies used seroconversion panels to assess the increasing phase of acute HBV infection. The difference may also be accounted for by differences in epidemiology of HBV genotypes in Japan, where genotype C predominates, whereas genotypes A and D are mainly observed in USA and Europe. In their study, kinetic differences were observed between genotypes A and B in that the doubling time of genotype A is shorter, and the post-peak viral load half-life of genotype A is longer than that of genotype B (Yoshikawa *et al.*, 2005).

Late stages of hepatitis B virus infection

In the above studies on the comparative sensitivity of quantitative NAT and qualitative HBsAg assays, it has been possible to extrapolate viral load at cut-off using linear regression models because of the linear relationship between the two in acute HBV infection (Kuhns *et al.*, 2004). No such relationship occurs in the late stages of HBV infection where HBV DNA levels in HBsAg positive, anti-HBc reactive blood donations can be extremely low. In a US report, only a weak correlation (correlation coefficient = 0.33) between HBsAg (Architect HBsAg, Abbott laboratories, Abbott Park, IL, sensitivity 0.28 ng/ml) and HBV DNA concentration was found in a study on 200 samples from HBsAg, anti-HBc reactive donors, 90% of whom had a serological profile consistent with chronic HBV infection (Kuhns *et al.*, 2004). Thirty-six per cent (72/200) of donor samples had DNA levels <400 copies/ml. Retesting of the 72 samples by more sensitive PCR assays showed that 60 out of 200 (30%) were positive by PCR with a sensitivity of 65 copies/ml, whereas 6 out of 200 (3%) required a PCR sensitivity of 1.3 copies/ml to give a positive result. Three per cent (6/200) were negative by all three NAT assays used in the study (Kuhns *et al.*, 2004).

Sato *et al.*, also reported that blood donor samples from probable chronic HBV carriers had CLIA-HBsAg sample to cut-off values that were disproportionately high compared to the low concentrations of HBV DNA (Sato *et al.*, 2001). In the German MP-NAT programme, only 298 out of 432 (69%) confirmed HBsAg positive donations had detectable HBV DNA using a combination of mini-pool and more sensitive single-sample PCR assays (Roth *et al.*, 2002) and another German study recorded a consistent HBV DNA detection in 87.5% of HBsAg positive blood donors (Hennig *et al.*, 2002). Furthermore, in the large multicentre Roche HBV AmpliScreen clinical trial in the USA, HBV DNA was detected by MP-NAT in 84% of the HBsAg positive, anti-HBc positive donations, versus a 94% detection rate by ID NAT (Kleinman *et al.*, 2005).

The above data from acute HBV infection and chronic carriers shows that the amount of circulating HBsAg relative to HBV DNA can vary enormously depending on the stage of infection (Kuhns *et al.*, 2004). It is therefore likely that in the foreseeable future even the introduction of an ID-NAT strategy would not allow discontinuation of HBsAg screening.

Problems with antibody to hepatitis B core antigen screening

There are a number of major problems with anti-HB core blood screening assays, which limit their usefulness for blood donor screening, due to high donor loss rates (Busch, 1998).

(1) The usefulness of anti-HBc screening as a safety measure in addition to HBsAg testing is probably limited to low-prevalence countries as the donor loss rates would be unacceptably high in HBV endemic regions in Southern and Eastern Europe, Asia and Africa, where anti-HBc seroprevalence rates are high, unless a modified anti-HBc screening programme as successfully adopted in Japan was implemented.

(2) The problem of poor specificity of anti-HBc testing (Busch, 1998; NIH, 1995; Stramer, 2005) is that many donors with isolated anti-HBc reactivity are falsely positive, as evidenced by a primary immune response when vaccinated and the

transience of anti-HBc positivity in many persons (Aoki *et al.*, 1993; Christensen *et al.*, 2001; Mosley *et al.*, 1995; Stramer, 2005).

Modifying the test algorithm for defining a positive result, for example positive in two anti-HBc assays preferably with different formats, can improve the specificity although may not necessarily be sufficient to identify true positivity (Allain, 2004). In the Danish study, 34% of 116 repeat reactives were deemed to be falsely positive and the number of donors testing positive for 'anti-HBc only' could be reduced from 45 (34% of all repeat reactives) to five by implementing a second EIA (Christensen *et al.*, 2001).

The UK study used three anti-HBc assays and a sample was considered to contain anti-HBc if it was reactive in at least two of the three assays performed. The prevalence of anti-HBc reactivity in one assay (Corzyme) of 1.33% was reduced to 0.56% after repeat testing performed with an alternative assay (Imx), which reduced the donation loss (Allain *et al.*, 1999). In this UK study, components made from donations that were anti-HBc positive with an anti-HBs level $\geq$0.1 IU/ml were issued for clinical use.

The Irish Blood Transfusion Service (IBTS) implemented anti-HBc testing in 2002 using the Abbott PRISM HBc assay. Repeat reactive rates of 0.55% in the first six months declined to 0.35% at the end of 2002 and by 2004 had declined to 0.13%, reflecting the deferral of donors with past HBV infection from the donor pool. Of 742 repeat reactive donors over three years of testing, 261 (35%) were negative on two further EIAs, and 328 (44%) had past HBV infection, 85% of whom had anti-HBs levels >100 IU/L and 122 (16%) had isolated anti-core reactivity (as defined by positivity by two or more anti-HBc assays). Hepatitis B virus DNA was not detected in 122 'core only' samples or 48 samples with anti-HBs <100 IU/L using the COBAS AMPLICOR HBV MONITOR Test (Roche Molecular Diagnostics, Branchburg, NJ, USA Pleasanton, CA) but the detection limit of the assay is 300 copies/ml. In Ireland, the new Abbott PRISM HBcore assay was recently implemented in 2005 with improved specificity due to addition of a mild reducing agent, cysteine. From April 2005 to May 2006, 130 266 donations have been screened with this assay, yielding a repeat reactive rate of 0.09%; 80% of reactive donors had past HBV infection, 15% were negative with two further EIAs and only 5% had isolated anti-HB core reactivity on two or more assays. Another problem with anti-HBc testing is the absence of an accepted confirmatory test strategy, which makes the management of donors problematic (Busch, 1998). In this author's experience, the availability of this more specific PRISM assay has contributed not only in terms of diminishing donor loss but in having smaller numbers of donors with weakly reactive isolated anti-HB core positive results to manage. A history of HBV vaccination, which is sometimes uncertain in donors, adds to the difficulty in interpretation of results. The availability of sensitive HBV DNA tests is now becoming an essential component in managing donors with anti-HBc reactive results.

To prevent high rates of donor loss in Germany, where anti-HBc screening is being introduced, the donation can be used provided that the anti-HBs level is at least 100 IU/L and there is no detectable HBV DNA (where a detection limit of 30 IU/ml or 150 qeq/ml is used) (Burger, 2005).

Conclusion

With the advent MP-NAT and even ID-NAT for HBV DNA, a reassessment of the role of anti-HBc screening in minimizing the risk of TT-HBV is timely. The conclusions of a review of the relationship between anti-HBc positivity and HBV DNA by Kleinman and Busch in 2001 still stand and are reinforced by more recent data (Kleinman and Busch, 2001):

(1) Hepatitis B surface antigen-negative, anti-HBc positive units can transmit HBV infection to recipients (Allain *et al.*, 1999; Burger, 2005; Matsumoto *et al.*, 2001; Mosley *et al.*, 1995; Roth *et al.*, 2002; Satake *et al.*, 2005; Wang *et al.*, 2002).

(2) Hepatitis B virus DNA has been detected in 1% or less of HBsAg negative, anti-HBc positive units (and therefore HBV transmission from these units may be possible). The HBV DNA concentration in these units is often low (Busch, 2004; Hennig *et al.*, 2002; Kleinman *et al.*, 2003; Roth *et al.*, 2002; Sato *et al.*, 2001; Wang *et al.*, 2002). Mini-pool-HBV NAT would not be sensitive enough to provide a level of risk reduction in chronic low-level carriers similar to that of anti-HBc testing (Kleinman and Busch, 2001; Kleinman *et al.*, 2003; Kleinman, 2005; Roth *et al.*, 2002; Sato *et al.*, 2001). Even if ID NAT for HBV were to be implemented, anti-HBc testing would still be required (Kleinman *et al.*, 2005; Matsumoto *et al.*, 2001; Stramer, 2005). With the effective implementation of MP-HBV NAT in Japan, a country endemic for HBV, screening out high-titre anti-HBc reactive donations in the absence of anti-HBs is maintained in order to avoid transmissions from donors in the later stages of HBV infection, who have a very low HBV load. Since the introduction of this anti-HBc testing strategy in 1989, reported cases of post-transfusion fulminant hepatitis B in Japan have become extremely rare (Mineghishi *et al.*, 2003).

The relative contributions of chronic low-level carriers versus donors in the early seroconversion window period to the residual risk of TT-HBV infection will depend on the epidemiology of HBV in different countries. Changes in the epidemiology, such as have been reported in the UK over the last decade, will have implications for strategies to reduce the risk of TT-HBV in a country that does not test for anti-HBc (Soldan *et al.*, 2002).

In recent times a number of low prevalence countries have introduced anti-HBc screening, including Ireland, 2002, Canada, 2005 and most recently Germany, even though the majority of donations in Germany are tested by MP-HBV NAT.

Although residual risk estimates for TT-HBV are declining in low prevalence countries, the incorporation of immigrants from high HBV endemic areas into the pool of blood donors might increase the number of HBsAg negative carriers who pass undetected through current blood donation screening protocols in low prevalence countries (Pereira, 2003). The changing demographics of the Irish population were a factor which influenced the decision of the Irish BTS to implement anti-HBc screening in 2002. This is illustrated by the fact that in 2005, 43% of all the anti-HB core reactive donors with past HBV infection were born outside Ireland (63% of whom came from Eastern Europe) even though such donors currently comprise less than 1% of the entire donor population in Ireland.

With the use of highly sensitive HBsAg tests, the impact of MP-NAT in reducing the risk from the primary pre-seroconversion HBV window period is marginal in areas of low HBV prevalence. Individual donor-NAT would have a higher yield and greater benefit but at a high cost. Cost-effectiveness analyses has shown that MP or ID- HBV NAT would provide a small health benefit at a very high cost relative to other blood safety measures in the European Union (EU) and the USA (Jackson et al., 2003; Pereira, 2003). The projected cost per life-year gained in the EU was estimated to be 53 million euros (95% CI, 16–127) for ID-NAT when compared to enhanced sensitivity HBsAg assays (Pereira, 2003).

The yield for MP- or ID-NAT is likely to be highest in countries where HBV is often highly endemic but many of these developing countries often lack the resources for its implementation. Implementation of novel approaches to blood safety in addition to vaccination in resource-poor settings may be required, such as pre-donation serology screening with rapid tests and post-donation small pool multiplex NAT screening of seronegative donors, as recently proposed arising out of a study in a hospital-based small collection unit in Ghana (Owusu-Ofori et al., 2005).

Anti-HBc positive, HBsAg neg donors, with protective anti-HBs titres, are considered non-infectious for HBV and there is limited clinical data to support this premise (Allain et al., 1999; Dreier et al., 2004; Matsumoto et al., 2001; Mosley et al., 1995). Hepatitis B virus DNA has been detected in a small number of such donors (Hennig et al., 2002; Roth et al., 2002). As the transfused inoculum is large, the question as to whether such donors are ever infectious can only be demonstrated by large look-back studies, particularly in immunosuppressed recipients as well as chimpanzee experiments. The German anti-HBc testing strategy allowing such donors to donate provided they are HBV DNA negative provides a useful model to limit donor loss whilst attempting to ensure safety.

One component in the risk assessment when considering strategies to reduce the risk of TT-HBV is the often cited fact that only 5% of (immunocompetent) adults who are infected with HBV become chronic carriers (Kleinman and Busch, 2001). This figure is much higher for small premature infants, an intensively transfused population who are also the longest living survivors of transfusion and for immunocompromised patients, who form an increasing proportion of the transfused recipient population.

REFERENCES

Allain, J.-P. (2004) Occult hepatitis B virus infection: implications in transfusion. Vox Sang, 86, 83–91.

Allain, J.-P., Hewitt, P. E., Tedder, R. S., et al. (1999) Evidence that anti-HBc but not HBV DNA testing may prevent some HBV transmission by transfusion. Br J Haematol, 107, 186–95.

Alvarez do Barrio, M., Gonzalez Diez, R., Hernandez Sanchez, J. M., et al. (2005) Residual risk of transfusion-transmitted viral infections in Spain, 1997–2002, and impact of nucleic acid testing. Euro Surveill, 10(2), 20–2.

Aoki, S. K., Finegold, D., Kuramoto, I. K., et al. (1993) Significance of antibody to hepatitis B core antigen in blood donors as determined by their serological response to hepatitis B vaccine. Transfusion, 33, 362–7.

Aymard, J. P., Janot, G., Gayet, S., et al. (1986) Post-transfusion non-A, non-B hepatitis after cardiac surgery. Prospective analysis of donor blood anti-HBc antibody as a predictive indicator of the occurrence of non-A, non-B hepatitis in recipients. Vox Sang, 51, 236–8.

Biswas, R., Tabor, E., Hsia, C. C., et al. (2003) Comparative sensitivity of HBV NATs and HBsAg assays for detection of acute HBV infection. Transfusion, 43, 788–98.

Blajchman, M. A., Bull, S. B. and Feinman, S. V. (1995) Post-transfusion hepatitis: impact of non-A, non-B hepatitis surrogate tests. Canadian Post-transfusion Hepatitis Prevention Study Group. Lancet, 345, 21–5.

Brojer, E. (2005) Implementation of donor screening for infectious agents transmitted by blood by nucleic acid technology in Poland. Vox Sang, 89, 267–8.

Burger, R. O. R. (2005) Mitteilung des Arbeidskreises Blut des Bundesministeriums fur Gesundheit und Soziale Sicherung. Vottum 31 beide 58. Sitzung des Arbeitskreis Blut.

Busch, M. P. (1998) Prevention of transmission of hepatitis B, hepatitis C and human immunodeficiency virus infections through blood transfusion by anti-HBc testing. Vox Sang, 74 (Suppl. 2), 147–54.

Busch, M. P. (2004) Should HBV DNA NAT replace HBsAg and/or anti-HBc screening of blood donors? Transfus Clin Biol, 11, 26–32.

Busch, M. P., Dodd, R. Y., Lackritz, E. M., et al. (1997) Value and cost-effectiveness of screening blood donors for antibody to hepatitis B core antigen as a way of detecting window-phase human immunodeficiency virus type 1 infections. Transfusion, 37, 1003–11.

Chambers, L. A. and Popovsky, M. A. (1991) Decrease in reported post-transfusion hepatitis. Contribution of donor screening for alanine aminotransferase and antibodies to hepatitis B core antigen and changes in the general population. Arch Intern Med, 151, 2445–8.

Christensen, P. B., Titlestad, I. L., Homburg, K. M., et al. (2001) Hepatitis B core antibodies in Danish blood donors: a surrogate marker of risk behaviour. Vox Sang, 81, 222–7.

Comanor, L. and Holland, P. (2006) Hepatitis B virus blood screening: unfinished agendas. Vox Sang, 91, 1–12.

Dhedin, N., Douvin, C., Kuentz, M., et al. (1998) Reverse seroconversion of hepatitis B after allogeneic bone marrow transplantation: a retrospective study of 37 patients with pretransplant anti-HBs and anti-HBc. Transplantation, 66, 616–9.

Dickson, R. C., Everhart, J. E., Lake, J. R., et al. (1997) Transmission of hepatitis B by transplantation of livers from donors positive for antibody to hepatitis B core antigen. The National Institute of Diabetes and Digestive and Kidney Diseases Liver Transplantation Database. Gastroenterology, 113, 1668–74.

Dodd, R. Y., Notari, IV, E. P. and Stramer, S. L. (2002) Current prevalence and incidence of infectious disease markers and estimated window-period risk in the American Red Cross blood donor population. Transfusion, 42, 975–9.

Dodson, S. F., Issa, S., Araya, V., et al. (1997) Infectivity of hepatic allografts with antibodies to hepatitis B virus. Transplantation, 64, 1582–4.

Douglas, D. D., Rakela, J., Wright, T. L., et al. (1997) The clinical course of transplantation-associated de novo hepatitis B infection in the liver transplant recipient. Liver Transpl Surg, 3, 105–11.

Dreier, J., Kroger, M., Diekman, J., et al. (2004) Low-level viraemia of hepatitis B virus in an anti-HBc- and anti-HBs-positive blood donor. Transfus Med, 14, 97–103.

Flanagan, P., Charlewood, G., Horder, S., et al. (2005) Reducing the risk of transfusion transmitted hepatitis B in New Zealand. Vox Sang, 89(Suppl. 2), 23 (abstract).

Glynn, S. A., Kleinman, S. H., Wright, D. J., et al. (2002) International application of the incidence rate/window period model. Transfusion, 42, 966–72.

Hennig, H., Puchta, I., Luhm, J., *et al.* (2002) Frequency and load of hepatitis B virus DNA in first-time blood donors with antibodies to hepatitis B core antigen. *Blood*, **100**, 2637–41.

Iizuka, H., Ohmura, K., Ishijima, A., *et al.* (1992) Correlation between anti-HBc titres and HBV DNA in blood units without detectable HBsAg. *Vox Sang*, **63**, 107–11.

Inaba, S., Miyata, Y., Ishii, H., *et al.* (2005) Hepatitis B transmission from an occult HB virus carrier. *Transfusion*, **45** (Suppl.), 94A (abstract).

Jackson, B. R., Busch, M. P., Stramer, S. L., *et al.* (2003) The cost-effectiveness of NAT for HIV, HCV and HBV in whole-blood donations. *Transfusion*, **43**, 721–9.

Japanese Red Cross non-A, non-B Hepatitis Research Group (1991) Effect of screening for hepatitis C virus and hepatitis B virus core antibody on incidence of post-transfusion hepatitis. *Lancet*, **338**, 1040–1.

Jongerius, J. M., Wester, M., Cuypers, H. T. M., *et al.* (1998) New hepatitis B virus mutant form in a blood donor that is undetectable in several hepatitis B surface antigen-screening assays. *Transfusion*, **38**, 56–9.

Kleinman, S. H. and Busch, M. P. (2001) HBV: amplified and back in the blood safety spotlight. *Transfusion*, **41**, 1081–5.

Kleinman, S. H., Kuhns, M. C., Todd, D. S., *et al.* (2003) Frequency of HBV DNA detection in US blood donors testing positive for the presence of anti-HBc: implications for transfusion transmission and donor screening. *Transfusion*, **43**, 696–704.

Kleinman, S., Strong, D. M., Tegtmeier, G. E., *et al.* (2005) Hepatitis B virus (HBV) DNA screening of blood donations in minipools with the COBAS AmpliScreen HBV test. *Transfusion*, **45**, 1247–57.

Koppelman, M., Assal, A., Chudy, M., *et al.* (2005) Multicenter performance evaluation of a transcription-mediated amplification assay for screening of human immunodeficiency virus-1 RNA, hepatitis C virus RNA, and hepatitis B virus DNA in blood donations. *Transfusion*, **45**, 1258–66.

Korelitz, J. J., Busch, M. P., Kleinman, S. H., *et al.* (1997) A method for estimating hepatitis B virus incidence rates in volunteer donors. *Transfusion*, **37**, 634–40.

Koziol, D. E., Holland, P. V., Alling, D. W., *et al.* (1986) Antibody to hepatitis B core antigen as a paradoxical marker for non-A, non-B hepatitis agents in donated blood. *Annals of Internal Medicine*, **104**, 488–95.

Kuhns, M. C., Kleinman, S. H., McNamara, A. L., *et al.* (2004) Lack of correlation between HBsAg and HBV DNA levels in blood donors who test positive for HBsAg and anti-HBc: implications for future HBV screening policy. *Transfusion*, **44**, 1332–9.

Marcellin, P., Giostra, E., Martinot-Peignoux, M., *et al.* (1991) Redevelopment of hepatitis B surface antigen after renal transplantation. *Gastroenterology*, **100**, 1432–4.

Matsumoto, C., Tadokoro, K., Fujimura, K., *et al.* (2001) Analysis of HBV infection after blood transfusion in Japan through investigation of a comprehensive donor specimen repository. *Transfusion*, **41**, 878–84.

Mine, H., Emura, H., Miyamoto, M., *et al.*, (2003) High throughput screening of 16 million serologically negative blood donors for hepatitis B virus, hepatitis C virus and human immunodeficiency virus type-1 by nucleic acid amplification testing with specific and sensitive multiplex reagent in Japan. *J Virol Methods*, **112**, 145–51.

Minegishi, K., Yoshikawa, A., Kishimoto, S., *et al.* (2003) Superiority of minipool nucleic acid amplification technology for hepatitis B virus over chemiluminescence immunoassay for hepatitis B surface antigen screening. *Vox Sang*, **84**, 287–91.

Mosley, J. W., Stevens, C. E., Aach, R. D., *et al.* (1995) Donor screening for antibody to hepatitis B core antigen and hepatitis B virus infection in transfusion recipients. *Transfusion*, **35**, 5–12.

Niederhauser, C., Schneider, P., Fopp, M., *et al.* (2005) Incidence of viral markers and evaluation of the estimated risk in the Swiss blood donor population from 1996 to 2003. *Euro Surveill*, **10**(2), 14–16.

NIH Consensus Statement. Infectious Disease Testing for Blood Transfusions (1995) NIH, Office of the Director, Jan 9–11, **13**(1), 1–29.

Offergeld, R., Faensen, D., Ritter, S., *et al.* (2005) Human immunodeficiency virus, hepatitis C and hepatitis B infections among blood donors in Germany 2000–2002: risk of virus transmission and the impact of nucleic acid amplification testing. *Euro Surveill*, **10**(2), 8–11.

Owusu-Ofori, S., Temple, J., Sarkodie, F., *et al.* (2005) Predonation screening of blood donors with rapid tests: implementation and efficacy of a novel approach to blood safety in resource-poor settings. *Transfusion*, **45**, 133–40.

Pereira, A. (2003) Health and economic impact of post-transfusion hepatitis B and cost-effectiveness analysis of expanded HBV testing protocols of blood donors: a study focused on the European Union. *Transfusion*, **43**, 192–201.

Pillonel, J., Laperche, S. and L'Etablissement Francais du sang. (2005) Trends in risk of transfusion-transmitted viral infections (HIV, HCV, HBV) in France between 1992 and 2003 and impact of nucleic acid testing (NAT) *Euro Surveill*, **10**(2), 5–8.

Pillonel, J., Laperche, S., Saura, C., *et al.* (2002) Trends in residual risk of transfusion-transmitted viral infections in France between 1992–2000. *Transfusion*, **42**, 980–88.

Prince, A., Lee, D.-H. and Brotman, B. (2001) Infectivity of blood from PCR-positive, HBsAg-negative, anti-HBs positive cases of resolved hepatitis B infection. *Transfusion*, **41**, 329–32.

Rehermann, B., Ferrari, C., Pasquinelli, C., *et al.* (1996) The hepatitis B virus persists for decades after patients' recovery from acute viral hepatitis despite active maintenance of a cytotoxic T-lymphocyte response. *Nat Med*, **2**, 1104–8.

Roth, W. K., Weber, M., Petersen, D., *et al.* (2002) NAT for HBV and anti-HBc testing increase blood safety. *Transfusion*, **42**, 869–75.

Satake, M., Taira, R., Yugi, H., *et al.* (2005) Lookback study for transfusion-related HBV infection in Japan. *Transfusion*, **45**(Suppl.), 9A (abstract).

Sato, S., Ohhashi, W., Ihara, H., *et al.* (2001) Comparison of the sensitivity of NAT using pooled donor samples for HBV and that of a serologic HBsAg assay. *Transfusion*, **41**, 1107–13.

Schreiber, G. B., Busch, M. P., Kleinman, S. H., *et al.* (1996) The risk of transfusion-transmitted viral infections. *N Eng J Med*, **334**, 1685–90.

Seed, C. R., Cheng, A., Ismay, S. L., *et al.* (2002) Assessing the accuracy of three viral risk models in predicting the outcome of implementing HIV and HCV NAT donor screening in Australia and the implications for future HBV NAT. *Transfusion*, **42**, 1365–72.

Serious Hazards of Transfusion Annual Report 2004 (2005), ISBN 0 9532 789 7 2, 21 November 2005, (available at: www.SHOT-uk.org).

Soldan, K., Barbara, J. A. J. and Dow, B. C. (2002) Transfusion-transmitted hepatitis B virus infection in the UK: a small and moving target. *Vox Sang*, **83**, 305–8.

Soldan, K., Barbara, J. A. J., Ramsay, M. E., *et al.* (2003) Estimation of the risk of hepatitis B virus, hepatitis C virus and human immunodeficiency virus infectious donations entering the blood supply in England, 1993–2001. *Vox Sang*, **84**, 274–86.

Soldan, K., Davison, K. and Dow, B. (2005) Estimates of the frequency of HBV, HCV and HIV infectious donations entering the blood supply in the United Kingdom, 1996 to 2003. *Euro Surveill*, **10**(2), 17–9.

Stramer, S., Brodsky, J., Preston, S., *et al.* (2001) Comparative sensitivities of HBsAg and HBV NAT. *Transfusion*, **41**(Suppl.), 8S (abstract).

Stramer, S. L. (2005) Pooled hepatitis B virus DNA testing by nucleic acid amplification: implementation or not. *Transfusion*, **45**, 1242–6.

Stramer, S. L., Glynn, S. A., Kleinman, S. H., *et al.* (2004) Detection of HIV-1 and HCV infections among antibody-negative blood donors by nucleic acid-amplification testing. *N Eng J Med*, **351**, 760–8.

Wachs, M. E., Amend, W. J., Ascher, N. L., *et al.* (1995) The risk of transmission of hepatitis B from HBsAg(−), HBcAb(+), HBIgM(−) organ donors. *Transplantation*, **59**, 230–4.

Wang, J.-T., Lee, C.-Z., Chen, P.-J., *et al.* (2002) Transfusion-transmitted HBV infection in an endemic area: the necessity of more sensitive screening for HBV carriers. *Transfusion*, **42**, 1592–7.

Yoshikawa, A., Gotanda, Y., Itabashi, M., *et al.* and the Japanese Red Cross NAT Screening Research Group (2005) Hepatitis B NAT virus-positive blood donors in the early and late stages of HBV infection: analyses of the window period and kinetics of HBV DNA. *Vox Sang*, **88**, 77–86.

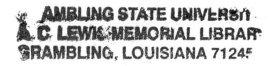

Yotsuyanagi, H., Yasuda, K., Moriya, K., *et al.* (2001) Frequent presence of HBV in the sera of HBsAg-negative, anti-HBc-positive blood donors. *Transfusion*, **41**, 1093–9.

Yugi, H., Hino, S., Satake, M., *et al.* (2005) Implementation of donor screening for infectious agents transmitted by blood by nucleic acid technology in Japan. *Vox Sang*, **89**, 265.

Yugi, H., Mizui, M., Tanaka, J., *et al.* (2006) Hepatitis B virus (HBV) screening strategy to ensure the safety of blood for transfusion through a combination of immunological testing and nucleic acid amplification testing – Japanese experience. *J Clin Virol*, **36**(Suppl.), S56–S64.

Zervou, E. K., Dalekos, G. N., Boumba, D. S., *et al.* (2001) Value of anti-HBc screening of blood donors for prevention of HBV infection: results of a 3-year prospective study in Northwestern Greece. *Transfusion*, **41**, 652–8.

Zuckerman, J. N. and Zuckerman, A. J. (2000) Current topics in hepatitis B. *J Infect*, **41**, 130–6.

3 HERPES VIRUSES

Eleftherios C. Vamvakas and Gary E. Tegtmeier

Human herpes viruses are highly successful intracellular parasites. With the exception of varicella-zoster virus (VZV), they cause asymptomatic or mildly symptomatic primary infection, establish latent infection, and persist lifelong. During the host's lifetime, they periodically reactivate and infect other susceptible individuals. As long as the host's immune system is not compromised, the balance between virus and host is maintained. However, immunosuppression induced by disease or therapy can alter the balance between virus and host, resulting in systemic virus infection and concomitant disease.

The human Herpesviridae includes three subfamilies (see Table 3.1). Transmission by transfusion does not appear to occur with herpes simplex virus (HSV) or VZV. Cytomegalovirus (CMV) is by far the most important herpes virus in transfusion medicine, and its relative significance increased greatly in the last two decades, due to increases in bone marrow transplantation, solid-organ transplantation and more aggressive chemotherapy for malignant disease. This chapter reviews the role of CMV and Epstein-Barr Virus (EBV) in transfusion medicine. Human herpes viruses 6, 7, and 8 (HHV-6, HHV-7, and HHV-8) are reviewed briefly but are covered in detail in the chapter on newly identified agents (Please refer to Chapter 28.).

Cytomegalovirus

Transfusion-acquired CMV infection has been the subject of numerous reviews (Blajchman et al., 2001; Gunter and Luban, 1996; Hillyer et al., 1994; Pamphilon et al., 1999b; Preiksaitis, 2000; Tegtmeier, 1989; 2001; Wong and Luban, 2002). The association between transfusion and CMV was first reported in 1960 by Kreel et al., who described a syndrome with fever, lymphocytosis, and splenomegaly occurring 3–8 weeks after cardiopulmonary bypass (Kreel et al., 1960). However, it was not until the 1980s that severe CMV disease was unequivocally linked to the transfusion of CMV-seropositive blood in premature infants (Yeager et al., 1981). It was more gradually recognized that transfused blood might be the source of CMV disease in bone marrow transplant (BMT) recipients (Meyers et al., 1986), particularly CMV-seronegative patients receiving bone marrow allografts from CMV negative donors (Bowden et al., 1986; 1987).

The efficacy of CMV-seronegative blood components in reducing the risk of transfusion-acquired CMV infection in such patients was then established (MacKinnon et al., 1988; Miller et al., 1991). Because it became difficult to maintain adequate CMV-seronegative inventories as the number of transfusion recipients at risk of CMV disease kept rising, attention shifted to the potential safety of white-blood-cell (WBC) reduced blood components. The efficacy of these components in lowering the risk of transfusion-acquired CMV infection was then established as well (Bowden et al., 1991; Brady et al., 1984).

Despite the promising results reported with both CMV-seronegative and WBC-reduced blood components, it remains unclear whether CMV-seronegative and WBC-reduced blood components are equivalent in reducing the risk of transfusion-acquired CMV infection (Malloy and Lipton, 2002; Pamphilon et al., 1999b; Preiksaitis, 2000; Smith, 1997; Vamvakas, 2005.) Moreover, the use of CMV-seronegative or WBC-reduced blood components has been generally successful in controlling transfusion-acquired CMV infection, although an intractable, small risk of CMV disease persists in BMT patients (Bowden et al., 1995; Nichols et al., 2003). Regardless of the interventions used to prevent CMV infection in these patients, 2–3% of them will develop CMV infection and 1–2% will suffer CMV disease. The origins of such 'breakthrough' infections and the strategies indicated for their prevention remain a matter for debate. Yet another controversy regards the appropriateness of transfusing WBC-reduced components to CMV-seropositive patients at risk of CMV disease. According to some investigators, WBC reduction is indicated in this case to prevent reactivation of CMV infection in the transfusion recipient (Hillyer et al., 1999; Preiksaitis, 2000).

Characteristics of cytomegalovirus

Along with vaccinia virus, CMV has the largest genome of any known animal virus. Like other herpes viruses, its genome consists of a linear, double-stranded DNA molecule. Cytomegalovirus is transmitted both vertically (from mother to her fetus or the newborn) and horizontally (through body fluids, sexual contact, transplantation and blood transfusion). Humans are the only hosts for human CMV, but other types of species-specific CMV have been well characterized.

Cytomegalovirus infection may manifest as a primary infection, a reactivation, or a secondary infection. Primary infection occurs in the seronegative person who is exposed to the virus for the first time. In immunocompetent hosts, this usually results in an asymptomatic or mildly symptomatic mononucleosis-like syndrome. Viraemia, viruria, and an IgM and then IgG CMV-specific serologic response are noted. The role of antibody in controlling primary infection is unclear. However, in the immunocompetent adult, the viraemia of primary infection is low-level and short-lived (Revello et al., 1998). Infectious virus can be isolated from both granulocytes and mononuclear cells, but infectivity is highest in the granulocyte fraction. High and persistent levels of viraemia have been documented in immunocompromised

Transfusion Microbiology, eds John A. J. Barbara, Fiona A. M. Regan and Marcela C. Contreras. Published by Cambridge University Press. © Cambridge University Press 2008.

Table 3.1 Pathogenic human herpes viruses.

	Subfamily
Herpes simplex virus (HSV) type 1 and type 2	α
Varicella-zoster virus (VZV)	α
Cytomegalovirus (CMV)	β
Human herpes virus 6 (HHV-6)	β
Human herpes virus 7 (HHV-7)	β
Epstein-Barr virus (EBV)	γ
Human herpes virus 8 (HHV-8)	γ

Table 3.2 CMV-Seronegative patient populations at high risk of serious (or organ- and/or life-threatening) CMV disease following transfusion-transmitted CMV infection.

(1) Fetuses receiving intrauterine transfusions (and pregnant women)
(2) Very low birthweight premature neonates or infants
(3) Recipients of CMV-seronegative allogeneic or autologous bone marrow transplants
(4) Patients who may need allogeneic or autologous bone marrow transplantation in the future
(5) Transplant recipients of organs from CMV-seropositive donors
(6) Patients with haematologic malignancies receiving intensive chemotherapy that produces severe neutropenia
(7) Patients with HIV infection

patients who experience primary CMV infection (Gerna *et al.*, 1992).

Following primary infection, active viral replication stops and CMV becomes latent. The site(s) of CMV latency have not been established, but recent evidence has identified one possible site. Soderberg-Naucler *et al.* have suggested that the virus may reside in a small subset of peripheral blood mononuclear cells that express both macrophage (CD14 and CD64) and dendritic-cell (CD83 and CD1a) markers (Soderberg-Naucler *et al.*, 1997). Latent virus can become reactivated in such cells, but the mechanisms of reactivation remain incompletely understood. During reactivation, active viral replication resumes, with viral shedding and a four-fold (or greater) rise in the titre of IgG antibodies.

Secondary infection (or reinfection) occurs in seropositive individuals who become infected with a different strain of the virus. It is demonstrated by an increase in IgG antibody titre, by isolation of shed virus, and – most definitively – by differences in the DNA genome that indicate presence of more than one strain of CMV by molecular techniques.

Recently, Soderberg-Naucler *et al.* reported the successful reactivation of CMV from seven healthy seropositive subjects who were subjected to allogeneic stimulation of their peripheral blood mononuclear cells (Soderberg-Naucler *et al.*, 1997). Virus was recovered after long-term culture from macrophages expressing dendritic-cell markers. This study suggested that CMV reactivation requires a specific cellular differentiation pathway that involves an allogeneic stimulus. Moreover, the frequency of peripheral blood mononuclear cells latently infected with CMV and capable of reactivating infectious virus in healthy subjects was estimated at 0.01% to 0.12%.

Based on such evidence, the following model of CMV latency and reactivation has been proposed (Hahn *et al.*, 1998). A primitive haematopoietic cell population is infected with CMV as a result of the viraemia during primary infection. The viral genome is maintained in these cells with limited gene expression as the cells reside quiescently in the bone marrow or self-renew. When these cells differentiate into lineage-committed progenitors, latency-associated transcripts and proteins are expressed in a subset of CD33 + cells that are progenitors of dendritic cells, granulocytes and macrophages. If these cells are exposed to a particular proinflammatory cytokine milieu as they differentiate along specific pathways, reactivation of lytic virus occurs, and CMV replication ensues in fully-differentiated tissue dendritic cells or macrophages. However, it remains unclear whether CD33 + progenitors of

dendritic cells and macrophages are the major, or only, site of CMV latency in healthy seropositive donors.

Clinical manifestations of transfusion-acquired cytomegalovirus disease

To interpret the voluminous literature on transfusion-acquired CMV, one has to distinguish between CMV *infection* and CMV *disease*. In the large majority of cases, CMV *infection* is asymptomatic and identified by means of seroconversion or direct detection of the virus. CMV *disease* is defined as laboratory evidence of infection coupled with signs and/or symptoms attributable to the virus (as opposed to the patient's underlying disease or other pathogens). The clinical manifestations of CMV disease can range from a heterophile-antibody negative, mononucleosis-like syndrome to disseminated disease. The mononucleosis-like syndrome can present with lymphocytosis, fever, pharyngitis, lymphadenopathy, and/or hepatitis, and may sometimes be associated with thrombocytopenia, hemolytic anaemia, interstitial pneumonitis, meningoencephalitis and/or polyneuropathy. Disseminated disease can further present with retinitis, colitis, gastritis, nephritis, or rash.

Cytomegalovirus infection in immunocompetent hosts is asymptomatic or manifests as the self-limiting mononucleosis-like syndrome described above. Specific categories of immunocompromised patients are at risk of severe (and potentially fatal) CMV disease, although CMV infection can be asymptomatic (or mildly symptomatic) in immunocompromised patients as well. In general, only fetuses, low-birth-weight neonates, BMT recipients, solid-organ transplant recipients, and patients infected with human immunodeficiency virus (HIV) are at risk of life (or organ-) threatening CMV disease (see Table 3.2). If these patients are CMV-seronegative, they should thus receive CMV-seronegative or WBC-reduced blood components to prevent transfusion-acquired CMV disease.

Moreover, patients likely to become candidates for bone marrow transplantation should also receive CMV-seronegative or WBC-reduced blood components if they are currently CMV-seronegative. Prevention of CMV infection in such patients could prevent life-threatening CMV disease in the future (if CMV were to be reactivated following receipt of the BMT).

Therefore, CMV negative patients with malignant disease, aplastic anaemia, thalassaemia, congenital immunodeficiency, or other genetic disease who may be treated with bone marrow transplantation, should receive CMV-seronegative or WBC-reduced blood components. Cytomegalovirus-seronegative pregnant women should similarly receive CMV-seronegative or WBC-reduced blood components to prevent CMV disease in the fetus or newborn. Primary CMV infection during pregnancy is associated with a 40% risk of vertical transmission of infection.

Infants born to mothers who had been transfused early in pregnancy developed fever, respiratory distress, hepatosplenomegaly, CMV viruria, and evidence of disseminated CMV disease on autopsy (McCracken et al., 1969; McEnery and Stern, 1970). Fatal CMV disease likely secondary to intrauterine transfusion has also been reported (Evans and Lyon, 1991).

A pivotal study carried out by Yeager et al. in the early 1980s showed that 10 of 74 seronegative infants who received at least one seropositive unit seroconverted (Yeager et al., 1981). Five of the ten infants developed pneumonia, hepatosplenomegaly, and various cytopenias; four of them died. There was little associated morbidity and mortality, however, when full-term infants underwent exchange transfusion from seropositive donors and seroconverted to CMV (Kumar et al., 1980; Pass et al., 1976; Tobin et al., 1975). It appears that only low-birthweight infants, weighing less than 1250 g, are at risk of transfusion-acquired CMV disease.

Bone marrow transplant recipients are at great risk of acquiring CMV from the marrow graft, from blood components, or from nosocomial infection. Cytomegalovirus disease occurring in seropositive BMT recipients post-transplant most likely represents reactivation of latent virus or secondary infection with another CMV strain. Those patients who are seronegative and receive a seronegative marrow allograft are at the highest risk of transfusion-acquired CMV infection and disease. A significant number of BMT recipients with CMV infection will develop interstitial pneumonia that often proves fatal. Acute graft versus host disease (GVHD), older age, lung irradiation, administration of granulocyte transfusions before transplantation, human leucocyte antigen (HLA)-incompatibility between donor and recipient, and pre-existing CMV seropositivity have been associated with an increased risk of CMV pneumonia following bone marrow transplantation.

Renal transplant recipients also suffer CMV disease, but acquisition of CMV tends to occur through reactivation of endogenous virus or from the renal allograft itself. Seropositive persons receiving seropositive kidneys sometimes shed their own reactivated strain, the donor strain, or both (Chou 1986). Cytomegalovirus can damage the renal allograft, leading to glomerulonephritis and rejection (Rubin et al., 1985). Cytomegalovirus disease also occurs in recipients of heart, heart/lung, or liver transplants. Moreover, accelerated atherosclerosis of transplanted hearts has been reported in association with primary CMV infection (Grattan et al., 1989).

Before the introduction of antiretroviral therapy, a large number of patients infected with HIV developed CMV disease. Chorioretinitis, esophagitis, colitis, pneumonia, and/or encephalitis caused significant morbidity and mortality in these patients,

and the risk of CMV disease in HIV infected patients still exists. Homosexual men are almost universally positive for CMV antibody before they receive transfusion for HIV disease, and CMV disease in this population likely results from CMV reactivation. However, HIV infected haemophiliacs are CMV-seropositive as often as the general population, and they could be at risk of primary, transfusion-acquired CMV infection if they received CMV-seropositive/non-WBC-reduced blood components.

Evidence of significant transfusion-acquired CMV disease is lacking in adult and paediatric cancer patients. For example, in the study of Stevens et al., one-third of 31 adult patients with solid tumours were infected with CMV, but the infections remained asymptomatic (Stevens et al., 1979). Two studies have suggested that splenectomy in the immunocompetent patient can exacerbate the morbidity and mortality associated with CMV disease (Baumgartner et al., 1982; Drew and Minor, 1982), whereas a third study has refuted this concept (Rader et al., 1985). Burn patients often experience CMV reactivation or primary infection, but CMV infection does not appear to contribute to morbidity or mortality in this setting (Bale et al., 1990; Kealey et al., 1987). Similarly, there was no association between increased mortality and CMV infection in trauma patients (Curtsinger et al., 1989).

Tests for detection of cytomegalovirus

Please refer to Chapter 11.

Donors are screened for the presence of CMV antibody, and components from CMV-seronegative donors are considered to be suitable for transfusion to patients who are at high risk of developing transfusion-acquired CMV disease. Because a small, but intractable risk of transfusion-acquired CMV infection persists, despite the use of CMV-seronegative or WBC-reduced components, detection of CMV DNA in donor samples by polymerase chain reaction (PCR) may be implemented in the future by blood centres. The purpose of such testing will be to detect donor units that are viraemic, despite having been subjected to the process of WBC reduction and/or despite having been collected from CMV-seronegative donors. Viral culture or other direct detection methods are not being used on donor samples, but they are readily available in clinical laboratories for use in the diagnosis of CMV disease in patients with signs and/or symptoms potentially attributable to CMV (Hodinka, 2003).

Cytomegalovirus-antibody screening tests

Early studies documenting the efficacy of CMV-seronegative blood components in preventing transfusion-acquired CMV infection used complement fixation and indirect haemagglutination assays to detect CMV antibody in blood donors (Luthardt et al., 1971; Monif et al., 1976; Yeager et al., 1981). The assays used in these studies were in-house, unstandardized assays of undetermined sensitivity and specificity. An indirect haemagglutination assay based on the one used by Yeager et al. in their study became the first commercially available assay in 1983.

Other commercially available assays soon appeared, including solid-phase fluorescence, enzyme immunoassay, and passive latex agglutination. Comparative evaluation of these assays followed, which reported test sensitivities and specificities ranging from 89% to 100% (Adler *et al.*, 1985a; Beckwith *et al.*, 1985; Booth *et al.*, 1982; Phipps *et al.*, 1983; Taswell *et al.*, 1986). However, these evaluations were carried out in the 1980s, and no reliable supplemental test was available to corroborate the positivity of reactive screening test results, that is, no 'gold standard' existed then (as no gold standard exists now). Nonetheless, studies showing the efficacy of CMV-seronegative blood components have been performed using complement fixation, indirect haemagglutination and latex agglutination assays with equal success, suggesting that most types of CMV antibody tests are capable of detecting potentially infectious donors (Tegtmeier, 1989).

Five types of CMV antibody tests are commercially available today: a particle agglutination assay from Olympus; an enzyme immunoassay from Abbott; a latex agglutination assay from Beckton Dickinson; a solid-phase red-cell adherence assay from Immucor; and a haemagglutination assay from Hemagen. Both the Olympus particle agglutination test and the Hemagen haemagglutination test are automated assays that can be run on the Olympus PK7200. The Abbott enzyme immunoassay and the Immucor solid-phase red-cell adherence assay are semi-automated. The Beckton Dickinson latex agglutination assay is manual. No comparative evaluation of these contemporary CMV-antibody assays has been published (Tegtmeier, 2001). In Europe, process control during routine testing (together with full automation) is increasingly becoming a prerequisite of donation testing. (Please refer to Chapter 20.) Assays such as latex agglutination (and haemagglutination, other than in automated systems) are therefore less commonly used.

Because IgM antibodies appear early after infection and drop to low concentrations or disappear within three to six months, they are generally indicative of recent infection that is more often associated with donor viraemia. Retrospective testing for CMV IgM antibody of blood given to patients who contracted CMV infection through transfusion showed that CMV infected patients were more likely to have received one or more IgM positive units compared with patients who did not acquire CMV infection from transfusion (see below). However, the positive and negative predictive values of the CMV IgM tests were too low to warrant implementation of CMV IgM tests for donor screening. Technical problems with such assays include: lack of specificity of commercially-available anti-human IgM; the presence of rheumatoid factor in sera, which may cause false-positive reactions; and the presence of high-titre IgG CMV antibody in sera, which may cause false-negative results.

Polymerase chain reaction tests for detection of Cytomegalovirus DNA

Several studies have used PCR techniques to detect CMV DNA in donors, but their results have been highly variable. From 0% (Urushibara *et al.*, 1995) to 100% (Stanier *et al.*, 1989; Taylor-Wiedeman *et al.*, 1991) of CMV-seropositive donors produced positive results. At the same time, from 0% (Urushibara *et al.*, 1995) to 50% (Stanier *et al.*, 1989) of CMV-seronegative donors produced positive results as well. Positive results in CMV-seronegative donors run counter to clinical experience, which indicates that CMV-

negative blood components do not transmit CMV to recipients. Thus, it would appear that the reports of CMV DNA identification in CMV-seronegative blood donors represent false-positive results attributable to poor specificity of the assays. Similarly, in asymptomatic seropositive individuals, the presence of CMV DNA may be due to non-viable virus, residual CMV genomic DNA, or latent CMV DNA (Ratnamohan *et al.*, 1992).

Because of the marked variation in the frequency of detection of CMV DNA in reported studies, a multicentre, blinded proficiency study was undertaken at five laboratories that had previously reported widely discordant results using different PCR tests that targeted various regions of the CMV genome. One laboratory prepared and distributed 61 coded samples to the other laboratories. Ten of these served as positive analytical controls, containing from 1 to 100 CMV genome equivalents in background DNA from 250 000 cells. Eleven served as negative analytical controls, containing only the DNA extraction solution. Twenty served as positive clinical controls, being pedigreed HIV-positive, CMV positive blood samples obtained from the Viral Activation Transfusion Study (VATS – see below). Twenty served as negative clinical controls, having been obtained from pedigreed CMV-seronegative apheresis donors.

The participating laboratories were instructed to assay the samples by their standard protocols. Seven CMV PCR assays were thus evaluated. Five assays displayed sufficient sensitivity for donor screening, as judged by consistent detection of a minimum of 25 CMV genome equivalents in the positive analytical controls. Three of these sensitive assays did not detect CMV DNA in samples from any of the 20 negative clinical controls. All 11 negative analytical controls and all 20 positive clinical controls were identified correctly, as negative or positive, by all assays. Of the three assays that had both sufficient sensitivity and good specificity, two were based on nested PCR directed at the UL93 and UL32 regions of the CMV genome; the third assay was the Roche Monitor Assay (Roback *et al.*, 2001).

The same team of investigators followed up with a large, multicentre, cross-sectional study of 1000 US blood donors (Roback *et al.*, 2003). To detect CMV DNA in the sera of donors, they used two CMV PCR assays that had been validated in the previous study: a nested PCR assay directed at the UL93 region of the CMV genome and the Roche Monitor Assay. All blood donors were screened with two tests for CMV antibody. Seventy donor samples produced discrepant results by serology; 416 tested consistently CMV-seropositive; and 514 tested consistently CMV-seronegative. Cytomegalovirus DNA could be reproducibly detected from only 2 of 1000 donor samples; both of these were CMV-seropositive. Cytomegalovirus DNA was not reproducibly detected in CMV-seronegative samples or in samples with discrepant results on CMV antibody testing.

The authors concluded that CMV DNA is detected only very rarely in US blood donors when previously validated PCR assays are used. Importantly, in this large study, the use of CMV PCR assays with optimal performance characteristics did not increase the detection of potentially infectious donor units beyond the detection ensured by current serologic screening assays. Thus, in an accompanying editorial, Preiksaitis concluded that the time to consider implementing PCR-based assays for CMV DNA for the prevention of transfusion-acquired CMV infection had not yet come (Preiksaitis, 2003).

Viral culture, antigen detection and molecular amplification

Viral culture is relatively insensitive, but it unequivocally determines whether or not infectious virus is present. Because of intermittent viral shedding, cultures of urine, blood, saliva, buffy coat and other body fluids are most effective when serial or weekly cultures are obtained from multiple sites. These cultures are used for the diagnosis of CMV disease in patients, and they are performed by inoculating a specimen onto human diploid fibroblast cell lines and examining the cultures for focal cytopathic effects within 1–2 weeks or on second passage. Cytomegalovirus grows very slowly, and 4–6 weeks of observation are needed before a culture can be read as negative. Thus, a more rapid cell culture method of diagnosis was developed in the spin-amplification shell vial assay that allows detection of CMV within 24 hours (Gleaves *et al.* 1984).

Surveillance for CMV antigenaemia is based on detection of the CMV tegument phosphoprotein pp65 in peripheral blood WBCs by immunofluorescence. It is used to monitor clinical infection in patients, and it permits much faster detection of CMV in high-risk populations such as BMT recipients (Landry *et al.*, 1996). Weekly monitoring using the pp65 antigenaemia assay permits pre-emptive ganciclovir therapy to be administered to such high-risk patients when there is a positive antigen test (Boeckh *et al.*, 1999). However, CMV antigenaemia assays are rather insensitive, technically demanding and low throughput. Thus, they are not practical to determine the CMV status of latently-infected blood donors. Molecular amplification methods, often in the form of PCR, have been developed more recently for CMV diagnosis and monitoring high risk patients (Hodinka, 2003). As with the antigenaemia assay, molecular amplification methods are most useful in predicting and/or diagnosing CMV disease when they are quantitative and blood is the specimen assayed.

Risk factors for cytomegalovirus infection

Rates of primary infection (CMV seroconversion) in immunocompetent seronegative health care workers have been found to vary from 0.6% to 3.3% per year (Dworsky *et al.*, 1983). Higher rates have been documented in women who have contact with young children. Middle-class women seroconvert at a rate of 4.6% to 6.3% per year between pregnancies (Stagno and Cloud 1994). The seroconversion rate in seronegative blood donors is expected to be low and is estimated to be approximately 1.0% per year.

Cytomegalovirus antibody prevalence increases with age, is inversely related to socio-economic status, varies widely between and within countries, and is higher among females within any particular age group. The wide variation in CMV antibody prevalence in blood donors around the world was highlighted in a 1973 study that reported prevalence figures ranging from 40% in Western Europe to 100% in third-world countries (Krech, 1973). Within the USA, this study showed variation in CMV

seroprevalence ranging from 45% in Albany to 79% in Houston. A 1985 telephone survey of seven US blood centres indicated CMV prevalence rates that ranged from 30% in Boston to 70% in Nashville (Tegtmeier, 1986).

A combination of factors (geography, coupled with age, gender and race) determine the prevalence of CMV seropositivity in a particular community, as well as in blood donors from that community. In Kansas City, Missouri, donors 17–25 years of age had a 30% CMV seroprevalence, as compared with an 80% prevalence for donors over 65 years old. Caucasians showed the lowest prevalence (46%), followed by African-Americans (64%) and Asians (76%).

Estimated risk of cytomegalovirus transmission by transfusion of cytomegalovirus-unscreened/non-white blood cell reduced components

There are no adequate estimates of the frequency of reactivation or secondary infection in transfusion-acquired CMV. Historically, estimates of the risk of primary infection from transfusion have ranged up to 67% per recipient, at least in studies published within the decade following the description of CMV-induced 'post-perfusion' syndrome (Preiksaitis, 1991). However, it is difficult to interpret the results of some of these studies, because some patients who were CMV-seropositive before transfusion were included in the calculation of the rate of primary CMV infection. Also, these studies were conducted mostly in immunocompetent, cardiac-surgery patients who had received large volumes of fresh heparinized blood.

The epidemiology of transfusion-acquired CMV infection changed as transfusion practice evolved from administration of fresh whole blood to use of blood component therapy in the 1970s and 1980s. In 1986 and 1988, a per-recipient post-transfusion CMV risk of only 1.2% and 0.9%, respectively, was observed in patients hospitalized for burns, major surgery, pregnancy and delivery, neonatal complications and oncologic treatment (Preiksaitis *et al.*, 1988b; Wilhelm *et al.*, 1986). These studies included a relatively high proportion of patients with normal immune function. Heavily transfused patients hospitalized for burns and major trauma were at increased risk of transfusion-acquired CMV infection.

Studies of low birthweight neonates published between 1981 and 1989 (Adler *et al.*, 1983; Gilbert *et al.*, 1989; Yeager *et al.*, 1981) showed a risk of transfusion-acquired primary CMV infection of 24% to 32% per infant. However, more recent studies published between 1988 and 2000 showed a risk of 0% to 5% per newborn (Galea and Urbaniak, 1992; Griffin *et al.*, 1988; Lamberson *et al.*, 1988; Ohto *et al.*, 1999; Preiksaitis *et al.*, 1988a; Snydman *et al.*, 1995). The frequency of donor CMV seropositivity in a particular geographic area, the number of donor exposures, the volume of transfused blood, and the length of storage of transfused components (vide infra) have been considered as possible explanations for the variation in the risk of transfusion-acquired CMV in these studies.

Donor seropositivity was likely not a factor, however, because it varied between 34% and 46% in the three studies that had reported a high risk of transmission, and between 38% and 47% in the studies that had reported a low risk of transmission. The number of donor exposures and the volume of transfused blood correlated with the risk of transmission in some (but not all) studies. In fact, in two studies (Gilbert *et al.*, 1989; Lamberson *et al.*, 1988), four low-birthweight infants acquired CMV infection after a single exposure to a relatively small volume of blood from a single seropositive donor. Thus, the reasons for the variation in the risk of transfusion-acquired CMV infection in studies of low-birthweight neonates remain obscure. Perhaps, the donor self-deferral criteria introduced for the prevention of transfusion-acquired HIV infection and the implementation of HIV antibody testing in 1985 also reduced the risk of transmission of CMV by transfusion.

Thirty-two per cent to 50% of CMV-seronegative allogeneic BMT recipients who received CMV-seronegative bone marrow allografts and were supported with routine (i.e. CMV-unscreened and non-WBC-reduced) blood components acquired CMV infection through transfusion (Bowden *et al.*, 1986; 1991; Miller *et al.*, 1991). The risk for CMV-seronegative autologous BMT recipients who were supported with routine blood components was 21% (Bowden *et al.*, 1986).

The risk of transfusion-acquired CMV infection in CMV-seronegative recipients of CMV-seronegative solid-organ transplants studied by Preiksaitis *et al.* over a 13-year period was only 2.4% (Preiksaitis *et al.*, 2002). The organ-specific risk was distributed as follows: kidney, 0/57 (0%); heart, 0/29 (0%); heart-lung/lung, 1/6 (16.7%); and liver, 2/20 (10%). The risk observed by Preiksaitis *et al.* in solid-organ transplant recipients receiving routine blood components in one Canadian centre has been lower than that reported from most other studies. Results of other studies of CMV-seronegative solid-organ transplant recipients have been exceedingly variable, reporting CMV rates ranging between 0% and 20% in renal transplant recipients, between 0% and 26% in heart transplant recipients, between 4.5% and 33% in heart/lung transplant recipients, and between 7% and 100% in liver transplant recipients (Preiksaitis, 2000; Tegtmeier, 2001).

Studies have documented CMV infection rates varying between 12% and 57% in paediatric oncology patients (Furukawa *et al.*, 1987; Ho, 1982). More recently, Preiksaitis *et al.* observed no case of transfusion-acquired CMV infection among 76 CMV-seronegative children with malignant disease who were randomized to receive CMV-seronegative or routine blood components (Preiksaitis *et al.*, 1997). Children allocated to receive routine blood components were given a median of 7 red blood cell and 11 platelet units. However, a number of children randomized to receive routine components in this study received relatively WBC-reduced components, for reasons other than CMV prevention.

Thus, a wide variation exists in the risk estimates of transfusion-acquired CMV that have been reported in different patient populations within relatively homogeneous groups of low birthweight neonates, BMT recipients, solid-organ transplant recipients, or oncology patients. This emphasizes that the pathogenesis of transfusion-acquired CMV infection is complex and involves multiple donor and recipient factors. As a result, the risk of CMV transmission per transfused CMV-seropositive (and/or CMV-

seronegative or WBC-reduced) unit is not constant, but depends on characteristics of both the donor and the recipient, as well as on the method(s) of preparation and length of storage of the transfused component(s). Consequently, a non-WBC-reduced, CMV-seropositive red blood cell unit may be 'safe' when it is administered to a CMV-seronegative patient who is undergoing uncomplicated, elective orthopedic surgery. In contrast, a WBC-reduced platelet unit may result in fatal CMV disease when it is administered to a CMV-seronegative allogeneic BMT transplant patient receiving aggressive immunosuppressive therapy for acute GVHD.

The relative contribution of donor, recipient and component preparation/storage factors to the risk of CMV transmission by blood components remains unresolved (Preiksaitis, 2003). One hypothesis holds that transmission of CMV results largely from receipt of cellular blood components from viraemic blood donors (i.e. recently infected donors or donors who are experiencing CMV reactivation associated with virion production). An alternative hypothesis holds that CMV infection occurring in CMV-seronegative recipients is the result of transfusion of latent virus in blood components that is subsequently reactivated in the circulation of the recipient. Moreover, reactivation of latent virus could occur in a cellular blood component during storage.

Factors related to the blood donor

Whether blood from all seropositive donors can transmit CMV or whether an *infectious subset* of donors can be identified remains unsettled. In 1969, CMV was isolated from buffy coats of 2 of 35 healthy blood donors (Diosi *et al.*, 1969). However, numerous subsequent studies failed to isolate CMV from the blood of over 1400 donors (Kane *et al.*, 1975; Mirkovic *et al.*, 1971; Perham *et al.*, 1971). More recently, CMV DNA could be reproducibly detected from the WBCs of only 2 of 416 seropositive blood donors (Roback *et al.*, 2003). If these observations were to be taken at face value, they would imply that:

(1) Asymptomatic blood donors are hardly ever viraemic.
(2) There are very few donors who are sources of truly infectious (i.e. viraemic) units.
(3) Either primary infection or CMV reactivation are rare events in blood donors, or – alternatively – such events in donors are not associated with viraemia.

If these inferences were shown to be correct, a search for an *infectious subset* of donors would be of limited utility, because such viraemic donors would be responsible for only a small proportion of cases of transfusion-acquired CMV infection.

Even if donors who are experiencing primary infection or CMV reactivation were not the only donors capable of transmitting CMV to recipients, however, it is possible that such donors could be more infectious than other CMV-seropositive donors, because they have either:

(1) Low-grade viraemia not detectable by standard isolation techniques
(2) A significantly greater proportion of WBCs that are *latently* infected with CMV.

Methods to isolate CMV or detect CMV DNA by PCR were developed for the diagnosis of CMV disease in immunosuppressed patients. It is possible that the sensitivity of such methods is not adequate when they are employed in asymptomatic blood donors, in whom both the viraemia and the proportion of infected WBCs are lower than in patients with CMV disease.

Thus, more work is needed to determine the frequency of acute infection or reactivation events in blood donors, and the relationship of such events to CMV transmission by blood components. Dumont *et al.* reported that a significant proportion of CMV-seropositive donors experienced transient CMV reactivation, sometimes associated with production of infectious virions, during periods characterized by high environmental pollen counts (Dumont, *et al.*, 2001). Whether donors experiencing primary infection or CMV reactivation had low-grade viraemia or a greater proportion of latently infected WBCs compared with other seropositive donors, individuals from these two categories would represent an *infectious subset* of donors, and their identification would be of great practical benefit. Virus isolation, screening for CMV-specific IgM, and (as discussed earlier) PCR testing for CMV DNA have been used to identify such infectious donors.

Studies of seroconverting pregnant women and adolescents support the thesis that recently infected donors may be the source of infectivity in some blood components. A study of recently infected pregnant women demonstrated WBC-associated CMV DNA by PCR in 100% of samples during the first month of infection, which fell to 90% during the second month, and to 0% by six months. Viral load fell even more rapidly (Revello *et al.*, 1998). Similar findings were reported from a study of seroconverting adolescents, where 75–85% of WBC samples were positive by PCR within 16 weeks of infection, but only 0–25% were still positive 48 weeks after infection. However, some samples were positive as late as 60 weeks after infection (Zhanghellini *et al.*, 1999). Using viruria as a measure of recent CMV infection, Lentz *et al.* found that 0.6% of blood donors shed CMV (Lentz *et al.*, 1988). In contrast, the figure had been 3% 13 years previously (Kane *et al.*, 1975).

Engelhard *et al.* studied the IgM and IgG responses to CMV in (previously seropositive) recipients of allogeneic BMTs. They found that IgM responses and a four-fold or greater rise in IgG titres correlated with viruria. Moreover, IgM responses preceded the rise in IgG and lasted 14 days (Engelhard *et al.*, 1991). Thus, CMV-specific IgM might identify a subset of seropositive donors who are experiencing either primary infection or CMV reactivation. The serologic prevalence of IgM in blood donors is far lower than that of IgG, ranging from <1% (Preiksaitis *et al.*, 1997) to 13% (Lentz *et al.*, 1988) depending, in part, on the assay used.

Increased risk of transfusion-acquired CMV following receipt of CMV IgM positive units has been reported (Beneke *et al.*, 1984; Demmler *et al.*, 1986). Lamberson *et al.* demonstrated a significant difference in the number of infections occurring in seronegative infants who received IgM positive blood, as compared with those who received IgM negative blood (7/222 vs. 1/141, respectively) (Lamberson *et al.*, 1988). Although such findings might suggest that IgM CMV-seropositive donors are sources of truly infectious units, the sensitivity and specificity of this marker for predicting the infectivity of a blood component is limited. Recently, Preiksaitis *et al.* were unable to detect an association between

receipt of IgM CMV positive components and increased risk of transfusion-acquired CMV infection (Preiksaitis *et al.*, 1997).

Factors related to the transfusion recipient

Transmission of infectious CMV from viraemic blood donors experiencing subclinical primary infection or CMV reactivation may be responsible for some cases of transfusion-acquired CMV infection. Such donors are uncommon, however, and they could not account for the very high incidence of CMV infection reported after exchange transfusion in neonates or after granulocyte transfusions in adults. In early studies, 10% to 30% of infants who received exchange transfusion from seropositive donors seroconverted to CMV (Kumar *et al.*, 1980; Pass *et al.*, 1976; Tobin *et al.*, 1975), and it would be most unlikely for 10–30% of the seropositive donors used in these reports to have been viraemic. Moreover, in a study of BMT recipients, there was a 77% CMV seroconversion rate in seronegative recipients of granulocytes harvested from at least some seropositive donors, as compared with a 32% seroconversion rate observed in seronegative recipients of granulocytes harvested exclusively from seronegative donors (Hersman *et al.*, 1982). As in the case of neonates undergoing exchange transfusion, even if multiple seropositive donors had been used for each BMT recipient, there could not have been enough viraemic donors among the CMV-seropositive donors used in the study to account for a 45% difference in seroconversion rates between the two groups.

Thus, these observations might suggest that CMV is most often transmitted in a latent form in donor WBCs and is reactivated after the transfusion in the circulation of the recipient. Allogeneic transfusion stimulates latent virus in donor WBCs to become reactivated. According to the previously discussed model of CMV reactivation, for reactivation to occur, latently infected cells would have to be induced to differentiate along specific pathways, and they would also have to be exposed to a pro-inflammatory cytokine milieu (Hahn *et al.*, 1998). The transfusion of allogeneic WBCs constitutes a profound immunologic stimulus to the recipient: it amounts to an in vivo analogue of a mixed lymphocyte reaction (Dzik, 1994). As already discussed, Soderberg-Naucler *et al.* recently demonstrated that an allogeneic stimulus both induces appropriate differentiation in mononuclear cells latently infected with CMV as well as providing a trigger for CMV reactivation (Soderberg-Naucler *et al.*, 1997).

Although results of animal models have been inconsistent, a mouse model demonstrated that CMV is reactivated when latently infected donor lymphocytes are stimulated into blastogenesis (Cheung and Lang, 1977). Histocompatibility differences between donor and recipient, transfusion of foreign protein, and/or alterations in T-cell immune function may act as stimuli for blastogenesis and viral reactivation. In the setting of BMT, acute GVHD and host-versus-graft reaction (a subclinical cell-mediated response against donor lymphocytes) alter T-cell immune function and may provoke CMV reactivation.

Longer survival of transfused donor lymphocytes might allow for longer opportunity for CMV reactivation. Immunocompetent hosts clear donor lymphocytes very rapidly, within a few days, and they may be at reduced risk of transfusion-acquired CMV infection for this reason. In contrast, fetuses and newborns, renal transplant recipients receiving donor-specific (HLA-matched) transfusions, and trauma victims experience much longer survival of donor lymphocytes compared with immunocompetent subjects, and – at least in some reports – they appear to be at increased risk of transfusion-acquired CMV infection. For example, CMV disease has been described in splenectomized trauma victims (Baumgartner *et al.*, 1982), and donor lymphocytes can survive for up to 1.5 years post-transfusion in such patients (Lee *et al.*, 1999). Compared with transfusions from random donors, donor-specific transfusions were associated with a higher risk of CMV infection (Chou and Kim, 1987). Recipients of exchange and intrauterine transfusions are at a much higher risk of CMV infection than immunocompetent recipients, and donor lymphocytes persist for long periods after exchange and intrauterine transfusions (Hutchinson *et al.*, 1971).

Receipt of large quantities of blood components is also associated with prolonged survival of donor lymphocytes (Adams *et al.*, 1992). Also, greater numbers of transfusions, with presumably greater numbers of circulating donor lymphocytes, may increase the risk of subclinical GVHD or host-versus-graft reaction. Accordingly, Preiksaitis *et al.* observed that patients who had received more than 30 cellular blood components had a significantly higher risk per transfused unit than those who had received fewer components (Preiksaitis *et al.*, 1988b). However, this observation has not been made consistently in all studies (Manez *et al.*, 1993).

Factors related to the transfused component

All cellular blood components (whole blood, red blood cells, platelets, and granulocytes, see Table 3.3) have been associated with CMV transmission, but there have been no reports of CMV infections acquired from fresh frozen plasma (Bowden and Sayers, 1990). This is probably because fresh frozen plasma contains few viable WBCs. Moreover, CMV antibody is administered passively in plasma from seropositive donors and could protect recipients from transfusion-acquired CMV infection.

Granulocyte concentrates and whole blood (i.e. the two components with the highest WBC content) have been associated with the highest rates of CMV transmission from seropositive donors in BMT recipients and in neonates undergoing exchange transfusion (Hersman *et al.*, 1982; Kumar *et al.*, 1980; Luthardt *et al.*, 1971; Pass *et al.*, 1976; Tobin *et al.*, 1975; Winston *et al.*, 1980). Moreover, the high rates of CMV transmission seen in early cardiac-surgery studies (Paloheimo *et al.*, 1968) suggested that fresh blood (containing many viable WBCs) may be more infectious than stored blood. As storage time increases, fewer WBCs can be isolated from either red blood cell (McCullough *et al.*, 1969) or platelet (Sherman and Dzik, 1988) units. The number of WBCs decreases in stored components, presumably as a result of cytolysis. Equally importantly, as the number of WBCs decreases during storage, the relative percentage of lymphocytes increases. If monocytes or granulocytes are the cells that harbour CMV, the infectivity of components stored for long periods should be reduced because monocytes and granulocytes are no longer intact.

The effect of the length of storage of transfused red blood cells on the risk of CMV reactivation was assessed in a group of 84

Table 3.3 Approximate WBC content of blood components in the USA[a].

Granulocyte concentrate	10^{10}
Whole blood	10^9
Red blood cell concentrate	5×10^8
Washed red blood cells	10^7–10^8
Frozen deglycerolized red blood cells	10^6–10^7
Red blood cells filtered at the bedside with WBC reduction filter	10^6
Red blood cells filtered before storage with WBC reduction filter	10^5
Whole blood derived platelet concentrate[b]	10^7
Whole blood derived platelet concentrate filtered at the bedside with WBC reduction filter[b]	10^5
Whole blood derived platelet concentrate filtered before storage with WBC reduction filter[b]	10^4
Single donor platelet concentrate whose WBC reduction is an integral part of the centrifugal apheresis process itself[c]	10^4–10^5

[a] Number of WBCs/unit of component compiled from various sources. The numbers shown are approximate and are intended to capture the average performance of US blood centres. The numbers vary over time, as well as across blood centres and filter manufacturers, and they thus often vary between published sources as well.

[b] Transfusion dose for adults consists of a pool of five or six whole blood derived platelet concentrates.

[c] Component WBC-reduced without use of a WBC reduction filter. The residual WBC content of the component can be device-dependent.

seropositive patients undergoing surgery (Adler and McVoy 1989). Patients receiving red blood cells stored for three to eight days did not differ from patients transfused with red blood cells stored for 20 to 42 days in terms of the noted rise in CMV antibody titre. Thus, the rate of reactivation events did not appear to differ between the two groups. However, two studies showed higher rates of seroconversion to CMV in recipients of fresh whole blood (Paloheimo *et al.*, 1968; Wilhelm *et al.*, 1986).

Pro-inflammatory cytokines are released in WBC-containing cellular blood components during storage (Nielsen *et al.*, 1997). Such cytokines may cause reactivation of latent CMV in donor cells during storage, because they may trigger cellular differentiation that promotes viral reactivation (Hahn *et al.*, 1998). Pre-storage WBC reduction significantly reduces the levels of such WBC-derived cytokines in stored blood components (Nielsen *et al.*, 1997). For this reason, pre-storage WBC reduction should be more effective than post-storage WBC reduction in preventing transfusion-acquired CMV infection. Post-storage WBC reduction can remove latently infected donor WBCs and prevent reactivation of CMV in the circulation of the recipient. Pre-storage WBC reduction can both remove latently infected donor cells and prevent accumulation of WBC-derived cytokines during storage. Therefore, pre-storage WBC reduction can prevent reactivation events from occurring either in the circulation of the recipient or in the stored blood component (Preiksaitis, 2000).

Table 3.4 CMV infections observed in patients receiving CMV-seronegative blood components in studies reported between 1971 and 1999.

Report (year)	Patient population	CMV infection: Infected/total	CMV infection: %
Luthardt *et al.* (1971)	Neonates	0/20	0
Kumar *et al.* (1980)	Neonates	1/7	14.3
Yeager *et al.* (1981)	Low-birth-weight neonates	0/90[a]	0
Preiksaitis *et al.* (1983)	Heart transplant recipients	0/8	0
Bowden *et al.* (1986)	BMT recipients	1/32[b]	3.1
MacKinnon *et al.* (1988)	BMT recipients	0/37	0
Miller *et al.* (1991)	BMT recipients	2/45[b]	4.4
Bowden *et al.* (1991)	BMT recipients	0/35	0
Bowden *et al.* (1995)	BMT recipients	2/252[b]	0.8
Preiksaitis *et al.* (1997)	Paediatric oncology patients	0/30	0
Pamphilon *et al.* (1999b)	BMT recipients	0/114	0

[a] For infants born to CMV-seronegative mothers. Twenty-three of 131 (17.6%) infants born to CMV-seropositive mothers developed evidence of CMV infection.

[b] No patient developed CMV disease.

Estimated risk of cytomegalovirus transmission by transfusion of cytomegalovirus-seronegative or white-blood-cell reduced components

Please refer to Chapter 19.

In some of the studies that established the efficacy of CMV-seronegative blood components in reducing the risk of transfusion-acquired CMV infection, there was a 1–4% risk of breakthrough infections (i.e. CMV infections occurring in CMV-seronegative patients despite the use of CMV-seronegative components, see Table 3.4). More specifically, between 1971 and 1999, 11 studies (including case-series, cohort comparisons, before/after comparisons and randomized controlled trials) reported on 670 patients who had been transfused with CMV-seronegative components (see Table 3.4). Six of these 670 (0.9%) patients developed CMV infection.

Many small studies that evaluated the efficacy of WBC reduction in preventing transfusion-acquired CMV infection observed no case of CMV infection in recipients of WBC-reduced red blood cells and/or platelets (see Table 3.5). However, studies that observed no case of CMV infection in such recipients had enrolled only 11 to 62 patients in the WBC-reduced group. Ohto *et al.* observed a CMV infection rate of 9% (3/33) in infants transfused with WBC-reduced components, although the route of transmission of CMV in this study is impossible to determine because infants born to CMV-seropositive mothers were breast-fed with milk not tested for CMV (Ohto *et al.*, 1999). Narvios *et al.* observed a CMV infection rate of 2.2% in recipients of WBC-reduced components. In this study, 1 out of 45 patients transfused with WBC-reduced components developed CMV pneumonia (Narvios *et al.*, 1998). The randomized trial of Bowden *et al.* (Bowden *et al.*, 1995) is discussed in detail below. When the study of Ohto *et al.* is included along with the other ten studies, the literature indicates that – between 1987 and 2000 – 618 patients had been included in 11 studies (encompassing case-series, cohort comparisons, before/after comparisons and randomized controlled trials).

Seven of 618 (1.1%) patients developed CMV infection following transfusion with WBC-reduced blood components.

Bowden *et al.* compared the efficacy of using WBC-reduced versus CMV-seronegative components for the prevention of transfusion-acquired CMV infection (Bowden *et al.*, 1995). They randomized 502 CMV-seronegative BMT recipients to receive either WBC-reduced or CMV-seronegative components, and they followed the patients for 100 days following entry into the study. Patients entered the study on the day that they received a CMV-seronegative bone marrow graft. Cytomegalovirus infection was defined as identification of CMV by viral culture or antigen-based assay in weekly urine, throat and blood cultures. Cytomegalovirus disease was defined as presence of CMV in tissue specimens or bronchoalveolar lavage fluid and associated clinical symptoms. Cytomegalovirus infections recorded after day 21 and until the end of the follow-up period were considered to have been contracted through transfusion. Infections occurring during the first three weeks of entry into the study were considered to have been acquired prior to entry into the study. (Although these latter infections were recorded in patients who had been CMV-seronegative when they entered the study, these subjects could still have acquired the infection prior to entry. It is possible that such patients might not have had the immunologic competence or the time to seroconvert by the time of entry into the study. Alternatively, they might have had so low an antibody titre upon entry into the study that their CMV antibody status could not be reproducibly determined at that time.)

Seronegative blood donors were identified by latex agglutination tests, and they were used as the source of CMV-seronegative red-blood-cell and platelet units. Platelets and red blood cells were filtered in-line at the bedside using Pall filters (Pall Biomedical Products Corporation, East Hills, NY). All employed filters were known to consistently remove more than 3 $\log_{10}$ of total WBCs (including granulocytes) and more than 4 $\log_{10}$ of B and T-cells and monocytes. Patients in either study arm received

Table 3.5 CMV infections observed in patients receiving WBC-reduced blood components in studies reported between 1987 and 1999.

Report (year)	Patient population	CMV infection: infected/total	CMV infection: %
Verdonck et al. (1987)	BMT recipients	0/29	0
Murphy et al. (1988)	Leukaemics	0/11	0
De Graan-Hentzen et al. (1989)	Haematologic malignancy patients	0/59	0
Bowden et al. (1989)	BMT recipients	0/17	0
Gilbert et al. (1989)	Low birth weight neonates	0/24	0
De Witte et al. (1990)	BMT recipients	0/28	0
Van Prooijen et al. (1994)	BMT recipients	0/60	0
Bowden et al. (1995)	BMT recipients	3/250	1.2
Narvios et al. (1998)	BMT recipients	1/45	2.2
Pamphilon et al. (1999b)	BMT recipients	0/62	0
Ohto et al. (1999)	Low birthweight neonates	3/33[a]	9.1

[a] See text.

a similar number of blood components during the 100-day follow-up period.

Between days 21 and 100 post-transplantation, there was a total of five CMV infections. Two CMV infections occurred among 252 recipients of CMV-seronegative components (CMV infection rate, 0.8%; 95% confidence interval [CI], 0.1% to 2.8%). Three CMV infections occurred among 250 recipients of WBC-reduced components (CMV infection rate, 1.2%; 95% CI, 0.3% to 3.5%). The difference in infection rate between the arms was not significant. The actuarial probability of developing CMV infection by day 100 post-transplantation was 1.3% among recipients of seronegative components and 2.4% among recipients of WBC-reduced components ($p = 1.0$).

Neither of the two infected recipients of CMV-seronegative components developed CMV disease, whereas all three infected recipients of WBC-reduced components developed CMV disease. The actuarial probability of developing CMV disease by day 100 post-transplantation was 0% among recipients of seronegative components and 1.2% among recipients of WBC-reduced components. The difference was not significant ($p = 0.25$).

In a secondary analysis, patients who had developed CMV infection within three weeks of entry into the study were added to the patients who had developed CMV infection between days 21 and 100 post-transplantation. Overall, four recipients of seronegative components and six recipients of WBC-reduced components developed CMV infection over 100 days of follow-up. Actuarial probabilities of CMV infection by day 100 were, respectively, 1.4% and 2.4%, and the difference between the arms was not significant ($p = 0.5$). However, there were no cases of CMV disease among recipients of seronegative components, whereas all six CMV infected recipients of WBC-reduced components developed CMV disease. Actuarial probabilities of CMV disease by day 100 were 0% and 2.4%, respectively, and the difference between the arms was significant ($p = 0.03$). Nonetheless, survival did not differ significantly between the arms on day 100, being 79% in recipients of seronegative components and 82% in recipients of WBC-reduced components ($p = 0.56$).

As already discussed, the earlier literature had indicated breakthrough infection rates of 1–4% in recipients of CMV-seronegative components. For this reason, before Bowden et al. began their study, they had determined that rates of CMV infection (and disease) of less than 5% in either arm of the trial would not be considered to represent clinically significant aberrations from the rate of CMV infection (and disease) that one would have expected to observe if one had conformed to the standard of care (i.e. if one had provided components collected from CMV-seronegative donors to all patients). Accordingly, in discussing their findings, the authors emphasized that the infection (and disease) rate in both arms of the study had not exceeded the 5% rate that could have been observed in the absence of any intervention. Since a <5% infection rate was observed in both arms of the study, the investigators concluded that WBC reduction was an effective alternative to the use of seronegative blood components for the prevention of transfusion-acquired CMV infection. The investigators also pointed out that four out of five patients who had developed CMV infection within three weeks of entering the study had had discrepant or equivocal CMV antibody test results at randomization. Therefore, these patients had probably been infected before they were transfused with WBC-reduced components during the study.

Some investigators believe that the report of Bowden et al. has overestimated the rate of CMV infection and disease in BMT patients who receive WBC-reduced components (Preiksaitis, 2003), because they had not optimized the provision of either CMV-seronegative or WBC-reduced components. A latex agglutination assay was used to identify CMV-seronegative donors, which requires subjective interpretation and is known to have poorer sensitivity than other commercially available assays. Moreover, bedside filtration was used to prepare WBC-reduced components for transfusion (which is inferior to pre-storage WBC reduction where better quality control and more reproducible WBC removal is achieved).

It is probably inappropriate to extrapolate the CMV infection rate observed by Bowden et al. in BMT recipients to other patient populations. Haemopoiesis is highly stimulated in bone marrow transplantation by an environment that often combines acute GVHD and sepsis. Repetitive blood transfusions that result in transient microchimerism in these immunosuppressed patients, coupled with a cytokine microenvironment that promotes CMV reactivation from latency within the transfused WBCs, may explain the high rate of transfusion-acquired CMV infection in BMT recipients. Before concluding that WBC-reduced and CMV-seronegative components are associated with a 1–3% rate of breakthrough infections in general, it will be essential to study the incidence of transfusion-acquired CMV infection in other at-risk populations. Importantly, optimal technology should be used in these future studies when either WBC-reduced or CMV-seronegative components are provided (Preiksaitis, 2003).

Is white blood cell reduction equivalent to the provision of cytomegalovirus-seronegative components?

In reviewing the results of Bowden *et al.* (Bowden *et al.*, 1995), Landaw *et al.* commented that Bowden *et al.* had demonstrated that using WBC-reduced, rather than CMV-seronegative, blood puts BMT patients at an unacceptably higher risk of CMV disease. These investigators pointed out that the presented data were consistent with the thesis that 2–5 additional deaths attributable to CMV pneumonia could be expected to occur per 250 BMT patients if WBC-reduced components were used in lieu of CMV-seronegative components. Over 100 days of follow-up, there had been six deaths from CMV disease in the arm that received WBC-reduced components, as compared with no deaths in the arm transfused with CMV-seronegative components. If Fisher's exact test had been used in lieu of actuarial analysis, the difference between the two arms of the trial would have been shown to be highly significant (p = 0.005) (Landaw, *et al.*, 1996).

In 2000, Canadian Blood Services and Héma-Québec convened a Consensus Conference to examine whether serologic testing for CMV could be abandoned in Canada following the implementation of universal WBC reduction. The consensus panel concluded that there was insufficient evidence on which to base a decision on this question. More specifically, one could favour abandoning serologic testing, because there was no evidence that serologic testing and WBC reduction employed together might be superior to WBC reduction alone. Alternatively, one could favour the concomitant use of both methods, because there was no evidence that abandoning serologic testing would not lead to a slight increase in the risk of CMV transmission through transfusion. Thus, the panel recommended the continued provision of both WBC-reduced and CMV-seronegative components to CMV-seronegative pregnant women, fetuses requiring intrauterine transfusion and allogeneic BMT recipients. In addition, the panel believed that continued use of CMV-seronegative blood in an era of universal WBC reduction was probably indicated for solid-organ transplant recipients, patients with HIV and patients with conditions likely to require allogeneic bone marrow transplantation in the future. However, because WBC reduction alone provides excellent protection from CMV, there was agreement that the administration of WBC-reduced components should not be delayed when CMV-seronegative components are not available (Blajchman *et al.*, 2001; Laupacis *et al.*, 2001).

In part, the conclusions of the Canadian Consensus Conference were driven by the ambiguity of the findings of the randomized trial of Bowden *et al.* (Bowden *et al.*, 1995; Landaw *et al.*, 1996). In contrast to the Canadian Consensus Conference, and following consideration of the same set of data, a US expert panel convened by the University Health System Consortium determined that components that have been processed by current WBC reduction methods and manufacturing standards are equivalent to CMV-seronegative components (Ratko *et al.*, 2001).

Moreover, in 2000, after reviewing the evidence from clinical trials and combining these data with theoretical considerations based on our current understanding of the pathogenesis of transfusion-acquired CMV infection, Preiksaitis concluded that pre-storage WBC reduction of blood components is the preferred method for providing CMV-'safe' blood components to patients at high risk of CMV disease. There is insufficient evidence to suggest that the additional screening of such WBC-reduced products for CMV antibody will add any significant incremental safety with respect to CMV transmission (Preiksaitis, 2000). In contrast, many of the patient populations for whom CMV-seronegative components are recommended would benefit from the other potential advantages of WBC-reduced blood components (i.e. prevention of febrile, non-haemolytic transfusion reactions, prevention of HLA-alloimmunization, and prevention of infection with other herpes viruses). The use of WBC-reduced components further permits the infusion of passive CMV-specific antibody from seropositive donors, which may have beneficial effects in some settings (e.g. in neonatal transfusions).

Thus, the American Association of Blood Banks subsequently concluded that although conclusive randomized trials proving the equivalence of CMV-seronegative components and components that have been WBC-reduced prior to storage are lacking, in the available studies, pre-storage WBC-reduced components had shown, at most, rates of CMV infection (1–3%) that had been equivalent to the rates reported previously among recipients of CMV-seronegative components (1–4%). Therefore, the available data supported the use of pre-storage WBC-reduced components, in lieu of CMV-seronegative components, for the prevention of transfusion-acquired CMV infection. Hospital transfusion services were encouraged to ensure that pre-storage WBC reduction (as opposed to bedside filtration) was used to provide CMV-unscreened components for patients at high risk of CMV disease (Malloy and Lipton, 2002).

To determine whether the risk of transfusion-acquired CMV infection was affected by the increasing use of WBC-reduced/CMV-unscreened components, Nichols *et al.* prospectively followed a cohort of 807 CMV-seronegative BMT recipients (Nichols *et al.*, 2003). The investigators recorded the incidence of transfusion-acquired CMV infection during two time periods. During the first period (May 1994 to November 1996), BMT recipients had been supported with CMV-seronegative or WBC-reduced components. During the second period (December 1996 to February 2000), WBC-reduced platelets obtained by plateletapheresis were also used. Importantly, however, the use of CMV-seronegative components declined over time, whereas the use of WBC-reduced and plateletapheresis components increased over time. Platelet units (either pooled or apheresis) were filtered after storage at the blood bank using Pall filters (Pall Biomedical Corporation, East Hills, NY), while red blood cell units were filtered before storage at the blood centre, also using Pall filters. All patients underwent weekly surveillance for CMV infection with the pp65 antigenaemia assay. The incidence of CMV infection was compared between the two time periods.

The risk of transfusion-acquired CMV infection was significantly higher during the second period than during the first period (4% versus 1.7%, respectively; p = 0.05). Multivariate analysis identified red blood cell units WBC-reduced by filtration (and not WBC-reduced platelet units obtained by plateletapheresis) as the primary predictor of transfusion-acquired CMV infection. Each additional red blood cell unit that had been collected from a CMV-seropositive donor and had been WBC-reduced by filtration was associated with a 32% increase in the odds of transfusion-acquired CMV infection (95% CI, 8% to 61%; p = 0.006). Pre-emptive therapy with ganciclovir after detection of pp65 antigenaemia prevented all but one case of CMV disease prior to day 100.

Nichols et al. concluded that:

(1) CMV-seronegative components may be superior to WBC-reduced components for the prevention of transfusion-acquired CMV disease.

(2) The abandonment of CMV-seronegative inventories in an era of universal WBC reduction may be premature.

In particular, the authors highlighted that the component most likely to transmit CMV in their study was a red blood cell unit that had been drawn from a CMV-seropositive donor and had been WBC-reduced by pre-storage filtration. Despite the better quality control of pre-storage WBC reduction, it was the red blood cell units that had been filtered pre-storage, rather than the platelet units that had been filtered post-storage, that were associated with transmission of CMV. This unexpected finding might be due to the fact that a unit of non-WBC-reduced red blood cells contains ten times more WBCs than a unit of non-WBC-reduced platelets. Therefore, even after WBC reduction, there can be a higher number of residual WBCs in pre-storage WBC-reduced red blood cells than in post-storage WBC-reduced platelets.

Nichols et al. also observed, however, that the risk of transfusion-acquired CMV infection in patients exclusively transfused with CMV-seronegative components was 2%. Thus, the authors concluded that transfusion of any blood component (whether CMV-seronegative or WBC-reduced) is associated with some small, residual risk of transmission of CMV. Although several studies had previously reported a 0% risk of CMV transmission in recipients of either CMV-seronegative or WBC-reduced components, those studies had not included sufficiently large patient populations to detect rare events. The study of Nichols et al. is the largest study reported to date, and it has other strengths, such as the use of prospective monitoring for pp65 antigenaemia. However, this study was not randomized, and it leaves open the possibility that the observed difference between the two periods might have been due to some other, unidentified factor that could have changed at the same time that the change in transfusion practice occurred. Moreover, the higher risk of CMV transmission in recipients of WBC-reduced components was associated with only one case of CMV disease in this large study. Prospective monitoring for pp65 antigenaemia, along with pre-emptive ganciclovir therapy, has greatly reduced the morbidity and mortality from CMV disease in contemporary BMT units.

Following publication of the study of Nichols et al., Vamvakas reviewed the literature pertaining to the question of whether the use of CMV-seronegative versus WBC-reduced components is equally efficacious in preventing transfusion-acquired CMV infection (Vamvakas, 2005). By the time of that review, a total of 829 recipients of CMV-seronegative components had been followed in 11 studies, and a total of 878 recipients of WBC-reduced components had been followed in 12 studies. (These numbers include 429 of the 807 patients of Nichols et al., on whom the numbers of patients developing CMV infection among recipients of CMV-seronegative or WBC-reduced components had been reported by the authors.) Twelve (1.45%) of 829 recipients of CMV-seronegative components and 24 (2.73%) of 878 recipients of WBC-reduced components had developed CMV infection in the reviewed studies. Among BMT recipients, the risk of CMV infection was, respectively, 1.63% (11/674) and 3.01% (21/697). Importantly, across three studies that compared CMV-seronegative and WBC-reduced components to each other (Bowden et al., 1995; Nichols et al., 2003; Pamphilon et al., 1999b), CMV-seronegative components were associated with a 58% reduction in the risk of CMV infection when the three studies were combined in a meta-analysis. The benefit from the use of CMV-seronegative (compared with WBC-reduced) components was statistically significant across the three studies (p < 0.05, see Figure 3.1).

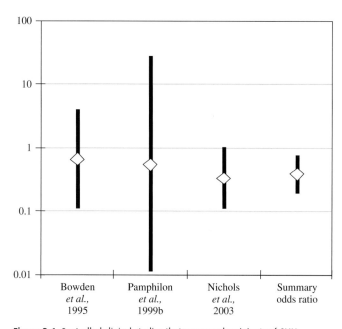

Figure 3.1 Controlled clinical studies that compared recipients of CMV-seronegative versus WBC-reduced components. For each study, the figure shows the odds ratio (OR) of CMV infection in recipients of CMV-seronegative versus WBC-reduced components. Each OR is surrounded by its 95% confidence interval (CI). If the 95% CI of the OR includes the null value of 1, the benefit from the use of CMV-seronegative (compared with WBC-reduced) components is not significant (i.e. p > 0.05). When OR < 1, a study favours CMV-seronegative (compared with WBC-reduced) components; when OR > 1, a study favours WBC-reduced (compared with CMV-seronegative) components. The figure also shows the summary OR across the three studies, as calculated by a meta-analysis that demonstrated a statistically significant (p < 0.05) benefit from the use of CMV-seronegative (compared with WBC-reduced) components (summary OR = 0.42; 95% CI, 0.22–0.79). (Modified with permission from Vamvakas, 2005).

Thus, a meta-analysis of the available studies comparing CMV-seronegative and WBC-reduced components has indicated that CMV-seronegative components are more efficacious than WBC-reduced components in preventing transfusion-acquired CMV infection.

In conclusion, the question whether WBC reduction is equivalent to the provision of CMV-seronegative components for the prevention of transfusion-acquired CMV infection remains unresolved. The data hitherto presented suggest that:

(1) A small, but real and intractable, risk of acquiring CMV infection through transfusion remains, whether CMV-seronegative or WBC-reduced components are used.

(2) The contemporary risk of CMV transmission through transfusion is small (2% to 4% per recipient in the setting of bone marrow transplantation).

(3) There are some data to indicate that the risk of CMV transmission may be slightly increased when WBC-reduced components (and especially WBC-reduced red-blood-cell units) are administered to BMT recipients in lieu of CMV-seronegative components.

No studies comparing WBC reduction alone with WBC reduction plus the use of CMV-seronegative blood components have been reported. Because the difference in the risk of transfusion-acquired CMV infection between these two arms would be expected to be very small, an extremely large study would be required to demonstrate a difference. For example, to show a decrease in the risk of transfusion-acquired CMV infection from 2.5% to 1.5%, a randomized controlled trial would have to enroll 6500 patients in order to have 80% power to detect a statistically significant (p = 0.05) difference (Blajchman et al., 2001).

Possible reasons for breakthrough infections from cytomegalovirus-seronegative or white blood cell reduced components

Failures of antibody screening of blood donors to prevent CMV transmission by transfusion can be attributed to window-period infections, seroreversion, or variant viral strains. Failures of WBC reduction can be caused by inadequate removal of WBCs or cell-free viraemia.

Window-period infections are the most likely source of failures of antibody screening of blood donors. The length of the CMV window period remains to be determined, but CMV DNA is readily detected in the plasma of donors with acute CMV infection (Zhangellini et al., 1999). Seroreversion refers to a decline in the levels of CMV antibody in the circulation of CMV-seropositive donors, so that seropositivity is not detected with the commercially-available assays. However, CMV establishes lifelong latent infection with periodic reactivations that provide an immune stimulus which ensures lifelong antibody positivity. Thus, seroreversion is unlikely to account for the failure of antibody screening of blood donors to prevent transfusion-acquired CMV infection, despite the fact that it has been documented in one early publication (Waner et al., 1973). Finally, although some variation among CMV strains does occur, there is no solid evidence that variant strains cause breakthrough infections. Strain AD169 that serves as the basis for most commercial assays has broad reactivity, making viral strains an unlikely explanation for the occasional failure of CMV-antibody tests.

Regarding cell-free viraemia, James et al. examined CMV-seropositive components for the presence of free infectious virus particles in the plasma (James et al., 1997). They showed that the plasma of seropositive red blood cells and platelets contained CMV DNA, but it also contained virus particles able to infect tissue culture cells in vitro. The presence of these virus particles was associated with an increased length of storage and was attributed to the release of infectious virus into the supernatant plasma due to the progressive breakdown of WBCs during storage.

A study of 168 seroconverting blood donors identified transient plasma viraemia in three (0.9%) of them during the peri-seroconversion phase of infection (Drew et al., 2003). A plausible, but unproven, hypothesis about the source of the residual risk of CMV transmission by transfusion is that the plasma of seroconverting donors might transmit CMV. If plasma DNA is infectious – and this remains to be proven – individuals early in the course of an asymptomatic infection would be potentially infectious, and they would also be missed by tests used to detect CMV antibody. Moreover, such donors could transmit CMV even if blood components were WBC-reduced. Although infected cells would be retained by the filter, CMV DNA in plasma would be unlikely to be retained. In theory, CMV PCR could detect such viraemic units; however, in the large, cross-sectional study of Roback et al. (Roback et al., 2003) CMV PCR did not increase the detection of potentially infectious blood components beyond the detection ensured by current serologic screening assays.

How much WBC reduction of a cellular blood component is required to eliminate the component's capacity to transmit CMV? In keeping with the definition of a 'WBC-reduced' component, the American Association of Blood Banks has suggested that residual WBC counts of less than 5×10^6 (per red blood cell or platelet apheresis unit or per pool of six whole-blood-derived platelet units) renders a blood component CMV-'safe' (Smith, 1997). However, the $< 5 \times 10^6$ residual WBCs/unit content of WBC-reduced components had been originally set because of experimental evidence relating to HLA alloimmunization. The precise degree of WBC removal that is required to prevent CMV transmission to transfusion recipients is unknown.

It is estimated that fewer than 0.2% of circulating WBCs of CMV-seropositive donors are latently infected with CMV. If blood components undergo a $\geq 3 \log_{10}$ WBC reduction, fewer than 1000 latently infected WBCs per unit would remain in WBC-reduced CMV-seropositive units (Hillyer et al., 1999). In theory, the infusion of a single latently infected donor WBC might be sufficient to infect a CMV-seronegative recipient. However, in practical terms, because the pathogenesis of transfusion-acquired CMV infection involves a complex interaction between donor and recipient, WBC reduction to less than 5×10^6 WBCs per component appears to make the sequence of events required to reactivate CMV from latency in almost all transfusion recipients so unlikely to occur that a component containing $< 5 \times 10^6$ WBCs can be considered CMV-'safe' (Preiksaitis, 2000).

Current WBC reduction filters remove in excess of $3 \log_{10}$ of total WBCs, including $4 \log_{10}$ of lymphocytes and monocytes

(Wenz and Burns, 1991). In fact, current methods for WBC reduction achieve much lower counts of residual total WBCs per component than the $<5 \times 10^6$ count required by North American standards (see Table 3.3). Recently, Hillyer *et al.* (2003) reported that approximately 1 million monocytes would be required for transmission of CMV to humans if the findings of a mouse model of transfusion-transmitted murine CMV were extrapolated to humans. Since there are only approximately 50 000 residual monocytes in WBC-reduced components, such components could be expected *not* to transmit CMV.

However, the current quality control requirements are insufficient to ensure that such low counts of residual WBCs are achieved in *all* WBC-reduced components issued for transfusion (Adams *et al.*, 2000). As a result, some cases of CMV transmission by WBC-reduced components are likely to occur due to administration of units that contain an unacceptably high ($>5 \times 10^6$) count of residual WBCs. Regulatory agencies in North America have not hitherto mandated stringent quality control of WBC reduction, because counting the number of residual WBCs in blood components had been difficult until recently. In contrast, UK guidelines mandate that WBC reduction must be shown to have been achieved, either by counting residual WBCs in all components or by using recognized methods of statistical process control. The latter take into account the mean count of residual WBCs in the tested units, the standard deviation, the specified upper limit (5×10^6/unit), and the number and percentage of units tested (Pamphilon *et al.*, 1999a).

Based on such input, one can calculate that there is 95% confidence that at least 95% of the released components will be WBC-reduced; or that there is 99% confidence that at least 99% of the released components will be WBC-reduced; and so on. Despite such very high confidence, however, unless residual WBCs are counted in each and every released component, one can never be 100% confident that each and every component that has been labelled as 'WBC-reduced' is indeed WBC-reduced. Thus, even in settings where appropriate statistical process control is performed, the question persists as to whether WBC reduction gives the same degree of protection as does testing of donors for CMV antibody.

Cytomegalovirus reactivation by allogeneic transfusion

Transfused donor WBCs encountering the recipient's foreign human leucocyte antigens induce immune activation of both recipient and donor lymphocytes. When blood from a latently infected (CMV-seropositive) donor is transfused to an uninfected (CMV-seronegative) recipient, it is thought that donor WBCs harbouring latent virus are stimulated and thereby induced to activate their virus with resultant transmission to the recipient. In a similar vein, when blood from a CMV-seronegative (or CMV-seropositive) donor is transfused to a CMV-seropositive recipient, recipient WBCs harbouring latent virus could also be induced to reactivate their virus and to trigger CMV proliferation and dissemination to uninfected recipient cells. In the former case, CMV carried in a latent form in blood components is believed to be reactivated by the process of allogeneic transfusion, resulting in exogenous CMV infection in the recipient. In the latter case, the mere act of allogeneic transfusion might similarly trigger endogenous CMV infection in a latently infected transfusion recipient (Preiksaitis, 2000).

Indirect evidence supports the thesis that in patients who are CMV-seropositive before the transfusion the vast majority of transfusion-associated CMV infections represent reactivation of latent virus as opposed to reinfection, and, for this reason, there is considerable agreement in the literature that CMV-seropositive patients do not benefit from the transfusion of CMV-seronegative components. Adler *et al.* randomized CMV-seropositive patients undergoing cardiac surgery to receive blood from CMV-unscreened or CMV-seronegative donors. Five of 46 (10.9%) patients who received CMV-seronegative blood exhibited more than a fourfold rise in CMV antibody titre, as compared to 7 of 48 (14.6%) patients who received CMV-unscreened blood (p = 0.8) (Adler *et al.*, 1985b). Cytomegalovirus-seropositive BMT patients receiving CMV-seronegative or CMV-unscreened blood also developed similar rates of transfusion-acquired/induced CMV infection (Bowden *et al.*, 1986; Miller *et al.*, 1991).

Furthermore, granulocyte transfusions from CMV-seropositive donors were not a significant risk factor for CMV infection in CMV-seropositive patients undergoing allogeneic bone marrow transplantation (Meyers *et al.*, 1986). Using restriction endonuclease analysis, Winston *et al.* observed no second-strain infections in a study of allogeneic bone marrow transplant patients who developed CMV infection during the course of treatment (Winston *et al.*, 1985). All these studies indicate that, although there is evidence for second-strain CMV transmission by solid-organ allografts (Chou, 1986; 1987; 1989; Grundy *et al.*, 1988) and sexual contacts (Chandler *et al.*, 1987; Spector *et al.*, 1984), there is no evidence of second-strain CMV transmission by allogeneic transfusion (Smith, 1997).

Tegtmeier tabulated the results of studies completed between 1966 and 1988 and reporting the prevalence of transfusion-acquired CMV infection in immunocompetent patients who had been CMV-seropositive before the transfusion (Tegtmeier, 1989). The overall incidence of infection among 1063 patients included in the reviewed studies was 10.3% (109/1063). Among 282 patients included in eight studies published prior to 1972, the incidence of CMV infection was 23.8% (67/282); among 781 patients included in seven studies published after 1972, the incidence of CMV infection was 5.4% (42/781). The majority of these studies had included patients undergoing open heart surgery; the decline in the incidence of post-transfusion CMV infection over time correlated with the decrease in the use of fresh blood in cardiac surgery and with a reduction in the number of red blood cell units transfused perioperatively.

Discussing the figures compiled by Tegtmeier, Busch and Lee highlighted the prevalence of CMV viraemia among transfused seropositive patients (10.3% is very high, compared to the [well under 3%] spontaneous CMV reactivation rates reported in seropositive blood donors or in untransfused patients). They observed that allogeneic transfusion appears to increase the prevalence of CMV reactivation by as much as five-fold, and they cited these figures as indirect evidence in support of the thesis of CMV reactivation by allogeneic transfusion (Busch and Lee, 1995).

While the studies reviewed by Tegtmeier suggest that transfusion may result in CMV reactivation in some transfused patients, transfusion may have been only a surrogate marker for other reactivation stimuli (Smith, 1997). Cytomegalovirus reactivation has been observed following immunosuppressive therapy, as well as with malignancy, various drug therapies, radiation therapy, transplantation, pregnancy, prematurity, HIV infection and other circumstances. Although these factors were probably absent in the studies of immunocompetent patients reviewed by Tegtmeier, it is possible that other (unknown) variables may have triggered the reactivation of CMV infection in a proportion of the included subjects. If clinical conditions likely to trigger CMV reactivation occur preferentially in transfused patients, it may be difficult to identify whether reactivation results from allogeneic transfusion or from other clinical circumstances shared by the transfused patients.

Furthermore, latently infected cells exposed to cytokines or to other inflammatory signals can be induced to undergo viral activation in vitro (Smith, 1997). For this reason, viral reactivation induced in CMV-seropositive recipients by allogeneic transfusion may (or may not) be the result of antigenic stimulation of the recipient's peripheral-blood mononuclear cells by allogeneic (donor) WBCs. In this regard, the findings of animal models have been conflicting, and they are reviewed in the next section.

Findings of animal models

The murine model of transfusion-acquired CMV infection developed by Cheung and Lang suggested that viral reactivation was not specifically related to exposure to allogeneic blood. When uninfected CH3 mice served as blood donors and allogeneic, latently infected BALB/c mice served as blood recipients, both allogeneic and syngeneic transfusions caused viral reactivation: CMV could be recovered from the salivary gland homogenates of the transfused mice whether donor blood had been administered to allogeneic (BALB/c) or to syngeneic (CH3) animals. When uninfected BALB/c mice served as blood donors and allogeneic, latently infected CH3 mice served as blood recipients, the results of the experiment were ambiguous. Allogeneic transfusion recipients experienced viral reactivation, and CMV could be recovered from their salivary gland homogenates. Cytomegalovirus could not be recovered from the salivary glands of the transfused syngeneic controls, but there was a more than four-fold rise in CMV antibody titre in these animals. The authors interpreted this serologic finding as evidence of viral reactivation in the syngeneic transfusion recipients (Cheung and Lang, 1977).

Although the transfusion of blood from an allogeneic, uninfected donor could alone trigger CMV reactivation in a latently infected animal in the murine model of Cheung and Lang, both stimulation by allogeneic mononuclear cells and recipient immunosuppression were required for the production of CMV reactivation in a rat model. Bruggerman intravenously administered whole blood, thoracic duct lymphocytes, or spleen cells from uninfected LEW rats to latently infected BN rats. When the BN

rats were immunocompetent, allogeneic transfusion did not trigger CMV reactivation in four separate experiments. However, when the BN rats were rendered immunocompromised by total body irradiation, allogeneic transfusion triggered CMV reactivation in three of three experiments. Activation did not occur after syngeneic transfusion (Bruggerman, 1991).

Olding et al. cultured lymphoid cells obtained from latently infected mice in the presence of allogeneic mouse embryo cells. They documented reactivation of murine CMV in vitro, in response to stimulation by allogeneic (but not syngeneic) embryo cells; reactivation in response to allogeneic WBCs was not tested in these experiments (Olding, et al., 1975). Mayo et al. recovered CMV from spleen cells of latently infected mice by cocultivation of spleen cells on either syngeneic (DBA/2) or allogeneic (CD1) embryonic fibroblast cultures (Mayo et al., 1978). Although these experiments have been cited in support of the hypothesis of CMV reactivation by allogeneic transfusion, the reactivation of latent virus observed in these studies did not occur in response to stimulation by allogeneic WBCs.

Findings of clinical studies

Sloand et al. studied whether allogeneic transfusion increases the likelihood of specific opportunistic infections in HIV-1-seropositive patients. They reviewed the records of all AIDS patients who had attended an HIV clinic between February 1990 and February 1992. All but 2 of the 196 patients were receiving antiretroviral therapy with zidovudine, dideoxyinosine, and/or dideoxycytodine. Patients were followed for 6–24 months (mean, 18 months). The frequencies of CMV infection (retinitis, gastritis, colitis, or pneumonitis) and other AIDS-defining opportunistic infections were calculated for each six months of follow-up. One hundred and thirty patients received transfusion during the follow-up period, and 30 developed CMV infection. Non-WBC-reduced red blood cells were transfused and an average transfusion dose of 13 units was administered.

There was a strong association (p < 0.01) between increased frequency of CMV infection and blood transfusion. There was no association between transfusion and other opportunistic infections. The association between CMV infection and blood transfusion persisted (p < 0.01) following stratification by CD4 + T-cell count. It also persisted following stratification by race and by risk factor for AIDS. Furthermore, transfused and untransfused patients were similar in terms of history of CMV infection, history of other opportunistic infections, and frequency of AIDS wasting syndrome at study entry. The authors concluded that the higher frequency of particular opportunistic infections in HIV-1-seropositive patients indicated a relationship between allogeneic blood transfusion and CMV reactivation in patients with AIDS (Sloand et al., 1994).

Vamvakas and Kaplan conducted a similar observational study, including 569 AIDS patients who had been discharged from their hospital between January 1985 and January 1988 without receiving antiretroviral therapy. Patients were followed for <1–96 months (mean, 10 months) following the diagnosis of AIDS. Transfused components were not WBC-reduced, and 158 patients received transfusion during the initial three months following the diagnosis of AIDS. A preferential occurrence of active CMV infection in the transfused group was not observed in this cohort (Vamvakas and Kaplan, 1993; 1994).

If allogeneic transfusion does cause viral reactivation in CMV-seropositive transfusion recipients owing to the antigenic stimulation of the recipient's peripheral blood mononuclear cells by the donor WBCs, the provision of WBC-reduced blood components should prevent viral reactivation in CMV-seropositive transfusion recipients (Preiksaitis, 2000). Cytomegalovirus is the most serious viral infection in AIDS patients, and it may be appropriate to administer WBC-reduced blood components to CMV-seropositive AIDS patients in order to prevent CMV reactivation. The Viral Activation Transfusion Study (VATS) was undertaken to investigate whether transfusion of non-WBC-reduced components to CMV-seropositive patients with HIV infection results in clinically significant CMV disease (Collier et al., 2001).

The VATS randomly allocated 531 patients, who were both HIV-1 and CMV-seropositive at the time of their first red blood cell transfusion, to receive non-WBC-reduced or WBC-reduced red blood cells for the duration of the trial (1–3 years). All transfused platelets underwent WBC reduction. Based on the assumption that CMV reactivation by allogeneic transfusion is probably mediated by intact, immunologically competent donor WBCs, relatively fresh red blood cells were administered to all transfusion recipients in this study. Recipients of WBC-reduced or non-WBC-reduced red blood cells did not differ in CMV viral load after transfusion, or in the time it took them to develop new CMV end-organ disease. Moreover, recipients of WBC-reduced or non-WBC-reduced red blood cells did not differ in any of the primary or secondary endpoints of the study, including the length of survival, the time to the first new serious HIV complication, the level of plasma cytokines, the HIV-1 viral load, or the CD4+ or activated CD8+ cell counts.

Thus, the VATS results did not support the use of WBC-reduced components in CMV-seropositive patients with HIV infection, at least not for the purpose of preventing CMV reactivation. Whether CMV-seropositive patients at risk of CMV disease should receive WBC-reduced components in order to prevent CMV reactivation, however, is still debated by some investigators. Because of the complex pathogenesis of CMV reactivation and its dependence on the nature of recipient immunosuppression, it may be difficult to generalize the findings of a single randomized trial conducted in one group of patients to other patient categories. Several studies enrolling different patient groups (e.g. allogeneic BMT recipients, solid-organ transplant recipients, etc.) may be needed, to determine if WBC-containing allogeneic transfusion causes CMV reactivation in all patient groups (Smith, 1997).

Epstein-Barr virus

Transfusion-acquired Epstein-Barr virus (EBV) infection has only *very* rarely been reported in the literature, mostly in multitransfused thalassaemic children and patients undergoing open-heart surgery. No serious morbidity from transfusion-acquired EBV disease has been reported, but, at least in theory, transfusion-acquired EBV disease could be catastrophic. This is because EBV can cause severe complications in a minority of immunosuppressed subjects, such as solid-organ transplant recipients treated with cyclosporin or patients with certain rare congenital immunodeficiency diseases. Epstein-Barr virus encephalitis, EBV-induced lymphoma, and EBV-induced lymphoproliferative disease have been described in transfused transplant recipients, but they have been ascribed to reactivation of endogenous virus rather than to primary infection originating in the transfused blood component or the transplanted organ.

Epstein-Barr virus establishes chronic, lifelong infection in B lymphocytes, and it can be isolated from 1 per 100 000 to 1 per million B-cells of asymptomatic EBV-seropositive donors who have IgG antibodies to viral capsid antigen (anti-VCA). Because EBV is readily transmitted by saliva and 90% of donors are EBV-seropositive, the rarity of transfusion-acquired EBV disease is somewhat of an enigma. In part, this is explained by the fact that B-lymphocytes deteriorate during blood component storage, and intact B-lymphocytes are cleared shortly after transfusion into the recipient. Moreover, protective EBV antibody is passively acquired with plasma transfusions, while most adult patients are already EBV-seropositive before the transfusion.

Because of the rarity of transfusion-acquired EBV disease, no recommendations for prevention have been made. Perhaps transplant recipients on cyclosporin and patients with congenital T-cell defects should be receiving WBC-reduced components if they are EBV-seronegative. Some investigators maintain that EBV-seropositive patients from these groups should also receive WBC-reduced components, because allogeneic transfusion might provoke EBV reactivation, along the lines discussed previously for CMV reactivation.

Characteristics of Epstein-Barr virus

Epstein-Barr virus infects the vast majority of humans, but it usually results in subclinical infection. Individuals who can transmit EBV have infectious virus in their saliva which is produced by B-lymphocytes of the oropharynx. Infection of the oropharyngeal epithelium by another person's saliva leads to lytic replication of EBV in the epithelial cells, with release of viral particles that subsequently infect B-lymphocytes expressing class II HLA antigens and CD21. (Such B-cells are present in the Waldeyer ring of the oropharynx.) Infected B-cells may remain latently infected in the oropharynx, or they may disseminate throughout the body and create a reservoir of latent EBV infection in the lymph nodes, spleen and bone marrow. Latent EBV within the oropharyngeal B-cells can become reactivated, with resulting cellular lysis and viral shedding into the saliva (Anagnostopoulos et al., 1995; Babcock et al., 1998; Masucci and Ernberg, 1994).

Clinical manifestations of transfusion-acquired Epstein-Barr virus disease

Epstein-Barr virus is the aetiologic agent of infectious mononucleosis, and it has been associated with a variety of other diseases, including Burkitt's lymphoma, nasopharyngeal carcinoma, and X-linked lymphoproliferative disease. It has also been linked to several non-malignant, but often fatal, diseases, such as chronic active EBV infection and virus-associated haemophagocytic syndrome. The role of EBV in the pathogenesis of these disorders remains to be elucidated.

Infectious mononucleosis is characterized by the clinical triad of fever, pharyngitis, and generalized lymphadenopathy, along with the demonstration of *atypical* lymphocytosis and the presence of heterophil antibodies. The IgM and IgG antibody responses to a panoply of EBV antigens are also detected, including IgM and IgG anti-VCA, IgG anti-early antigen (anti-EA), and IgG anti-Epstein Barr nuclear antigen (anti-EBNA) (Linde, 2003). However, the serologic diagnosis of infectious mononucleosis rests on the demonstration of heterophil antibodies, that is, antibodies directed against sheep red cells. Moreover, at least 10% of lymphocytes are atypical, showing striking pleomorphism. Only in the minority of cases of heterophil-antibody-negative, EBV-induced infectious mononucleosis is EBV-specific serology required to make the diagnosis.

As in the case of CMV, transfusion-acquired EBV disease was initially described in open-heart surgery in the 1960s when large volumes of fresh blood, presumably containing intact B-cells, were administered to patients having cardiac surgery. Most cases of 'post-perfusion' syndrome described at that time were attributed to CMV, although occasional cases were linked to EBV (Gerber et al., 1969; Henle et al., 1970; Kapsenberg et al., 1970; Paloheimo et al., 1968; Purcell et al., 1971; Solem and Jörgensen, 1969; Turner et al., 1972). The diagnosis of EBV-associated disease was often not confirmed by heterophil-antibody tests in these early studies, however, and the possibility of a CMV-associated 'post-perfusion' syndrome was sometimes not excluded. Moreover, the clinical picture did not mimic infectious mononucleosis in many cases, because pharyngitis was often absent and lymphadenopathy was often absent or minimal. Thus, most transfusion-acquired cases presented as febrile syndromes resembling the so-called 'typhoidal' type of infectious mononucleosis.

Gerber et al. reported on 54 cardiac-surgery patients, 49 of whom were EBV-seropositive before the transfusion. One of five EBV-seronegative patients developed clinical and laboratory findings of heterophil antibody positive infectious mononucleosis post-operatively, while two of the remaining patients demonstrated seroconversion. Thus, three of five (60%) EBV-seronegative patients contracted EBV perioperatively, apparently through transfusion (Gerber et al., 1969). In the study of Henle et al., 6 of 229 cardiac-surgery patients seroconverted, and 11 EBV-seropositive patients developed four-fold or greater increases in EBV antibody titre. However, none of the 17 patients developed signs or symptoms of a 'post-perfusion' syndrome (Henle et al., 1970).

Kapsenberg et al. described a case of 'post-perfusion' syndrome that was initially heterophil antibody negative and was thought to be due to CMV. Several weeks later, occipital lymphadenopathy developed and a high-titre heterophil antibody was detected. These authors further reviewed records of 104 patients with a diagnosis of 'post-perfusion' syndrome, and they noted that 11 (10.5%) had positive heterophil-antibody reactions

(Kapsenberg et al., 1970). Other isolated cases of the heterophil antibody positive, EBV-associated syndromes have been reported, not only after open-heart surgery but also following blood transfusion of non-surgical patients (Blacklow et al., 1971; Purtilo et al., 1980; Turner et al., 1972).

McMonigal et al. reported on two cases of heterophil-antibody-positive infectious mononucleosis that presented predominantly as febrile illnesses. Initial blood samples lacked both atypical lymphocytes and heterophil antibodies, and infectious mononucleosis was not considered in the differential diagnosis. When atypical lymphocytes appeared 8–9 days later, CMV was thought to be the cause of the 'post-perfusion' syndrome, because of the absence of pharyngitis and cervical lymphadenopathy. Only when heterophil antibodies became positive, 35 and 48 days after surgery, was the diagnosis of EBV-associated infectious mononucleosis established (McMonigal et al., 1983).

Studies of paediatric transfusion recipients have shown that transfusion-acquired EBV infection is rare, and, when it does occur, it is generally asymptomatic. Pearson et al. found an EBV seroprevalence of 82% among 25 thalassaemic children, and they interpreted this prevalence to be age-appropriate rather than transfusion-related (Pearson et al., 1986). Papaevangelou et al. found an EBV seroprevalence of 76% in polytransfused thalassaemic children, which was only slightly higher than the 70% seroprevalence found in age-matched controls. The investigators found no evidence of mononucleosis-like illness in their patient population, and they concluded that the incidence of transfusion-acquired EBV infection is very low (Papaevangelou et al., 1979). Henle and Henle followed paediatric patients having open-heart surgery over 6 to 12 months post-discharge. All 25 patients were CMV-seronegative when they underwent surgery, and only one developed likely EBV seroconversion 63 days after transfusion (Henle and Henle, 1985).

Rare cases of transfusion-acquired EBV infection have continued to be reported (Alfieri et al., 1996; Tattevin et al., 2002). Alfieri et al. recovered the same EBV strain from a unit of donor blood and the oropharynx of the recipient. Because the recipient was a transplant patient, the potential for serious transfusion-acquired EBV infection in this patient population was raised. Tattevin et al. reported a case of transfusion-related infectious mononucleosis in 2002. The case was reported from France after universal WBC reduction had been implemented, although the report did not state whether the blood components administered to this patient had been WBC-reduced.

Prevention of transfusion-acquired Epstein-Barr virus infection

Because of the rarity of transfusion-acquired EBV infection, and the lack of significant morbidity when transmission by transfusion does occur, no specific preventive measures have been recommended. Testing of donors for EBV IgG anti-VCA or EBV DNA is not performed. Because EBV is B-cell-associated, WBC reduction should be able to remove the cells that harbour EBV and should thus render components EBV-'safe'. (Current filters are known to remove more than 4 $\log_{10}$ of B-cells (Wenz and

Burns, 1991).) Some evidence of the relative safety of frozen deglycerolized blood in preventing transmission of EBV has been reported (Jacobs, 1986). The red blood cells of a donor who developed a mononucleosis-like syndrome three days after donation were frozen and deglycerolized (and thus WBC-reduced), and they were then transfused to three neonates. No recipient developed serologic evidence of EBV infection over a follow-up period of three months.

Although the efficacy of components WBC-reduced by filtration in preventing transmission of EBV has not been demonstrated, one might extrapolate from the efficacy of filtered components in preventing transmission of CMV, and conclude that such components can probably be regarded as EBV-'safe'. Recently, Qu *et al.* demonstrated efficient, 4 $\log_{10}$ removal of EBV from filtered red blood cell units (Qu *et al.*, 2005). Units were WBC-reduced before storage, and pre- and post-WBC-reduction samples from each unit were assayed for EBV DNA. Epstein-Barr virus genomes were detected in B-cells in 14 of 16 pre-WBC-reduction samples, as compared with only one post-WBC-reduction sample. The lone PCR positive unit following WBC reduction was the unit that had had the highest EBV viral load before WBC reduction. The authors concluded that WBC reduction renders most red-blood-cell units EBV DNA negative. However, clinical studies are needed to determine to what extent the risk of transfusion-acquired EBV infection decreases thanks to WBC reduction.

Clinicians can opt to provide WBC-reduced components to patients deemed to be at high risk of EBV disease even though no significant morbidity from transfusion-acquired EBV infection has hitherto been reported in such patients. Some investigators believe that all patients at high risk of EBV disease should receive WBC-reduced components, regardless of whether their pre-transfusion status is EBV-seropositive or EBV-seronegative (Hillyer *et al.*, 1999). Regardless of the recipient's EBV serostatus, the justification for using WBC-reduced components is theoretical. However, the consequences of transfusion-acquired infection in such patients can, in theory, be catastrophic. Moreover, many of these patients are already receiving WBC-reduced components for other reasons. An additional action to reduce the risk of transfusion-acquired EBV infection in vulnerable patients would be the provision of blood components from donors who are seronegative for IgG anti-VCA. An alternative school of thought holds that our knowledge of the relevance of EBV to blood transfusion safety is incomplete. Until the pathogenicity of the virus in transfusion recipients is known, recommendations about special processing of blood components because of concern about transfusion-acquired EBV disease are premature (Sayers, 1994).

Human herpes viruses 6 and 7

Human herpesvirus 6 (HHV-6) is a T-lymphotropic herpes virus that was identified in 1986 from lymphocytes of patients with various lymphoproliferative disorders (Salahuddin *et al.*, 1986). It infects almost all children by the age of two years and persists lifelong. It is a common cause of acute febrile illnesses in young children, including exanthem subitum (roseola infantum)

(Yamanishi *et al.*, 1988; Zerr *et al.*, 2005). Human herpes virus 6 infection has also been described in BMT recipients (Asano *et al.*, 1991). Human herpes virus 6 reactivation is frequent in such patients, but many patients with reactivation remain asymptomatic (Cone *et al.*, 1999). Human herpes virus 6-associated pneumonitis and encephalitis have been reported in such patients (Cone *et al.*, 1993; Drobyski *et al.*, 1994; Zerr *et al.*, 2001), but whether HHV-6 is actually the cause of the pneumonitis or encephalitis remains uncertain. HHV-6 has also been implicated in viral illnesses in solid-organ transplant recipients (Ratnamolan *et al.*, 1998), and it has been associated with a number of neurological disorders including multiple sclerosis (Dewhurst *et al.*, 1997a).

Human herpes virus 7 is a T-lymphotropic herpes virus first identified in 1990 from lymphocytes of a healthy individual. It is similar to HHV-6 in its genetic make-up and in many of its properties, including the ability to cause at least some cases of exanthem subitum. Despite these similarities, there are important differences between HHV-6 and HHV-7, including the cellular receptors to which the viruses attach on T-lymphocytes. Primary infection with HHV-7 occurs later in life than primary infection with HHV-6. Like EBV and HHV-6, HHV-7 is ubiquitous, with a greater than 85% prevalence in the US population. Human herpes virus 7 was isolated from a patient with hepatosplenomegaly and pancytopenia who lacked both EBV and CMV (Ablashi *et al.*, 1995; Dewhurst *et al.*, 1997b).

No case of overt transfusion-acquired infection has been reported in association with HHV-6 or HHV-7. However, because these two viruses are T-lymphotropic and might potentially cause significant morbidity in transplant recipients, the possibility of significant transfusion-acquired disease remains a consideration. As in the case of EBV, virtually all transfusion recipients are already HHV-6 or HHV-7-seropostive pre-transfusion. Thus, no recommendations for prevention of transfusion-acquired HHV-6/HHV-7 infection have been made.

Blood donors are not screened for HHV-6/HHV-7 antibody or DNA. Recently, 150 Latvian blood donors were tested by PCR for HHV-6/HHV-7 DNA in peripheral-blood WBCs. No active HHV-6 infections were found, but HHV-7 DNA was present in 10.6% of the donors (Kozireva *et al.*, 2001). The efficacy of WBC reduction in preventing transmission or reactivation of these viruses by transfusion has not been demonstrated. However, current filters are known to remove more than 4 $\log_{10}$ of T-cells (Wenz and Burns, 1991). Thus, one might extrapolate to these viruses the results of studies establishing the efficacy of WBC reduction in preventing CMV transmission by transfusion. Some clinicians may opt to administer WBC-reduced components to patients at risk of significant HHV-6 or HHV-7 disease, for example following bone marrow or solid-organ transplantation, in an effort to prevent transfusion-acquired HHV-6 or HHV-7 infection (Hillyer *et al.*, 1999). Others feel that special processing of blood components in order to prevent such a risk is premature (Sayers, 1994).

Human herpes virus 8

Discovered in 1994, human herpesvirus 8 (HHV-8) is known as Kaposi's sarcoma (KS)-associated herpes virus. It has been shown to cause all forms of KS. It has also been associated with primary effusion lymphoma in patients with HIV infection and with multicentric Castleman's disease (Cannon *et al.*, 2003). Human herpes virus 8 does not appear to cause disease in immunocompetent individuals unless certain co-factors are present. Kaposi's sarcoma develops only in those who become immunosuppressed because of HIV disease, transplantation, or older age. Primary infection with HHV-8 is sometimes associated with a febrile viral syndrome.

Human herpes virus 8 is akin to EBV in that it can produce either lytic or latent infection in a variety of cells, including B-lymphocytes, monocytes, endothelial and epithelial cells. In HHV-8-seropositive individuals, the virus is probably latently maintained at undetectable levels in peripheral-blood B-lymphocytes and monocytes. Despite a large number of epidemiologic and virologic studies, the exact modes of transmission of HHV-8 are yet to be fully elucidated. Human herpes virus 8 transmission modalities may differ between countries where the virus is prevalent and countries where the virus is sporadic (Dukers and Rezza, 2003).

In endemic countries, HHV-8 is mainly transmitted by a non-sexual route(s) among family members and close contacts. In countries where the prevalence of HHV-8 infection is low, HHV-8 is probably transmitted sexually or through needle sharing among injecting drug users. Heterosexual transmission is probably infrequent. In contrast, many investigators agree that sexual transmission occurs between homosexual men (Atkinson *et al.*, 2003; Cannon *et al.*, 2001; Diamond *et al.*, 2001; Goedert *et al.*, 2003).

Human herpes virus 8 seroprevalence rates in sub-Saharan Africa vary from 22% in Central Africa to 87% in the Republic of Congo and Botswana. Mediterranean countries, where 'classical' KS occurs rather frequently in older males, have higher prevalence of HHV-8 compared with Northern European countries. For example, the prevalence of HHV-8 is 20% in southern Italy compared to <10% in northern Italy. In Northern Europe, the USA, Latin America and Asia, the prevalence of HHV-8 has been reported to range from 0% to 5%. In patients with HIV infection, the prevalence of HHV-8 corresponds to the occurrence of KS among HIV risk groups. Homosexual men have higher prevalence than injecting drug users, heterosexuals, haemophiliacs, or children (Dukers and Rezza, 2003).

In countries where the prevalence of HHV-8 infection is low, risk factors for HHV-8 overlap with risk factors for HIV, hepatitis B virus (HBV) and hepatitis C virus (HCV). Human herpes virus 8 transmission has been traced to transplantation of infected organs (Luppi *et al.*, 2003), and the possibility of transmission by blood components was raised when HHV-8 was isolated from five of seven donations from one blood donor (Blackbourn *et al.*, 1997).

Studies in Uganda and Tanzania where both HHV-8 and KS are prevalent, found HHV-8 DNA in blood donors and observed that HHV-8 seropositivity in children correlates with the number of transfusions they have received (Enbom *et al.*, 2002; Mbulaiteye *et al.*, 2003). In North America, however, none of 138 HHV-8-seropositive blood donors had HHV-8 DNA in their peripheral-blood mononuclear cells (Pellett *et al.*, 2003). Moreover, none of ten recipients of blood components from 14 HHV-8 seropositive

donors developed antibodies to HHV-8 (Operskalski *et al.*, 1997). Similarly, negative results were reported from Jamaica (Engels *et al.*, 1999).

Recently, however, evidence of transmission of HHV-8 by transfusion was reported from Baltimore, Maryland. Serum specimens collected before and after surgery from 406 patients enrolled in the Frequency of Agents Communicable by Transfusion Study (FACTS) between 1986 and 1990 were tested for HHV-8 antibody. Of 284 patients who were initially HHV-8 seronegative and who received transfusions, two seroconverted. These patients had received 12 and 13 units of blood. If seroconversion had been caused by the transfused blood, the risk of transmission of HHV-8 through transfusion would have been 0.082% per unit. Because linked donor specimens were not available, other routes of HHV-8 transmission were not excluded. None of the HHV-8-seronegative patients who had not received transfusions seroconverted, although there were only 75 patients in this group and the difference between 2/284 and 0/75 did not attain statistical significance. The authors concluded that the presented evidence supported the thesis that HHV-8 infection had been acquired from the transfusion (Dollard *et al.*, 2005).

Subsequently, stronger evidence of transmission of HHV-8 by transfusion was presented by Hladik *et al.* from Uganda, where HHV-8 is endemic (Hladik *et al.*, 2006). These investigators followed 1811 transfusion recipients, 991 of whom were HHV-8-seronegative before transfusion and completed all requisite follow-up. Human herpes virus 8 seroconversion occurred in 41 (4.1%) of the 991 transfusion recipients. The risk of seroconversion was significantly higher among recipients of HHV-8 seropositive blood than among recipients of HHV-8 seronegative blood (excess risk, 2.8%; $p < 0.05$), and the increase in risk was seen mainly among patients in whom seroconversion occurred three to ten weeks after transfusion – a result consistent with transmission of HHV-8 by transfusion. Red blood cell units stored for up to four days were more often associated with seroconversion than RBC units stored for more than four days – a result consistent with transmission of a herpes virus that resides in WBCs that deteriorate during storage.

Hudnall *et al.* tested 100 random blood donors in south-east Texas for HHV-8 antibody and DNA. Twenty-three per cent of them were HHV-8 seropositive, although none was found to carry HHV-8 DNA (Hudnall *et al.*, 2003). These results contrast with the findings reported from the Retrovirus Epidemiology Donor Study group that tested 1000 donor samples collected in 1994–1995 from five geographically dispersed areas of the USA by a variety of assays for HHV-8 antibodies. Seroprevalence was 3.5%, based on several statistical analyses that required concordance of multiple serologic tests to establish seropositivity. Importantly, none of 138 seropositive donors assayed by PCR was found to carry HHV-8 DNA (Pellett *et al.*, 2003).

Although all of the following statements need further corroboration, it appears that:

(1) Infectious HHV-8 can be present in blood donors.

(2) Human herpes virus 8 can be transmitted by transfusion.

(3) Human herpes virus 8 may have the potential to cause serious disease in immunocompromised transfusion recipients.

However, it is important to note that HHV-8 is not a new agent; rather, it is newly described. Presumably, blood for HHV-8 seropositive donors has been transfused for many years, without any well documented report(s) of cases of KS occurring in patients who developed KS after contracting HHV-8 through transfusion (Blajchman and Vamvakas, 2006).

Prior to the discovery of HHV-8 in 1994, isolated case reports and case series had appeared that mentioned the development of KS in transfused patients not infected with HIV (Bendsoe et al., 1990; Friedman-Kien et al., 1990; Roujeau et al., 1988) or in patients with transfusion-associated AIDS (Aboulafia et al., 1991; Cockerill et al., 1986; Padilla et al., 1990; Velez-Garcia et al., 1985). Of 63 patients who developed KS in the absence of HIV in the case series of Bendsoe et al. (1990), four had previous transfusion documented in their medical records. These authors stated that transfusion deserves further study as an aetiologic factor of KS; however, they cautioned that clinical indications for transfusion often exist in diseases that cause immunosuppression and are themselves associated with development of KS.

Padilla et al. (1990) reviewed the literature on the frequent co-existence of KS and CMV in patients with AIDS, as well as the literature on five cases of KS occurring in patients with transfusion-associated AIDS, and they speculated that these five patients might have received blood products infected with both CMV and HIV, or might have been exposed to CMV elsewhere, so that their simultaneous exposure to both viruses could have accounted for the development of KS. Thus, the possibility that KS may be due to an oncogenic virus transmissible by transfusion had been raised before the discovery of HHV-8. In a similar vein, Aboulafia et al. (1991) had proposed that the far higher incidence of KS in male homosexuals with AIDS – as compared with female AIDS patients or AIDS patients acquiring the infection through IVDU, transfusion, or infusion of clotting-factor concentrates – might suggest that KS is attributable to a sexually-transmitted virus. If that were the case, a sexually-transmitted virus like HIV might also be transmitted by transfusion, and transfusion-transmission of such a virus might lead to the development of KS either in the presence or in the absence of HIV.

To our knowledge, there have been no reports of KS in patients who developed it after acquiring HHV-8 infection through transfusion. However, it is unclear whether this possibility has been adequately investigated (Blajchman and Vamvakas, 2006), and the earlier reports of development of KS in transfused patients not infected with HIV or in patients with transfusion-associated AIDS suggest that it is possible for patients who acquire HHV-8 infection through transfusion to develop KS. Given the evidence for transmission of HHV-8 through transfusion hitherto accumulated, especially the strong evidence for transfusion-transmission reported by Hladik et al. (2006), we feel that it is now necessary to investigate the best approach(es) to the prevention of the transfusion-transmission of HHV-8, especially to immunocompromised patients.

Any current risk of transfusion-acquired HHV-8 infection in the USA, however, would be less than the 0.082% per-unit risk that was estimated from the FACTS Study (Nelson et al., 2004). Since the FACTS was conducted in 1986–1990, donor deferral criteria have become more stringent and further tests for HIV

and HCV have been added. More importantly, red blood cell and platelet units that are issued for transfusion today are often WBC-reduced. Although the efficacy of WBC reduction in preventing transmission of HHV-8 has not been demonstrated, one might extrapolate from the efficacy of WBC-reduced components in preventing transmission of CMV and EBV, and infer that such components can probably be regarded as relatively HHV-8-'safe'.

Proposals to screen donated blood for HHV-8 should consider the magnitude of the risk of HHV-8 transmission by transfusion, the feasibility of screening, and the potential impact of screening on the availability of blood components. No suitable screening assay is available for the detection of either HHV-8 antibody or HHV-8 DNA, and screening for HHV-8 antibody may disqualify a significant proportion of current blood donors. No gold standard for the detection of HHV-8 antibodies exists, and the performance characteristics of the available tests differ considerably and do not seem to correlate with the presence of viral DNA (Pellett et al., 2003). Universal WBC reduction, or WBC reduction of cellular blood components intended for transfusion to immunocompromised patients, might be another approach to ensuring the safety of the blood supply if its efficacy in preventing transmission of HHV-8 is demonstrated in the future.

REFERENCES

Ablashi, D. V., Berneman, Z. N., Kramarsky, B., et al. (1995) Human herpes virus-7 (HHV-7): current status. Clin Diagn Virol, 4, 1–13.

Aboulafia, D., Mathisen, G. and Mitsuyasu, R. (1991) Case report: Aggressive Kaposi's sarcoma and Campylobacter bacteremia in a female with transfusion-associated AIDS. Am J Med Sci, 301, 256–8.

Adams, M. R., Fisher, D. M., Dumont, L. J., et al. (2000) Detecting failed WBC-reduction processes: computer simulations of intermittent and continuous process failure. Transfusion, 40, 1427–33.

Adams, P. T., Davenport, R. D., Reardon, D. A., et al. (1992) Detection of circulating donor white blood cells in patients receiving multiple transfusions. Blood, 80, 551–5.

Adler, S. P. and McVoy, M. M. (1989) Cytomegalovirus infections in seropositive patients after transfusion. Transfusion, 29, 667–71.

Adler, S. P., Baggett, J. and McVoy, M. (1985a) Transfusion-associated cytomegalovirus infections in seropositive cardiac-surgery patients. Lancet, 2, 743–6.

Adler, S. P., Chandrika, T., Lawrence, L., et al. (1983) Cytomegalovirus infections in neonates acquired by blood transfusions. Pediatr Infect Dis J, 2, 114–18.

Adler, S. P., McVoy, M. and Biro, V. G. (1985b) Detection of cytomegalovirus antibody with latex agglutination. J Clin Microbiol, 22, 68–70.

Alfieri, C., Tanner, J., Carpentier, L., et al. (1996) EBV transmission from a blood donor to an organ transplant recipient with recovery of the same virus strain from the recipient blood and oropharynx. Blood, 87, 812–817.

Anagnostopoulos, I., Hummel, M., Kreschel, C., et al., (1995) Morphology, immunophenotype, and distribution of latently and/or productively Epstein-Barr virus-infected cells in acute mononucleosis: implications for the interindividual infection route of Epstein-Barr virus. Blood, 85, 744–50.

Asano, Y., Yoshikawa, T., Suga, S., et al. (1991) Reactivation of herpes virus type 6 in children receiving bone marrow transplants for leukemia. N Engl J Med, 324, 634–635.

Atkinson, J., Edlin, B. R., Engels, E. A., et al. (2003) Seroprevalence of human herpes virus 8 among injection drug users in San Francisco. J Infect Dis, 187, 974–81.

Babcock, G. J., Decker, L. L., Volk, M., et al. (1998) EBV persistence in memory B-cells in vivo. Immunity, 9, 395–404.

Bale, J. F. Jr., Kealey, G. P., Massanari, R. M., et al. (1990) The epidemiology of cytomegalovirus infection among patients with burns. Infect Control Hosp Epidemiol, 11, 17–22.

Baumgartner, J. D., Glauser, M. P., Burgo-Black, A. L., *et al.* (1982) Severe cytomegalovirus infection in multiply transfused, splenectomized, trauma patients. *Lancet*, **2**, 63–6.

Beckwith, D. G., Halstead, D. C., Alpaugh, K., *et al.* (1985) Comparison of a latex agglutination test with five other methods for determining the presence of antibody against cytomegalovirus. *J Clin Microbiol*, **21**, 328–31.

Bendsoe, N., Dictor, M., Blomberg, J., *et al.* (1990) Increased incidence of Kaposi sarcoma in Sweden before the AIDS epidemic. *Eur J Cancer*, **26**, 699–702.

Beneke, J. S., Tegtmeier, G. E., Alter, H. J., *et al.* (1984) Relation of titers of antibodies to CMV in blood donors to the transmission of cytomegalovirus infection. *J Infect Dis*, **150**, 883–8.

Blackbourn, D. J., Ambroziak, J., Lennette, E., *et al.* (1997) Infectious human herpes virus 8 in a healthy North American blood donor. *Lancet*, **349**, 609–11.

Blacklow, N. R., Watson, B. K., Miller, G., *et al.* (1971) Mononucleosis with heterophil antibodies and EB virus infection: acquisition by an elderly patient in hospital. *Am J Med*, **51**, 549–52.

Blajchman, M. A. and Vamvakas, E. C. (2006) The continuing risk of transfusion-transmitted infections. *N Eng J Med*, **355**, 1303–5.

Blajchman, M. A., Goldman, M., Freedman, J. F., *et al.* (2001) Proceedings of a consensus conference: prevention of post-transfusion CMV in the era of universal leukoreduction. *Transfus Med Rev*, **15**, 1–20.

Boeckh, M., Bowden, R. A., Gooley, T., *et al.* (1999) Successful modification of a pp65 antigenemia-based early treatment strategy for prevention of cytomegalovirus disease in allogeneic marrow transplant recipients. *Blood*, **93**, 1781–2.

Booth, J. C., Hannington, G., Bakir, T. M. F., *et al.* (1982) Comparison of enzyme linked immunoabsorbent assay, radio-immunoassay, complement function, anti-complement immunofluorescence and passive hemagglutination techniques for detecting cytomegalovirus IG antibody. *J Clin Pathol*, **35**, 1345–8.

Bowden, R. and Sayers, M. (1990) The risk of transmitting cytomegalovirus infection by fresh frozen plasma. *Transfusion*, **30**, 762–3.

Bowden, R. A., Sayers, M. H., Cays, M., *et al.* (1989) The role of blood product filtration in the prevention of transfusion-associated cytomegalovirus (CMV) infection after marrow transplant. *Transfusion*, **29** (Suppl. 1), 57S.

Bowden, R. A., Sayers, M., Flournoy, N., *et al.* (1986) Cytomegalovirus immune globulin and seronegative blood products to prevent primary cytomegalovirus infection after marrow transplantation. *N Eng J Med*, **314**, 1006–10.

Bowden, R. A., Sayers, M., Gleaves, C. A., *et al.* (1987) Cytomegalovirus-seronegative blood components for the prevention of primary cytomegalovirus infection after marrow transplant: considerations for blood banks. *Transfusion*, **27**, 478.

Bowden, R. A., Slichter, S. J., Sayers, M. H., *et al.* (1991) Use of leukocyte-depleted platelets and cytomegalovirus-seronegative red blood cells for prevention of primary cytomegalovirus infection after marrow transplant. *Blood*, **79**, 246–50.

Bowden, R. A., Slichter, S. J., Sayers, M. H., *et al.* (1995) A comparison of filtered leukocyte reduced and cytomegalovirus (CMV) seronegative blood products for the prevention of transfusion-associated CMV infection after marrow transplant. *Blood*, **86**, 3598–606.

Brady, M. T., Milam, J. D., Anderson, D. C., *et al.* (1984) Use of deglycerolized red blood cells to prevent post-transfusion infection with cytomegalovirus in neonates. *J Infect Dis*, **150**, 334–9.

Bruggeman, C. A. (1991) Reactivation of latent CMV in the rat. *Transplant Proc*, **23** (Suppl.3), 22–4.

Busch, M. P. and Lee, T. H. (1995) Role of donor leukocytes and leukodepletion in transfusion-associated viral infections. In *Clinical Benefits of Leukodepleted Blood Products*, eds J. Sweeney and W. A. Heaton, pp. 97–112. Austin, TX, R.G. Landes Co.

Cannon, M. J., Dollard, S. C., Smith, D. K., *et al.* (2001) Blood-borne and sexual transmission of human herpes virus 8 in women with or at risk for human immunodeficiency virus infection. *N Eng J Med*, **344**, 637–43.

Cannon, M. J., Laney, A. S. and Pellett, P. E. (2003) Human herpes virus 8: current issues. *Clin Infect Dis*, **37**, 82–7.

Chandler, S. H., Handsfield, H. H. and McDougall, J. K. (1987) Isolation of multiple strains of cytomegalovirus from women attending a clinic for sexually transmitted diseases. *J Infect Dis*, **155**, 655–60.

Cheung, K. S. and Lang, D. J. (1977) Transmission and activation of cytomegalovirus with blood transfusion: a mouse model. *J Infect Dis*, **135**, 841–5.

Chou, S. (1986) Acquisition of donor strains of cytomegalovirus by renal transplant recipients. *N Eng J Med*, **314**, 1418–23.

Chou, S. (1987) Cytomegalovirus infection and reinfection transmitted by heart transplantation. *J Infect Dis*, **155**, 1054–5.

Chou, S. (1989) Neutralizing antibody responses to reinfecting strains of cytomegalovirus transplant patients. *J Infect Dis*, **160**, 16–21.

Chou, S. and Kim, D. Y. (1987) Transmission of cytomegalovirus by pre-transplant leukocyte transfusions in renal transplant candidates. *J Infect Dis*, **155**, 565–67.

Cockerill, F. R., Hurley, D. V., Miglagelada, J. R., *et al.* (1986) Polymicrobial cholangitis and Kaposi's sarcoma in blood product transfusion-related acquired immune deficiency syndrome. *Am J Med*, **80**, 1237–41.

Collier, A., Kalish, L., Busch, M., *et al.* (2001) Leukocyte-reduced red blood cell transfusions in patients with anemia and human immunodeficiency virus infection. *JAMA*, **285**, 1592–601.

Cone, R. W., Hackman, R. C., Huang, M.-L. W., *et al.* (1993) Human herpes virus 6 in lung tissue from patients with pneumonitis after bone marrow transplantation. *N Eng J Med*, **329**, 156–61.

Cone, R. W., Huang, M.-L. W., Corey, L., *et al.* (1999) Human herpes virus 6 infections after bone marrow transplantation: clinical and virologic manifestations. *J Infect Dis*, **179**, 311–8.

Curtsinger, L. J., Cheadle, W. G., Hershman, M. J., *et al.* (1989) Association of cytomegalovirus infection with increased morbidity is independent of transfusion. *Am J Surg*, **158**, 606–10.

De Graan-Hentzen, Y. C. E., Gratama, J. W., Mudde, G. C., *et al.* (1989) Prevention of primary cytomegalovirus infection in patients with hematologic malignancy by intensive white cell depletion of blood products. *Transfusion*, **29**, 757–60.

Demmler, G. J., Brady, M. T., Bijou, H., *et al.* (1986) Post-transfusion cytomegalovirus infection in neonates: role of saline-washed red blood cells. *J Pediatr*, **108**, 762–5.

Dewhurst, S., Skrincosky, D. and van Loon, N. (1997a) (5 Nov) Human herpes virus 6. *Expert Rev Mol Med*, pp. 1–17.

Dewhurst, S., Skrincosky, D. and van Loon, N. (1997b) (18 Nov) Human herpes virus 7. *Expert Rev Mol Med*, pp. 1–10.

DeWitte, T., Schattenberg, A., Van Dijk, B. A., *et al.* (1990) Prevention of primary cytomegalovirus infection after allogeneic bone marrow transplantation by using leukocyte-poor random blood products from cytomegalovirus unscreened blood bank donors. *Transplantation*, **50**, 964–8.

Diamond, C., Thiede, H., Perdue, T., *et al.* (2001) Seroepidemiology of human herpes virus 8 among young men who have sex with men. The Seattle Young Men's Survey Team. *Sex Transm Dis*, **28**, 176–83.

Diosi, P., Moldovan, E. and Tomescu, N. (1969) Latent cytomegalovirus infection in blood donors. *Br Med J*, **4**, 660–2.

Dollard, S. C., Nelson, K. E., Ness, P. M., *et al.* (2005) Possible transmission of human herpes virus 8 by blood transfusion in a historical United States cohort. *Transfusion*, **45**, 500–3.

Drew, N. L. and Minor, R. C. (1982) Transfusion-related cytomegalovirus infection following noncardiac surgery. *JAMA*, **247**, 2389–91.

Drew, W. L., Tegtmeier, G. E., Alter, H. J., *et al.* (2003) Frequency and duration of plasma CMV viremia in seroconverting blood donors and recipients. *Transfusion*, **43**, 309–13.

Drobyski, W. R., Knox, K. K., Majewski, D., *et al.* (1994) Brief report: fatal encephalitis due to variant B human herpes virus-6 infection in a bone marrow-transplant recipient. *N Eng J Med*, **330**, 1356–60.

Dukers, N. H. T. M. and Rezza, G. (2003) Human herpes virus 8 epidemiology: what we do and do not know. *AIDS*, **17**, 1717–30.

Dumont, L. J., Janos, L., VandenBroeke, T., *et al.* (2001) The effect of leukocyte-reduction method on the amount of human cytomegalovirus in blood products: a comparison of apheresis and filtration methods. *Blood*, **97**, 3640–7.

Dworsky, M. E., Welch, K., Cassady, G., *et al.* (1983) Occupational risk of primary cytomegalovirus infection among pediatric health-care workers. *N Eng J Med*, **309**, 950–3.

Dzik, W. H. (1994) Mononuclear cell microchimerism and the immunomodulatory effect of transfusion. *Transfusion*, **34**, 1007.

Enbom, M., Urassa, W., Massambu, C., *et al.* (2002) Detection of human herpes virus 8 DNA in serum from blood donors with HHV-8 antibodies indicates possible blood borne virus transmission. *J Med Virol*, **68**, 264–67.

Engelhard, D., Weinberg, M., Or, R., *et al.* (1991) Immunoglobulins A, G, and M to cytomegalovirus during recurrent infection in recipients of allogeneic bone marrow transplantation. *J Infect Dis*, **163**, 628–30.

Engels, E.A., Eastman, H., Ablashi, D.V., *et al.* (1999) Risk of transfusion-associated transmission of human herpes virus 8. *J Natl Cancer Inst*, **91**, 1773–5.

Evans, D.G.R. and Lyon, A.J. (1991) Fatal congenital cytomegalovirus infection acquired by an intra-uterine transfusion. *Eur J Pediatr*, **150**, 780–1.

Friedman-Kien, A.E., Saltzman, B.R., Cao, Y., *et al.* (1990) Kaposi's sarcoma in HIV-negative homosexual men. *Lancet*, **335**, 168–9.

Furukawa, T., Funamoto, Y., Ishida, S., *et al.* (1987) The importance of primary cytomegalovirus infection in childhood cancer. *Eur J Pediatr*, **146**, 34–7.

Galea, G. and Urbaniak, S.J. (1992) The incidence and consequences of cytomegalovirus transmission via blood transfusion to low birthweight, premature infants in North East Scotland. *Vox Sang*, **62**, 200–7.

Gerber, P., Walsh, J.H., Rosenblum, E.N., *et al.* (1969) Association of EB-virus infection with the post-perfusion syndrome. *Lancet*, **1**, 593–6.

Gerna, G., Zipeto, D., Percivalle, E., *et al.* (1992) Human cytomegalovirus infection of the major leukocyte subpopulations and evidence for initial viral replication in polymorphonuclear leukocytes from viremic patients. *J Infect Dis*, **166**, 1236–44.

Gilbert, G.L., Hayes, K., Hudson, I.L., *et al.* (1989) Prevention of transfusion-acquired cytomegalovirus infection in infants by blood filtration to remove leukocytes. Neonatal Cytomegalovirus Infection Study Group. *Lancet*, **1**, 1228–31.

Gleaves, C.A., Smith, T.F., Schuster, E.A., *et al.* (1984) Rapid detection of cytomegalovirus in MRC-5 cells inoculated with urine specimens by using low-speed centrifugation and monoclonal antibody to an early antigen. *J Clin Microbiol*, **19**, 917–9.

Goedert, J.J., Charurat, M., Blattner, W.A., *et al.* (2003) Risk factors for Kaposi's sarcoma-associated herpes virus infection among HIV-1 infected pregnant women in the USA. *AIDS*, **17**, 425–33.

Grattan, M.T., Moreno-Cabral, E., Starnes, V.A., *et al.* (1989) Cytomegalovirus infection is associated with cardiac allograft rejection and atherosclerosis. *JAMA*, **261**, 3561–66.

Griffin, M.P., O'Shea, M., Brazy, J.E., *et al.* (1988) Cytomegalovirus infection in a neonatal intensive care unit. *Am J Dis Child*, **142**, 1188–93.

Grundy, J.E., Super, M., Sweny, P., *et al.* (1988) Symptomatic cytomegalovirus infection in seropositive kidney recipients: reinfection with donor virus rather than reactivation of recipient virus. *Lancet*, **2**, 132–5.

Gunter, K.C., and Luban, N.L. (1996) Transfusion-transmitted cytomegalovirus and Epstein-Barr virus diseases. In *Principles of Transfusion Medicine*, eds E.C. Rossi, T.L. Simon, G.S. Moss and S.A. Gould, 2nd edn, pp. 717–31. Baltimore, MD, Williams & Wilkins

Hahn, G., Jores, R. and Mocarski, E.S. (1998) Cytomegalovirus remains latent in a common precursor of dendritic and myeloid cells. *Proc Natl Acad Sci*, **95**, 3937–42.

Henle, W. and Henle, G. (1985) Epstein-Barr virus and blood transfusion. In *Infection, Immunity and Blood Transfusion*, eds R.Y. Dodd and L.F. Barker, pp. 201–209. New York, Alan R. Liss.

Henle, W., Henle, G., Scriba, M., *et al.* (1970) Antibody responses to the Epstein-Barr virus and cytomegalovirus after open-heart and other surgery. *N Eng J Med*, **282**, 1068–74.

Hersman, J., Meyers, J.D., Thomas, E.D., *et al.* (1982) The effect of granulocyte transfusions on the incidence of cytomegalovirus infection after marrow transplantation. *Ann Intern Med*, **96**, 149–52.

Hillyer, C.D., Lankford, K.V., Roback, J.D., *et al.* (1999) Transfusion of the HIV-seropositive patient: immunomodulation viral reactivation, and limiting exposure to EBV (HHV-4), CMV (HHV-5), and HHV-6, 7, and 8. *Transfus Med Rev*, **13**, 1–17.

Hillyer, C.D, Roback, J.D., Saakadze, N., *et al.* (2003) Transfusion-transmitted cytomegalovirus (CMV) infection: elucidation of role and dose of monocytes in a murine model. *Blood*, **102**, 57a(Abstract no. 189).

Hillyer, C.D., Snydman, D.R. and Berkman, E.M. (1994) The risk of cytomegalovirus infection in solid organ and bone marrow transplant recipients: transfusion of blood products. *Transfusion*, **30**, 659–66.

Hladik, W., Dollard, S.C., Mermin, J., *et al.* (2006) Transmission of human herpes virus 8 by blood transfusion. *N Eng J Med*, **355**, 1331–38.

Ho, M. (1982) Human cytomegalovirus infections in immunosuppressed patients. In *Cytomegalovirus, Biology and Infection*, eds W.M. Greenough and T.C. Merigan, pp. 171–204. New York, NY, Plenum.

Hodinka, R.L. (2003) Human Cytomegalovirus. In *Manual of Clinical Microbiology*, eds P.R. Murray, E.J. Baron, J.H. Jorgensen, M.A. Pfaller and R.H. Yolken, 8th edn, pp. 1304–18. Washington, DC, American Society of Microbiology Press.

Hudnall, S.D., Chen, T., Rady, P., *et al.* (2003) Human herpes virus 8 seroprevalence and viral load in healthy adult blood donors. *Transfusion*, **43**, 85–90.

Hutchinson, D.L., Turner, J.H. and Schlesinger, E.R. (1971) Persistence of donor cells in neonates after fetal and exchange transfusion. *Am J Obstet Gynecol*, **109**, 281–4.

Jacobs, R.F. (1986) Frozen deglycerolized blood and transmission of Epstein-Barr virus. *J Infect Dis*, **153**, 800.

James, D.J., Sikotra, S., Sivakumaran, M., *et al.* (1997) The presence of free infectious cytomegalovirus (CMV) in the plasma of donated CMV-seropositive blood and platelets. *Transfus Med*, **7**, 123–6.

Kane, R.C., Rousseau, W.E., Noble, G.R., *et al.* (1975) Cytomegalovirus infection in a volunteer blood donor population. *Infect Immun*, **11**, 719–23.

Kapsenberg, J.G., Langenhuysen, M.M.A.C., Nieweg, H.O., *et al.* (1970) Post-transfusion mononucleosis with heterophil antibodies. *Acta Med Scand*, **187**, 79–82.

Kealey, G.P., Bale, J.F., Strauss, R.G., *et al.* (1987) Cytomegalovirus infection in burn patients. *J Burn Care Rehabil*, **8**, 543–5.

Kozireva, S., Nemceva, G., Ganilane, I., *et al.* (2001) Prevalence of blood-borne viral infections (cytomegalovirus, human herpes virus-6, human herpes virus-7, human herpes virus-8, human T-cell lymphotropic virus-I/II, human retro-virus-5) among blood donors in Latvia. *Ann Hematol*, **80**, 669–73

Krech, U. (1973) Complement-fixing antibodies against cytomegalovirus in different parts of the world. *Bull WHO*, **49**, 103–6.

Kreel, I., Zarroff, L.I. and Canter, J.W. (1960) A syndrome following total body perfusion. *Surg Gynecol Obstet*, **111**, 317–21.

Kumar, A., Nankervis, G.A., Cooper, R.A., *et al.* (1980) Acquisition of cytomegalovirus infection in infants following exchange transfusion: a prospective study. *Transfusion*, **20**, 327–31.

Lamberson, H.V., McMillan, J.A., Weiner, L.B., *et al.* (1988) Prevention of transfusion-associated cytomegalovirus (CMV) infection in neonates by screening blood donors for IgM to CMV. *J Infect Dis*, **157**, 820–3.

Landaw, E.M., Kanter, M. and Petz, L.D. (1996) Safety of filtered leukocyte-reduced blood products for prevention of transfusion-associated cytomegalovirus infection. *Blood*, **87**, 4910.

Landry, M.L., Ferguson, D., Stevens-Ayers, T., *et al.* (1996) Evaluation of CMV Brite kit for detection of cytomegalovirus pp65 antigenemia in peripheral blood leukocytes by immunofluorescence. *J Clin Microbiol*, **34**, 1337–39.

Laupacis, A., Brown, J., Costello, B., *et al.* (2001) Prevention of post-transfusion CMV in the era of universal leukoreduction: a consensus statement. *Transfusion*, **41**, 560–69.

Lee, T-H., Paglieroni, T., Ohto, H., *et al.* (1999) Survival of donor leukocyte subpopulations in immunocompetent transfusion recipients: frequent long-term microchimerism in severe trauma patients. *Blood*, **93**, 3127–39.

Lentz, E.B., Dock, N.L., McMahon, C.A., *et al.* (1988) Detection of antibody to cytomegalovirus-induced early antigens and comparison with four serologic assays and presence of viruria in blood donors. *J Clin Microbiol*, **26**, 133–5.

Linde, A. (2003) Epstein-Barr Virus. In *Manual of Clinical Microbiology*, 8th edn, eds P.R. Murray, E.J. Baron, J.H. Jorgensen, M.A. Pfaller and R.H. Yolken, pp. 1331–40. Washington, DC, American Society of Microbiology Press.

Luppi, M., Barozzi, P., Guaraldi, G., *et al.* (2003) Human herpes virus 8 associated diseases in solid-organ transplantation: importance of viral transmission from the donor. *Clin Infect Dis*, **37**, 606–607.

Luthardt, T., Siebert, H., Lösel, I., *et al.* (1971) Cytomegalovirus-infektionen bei Kindern mit Blutaustausch-transfusion im Neugeborenenalter. *Klin Wochenschr*, **49**, 81–6.

MacKinnon, S., Burnett, A. K., Crawford, R. J., *et al.* (1988) Seronegative blood products prevent primary cytomegalovirus infection after bone marrow transplantation. *J Clin Pathol*, **41**, 948–50.

Malloy, D. and Lipton, K. S. (2002) *Update on Provision of CMV-reduced-risk Cellular Blood Components. Association Bulletin no. 02–4.* Bethesda, MD, American Association of Blood Banks.

Manez, R., Kusne, S., Martin, M., *et al.* (1993) The impact of blood transfusion on the occurrence of pneumonitis in primary cytomegalovirus infection after liver transplantation. *Transfusion*, **33**, 594–7.

Masucci, M. G. and Ernberg, I. (1994) Epstein-Barr virus: adaptation to a life within the immune system. *Trends Microbiol*, **2**, 125–130.

Mayo, D., Armstrong, J. A. and Ho, M. (1978) Activation of latent murine cyto-megalovirus infection: cocultivation, cell transfer, and the effect of immu-nosuppression. *J Infect Dis*, **138**, 890–96.

Mbulaiteye, S. M., Biggar, R. J., Bakaki, P. M., *et al.* (2003) Human herpes virus 8 infection and transfusion history in children with sickle-cell disease in Uganda. *J Natl Cancer Inst*, **95**, 1330–35.

McCracken, G. H., Shinefield, H. R., Cobb, K., *et al.* (1969) Congenital cytome-galic inclusion disease. *Am J Dis Child*, **117**, 522–39.

McCullough, J., Yunis, E. J., Benson, S. J., *et al.* (1969) Effect of blood bank storage on leukocyte function. *Lancet*, **1**, 1333.

McEnery, G. and Stern, H. (1970) Cytomegalovirus infection in early infancy: five atypical cases. *Arch Dis Child*, **45**, 669–73.

McMonigal, M., Horwitz, C. A., Henle, W., *et al.* (1983) Post-perfusion syndrome due to Epstein-Barr virus: report of two cases and review of the literature. *Transfusion*, **23**, 331–5.

Meyers, J. D., Flournoy, N. and Thomas, E. D. (1986) Risk factors for cytomega-lovirus infection after human marrow transplantation. *J Infect Dis*, **153**, 478–88.

Miller, W. J., McCullough, J., Balfour, H. H. Jr., *et al.* (1991) Prevention of cytome-galovirus infection following bone marrow transplantation: a randomized trial of blood product screening. *Bone Marrow Transplant*, **7**, 227–34.

Mirkovic, R., Werch, J., South, M. A., *et al.* (1971) Incidence of cytomegaloviremia in blood bank donors and in infants with congenital cytomegalic inclusion disease. *Infect Immun*, **3**, 45–50.

Monif, G. R. G., Daicoff, G. I. and Flory, L. F. (1976) Blood as a potential vehicle for the cytomegaloviruses. *Am J Obstet Gynecol*, **126**, 445–8.

Murphy, M. F., Grint, P. C., Hardiman, A. E., *et al.* (1988) Use of leukocyte-poor blood components to prevent primary cytomegalovirus (CMV) infection in patients with acute leukemia. *Br J Hematol*, **70**, 253–4.

Narvios, A. B., Przepiorka, D., Tarrand, J., *et al.* (1998) Transfusion support using filtered unscreened blood products for cytomegalovirus-negative allo-geneic marrow transplant recipients. *Bone Marrow Transplant*, **22**, 575–7.

Nelson, K. E., Dovaid, S. C., Cannon, M. J., *et al.* (2004) Probable transmission of human herpes virus 8 (HHV-8) by blood transfusion among cardiac surgery patients. *Transfusion*, **44**(Suppl.), 96A.

Nichols, W. G., Price, T. H., Gooley, T., *et al.* (2003) Transfusion-transmitted cytomegalovirus infection after receipt of leukoreduced blood products. *Blood*, **101**, 4195–00.

Nielsen, H. J., Skov, F., Dybkjaer, E., *et al.* (1997) Leucocyte and platelet-derived bioactive substances in stored blood: effect of prestorage leucocyte filtra-tion. *Eur J Haematol*, **58**, 273–8.

Ohto, H., Ujiie, N. and Hirai, H. (1999) Lack of difference in cytomegalovirus transmissions via the transfusion of filtered-irradiated and nonfiltered-irradiated blood to newborn infants in an endemic area. *Transfusion*, **39**, 201–5.

Olding, L. B., Jensen, F. C. and Oldstone, M. B. (1975) Pathogenesis of cytome-galovirus infection: 1. Activation of virus from bone marrow derived lym-phocytes by in vitro allogeneic reaction. *J Exp Med*, **141**, 561–572.

Operskalski, E. A., Busch, M. P., Mosley, J. W., *et al.* (1997) Blood donations and viruses. *Lancet*, **349**, 1327–31.

Padilla, S., Rivera-Perlman Z. and Solomon, L. (1990) Kaposi's sarcoma in transfusion-associated acquired immunodeficiency syndrome. *Arch Pathol Lab Med*, **114**, 40–42.

Paloheimo, J. A., von Essen, R., Klemola, E., *et al.* (1968) Subclinical cytomega-lovirus infections and cytomegalovirus mononucleosis after open heart surgery. *Am J Cardiol*, **22**, 624–30.

Pamphilon, D. H., Foot, A. B. M., Adeodu, A., *et al.* (1999a) Prophylaxis and prevention of CMV infection in BM allograft recipients: leukodepleted platelets are equivalent to those from CMV-seronegative donors. *Bone Marrow Transplant* **23**(Suppl. 1), S66.

Pamphilon, D. H., Rider, J. R., Barbara J. A. J., *et al.* (1999b) Prevention of transfusion-transmitted cytomegalovirus infection. *Transf Med*, **9**, 115–23.

Papaevangelou, G., Economidou, J., Roumetiotou, A., *et al.* (1979) Epstein-Barr infection in polytransfused patients with homozygous β-thalassaemia. *Vox Sang*, **37**, 305–9.

Pass, M. A., Johnson, J. D., Schulman, I. A., *et al.* (1976) Evaluation of a walking-donor blood transfusion program with intensive care nursery. *J Pediatr*, **89**, 646–51.

Pearson, H. A., Wood, C., Andeman, W., *et al.* (1986) Low risk of hepatitis B from blood transfusions in thalassaemic patients in Connecticut. *J Pediatr*, **108**, 252–3.

Pellett, P. E., Wright, D. J., Engels, E. A., *et al.* (2003) Multicenter comparison of serologic assays and estimation of human herpesvirus 8 seroprevalence among US blood donors. *Transfusion*, **43**, 1260–68.

Perham, T. G. M., Carl, E. W., Conway, P. J., *et al.* (1971) Cytomegalovirus infection in blood donors – a prospective study. *Br J Haematol*, **20**, 307–20.

Phipps, P. H., Gregoire, L., Rossier, E., *et al.* (1983) Comparison of five methods of cytomegalovirus antibody screening of blood donors. *J Clin Microbiol*, **18**, 1296–300.

Preiksaitis, J. K. (1991) Indications for the use of cytomegalovirus-seronegative blood products. *Transfus Med Rev*, **5**, 1–17.

Preiksaitis, J. K. (2000) The Cytomegalovirus-'safe' blood product: is leukore-duction equivalent to antibody screening? *Transf Med Rev*, **14**, 112–36.

Preiksaitis, J. K. (2003) Prevention of transfusion-acquired CMV infection: is there a role for NAT? *Transfusion*, **43**, 302–5.

Preiksaitis, J. K., Brown, L. and McKenzie, M. (1988b) The risk of cytomegalo-virus infection in seronegative transfusion recipients not receiving exogen-ous immunosuppression. *J Infect Dis*, **157**, 523–9.

Preiksaitis, J. K., Brown, L., McKenzie, M., *et al.* (1988a) Transfusion-acquired cytomegalovirus infection in neonates: a prospective study. *Transfusion*, **28**, 205–9.

Preiksaitis, J. K., Desai, S., Vaudry, W., *et al.* (1997) Transfusion-and community-acquired cytomegalovirus infection in children with malignant disease: a prospective study. *Transfusion*, **37**, 941–6.

Preiksaitis, J. K., Rosno, S., Grumet, C., *et al.* (1983) Infections due to herpes viruses in cardiac transplant recipients: role of the donor heart and immu-nosuppressive therapy. *J Infect Dis*, **147**, 974.

Preiksaitis, J. K., Sandhu, J. and Strautman, M. (2002) The risk of transfusion-acquired CMV infection in seronegative solid-organ transplant recipients receiving non-WBC-reduced blood components not screened for CMV antibody (1984 to 1996): experience at a single Canadian center. *Transfusion*, **42**, 396–402.

Purcell, R. H., Walsh, J. H., Holland, P. V., *et al.* (1971) Seroepidemiological studies of transfusion-associated hepatitis. *J Infect Dis*, **123**, 406–13.

Purtilo, D. T., Paquin, L. A., Sakamoto, K., *et al.* (1980) Persistent transfusion-associated infectious mononucleosis with transient acquired immunode-ficiency. *Am J Med*, **68**, 437–40.

Qu, L., Xu, S., Rowe, D. and Triulzi, D. (2005) Efficacy of Epstein-Barr virus removal by leukoreduction of red blood cells. *Transfusion*, **45**, 591–5.

Rader, D. C., Nucha, P., Moore, S. B., *et al.* (1985) Cytomegalovirus infection in patients undergoing non-cardiac surgical procedures. *Surg Gynecol Obstet*, **160**, 13–6.

Ratko, A., Cummings, J. P., Oberman, H., *et al.* (2001) Evidence-based recom-mendations for the use of WBC-reduced cellular blood components. *Transfusion*, **41**, 1310–19.

Ratnamohan, V. M., Chapman, J., Howse, H., *et al.* (1998) Cytomegalovirus and human herpes virus 6 both cause viral disease after renal transplantation. *Transplantation*, **66**, 877–82.

Ratnamohan, V. M., Mathys, J. M., McKenzie, A., *et al.* (1992) HCMV-DNA is detected more frequently than infectious virus in blood leukocytes of immunocompromised patients: a direct comparison of culture-immuno-fluorescence and PCR for detection of HCMV in clinical specimens. *J Med Virol*, **38**, 252–9.

Revello, M. G., Zavattoni, M., Sarasini, A., *et al.* (1998) Human cytomegalovirus in blood of immunocompetent persons during primary infection: prognostic implications for pregnancy. *J Infect Dis*, **177**, 1170–75.

Roback, J. D., Drew, W. L., Laycock, M. E., *et al.* (2003) CMV DNA is rarely detected in healthy blood donors using validated PCR assays. *Transfusion*, **43**, 314–21.

Roback, J. D., Hillyer, C. D., Drew, W. L., *et al.* (2001) Multicenter evaluation of PCR methods for detecting CMV DNA in blood donors. *Transfusion*, **41**, 1249–57.

Roujeau, J. C., Brun-Buisson, C., Penso, D., *et al.* (1988) Non-acquired immune deficiency syndrome-related Kaposi's sarcoma after severe infection. *J Am Acad Dermatol*, **18**, 378.

Rubin, R. H., Tolkoff-Rubin, N. E., Oliver, D., *et al.* (1985) Multicenter seroepidemiologic study of the impact of cytomegalovirus infection on renal transplantation. *Transplantation*, **40**, 243–9.

Salahuddin, S. Z., Ablashi, D. V., Markham, P. D., *et al.* (1986) Isolation of a new virus, HBLV, in patients with lymphoproliferative disorders. *Science*, **234**, 596–601.

Sayers, M. H. (1994) Transfusion-transmitted viral infections other than hepatitis and human immunodeficiency virus infection. Cytomegalovirus, Epstein-Barr virus, human herpesvirus 6, and human parvovirus B19. *Arch Pathol Lab Med*, **118**, 346–9.

Sherman, M. E. and Dzik, W. H. (1988) Stability of antigens in leukocytes in banked platelet concentrates: decline in HLA-DR antigen expression and mixed lymphocyte culture stimulating capacity following storage. *Blood*, **72**, 867–72.

Sloand, E., Kumar, P., Klein, H. G., *et al.* (1994) Transfusion of blood components to persons infected with human immunodeficiency virus type 1: relationship to opportunistic infection. *Transfusion*, **34**, 48–53.

Smith, D. M. Jr. (1997) *Leukocyte reduction for the Prevention of Transfusion-transmitted Cytomegalovirus (TT-CMV). Association Bulletin no. 97–2.* Bethesda, MD, American Association of Blood Banks.

Snydman, D. R., Werner, B. G., Meissner, H. C., *et al.* (1995) Use of cytomegalovirus immunoglobulin in multiply transfused premature neonates. *Pediatr Infect Dis J*, **14**, 34–40.

Soderberg-Naucler, C., Fish, K. N. and Nelson, J. A. (1997) Reactivation of latent human cytomegalovirus by allogeneic stimulation of blood cells from healthy donors. *Cell*, **91**, 119–26.

Solem, J. H. and Jörgensen, W. (1969) Accidentally transmitted infectious mononucleosis. *Acta Med Scan*, 186–433.

Spector, S. A., Kirata, K. K. and Newman, T. R. (1984) Identification of multiple cytomegalovirus strains in homosexual men with acquired immunodeficiency syndrome. *J Infect Dis*, **150**, 953–6.

Stagno, S. and Cloud, G. A. (1994) Working parents: the impact of day care and breast-feeding on cytomegalovirus infections in offspring. *Proc Natl Acad Sci*, **91**, 2384–89.

Stanier, P., Taylor, D. L., Kitchen, A. D., *et al.* (1989) Persistence of cytomegalovirus in mononuclear cells in peripheral blood from blood donors. *Br Med J*, **299**, 897–8.

Stevens, D. P., Barker, L. F., Ketcham, A. S., *et al.* (1979) Asymptomatic cytomegalovirus infection following blood transfusion in tumor surgery. *JAMA*, **211**, 1341–44.

Taswell, H. F., Reisner, R. K, Rabe, D. E., *et al.* (1986) Comparison of three methods for detecting antibody to cytomegalovirus. *Transfusion*, **26**, 285–9.

Tattevin, P., Cremieux, A. C., Descamps, D., *et al.* (2002) Transfusion-related infectious mononucleosis. *Scand J Infect Dis*, **34**, 777–8.

Taylor-Wiedeman, J., Sissons, J. G. P., Borysiewicz, L. K., *et al.* (1991) Monocytes are a major site of persistence of human cytomegalovirus in peripheral blood mononuclear cells. *J Gen Virol*, **72**, 2059–64.

Tegtmeier, G. E. (1986) Transfusion-transmitted cytomegalovirus infections: significance and control. *Vox Sang*, **51**(Suppl. 1): 30–33.

Tegtmeier, G. E. (1989) Post-transfusion cytomegalovirus infections. *Arch Pathol Lab Med*, **113**, 236–45.

Tegtmeier, G. E. (2001) Transfusion-acquired cytomegalovirus infection: Approaching resolution. In *Blood Safety and Surveillance*, eds J. V. Linden and C. Bianco, pp. 315–33. New York, NY, Marcel Dekker, Inc.

Tobin, J. O. H., MacDonald, H. and Brayshay, M. (1975) Cytomegalovirus infection and exchange transfusion (letter). *Br Med J*, **2**, 404.

Turner, A. R., MacDonald, R. N. and Cooper, B. A. (1972) Transmission of infectious mononucleosis by transfusion of pre-illness plasma. *Ann Intern Med*, **77**, 751–3.

Urushibara, N., Kwon, K.-W., Takahashi, T. A., *et al.* (1995) Human cytomegalovirus DNA is not detectable with nested double polymerase chain reaction in healthy blood donors. *Vox Sang*, **68**, 9–14.

Vamvakas, E. (2005) Is white-blood-cell reduction equivalent to antibody screening in preventing transmission of cytomegalovirus by transfusion? A review of the literature and meta-analysis. *Transfus Med Rev*, **19**, 181–99.

Vamvakas, E. and Kaplan, H. S. (1993) Early transfusion and length of survival in acquired immune deficiency syndrome: experience with a population receiving medical care at a public hospital. *Transfusion*, **33**, 111–8.

Vamvakas, E. and Kaplan, H. S. (1994) Blood transfusion to AIDS patients: relationship to opportunistic infection. *Transfusion*, **34**, 740.

Van Prooijen, H. C., Visser, J. J., van Oostendorp, W. R., *et al.* (1994) Prevention of primary transfusion-associated CMV infection after marrow transplant recipients by the removal of white cells from blood components with high affinity filters. *Br J Haematol*, **87**, 144–7.

Velez-Garcia, E., Robles-Cardona, N. and Fradera, J. (1985) Kaposi's sarcoma in transfusion-associated AIDS. *N Eng J Med*, **312**, 648.

Verdonck, L. F., De Graan-Hentzen, Y. C., Dekker, A. W., *et al.* (1987) Cytomegalovirus seronegative platelets and leukocyte poor red blood cells can prevent primary cytomegalovirus infection after bone marrow transplantation. *Bone Marrow Transplant*, **2**, 73–8.

Waner, J. L., Weller, T. H. and Kevy, S. V. (1973) Patterns of cytomegalovirus complement fixing antibody activity: a longitudinal study of blood donors. *J Infect Dis*, **127**, 538–43.

Wenz, B. and Burns, E. R. (1991) Phenotypic characterization of white cells in white cell reduced red cell concentrate using flow cytometry. *Transfusion*, **31**, 829–35.

Wilhelm, J. A., Matter, L. and Schopfer, K. (1986) The risk of transmitting cytomegalovirus to patients receiving blood transfusion. *J Infect Dis*, **154**, 169–71.

Winston, D. J., Ho, W. G., Howell, C. L., *et al.* (1980) Cytomegalovirus infections associated with leukocyte transfusions. *Ann Intern Med*, **93**, 671–5.

Winston, D. J., Huang, E. S., Miller, M. J., *et al.* (1985) Molecular epidemiology of cytomegalovirus infections associated with bone marrow transplantation. *Ann Intern Med*, **102**, 16–20.

Wong, E. C., and Luban, L. N. (2002) Cytomegalovirus and parvovirus transmission by transfusion. In *Rossi's Principles of Transfusion Medicine*, 3rd edn, eds T. L. Simon, W. H. Dzik, E. L. Snyder, C. P. Stowell and R. G. Strauss, pp. 757–71. Philadelphia, PA, Lippincott Williams & Wilkins.

Yamanishi, K., Okuno, T., Shiraki, K., *et al.* (1988) Identification of human herpes virus 6 as a causal agent for exanthem subitum. *Lancet*, **1**, 1065–67.

Yeager, A. S., Grumet, F. C., Hafleigh, E. B., *et al.* (1981) Prevention of transfusion-acquired cytomegalovirus infections in newborn infants. *J. Pediatr*, **98**, 281–7.

Zerr, D. M., Gooley, T. A., Yeung, L., *et al.* (2001) Human herpes virus 6 reactivation and encephalitis in allogeneic bone marrow transplant recipients. *Clin Infect Dis*, **33**, 763–71.

Zerr, D. M., Meier, A. S., Selke, S. S., *et al.* (2005) A population-based study of primary human herpes virus 6 infection. *N Eng J Med*, **352**, 768–76.

Zhanghellini, F., Boppana, S. B., Emery, V. C., *et al.* (1999) Asymptomatic primary cytomegalovirus infection: virologic and immunologic features. *J Infect Dis*, **180**, 702–7.

4 RETROVIRUSES

Brian C. Dow, Eberhard W. Fiebig and Michael P. Busch

Retroviruses have a wide distribution in nature, with examples in insects, reptiles and nearly all mammals. The human retrovirus, human immunodeficiency virus (HIV 1 and 2), belongs to the lentivirus group of the retrovirus family, whilst human T-cell lymphotropic virus (HTLV I and II) belongs to the oncorna group. Human T-cell lymphotropic virus I and II are thought to have evolved from simian T-lymphotropic retroviruses that were transmitted to humans over the past centuries or millenia. Human immunodeficiency virus is thought to have derived from simian immunodeficiency viruses that are endemic in chimpanzees in Central Africa, and probably infected natives over the past century (Sharp et al., 2001).

Retroviruses are membrane-coated, single stranded RNA viruses that have a distinct genomic organization and require the presence of reverse transcriptase in their replication cycle. In a typical infection, retrovirus particles attach to the cell membrane, reverse transcriptase copies viral RNA into complementary double stranded DNA and this is integrated into the host cell chromosome. Host cell enzymes help virus and host regulatory genes complete the retrovirus lifecycle by producing virions that bud from the plasma membrane to infect other cells or organisms.

Human immunodeficiency viruses 1 and 2

Definition and characteristics of agent

Human immunodeficiency virus was discovered in the early 1980s by two groups of workers, Montagnier in France and Gallo in the USA. Originally described as human T cell lymphotropic virus type III (HTLV-III), the virus was shown to infect T-cell lymphocytes. Following infection, the virus integrates into the host cell DNA by reverse transcription. The infected individual usually has a 'glandular fever' like illness within two to three weeks of infection, then develops antibodies and is asymptomatic sometimes for many years. However, during this asymptomatic period the virus replicates actively in lymphoid tissues, macrophages and other tissues and gradually causes a dramatic decrease in CD4 + lymphocytes, such that the infected individual becomes increasingly prone to opportunistic infections. This marks the start of the acquired immunodeficiency syndrome (AIDS). In the Western world the use of combination drug therapy can considerably prolong life expectancy, but those denied such treatment generally die within a year or so after reaching this stage of the disease.

The HIV viral genome contains *gag* (group-specific core antigens), *pol* (polymerase and integrase enzymes) and *env* (envelope) genes that code for the main structural viral proteins and are found in all retroviruses. HIV also has an additional six genes that code for regulatory proteins and virulence factors. Human immunodeficiency virus replicates at extraordinarily high rates in infected persons, and its reverse transcriptase is error prone. Consequently, during each cycle of HIV replication around five to ten of the 10 000 nucleotides in each viral genome will be mistakenly copied. The resultant generation of variants leads to the development of a complex mixture of viral sequences, termed a quasispecies. During persistent infection the quasispecies evolves rapidly in response to viral fitness constraints and host immunological selection pressure. This propensity to mutation and selection also explains how HIV can break through drug therapy.

The HIV-1 family consists of M (main) and O (outlier) groups with 11 (A–K) subtypes of group M. Group B is common in the USA and Europe. Central Africa, the presumed origin of the pandemic, shows the greatest diversity (Janssens et al., 1997) (see Figure 4.1). Europe, and to a lesser extent the Americas and Asia, are now identifying increasing numbers of non-group B strains in recently diagnosed HIV positive patients, as well as among seropositive blood donors (Delwart et al., 2003; Parry et al., 2001; Simon et al., 1996). Group O strains were originally found in Cameroon and it is estimated that around 1–2% of West African HIV positives are infected with viral strains of this group. During the mid-1990s a number of group O isolates were detected in Europe. The then current commercial assays were deficient in the detection of these isolates (Apetrei et al., 1996; Schable et al., 1994), but within a year most manufacturers had introduced group O recombinant proteins within their test systems to facilitate the detection of individuals infected with HIV-1 group O.

Human immunodeficiency virus-2 was discovered in 1985 in West African countries and remains uncommon outside this geographical area. There is considerable sequence homology between HIV-1 and HIV-2 and both viruses cause a similar clinical picture, although HIV-2 disease tends to be milder. Early HIV-1 antibody tests were capable of detecting around 90% of HIV-2 isolates. Following the introduction of combined HIV-1/HIV-2 screening tests, only three US HIV-2 positive blood donors have been detected amongst 50 million blood donations, compared with around 4000 HIV-1 positive donors. Only two HIV-2 positive blood donors have been detected in the UK, while larger numbers of persons with HIV-2 have been identified in continental Europe.

Viral transmission

Human immunodeficiency virus has been isolated from blood, semen, cervical secretions, cerebrospinal fluid, tears, saliva, urine

Transfusion Microbiology, eds John A. J. Barbara, Fiona A. M. Regan and Marcela C. Contreras. Published by Cambridge University Press. © Cambridge University Press 2008.

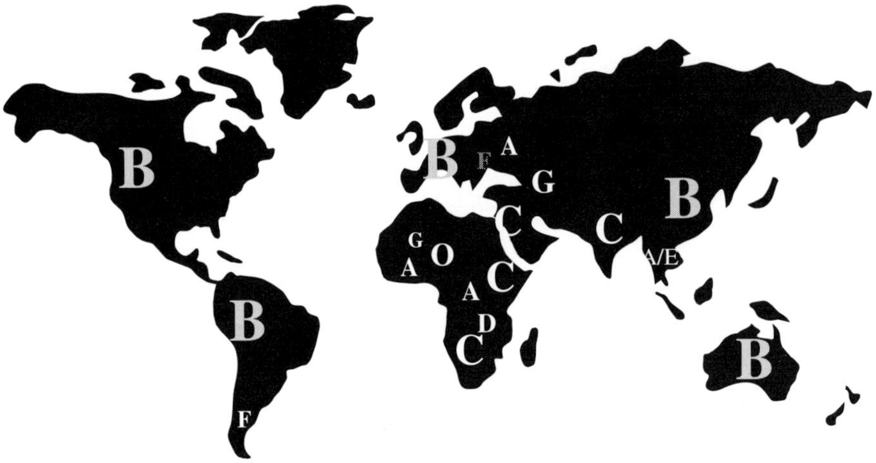

Figure 4.1 Predominant HIV-1 subtypes.

and breast milk. Transfusion-transmission has infected only 4% of those with HIV in the UK and USA, and between 2–5% world-wide (Adler, 2001). Seropositive units infect recipients at a 90% rate, with non-transmission explained by extremely low viral load in the donation, prolonged storage of the component prior to transfusion, and in rare cases by recipient mutations in viral receptor genes (Busch et al., 1996). Secondary transmission from infected transfusion recipients to sexual partners or a fetus or newborn is well documented and multifactorial, with viral load in the recipient a significant determinant of secondary transmission (Operskalski et al., 1997).

Testing

Detection of specific antibodies against HIV viral proteins and/or identification of HIV nucleic acid sequences form the basis for screening and confirmatory assays used in HIV diagnosis and blood donor screening. Many improvements have occurred in serological tests since they first became available in the early 1980s. Early antibody tests utilized viral lysates as the source of HIV antigenic material and enzyme-linked immunosorbent assay (EIA) based formats; these early tests proved to have significant batch to batch variation. Recombinant and peptide antigens were then used in second-generation tests to help provide more stable and sensitive test systems. The introduction of combined HIV-1/HIV-2 tests, and subsequent incorporation of HIV-1 group O components, into the EIA tests further spread the detection net to ensure that less frequent HIV strains or subtypes were detectable. Third-generation assays utilized the antigen-sandwich principle that required less dilution of test sample and improved detection of IgM antibodies, thereby considerably improving sensitivity for early seroconversion. In the USA p24 antigen testing was implemented mainly for blood donor screening as a means to detect early seroconverters, but failed to detect predicted numbers. In the first five years of testing only seven 'window-period' donations were obtained, referring to blood donations given by volunteer donors during the interval from the beginning of

infectiousness to assay reactivity, producing a yield of 1 in 10 million (Busch and Stramer, 1998). The comparatively recent development of fourth-generation HIV antigen/antibody 'combi' assays combined the theoretical advantages of individual antibody and p24 antigen assays in the one system (Weber et al., 2003). Figure 4.2 illustrates the abilities of various commercial HIV assays in detecting early HIV infection, based on testing several commercial HIV seroconversion panels. All manufacturers' fourth-generation assays detect HIV infection between 1 and 14 days earlier than third-generation assays. Indeed, fourth generation assays can differ by up to seven days in their abilities to detect early HIV infection. Manufacturers continue to strive to leapfrog their competitors by improving their test sensitivity, with some fourth-generation assays being particularly sensitive for p24 antigen (e.g. Murex HIV Ag/Ab), anti-HIV-1 (Genscreen HIV Ag/Ab) or anti-HIV-2 (Vironostika Ag/Ab). (Please refer to Chapter 17.)

The widespread adoption of HCV nucleic acid testing (NAT) in the late 1990s precipitated the use of HIV NAT in some countries to reduce the infectious window period. In the first three years of HIV NAT in the USA, 12 HIV-1 RNA positive, serology (p24 and antibody) negative donations were detected in 37 million donations (Stramer et al., 2004). In the UK, the Scottish and Northern Ireland blood services introduced HIV NAT at the end of 2002 and found one HIV-1 RNA positive, serology (p24 and antibody), negative donation (Morris et al., 2005) in around 900 000 donations tested. Despite the exquisite sensitivity of current assays, including NAT, reports of transfusion-transmitted HIV infection have continued to occur (Delwart et al., 2004; Ling et al., 2000) demonstrating that there remains minimal residual risk.

The situation outside Europe and North America varies considerably throughout the world. For many years, some countries ignored the threat of HIV and failed to use even simple HIV screening tests on their blood donations. Even today, many poor African countries are still unable to provide a basic HIV screen on their donated material despite a significant portion of their population being infected. In many African countries,

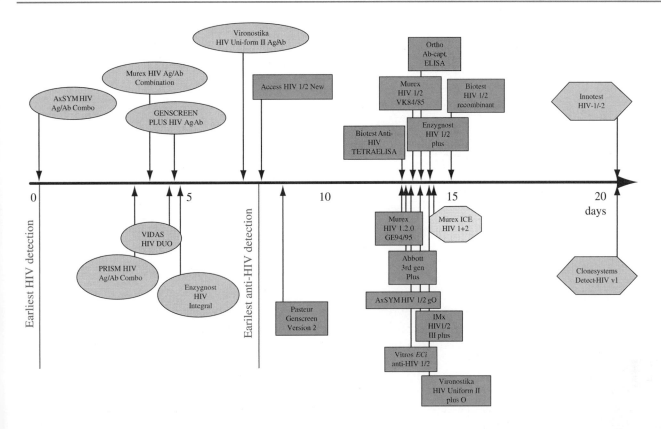

Note: This figure is based on data generated by testing 36 HIV seroconversion panels in each of the HIV screening tests shown

⬭ = 'fourth generation';   ▢ = immunometric ;   ⬭ = class specific antibody capture;   ⬡ = antiglobulin assay.

Figure 4.2 Comparative timing of HIV detection in primary infection based on 36 HIV seroconversion panels (courtesy of Drs J. Parry and K. Perry, Health Protection Agency, London, UK).

testing remains rudimentary and is often based on varied screening methods. Whilst efforts are being made in such countries to develop centralized blood services with access to the latest generations of assays several countries have still not achieved this. Furthermore in certain areas in Africa testing remains inconsistent or even absent. (Please refer to Chapter 28.) Thankfully, more and more of these countries are now able to use some form of HIV testing to screen donated blood.

In the developed world, 95 to 99% of antibody screen test reactive donation samples will be false-positive. Supplemental or confirmatory testing should be performed on any donation found to be screen test reactive. Other than the use of further EIAs of equivalent sensitivity, the main confirmatory test used throughout the world is Western blot (see Figure 4.3). (Please refer to Chapter 12.) Positive confirmation generally relies on the detection of p24, gp120, gp160 and a further viral specific band. Any banding pattern other than this is considered 'indeterminate' and confirmatory laboratories should know the proportion of negative screen samples that will exhibit this non-specific reactivity (varies from 10–50%). Weak positive reactions should be confirmed by a follow-up sample to ensure donor identity and also rule out the possibility of sample contamination. More recently, immunoblots have become available that utilize recombinant proteins painted on to nitrocellulose strips. Transfusion

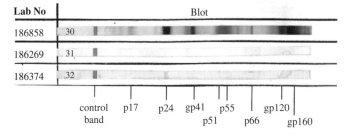

Figure 4.3 HIV Western blot (genelabs HIV 2.2) strip 30 confirmed positive, strip 31 negative, strip 32 indeterminate (p24). (See colour plate section).

microbiologists have to be cautious with the use of EIA-based confirmatory algorithm strategies as commercial assays often share similar (if not identical) antigenic components that can cross-react, resulting in (false) positive interpretation with dual EIA confirmatory strategies. Thus, a supplemental immunoblot or NAT assay should always be employed prior to notifying low-risk donors of HIV infection.

Although the finding of p24 antigen reactivity can be confirmed by a neutralization test, this is not always accurate; unlike the situation with HBV where HBsAg is produced in excess. In early acute HIV infection p24 antigen is often only produced at the limits of sensitivity of p24 antigen assays. Therefore, isolated HIV p24 antigen or NAT reactivity should always be confirmed

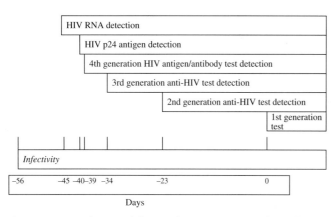

Figure 4.4 HIV window-period detection by various HIV assays (generalized) with first generation anti-HIV assays being detected at day 0.

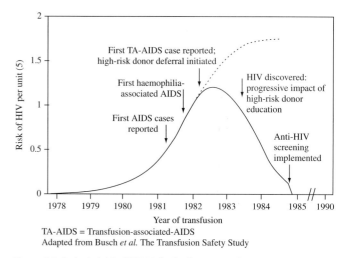

TA-AIDS = Transfusion-associated-AIDS
Adapted from Busch *et al.* The Transfusion Safety Study

Figure 4.5 Projected risk of HIV-I infection in San Francisco.

with a follow-up sample that demonstrates development of further HIV markers.

The immediate previous donation from a newly confirmed HIV positive regular donor should be thoroughly investigated in a look-back procedure (Learmont *et al.*, 2002). (Please refer to Chapter 24.) If an archived sample is available, this should be subject to HIV NAT, p24 antigen and EIA/Western blot testing to establish possible infection; regardless of test results on archived samples, recipients of components should be traced and offered testing. (Please refer to Chapter 14.)

Window period

Improvements in assay performance have incrementally narrowed the infectious window period associated with first, second and third-generation HIV antibody tests from an estimated 56 days to 33 days and 22 days, respectively. The p24 antigen or 'combi' tests may reduce the window period further to approximately 16 days, while detection of HIV RNA by NAT, as currently performed on mini-pools, is associated with a residual window period of only approximately 11 days (Glynn *et al.*, 2002) (see Figure 4.4). The infectivity of transfusions from donors in this residual window period may not be as high as in later stages of primary infection due to the exceedingly low levels of virus during this so-called pre-eclipse phase (Fiebig *et al.*, 2003).

Risk factors

In the late 1970s and early 1980s, HIV silently spread through groups of homosexual and bisexual men in the USA. By 1981, a number of Kaposi's sarcoma and *Pneumocystis carinii* pneumonia cases had occurred in these groups and shortly thereafter AIDS was recognized in haemophiliac patients and some blood recipients. In the UK, early HIV antibody tests revealed infection in a significant proportion of intravenous illicit drug users in Edinburgh. These population groups and immigrants from sub-Saharan Africa formed the main high-risk groups at the beginning of the epidemic. Potential blood donors were asked if they were members of any of those risk groups, with the understanding that they would seriously consider self-deferral. This was the only

means of preventing transfusion-transmission of HIV before early antibody tests became commercially available in the mid-1980s and was very effective. (See Figure 4.5) The donor questionnaire has been significantly enhanced over the past two decades, based on information gleaned from interviews of infected donors.(Please refer to Chapters 10 and 17.) Nevertheless, the donor selection process involves a great deal of honesty from donors so that those at risk do actually defer themselves. Early in the epidemic, if risk questions were answered absolutely truthfully, almost all HIV positive donors in certain areas of the world would have been barred from donating. Unfortunately, as the HIV epidemic has spread, and homosexual men have generally excluded themselves, heterosexual transmission has become the major mode of transmission throughout the world. The consequence of this is that our risk questions have a lessened effect of barring potential HIV positive donors, placing greater reliance on testing to interdict infected units.

Estimated risk of transfusion-transmission

Haemophiliac patients are probably the most vulnerable group of blood product recipients. Busch *et al.* (1994a) estimated that approximately 50% of North American haemophiliacs treated with factor VIII or IX in the early 1980s had seroconverted (i.e. developed anti-HIV). The rate approached 100% in haemophiliacs who were treated with high doses of factor concentrates. This indicates that given a large enough dose, virtually all recipients are susceptible to infection. Initially, it was hoped that seroconversion might have been, in effect, the result of vaccination by denatured HIV proteins, but experience has shown that all seropositive haemophiliacs have shown HIV NAT activity and the majority have gone on to develop AIDS (Busch *et al.*, 1994a; Operskalski *et al.*, 1995). Fortunately, the combination of donor screening and inactivation methods applied to plasma derivatives has eliminated the risk of HIV transmission by these products. (Please refer to Chapter 20.)

Residual risk estimates for standard blood components depend on a number of interacting factors, including incidence and prevalence of infection in donors, infectious window-period estimates in the context of serological or NAT assay sensitivities and testing error rates. The trend of the past ten years, where risk estimates have been progressively declining because of improved deferral of at-risk donors and introduction of more sensitive assays, is likely to be reversed because of increased heterosexual HIV transmission rates. Complex mathematical models predicting the risk of transfusion-transmitted HIV infections (Weusten et al., 2002) cannot realistically capture all the imponderables, and therefore these risk estimates should be considered to be the minimum level that may occur.

In the USA, around 1 in 400 donations were HIV infectious just prior to the introduction of testing. First-generation antibody testing reduced this risk 300-fold to a level of 7.7 per million. Second-generation antibody testing reduced this further to 4.5 per million and third-generation antibody testing alone would give a residual risk of 2 per million. The use of p24 antigen testing reduced the risk to 0.7 per million, whilst introduction of HIV mini-pool NAT has created the current residual risk of 0.5 per million (Dodd et al., 2002). Slightly lower risks (0.2 per million) have been expressed for Europe and other developed countries (Glynn et al., 2002).

Sadly, the WHO estimates that at least one-sixth of the 75 million blood donations collected in the world each year are not completely tested using even the most basic serological assay. It should also be remembered that some of these countries do not have the systems in place to prevent the release of screen positive blood donations (Bharucha, 2002). Thus, the risk of transfusion-transmitted HIV disease in such countries can only be estimated by the prevalence of HIV infection in the general population. In the developing world, voluntary non-remunerated blood donation and effective donor selection procedures can dramatically lower the prevalence of transfusion-transmitted HIV. For example, in Zimbabwe during the period 1998–1999, the HIV prevalence in the general adult population was 25%, while 2.3% of new blood donors and 0.7% of regular blood donors were infected (WHO, 2001).

Human T-cell leukaemia viruses I and II

Definition and characteristics of agent

In 1978, the first retrovirus, human T-cell leukaemia virus (HTLV-I), was found in a Japanese patient. The virus was found to cause adult T-cell leukaemia and lymphoma (ATL), and tropical spastic paraperesis (TSP), also known as HTLV-I associated myelopathy (HAM). Although the distribution of HTLV-I is worldwide, the virus is endemic in Japan, the Caribbean, South America, West and Central Africa, with infection rates well over 1%. A close relative, HTLV-II, was originally identified in 1982 in a case of hairy-cell leukaemia. This virus shows 65% homology with HTLV-I; HTLV-II is found in various American Indian populations and a proportion of users of illicit intravenous drugs throughout the world. More recently, HTLV-II has been found in some individuals exhibiting myelopathies (Murphy et al., 1997).

Both viruses establish an asymptomatic carrier state in close to 100% of seropositive persons. Adult T cell leukaemia can occur up to 40 years after infection in a small percentage (2–4%) of those infected. Tropical spastic paraperesis/HAM, characterized by spinal cord degeneration leading to immobility, bladder dysfunction and other neural dysfunctions, has a shorter incubation period, developing in a few (1.5–3%) HTLV-I and HTLV-II infected people. Human T-cell leukaemia virus I has also been associated with uveitis, marked by involvement of retinal vessels with characteristic granular grey-white deposits. Infection may progress to macular degeneration and blindness.

Viral transmission

As HTLV is cell associated, transmission is mainly by cellular blood products. Transmission occurs in approximately one-third of recipients given non-filtered cellular blood components stored for less than three weeks. Cell-free products such as fresh frozen plasma and plasma derivatives do not transmit infection. The process of white blood cell depletion by filtration (leucofiltration) is thought to reduce the transmission of HTLV-I through cellular blood components. Filtration has been shown to reduce the HTLV viral load by around 2 to 6 logs depending on component and type of filter used (Cesaire et al., 2002; Pennington et al., 2002). Although blood transfusion and other parenteral exposures are the most important modes of spread, sexual transmission is possible, as is spread from mother to infant via breast milk.

Testing

Antibody testing for anti-HTLV-I and anti-HTLV-II is the principal means of detecting individuals who have been infected with HTLV-I or HTLV-II. The first screening assays for HTLV-I were either EIA based or used particle-agglutination. Both systems used viral lysate as their source of antigen. Eventually these antigens have been replaced with recombinant materials such as are utilized in the current Abbott/Murex assay, a highly sensitive test system in a sandwich EIA format. Most, if not all, current antibody assays include HTLV-II components to facilitate the detection of either HTLV-I or HTLV-II.

Serological testing has been undertaken for some time in those areas of the world where the virus is thought to be endemic, such as Japan and the Caribbean. The USA and Canada introduced blood donor screening in 1988. Australia started donor screening in 1993. Many countries in Europe (France, the Netherlands, Germany, Spain, Ireland and Sweden) have introduced serological testing (France started in 1991; Sweden in 1994) and following a period of screening their donor population, some decided to revert to testing only previously untested donors. In the UK, mini-pool testing by serology was introduced during the summer of 2002 following an extensive pilot trial performed with Scottish and Irish blood donations (Dow et al., 2001). Mini-pool testing lent itself to one particular commercial EIA (from Abbott/Murex) that was shown to have considerably better dilutional sensitivity than assays from other manufacturers. The use of a pooled screening strategy reduced the rate of detection of false-positive samples,

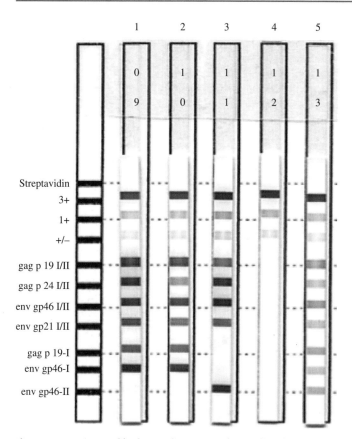

Figure 4.6 HTLV immunoblot (INNOLIA) strips 09 and 10 confirmed anti-HTLV-I positive, strip 11 confirmed anti-HTLV-II positive, strip 12 negative, strip 13 positive control. (See colour plate section).

so that in practice the use of mini-pooling has proven to be extremely specific.

Confirmatory testing has been mainly by immunoblot techniques. The earlier version of the Genelabs Western blot (v2.3) showed indeterminate band(s) with around 50% of serology reactive samples. A later version (v2.4) showed improved sensitivity and specificity. In addition, this later version was capable of identifying HTLV-I and HTLV-II. A line immunoassay (InnoLIA) (see Figure 4.6) recently became available and this has proven to be as sensitive and discriminatory as the Western blot, but has greatly improved specificity; it has generated less indeterminate samples (Thorstensson *et al.*, 2002). Indeterminate results can be further tested by a HTLV specific PCR assay, but few show positive reactivity (Busch *et al.*, 1994b). (Please refer to Chapter 12.)

Donor NAT for HTLV DNA is not currently under consideration due to the low residual risk and the need to develop sample processing methods targeting cell-associated, in addition, to plasma viruses.

Window period

It is thought that the infectious window period for HTLV preceding seroconversion is in the range of one to three months. In recipients of transfused products, the mean infectious window period was estimated at 51 days (range 36–72 days). There is essentially no data on the levels of infected cells, or the possible existence of plasma viraemia, during this window period.

Risk factors

In the UK, the majority of HTLV-I infected individuals had risk factors associated with being born in an endemic country, having had heterosexual sex with a high risk partner or having received a transfusion. Around 0.1 to 0.6% of Afro-Caribbean donors in the UK were found to be HTLV-I infected (Vrielink and Reesink, 2004).

Human T-cell leukaemia virus II has been mostly found amongst intravenous illicit drug users.

Estimated risk of transfusion-transmission

Countries in the developed world have an HTLV-I or -II prevalence of between 1 in 10 000 and 1 in 100 000. Infectivity rates from seropositive units vary, with an average around 27% (Whyte, 1997), some reports claiming transmission rates of 20–63% (Vrielink and Reesink, 2004). In the absence of antibody screening or leucoreduction, the risk of transmission would thus be around 2 to 63 per million. Introduction of donor screening should have reduced this figure by 99%, while leucoreduction probably reduces risk by 90%. An ongoing look-back in the UK has so far identified ten recipients positive for HTLV, who received transfusions from donors who subsequently tested positive for HTLV. Preliminary evidence suggests that leucodepletion procedures reduce the likelihood of HTLV transmission. The current risk for transfusion-transmitted HTLV has been estimated at approximately 1 in 3 million in the USA (Pomper *et al.*, 2003).

Conclusion

This chapter has been devoted to the clinically significant HIV and HTLV human retroviruses that originated from less-pathogenic simian counterparts. Humans also harbour endogenous retroviruses sequences and spumaviruses, but these are non-pathogenic and have not been demonstrated to be transmissible by blood components. Other simian retroviruses that might be transmitted to humans are of greater concern, and justify ongoing surveillance for zoonotic transmission to humans and prevalence in donors, as well as studies to investigate transfusion-transmissibility and disease causality. There are a number of divergent primate T-lymphotropic viruses (PTLVs), distantly related to HTLVs; however, studies have failed to document transmission to humans or presence of nucleic acid sequences in blood donors (Busch *et al.*, 2000). A further retrovirus, simian foamy virus (SFV) or spumaretrovirus, is endemic in most Old World primates and is known to readily transmit to research and zoo workers. A recent study (Wolfe *et al.*, 2004) identified human infection with SFV in several geographically isolated locations in Cameroon where people had exposure to non-human primate bushmeat. Whilst foamy viruses have no human disease association as yet (Peeters, 2004), this study suggests that simian retroviral zoonoses are more widespread than previously experienced. Who knows when a further cross-species transmission of a simian retrovirus or other pathogen will result in a further AIDS-like epidemic?

REFERENCES

Adler, M. W. (2001) ABC of AIDS: development of the epidemic. *BMJ*, **322**, 1226–9.

Apetrei, C., Loussert-Ajaka, I., Descamps, D., *et al.* (1996) Lack of screening test sensitivity during HIV-1 non-subtype B seroconversions. *AIDS*, **10**, F57–60.

Bharucha, Z. S. (2002) Risk management strategies for HIV in blood transfusion in developing countries. *Vox Sang*, **83** (Suppl. 1), 167–71.

Busch, M. P. and Stramer, S. L. (1998) The efficiency of HIV p24 antigen screening of US blood donors: projections versus reality. *Infusionsther und Transfusionmed*, **25**, 194–7.

Busch, M. P., Laycock, M., Kleinman, S. H., *et al.* and the Retrovirus Epidemiology Donor Study (REDS) (1994b) Accuracy of supplemental serological testing for human T-lymphotropic virus (HTLV) types I and II in US blood donors. *Blood*, **83**, 1143–8.

Busch, M. P., Operskalski, E. A., Mosley, J. W., *et al.* and the Transfusion Safety Study Group (1994a) Epidemiological background and long-term course of disease in human immunodeficiency virus type 1-infected blood donors identified before routine laboratory screening. *Transfusion*, **34**, 858–64.

Busch, M. P., Operskalski, E. A., Mosley, J. W., *et al.* and the Transfusion Safety Study Group (1996) Factors influencing HIV-1 transmission by blood transfusion. *J Infect Dis*, **174**, 26–33.

Busch, M. P., Switzer, W. M., Murphy, E. L., *et al.* (2000) Absence of evidence of infection with divergent primate T-lymphotropic viruses in US blood donors who have seroindeterminate HTLV test results. *Transfusion*, **40**, 443–9.

Cesaire, R., Kerob-Bauchet, B., Bourdonne, O., *et al.* (2002) Evaluation of HTLV-I removal by filtration of blood cell components in a routine setting. *Transfusion*, **44**, 42–8.

Delwart, E. L., Kalmin, N. D., Jones, T. S., *et al.* (2004) First case of HIV transmission by an RNA-screened blood donation. *Vox Sang*, **86**, 171–7.

Delwart, E. L., Orton, S., Parekh, B., *et al.* (2003) Two per cent of HIV-positive US blood donors are infected with non-subtype-B strains. *AIDS Res & Hum Retrovir*, **19**, 1065–70.

Dodd, R. Y., Notari, E. P. IV. and Stramer, S. L. (2002) Current prevalence and incidence of infectious disease markers and estimated window-period risk in the American Red Cross blood donor population. *Transfusion*, **42**, 975–9.

Dow, B. C., Munro, H., Ferguson, K., *et al.* (2001) HTLV antibody screening using mini-pools. *Transfus Med*, **11**, 419–22.

Fiebig, E. W., Wright, D. J., Rawal, B. D., *et al.* (2003) Dynamics of HIV viraemia and antibody seroconversion in plasma donors: implications for diagnosis and staging of primary HIV infection. *AIDS*, **17**, 1871–9.

Glynn, S. A., Kleinman, S. H., Wright, D. J., *et al.* (2002) International application of the incidence rate/window period model. *Transfusion*, **42**, 966–72.

Janssens, W., Buve, A. and Nkengasong, J. N. (1997) The puzzle of HIV-1 subtypes in Africa. *AIDS*, **11**, 705–12.

Learmont, J. C., Phillips, R. S. and Bickerton, I. J. (2002) The value of lookback to understanding blood-borne infectious diseases: the New South Wales' HIV experience. *Transfus Med Rev*, **16**, 315–24.

Ling, A. E., Robbins, K. E., Brown, T. M., *et al.* (2000) Failure of routine HIV-1 tests in a case involving transmission with preseroconversion blood components during the infectious window period. *JAMA*, **284**, 210–4.

Morris, K., Webb, B., Dow, B., *et al.* (2005) First HIV 'window-period' donation in a UK blood donor. *Transfus Med*, **15**, 249–50.

Murphy, E. L., Fridey, J., Smith, J. W., *et al.* (1997) HTLV-associated myelopathy in a cohort of HTLV-I and HTLV-II-infected blood donors. The REDS investigators. *Neurology*, **48**, 315–20.

Operskalski, E. A., Stram, D. O., Busch, M. P., *et al.* (1997) Role of viral load in heterosexual transmission of human immunodeficiency virus type 1 by blood transfusion recipients. *Amer J Epid*, **146**, 655–61.

Operskalski, E. A., Stram, D. O., Lee, H., *et al.* (1995) Human immunodeficiency virus type 1 infection: Relationship of risk group and age rate of progression to AIDS. Transfusion Safety Study Group. *J Infect Dis*, **172**, 648–55.

Parry, J. V., Murphy, G., Barlow, K. L., *et al.* (2001) National surveillance of HIV-1 subtypes for England and Wales: design, methods and initial findings. *J Acquir Immune Defic Syndr*, **26**, 381–8.

Peeters, M. (2004) Cross-species transmissions of simian retroviruses in Africa and risk for human health. *Lancet*, **363**, 911–2.

Pennington, J., Taylor, G. P., Sutherland, J., *et al.* (2002) Persistence of HTLV-I in blood components after leukocyte depletion. *Blood*, **100**, 677–81.

Pomper, G. J., Wu, Y. Y. and Snyder, E. L. (2003) Risks of tranfusion-transmitted infections: 2003. *Curr Opin Haematol*, **10**, 412–8.

Schable, C., Zekeng, L., Pau, C. P., *et al.* (1994) Sensitivity of US HIV antibody tests for detection of HIV-1 group O infections. *Lancet*, **344**, 1333–4.

Sharp, P. M., Bailes, E., Chaudhuri, R. R., *et al.* (2001) The origins of acquired immune deficiency syndrome viruses: where and when? *Philos Trans R Soc Lond B Biol Sci*, **356**, 867–76.

Simon, F., Loussert-Ajaka, I., Damond, F., *et al.* (1996) HIV type 1 diversity in northern Paris, France. *Aids Res Hum Retroviruses*, **12**, 1427–33.

Stramer, S. L., Glynn, S. A., Kleinman, S. H., *et al.* (2004) Detection of HIV and HCV infections among antibody-negative blood donors by nucleic acid-amplification testing. *NEJM*, **351**, 760–8.

Thorstensson, R., Albert, J. and Andersson, S. (2002) Strategies for diagnosis of HTLV-I and -II. *Transfusion*, **42**, 780–91.

Vrielink, H. and Reesink, H. W. (2004) HTLV-I/II prevalence in different geographic locations. *Transfus Med Rev*, **18**, 46–57.

Weber, B., Thorstensson, R., Tanprasert, S., *et al.* (2003) Reduction of the diagnostic window in three cases of human immunodeficiency-1 subtype E primary infection with fourth-generation HIV screening assays. *Vox Sang*, **85**, 73–9.

Weusten, J. J. A. M., van Drimmelen, H. A. J. and Lelie, P. N. (2002) Mathematic modeling of the risk of HBV, HCV and HIV transmission by window-phase donations not detected by NAT. *Transfusion*, **42**, 537–48.

Whyte, G. S. (1997) Is screening of Australian blood donors for HTLV-I necessary? *Med J Austral*, **166**, 478–81.

Wolfe, N. D., Switzer, W. M., Carr, J. K., *et al.* (2004) Naturally acquired simian retrovirus infections in central African hunters. *Lancet*, **363**, 932–7.

World Health Organization (2001) Global Database on Blood Safety, summary report 1998–1999. Available at: http//www.who.int/bloodsafety/global_database/en/SumRep_English.pdf

5 PARVOVIRUS B19 (HUMAN ERYTHROVIRUSES)

Kevin E. Brown

Parvovirus B19 (B19V)

Definition and characteristics of agent

Parvoviruses are small, 20–25 nm icosahedral viruses (see Figure 5.1), encapsidating a linear single stranded DNA genome of approximately 4000–6000 nucleotides. The family (*Parvoviridae*) is divided into two subfamilies based on their host species and viral coding strategies, the *Parvovirinae* that infect vertebrates, including fish, birds, reptiles and mammals, and the *Densovirinae* that infect insects. The *Parvovirinae* are similarly divided into five genera, Parvovirus, Dependovirus, Erythrovirus, Bocavirus and Amdovirus, based on the number of promoters, their transcription map, the similarity of the 5' and 3' terminal repeat sequences, and their sequence homology (Fauquet *et al.*, 2005). Several different parvoviruses have been identified in humans, including adeno-associated viruses (AAVs), Parv4 (Jones *et al.*, 2005) and Parv5 (Fryer *et al.*, 2006), human bocavirus (Allander *et al.*, 2005), and parvovirus B19 (B19V) (Cossart *et al.*, 1975), but only parvovirus B19 has definitively been shown to be a human pathogen.

B19V was the first member to be described and is the type species of the genus *Erythrovirus*. The virus has a genome of 5596 nucleotides, consisting of an internal coding sequence of 4830 nucleotides, flanked by identical terminal repeat sequences at the 5' and 3' end of 383 nucleotides which form the imperfect palindrome and hairpin structures necessary for DNA replication and encapsidation.

Sequence conservation and parvovirus B19 genotypes

The B19V genome is relatively well conserved, with approximately 10% sequence variation between isolates, but has three distinct genotypes (Servant *et al.*, 2002). Genotype 2 (A6- or Lali-like sequences (Hokynar *et al.*, 2002; Nguyen *et al.*, 2002; Servant *et al.*, 2002)) and genotype 3 (V9-like (Nguyen *et al.*, 1999)) have only been recognized in recent years, and almost all the studies in the literature relate to genotype 1. There is no evidence of different B19 serotypes, with most studies (Corcoran *et al.*, 2005; Heegaard *et al.*, 2002a; 2002b) suggesting that current serological assays can detect all three genotypes. Genotype 1 isolates have less than 5% sequence variation, and have a worldwide circulation, with isolates being found in different parts of the world and in different time periods. In contrast, the other genotypes appear to be much rarer, especially in most parts of Europe and America. Genotype 3 infection may be common in some parts of Africa (Candotti *et al.*, 2004).

Although most primer pairs based on the B19-Au isolate (GenBank M13178) are able to detect temporally and geographically diverse genotype 1 B19V isolates (Durigon *et al.*, 1993) they do not routinely detect the other two genotypes (Heegaard *et al.*, 2001; Nguyen *et al.*, 2002; Servant *et al.*, 2002). However, commercial assays are available that can detect all three genotypes (Baylis *et al.*, 2004; Braham *et al.*, 2004; Hokynar *et al.*, 2004).

Parvovirus B19 genome

The B19V genome encodes three major proteins, two capsid proteins, VP1 and VP2, and a multi-functional non-structural phosphoprotein, NS1. Each virus consists of 60 capsid proteins, and the major capsid protein, VP2, of 554 amino acids, makes up 95% of the capsid structure. The capsid protein VP1 has an additional 227 amino acids at the amino terminus (VP1u sequence), and the main neutralizing epitopes (Saikawa *et al.*, 1993) and a phospholipase motif (Dorsch *et al.*, 2002; Zadori *et al.*, 2001) thought to be important for viral entry are localized to this unique region. In contrast to VP1, VP2 proteins can self-assemble to form viral-like particles (Kajigaya *et al.*, 1991), and on permissive cells bind to the B19V receptor, globoside, also known as blood group P antigen (Brown *et al.*, 1993). The NS1 protein upregulates its own promoter (Doerig *et al.*, 1990) and is required for viral replication and encapsidation of the viral genome within the virus. It is cytotoxic, and induces cell cycle arrest and caspase activation in infected cells (Moffatt *et al.*, 1998).

Parvovirus B19 infectivity

Parvovirus B19 is highly erythrotropic, replicates to high titre and is cytotoxic to erythroid progenitor cells (BFU-E and CFU-E) in peripheral blood and bone marrow (Mortimer *et al.*, 1983a). In healthy individuals, at the height of the transient viraemia, viral titres as high as 10^{13} genome equivalents (ge)/ml are detectable. Although B19V has been shown to replicate in vitro in primary erythroid progenitor cells from bone marrow (Mortimer *et al.*, 1983a), peripheral blood (Ozawa *et al.*, 1986) and fetal liver (Brown *et al.*, 1991; Yaegashi *et al.*, 1989), only a few specialized cell lines have been found to be permissive for B19V infection (Miyagawa *et al.*, 1999; Morita *et al.*, 2001; Shimomura *et al.*, 1992) and even in these, viral replication is inefficient. So, assays for detecting infectious virus are extremely limited.

Transfusion Microbiology, eds John A. J. Barbara, Fiona A. M. Regan and Marcela C. Contreras. Published by Cambridge University Press. © Cambridge University Press 2008.

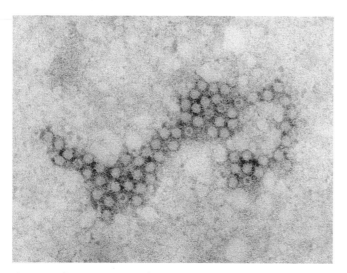

Figure 5.1 Electron microscopy of parvovirus B19 particles, demonstrating the typical ~ 22 nm diameter icosahedral virions. Figure courtesy of Dr Hazel Appleton, Virus Reference Department, HPA.

Table 5.1 Disease associations of parvovirus B19.

Host	Disease	Acute/chronic Infection
Children	Fifth disease	Acute
Adults	Polyarthropathy syndrome	Acute/chronic
Patients with increased erythropoiesis	Transient aplastic crisis	Acute
Immunodeficient/ immunocompromised patients	Pure red cell aplasia	Chronic
Fetus (<20 weeks)	Hydrops fetalis/ congenital anaemia	Acute/chronic

Parvovirus B19 stability

As a consequence of its small DNA genome and non-enveloped structure, B19V is resistant to many procedures used to inactivate viruses (Mortimer *et al.*, 1983b; Sayers, 1994). It is stable in lipid solvents (ether, chloroform) but can be inactivated by formalin, β-propiolactone and oxidizing agents. Gamma irradiation will also inactivate B19V, with 1.4 Mrad producing a 10 $\log_{10}$ reduction in infectivity (Cohen and Brown, 1992). The heat stability varies widely, depending on the environment. Although it is not quite as resistant to heat as other parvoviruses (Schwarz *et al.*, 1992), transmission of B19V by heat-treated blood products has been well documented (Blumel *et al.*, 2002a), and B19V can survive heat treatment at 48°C for 30 minutes. In blood products, B19V retained infectivity after heating at 56°C for 60 minutes, although in one report there was diminished B19 infectivity after 30 minutes at 56°C (Mortimer *et al.*, 1983a). However, the heat sensitivity varies depending on the diluent used, and the residual amount of moisture (Prikhod'ko *et al.*, 2005), and although B19V is inactivated by >4 logs at 60°C when diluted in 25% albumin (Blumel *et al.*, 2002b; Yunoki *et al.*, 2003), it is virtually resistant to 60°C heat for more than one hour when suspended in 60% sucrose (Yunoki *et al.*, 2003).

Consequences of transmission

The consequences of B19V virus infection range from asymptomatic to serious and potentially fatal conditions in the minority of the population that is particularly susceptible, either through immunosuppression, decreased erythropoietic reserve, or both (Young and Brown, 2004) (see Table 5.1).

Non-haematological disease

Although perhaps 50–75% of B19V infections are asymptomatic (or so minor as to not warrant medical attention), the most common presentation of infection is as the rash illness erythema infectiosum, also known as fifth disease or 'slapped cheek' disease, so named for the characteristic facial appearance. The infection is generally innocuous, with a minor febrile illness beginning approximately eight days after acquisition of virus, with mild haematological abnormalities during the second week, and the classical facial rash at 17 to 18 days (see Figure 5.2). The rash may spread to involve extremities in a lacy reticular pattern, but there can be great variation in the appearance of the erythema. Especially in adults the 'slapped cheek' may not be apparent. The rash may be difficult to distinguish from other viral exanthems such as rubella, and difficult to appreciate in dark-skinned individuals.

Although in children B19V infection is usually mild and of short duration, in adults, and especially in women, there may be arthropathy in approximately 50% of patients (Woolf, 1990). The joint distribution is often symmetrical, with arthralgia and even frank arthritis affecting the small joints of the hands and occasionally the ankles, knees and wrists. Resolution usually occurs within a few weeks, but persistent or recurring symptoms can continue for years (White *et al.*, 1985).

The role of parvovirus B19 in the aetiology of chronic arthritis is controversial, as although B19V DNA can be detected in synovial fluid or cells of patients with 'reactive arthritis', B19V DNA can also be found in approximately 50% of non-arthropathy controls (Soderlund *et al.*, 1997). Similarly, although it has been postulated that B19V is involved in the initiation and perpetuation of rheumatoid arthritis, leading to joint lesions (Takahashi *et al.*, 1998), these results have not been reproducible by other groups (Speyer *et al.*, 1998), and it seems unlikely that B19V plays a role in classic erosive rheumatoid arthritis.

Patients with haemolytic disease or decreased red cell reserve

Parvovirus B19 infection is the aetiological agent of transient aplastic crisis (TAC): the abrupt onset of severe anaemia with absent reticulocytes, and originally described in patients with hereditary spherocytosis. Transient aplastic crisis has now been described in a wide range of haemolytic disorders, including

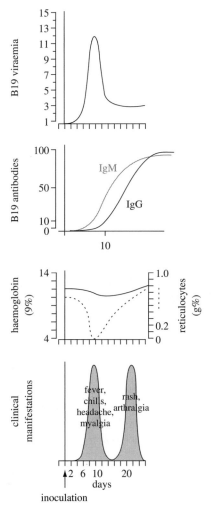

Figure 5.2 Time course of B19 infection following inoculation, showing the time course of viraemia and associated cessation of red cell production, and antibody production with development of the rash and arthralgia symptoms of fifth disease (first published in Young and Brown, 2004).

hereditary spherocytosis, thalassaemia, red cell enzymopathies like pyruvate kinase deficiency, and auto-immune haemolytic anaemia (Young, 1988). It can also occur under conditions of increased erythropoiesis, such as haemorrhage, iron deficiency anaemia, and following kidney or bone marrow transplantation. Although suffering from an ultimately self-limiting disease, patients with an aplastic crisis can be severely ill (Smith-Whitley *et al.*, 2004). Symptoms include dyspnoea, lassitude and confusion due to the worsening anaemia; congestive heart failure and bone marrow necrosis may develop, and the TAC can be fatal. Transient aplastic crisis and B19V infection in haematologically normal patients may also be associated with changes in the other blood lineages, with varying degrees of neutropenia, thrombocytopenia, haemophagocytosis and even pancytopenia.

Pure red cell aplasia

Patients who cannot mount a neutralizing immune response to B19V develop a persistent B19V infection resulting in pure red cell aplasia (PRCA). This can occur in a wide variety of immunosuppressed states, including congenital immunodeficiency (Kurtzman *et al.*, 1987), acquired immunodeficiency (HIV infection or frank AIDS) (Frickhofen *et al.*, 1990), lymphoproliferative disorders (Kurtzman *et al.*, 1988), and after organ transplantation. The immunosuppression may be subtle, and PRCA may be the presenting illness of patients with HIV infection or with very limited immune dysfunction (Kurtzman *et al.*, 1989). In all cases, the typical presentation is persistent anaemia associated with reticulocytopenia, but other blood lineages may also be affected, and patients rarely may present with pancytopenia.

Fetal infection

Maternal infection with parvovirus B19V during pregnancy, especially in the first half of pregnancy, can lead to either fetal loss or the development of hydrops fetalis. Prospective studies indicate that the risk of transplacental fetal infection is about 30%, and that the risk of fetal loss, predominantly in the early second trimester of pregnancy (before week 20), is about 9% (Public Health Laboratory Service Working Party on Fifth Disease, 1990). Follow-up studies of surviving infants indicated no long-term sequelae following fetal infection in the vast majority of individuals, and estimated the risk of congenital infection following B19V infection as less than 1% (Miller *et al.*, 1998). It has been estimated that B19V infection probably causes 10–20% of all cases of non-immune hydrops fetalis (Jordan, 1996).

Although parvovirus B19 does not appear to be teratogenic, some case reports of possible eye damage and CNS abnormalities following maternal B19V infection have been reported (Weiland *et al.*, 1987), and in addition several cases of congenital anaemia following maternal infection have been described (Brown *et al.*, 1994; Heegaard *et al.*, 2000).

Other suspected parvovirus B19 syndromes

A large number of unusual clinical presentations have been reported in the literature, usually either as case reports or small series with B19V detectable only by PCR, and the significance of which remain uncertain (Török, 1997). These complications of infection include hepatitis, myocarditis, encephalitis, meningitis, brachial plexus neuropathy and a collection of vasculitides.

Treatment and prevention

Fifth disease and symptoms of arthralgia/arthropathy are managed with symptomatic treatment only. Similarly, transient aplastic crises are treated symptomatically with blood components, if required. Pure red cell aplasia caused by B19V infection is due to the inability to mount a neutralizing antibody response, and can be treated with immunoglobulin (Frickhofen *et al.*, 1990; Kurtzman *et al.*, 1989).

Vaccines for the prevention of B19V are being developed, and are recombinant viral-like particles with increased levels of VP1 to enhance the neutralizing antibody response (Bansal *et al.*, 1993). The vaccine was shown to effectively induce neutralizing

Table 5.2 Published prevalence of B19V in cohorts of blood donors.

Reference	No of samples	Method[a]	B19V positive samples	Frequency	Prevalence %
(Mortimer et al., 1983b)	500 000	CIE	11	1:45 000	0.002
(Courouce et al., 1985)	2349	CIE	7	1:3356	0.030
(da Silva Cruz et al., 1989)	6400	CIE	1	1:6400	0.015
(Cohen et al., 1990)	24 000	CIE	1	1:24 000	0.004
(O'Neill and Coyle, 1992)	7580	CIE	2	1:3790[b]	0.026
(Tsujimura et al., 1995)	560 000	DID	16	1:35 000	0.003
(Wakamatsu et al., 1999)	257 710	RHA	31	1:8313	0.012
(McOmish et al., 1993)	100 000	PCR	17	1:5882	0.017
(Jordan et al., 1998)	9568	PCR	11	1:870	0.115
(Yoto et al., 1995)	1000	PCR	6	1:167[b]	0.6[b]
(Hitzler and Runkel, 2002)	28 972	RHA + PCR	4	1:7243	0.014
(Candotti et al., 2004)	2440	PCR	22[c]	1:111	0.90

[a] CIE, counter-immune electrophoresis, sensitivity $\sim 10^9$ IU/ml

DID, double immune diffusion, sensitivity $\sim 10^9$ IU/ml

RHA, receptor-mediated haemagglutination assay, $\sim 10^4$ IU/ml

PCR, polymerase chain reaction, $\sim 10^2$–10^4 IU/ml

[b] At the time of an outbreak of fifth disease

[c] Includes 12 from Ghana that were genotype 3 sequences

antibodies in normal volunteers (Ballou et al., 2003), and is about to go into phase 2 testing.

Risk factors for transmission

Epidemiology

Parvovirus B19 infection is a common illness of childhood, and although by the age of 15 years approximately 50% of children have detectable IgG (Cohen and Buckley, 1988), based on the data from studies of susceptible women, approximately 1% of adult blood donors will seroconvert each year (Koch and Adler, 1989). In temperate climates most infections occur in the spring, with mini-epidemics occurring at regular intervals several years apart. Although there are no direct studies of the risk factors associated with B19V infection in blood donors, studies of the risk factors among pregnant women suggest increased risk for those with contact with children, either in the household setting, as teachers, or day care workers, (Cartter et al., 1991; Chorba et al., 1986). Transmission is predominantly by the respiratory route, probably by droplet spread, and is highest at the time of viraemia, prior to the onset of rash or arthralgia.

Infection with B19V occurs only once, with the production of lifelong neutralizing antibodies. Development of a second infection of B19V has only rarely been documented, although boosting of the antibody response may occur, presumably due to subclinical infection (Anderson et al., 1985).

Prevalence of parvovirus B19 in blood donors

As in healthy asymptomatic individuals, at the height of the transient viraemia viral titre as high as 10^{14} genome equivalents (or IU)/ml are detectable, therefore contamination of blood and

blood products is not infrequent. In addition, in immunocompetent, healthy individuals low levels of B19V DNA may be detectable in serum by PCR for more than four months following acute infection (Musiani et al., 1995; Patou et al., 1993), and as the PCR tests become more sensitive, it may be detectable even for years (Brown and Yu, unpublished data). It is not known if this reflects full-length virus, intact virions, or even infectious virus. Polymerase chain reaction testing of serum or plasma indicates that low levels of B19V DNA can be detected in approximately 0.01%–0.1% of healthy blood donors (see Table 5.2) (Jordan et al., 1998), even rising to 0.6% when B19V is circulating in the community (Yoto et al., 1995). Almost all of the published studies tested for B19 genotype 1 only, but in one study of prevalence of viruses in the UK and Africa, all three genotypes were tested for, and B19V genotype 3 was detected in 12/1000 blood donors from Ghana (Candotti et al., 2004).

Prevalence of parvovirus B19 in blood products

Not surprisingly given the high rates of B19V in blood donors, prior to the screening of plasma pools for high titre B19V, contamination of plasma pools and blood products and especially factor concentrates with B19 DNA was almost universal (Azzi et al., 1999). In one early PCR-based study, B19 DNA was found in 3 of 12 albumin samples, in 7 of 7 factor VIII samples, 3 of 15 IVIG samples and 3 of 4 IMIG samples (Saldanha and Minor, 1996). Although not usually tested for, both genotypes 1 and 2 have been detected in coagulation factor concentrates (Schneider et al., 2004), although genotype 2 was much rarer (2.5%) than genotype 1 (81%), consistent with the much lower prevalence of genotype 2 in European donors (Hokynar et al., 2004; Nguyen et al., 2002).

Transmission of parvovirus B19 by blood and blood products

Transmission of B19V infection as a result of transfusion of blood or blood products, especially factor VIII and IX concentrates has been well documented in the literature (Azzi *et al.*, 1999), and even the use of high purity factor concentrates has not prevented transmission (Wu *et al.*, 2005). In addition to factor concentrates, B19V has been transmitted by solvent-detergent (S/D) treated plasma (Koenigbauer *et al.*, 2000), IVIG (Erdman *et al.*, 1997; Hayakawa *et al.*, 2002) and fibrin products (Hino *et al.*, 2000; Kawamura *et al.*, 2002).

Although less often, B19V infection has also been transmitted by cellular products including red cells (Jordan *et al.*, 1998; Yoto *et al.*, 1995; Zanella *et al.*, 1995), platelets (Cohen *et al.*, 1997) and peripheral blood stem cells (Arnold *et al.*, 2005)

Reducing the risk of transmission
Blood products

Although plasma pools invariably contain parvovirus B19 DNA, for many years it was considered that the high titre of neutralizing antibodies present in plasma pools would prevent transmission of infectious virus (Solheim *et al.*, 2000). In a post-market surveillance study of S/D treated plasma in B19V seronegative plasma pool recipients it was shown that only those recipients who received plasma containing $>10^7$ IU/mL became infected or seroconverted, whereas there was no seroconversion in those who received products containing $<10^4$ IU/mL (Brown *et al.*, 2001; Tabor and Epstein, 2002). In the USA, the FDA has proposed a limit of $<10^4$ IU/mL for manufacturing pools destined for all plasma derivatives (Tabor and Epstein, 2002; Wu *et al.*, 2005), and in Europe the European Pharmocopoeia (5.0) now requires that all human plasma (pooled and treated for virus inactivation, S/D plasma,) and human plasma pools used for the manufacture of anti-D has a B19V viral titre of $<10^4$ IU/mL (Council of Europe 2005a; 2005b; 2005c; Nubling *et al.*, 2004).

Cellular blood components

In addition, the Health Council of the Netherlands makes a distinction between cellular blood products and plasma products. As well as the plasma pool recommendations, the committee recommends an approach similar to that used to reduce CMV infection, namely the availabililty of 'B19-virus safe' blood products to be administered to risk groups. 'B19-virus safe' cellular blood products are defined as 'those from a blood donor in which IgG antibodies against B19V have been detected in two separate blood samples, one taken at least six months after the other' (Groeneveld and van der Noordaa, 2003). The rationale for the six-month delay is to allow viral titre to fall, and for the presence of high titre B19V neutralizing antibody, and the committee recommends these cellular products for administration to pregnant women, and B19-seronegative patients with either haemolytic anaemia or immunodeficiency. This initiative has not been emulated elsewhere in Europe because of a perception that there is little demand for such a product.

Testing of blood and blood products

Parvovirus B19 agglutinates primate and human red cells (Brown and Cohen, 1992), and haemagglutination-based assays (Hitzler and Runkel, 2002; Sakata *et al.*, 1999; Wakamatsu *et al.*, 1999) have been developed to detect viral antigen in blood and blood products. Similarly, EIA-based assays are being developed to detect B19V capsids. However, both types of assays are relatively insensitive, especially in the presence of B19V antibodies, and for most manufacturers screening for B19V is based on detection of viral DNA, generally by NAT. In most countries testing of plasma for fractionation is done on mini-pools and, at least in the USA, testing is considered an 'in-process' control testing, and not donor screening (Tabor and Epstein, 2002). Hence the individual B19V-positive donors are not identified.

Other parvoviruses

Although other parvoviruses have been detected in human blood and tissues, the risks of transmission by blood and blood products are unknown. No disease has been associated with adeno-associated viruses, although AAV sequences can be detected in peripheral blood monocytes (Grossman *et al.*, 1992). The newly described Parv4 (Jones *et al.*, 2005), and the closely related Parv5 (Fryer *et al.*, 2006) viruses can be detected in plasma pools, but at low levels, and relatively infrequently compared to B19V sequences (Fryer *et al.*, 2006 and own unpublished data). Less is known about the recently described human bocavirus (Allander *et al.*, 2005), although preliminary studies also suggest that it is a rare contaminant of plasma pools. Finally, erythroviruses closely related to B19V have been detected in other primates (Brown and Young, 1997), and animal handlers can have antibodies against these primate viruses, although they have not been shown to be pathogenic to humans (Brown *et al.*, 2004).

REFERENCES

Allander, T., Tammi, M. T., Eriksson, M., *et al.* (2005) Cloning of a human parvovirus by molecular screening of respiratory tract samples. *Proc. Natl. Acad. Sci. U.S.A*, **102** (36), 12891–6.

Anderson, M. J., Higgins, P. G., Davis, L. R., *et al.* (1985) Experimental parvoviral infection in humans. *Journal of Infectious Diseases*, **152**, 257–65.

Arnold, D. M., Neame, P. B., Meyer, R. M., *et al.* (2005) Autologous peripheral blood progenitor cells are a potential source of parvovirus B19 infection. *Transfusion*, **45**, 394–8.

Azzi, A., Morfini, M. and Mannucci, P. M. (1999) The transfusion-associated transmission of parvovirus B19. *Transfus. Med. Rev*, **13**, 194–204.

Ballou, W. R., Reed, J. L., Noble, W., *et al.* (2003) Safety and immunogenicity of a recombinant parvovirus B19 vaccine formulated with MF59 C.1. *J Infec Dis*, **187**, 675–8.

Bansal, G. P., Hatfield, J. A., Dunn, F. E., *et al.* (1993) Candidate recombinant vaccine for human B19 parvovirus. *J Infect Dis*, **167**, 1034–44.

Baylis, S. A., Shah, N. and Minor, P. D. (2004) Evaluation of different assays for the detection of parvovirus B19 DNA in human plasma. *J Virol Methods*, **121**, 7–16.

Blumel, J., Schmidt, I., Effenberger, W., *et al.* (2002a) Parvovirus B19 transmission by heat-treated clotting factor concentrates. *Transfusion*, **42**(11), 1473–81.

Blumel, J., Schmidt, I., Willkommen, H., *et al.* (2002b) Inactivation of parvovirus B19 during pasteurization of human serum albumin. *Transfusion*, **42**, 1011–18.

Braham, S., Gandhi, J., Beard, S., *et al.* (2004) Evaluation of the Roche LightCycler parvovirus B19 quantification kit for the diagnosis of parvovirus B19 infections. *J Clin Virol*, **31**, 5–10.

Brown, K. E. and Cohen, B. J. (1992) Haemagglutination by parvovirus B19. *J Gen Virol*, **73**, 2147–9.

Brown, K. E. and Young, N. S. (1997). The simian parvoviruses. *Rev Med Virol*, **7**, 211–8.

Brown, K. E., Anderson, S. M. and Young, N. S. (1993) Erythrocyte P antigen: cellular receptor for B19 parvovirus. *Science*, **262**, 114–7.

Brown, K. E., Green, S. W., Antunez de Mayolo, J., *et al.* (1994) Congenital anaemia after transplacental B19 parvovirus infection. *Lancet*, **343**, 895–6.

Brown, K. E., Liu, Z., Gallinella, G., *et al.* (2004) Simian parvovirus infection: a potential zoonosis. *J Infec Dis*, **190**, 1900–7.

Brown, K. E., Mori, J., Cohen, B. J., *et al.* (1991) In vitro propagation of parvovirus B19 in primary foetal liver culture. *J Gen Virol*, **72**, 741–45.

Brown, K. E., Young, N. S., Alving, B. M., *et al.* (2001) Parvovirus B19: implications for transfusion medicine. Summary of a workshop. *Transfusion*, **41**(1), 130–5.

Candotti, D., Etiz, N., Parsyan, A., *et al.* (2004) Identification and characterization of persistent human erythrovirus infection in blood donor samples. *J Virol*, **78**, 12169–178.

Cartter, M. L., Farley, T. A., Rosengren, S., *et al.* (1991) Occupational risk factors for infection with parvovirus B19 among pregnant women. *J Infect Dis*, **163**, 282–5.

Chorba, T., Coccia, P., Holman, R. C., *et al.* (1986) The role of parvovirus B19 in aplastic crisis and erythema infectiosum (fifth disease). *J Infect Dis*, **154**, 383–93.

Cohen, B. J. and Brown, K. E. (1992) Laboratory infection with human parvovirus B19 (letter). *J Infect*, **24**, 113–4.

Cohen, B. J. and Buckley, M. M. (1988) The prevalence of antibody to human parvovirus B19 in England and Wales. *J Med Microbiol*, **25**, 151–3.

Cohen, B. J., Beard, S., Knowles, W. A., *et al.* (1997) Chronic anemia due to parvovirus B19 infection in a bone marrow transplant patient after platelet transfusion. *Transfusion*, **37**, 947–52.

Cohen, B. J., Field, A. M., Gudnadottir, S., *et al.* (1990) Blood donor screening for parvovirus B19. *J Virol Methods*, **30**, 233–8.

Corcoran, A., Doyle, S., Allain, J. P., *et al.* (2005) Evidence of serological cross-reactivity between genotype 1 and genotype 3 erythrovirus infections. *J Virol*, **79**, 5238–9.

Cossart, Y. E., Field, A. M., Cant, B., *et al.* (1975) Parvovirus-like particles in human sera. *Lancet*, **i**, 72–3.

Council of Europe (2005a) Human anti-D immunoglobulin. No. 0557. *European Pharmacopoeia*, **5**, 1732–3.

Council of Europe (2005b) Human anti-D-immunoglobulin for intravenous administration. No. 1527. *European Pharmacopoeia*, **5**, 1733.

Council of Europe (2005c) Human plasma (pooled and treated for virus inactivation). No. 1646. *European Pharmacopoeia*, **5**, 1747–8.

Courouce, A. M., Beaulieu, M. J., Bouchardeau, F., *et al.* (1985) Viraemia with human parvovirus (letter). *Lancet*, **i**, 1218–19.

Cruz, A. da Silva, Serpa, M. J., Barth, O. M., *et al.* (1989) Detection of the human parvovirus B19 in a blood donor plasma in Rio de Janeiro. *Mem Inst Oswaldo Cruz*, **84**, 279–80.

Current Trends risks associated with human parvovirus B19 infection. (1989). *MMWR Morb Mortal Wkly Rep*, **38**, 81–97.

Doerig, C., Hirt, B., Antonietti, J. P., *et al.* (1990) Non-structural protein of parvoviruses B19 and minute virus of mice controls transcription. *J Virol*, **64**, 387–96.

Dorsch, S., Liebisch, G., Kaufmann, B., *et al.* (2002) The VP1 unique region of parvovirus B19 and its constituent phospholipase A2-like activity. *J Virol*, **76**, 2014–18.

Durigon, E. L., Erdman, D. D., Gary, G. W., *et al.* (1993) Multiple primer pairs for polymerase chain reaction (PCR) amplification of human parvovirus B19 DNA. *J Virol Methods*, **44**, 155–65.

Erdman, D. D., Anderson, B. C., Torok, T. J., *et al.* (1997) Possible transmission of parvovirus B19 from intravenous immune globulin. *J Med Virol*, **53**, 233–6.

Fauquet, C. M., Mayo, M. A., Maniloff, J., *et al.* (2005) *Virus Taxonomy: Classification and Nomenclature of Viruses: Eighth Report of the International Committee on Taxonomy of Viruses*. New York, Elsevier Academic Press.

Frickhofen, N., Abkowitz, J. L., Safford, M., *et al.* (1990) Persistent B19 parvovirus infection in patients infected with human immunodeficiency virus type 1 (HIV-1): a treatable cause of anemia in AIDS. *Ann Intern Med*, **113**, 926–33.

Fryer, J. F., Kapoor, A., Minor, P. D., *et al.* (2006) Novel parvovirus and related variant in human plasma. *Emerg Infect Dis* **12**(1): 151–4.

Groeneveld, K. and van der Noordaa, J. (2003) Blood products and parvovirus B19. *Neth J Med*, **61**(5), 154–6.

Grossman, Z., Mendelson, E., Brok-Simoni, F., *et al.* (1992) Detection of adeno-associated virus type 2 in human peripheral blood cells. *J Gen Virol*, **73**, 961–6.

Hayakawa, F., Imada, K., Towatari, M., *et al.* (2002) Life-threatening human parvovirus B19 infection transmitted by intravenous immune globulin. *Br J Haematol*, **118**, 1187–9.

Heegaard, E. D., Hasle, H., Skibsted, L., *et al.* (2000) Congenital anemia caused by parvovirus B19 infection. *Pediatr Infect Dis J*, **19**, 1216–8.

Heegaard, E. D., Panum, J. I. and Christensen, J. (2001) Novel PCR assay for differential detection and screening of erythrovirus B19 and erythrovirus V9. *J Med Virol*, **65**, 362–7.

Heegaard, E. D., Petersen, B. L., Heilmann, C. J., *et al.* (2002a) Prevalence of parvovirus B19 and parvovirus V9 DNA and antibodies in paired bone marrow and serum samples from healthy individuals. *J Clin Microbiol*, **40**, 933–6.

Heegaard, E. D., Qvortrup, K. and Christensen, J. (2002b) Baculovirus expression of erythrovirus V9 capsids and screening by ELISA: serologic cross-reactivity with erythrovirus B19. *J Med Virol*, **66**, 246–52.

Hino, M., Ishiko, O., Honda, K. I., *et al.* (2000) Transmission of symptomatic parvovirus B19 infection by fibrin sealant used during surgery. *Br J Haematol*, **108**, 194–5.

Hitzler, W. E. and Runkel, S. (2002) Prevalence of human parvovirus B19 in blood donors as determined by a haemagglutination assay and verified by the polymerase chain reaction. *Vox Sang*, **82**, 18–23.

Hokynar, K., Norja, P., Laitinen, H., *et al.* (2004) Detection and differentiation of human parvovirus variants by commercial quantitative real-time PCR tests. *J Clin Microbiol*, **42**, 2013–9.

Hokynar, K., Soderlund-Venermo, M., Pesonen, M., *et al.* (2002) A new parvovirus genotype persistent in human skin. *Virology*, **302**(2), 224–8.

Jones, M. S., Kapoor, A., Lukashov, V. V., *et al.* (2005) New DNA viruses identified in patients with acute viral infection syndrome. *J Virol*, **79**(13), 8230–6.

Jordan, J., Tiangco, B., Kiss, J., *et al.* (1998) Human parvovirus B19: prevalence of viral DNA in volunteer blood donors and clinical outcomes of transfusion recipients. *Vox Sang*, **75**, 97–102.

Jordan, J. A. (1996) Identification of human parvovirus B19 infection in idiopathic non-immune hydrops fetalis. *Am J Obstet Gynecol*, **174**, 37–42.

Kajigaya, S., Fujii, H., Field, A., *et al.* (1991) Self-assembled B19 parvovirus capsids, produced in a baculovirus system, are antigenically and immunogenically similar to native virions. *Proceedings of the National Academy of Science USA*, **88**, 4646–50.

Kawamura, M., Sawafuji, M., Watanabe, M., *et al.* (2002) Frequency of transmission of human parvovirus B19 infection by fibrin sealant used during thoracic surgery. *Ann Thorac Surg*, **73**, 1098–100.

Koch, W. C. and Adler, S. P. (1989) Human parvovirus B19 infections in women of childbearing age and within families. *Pediatr Infect Dis J*, **8**, 83–7.

Koenigbauer, U. F., Eastlund, T. and Day, J. W. (2000) Clinical illness due to parvovirus B19 infection after infusion of solvent/detergent-treated pooled plasma. *Transfusion*, **40**, 1203–6.

Kurtzman, G., Frickhofen, N., Kimball, J., *et al.* (1989) Pure red-cell aplasia of 10 years' duration due to persistent parvovirus B19 infection and its cure with immunoglobulin therapy. *New Eng J Med*, **321**, 519–23.

Kurtzman, G. J., Cohen, B., Meyers, P., *et al.* (1988) Persistent B19 parvovirus infection as a cause of severe chronic anaemia in children with acute lymphocytic leukaemia. *Lancet*, **ii**, 1159–62.

Kurtzman, G. J., Ozawa, K., Cohen, B., *et al.* (1987) Chronic bone marrow failure due to persistent B19 parvovirus infection. *New Eng J Med*, **317**, 287–94.

McOmish, F., Yap, P. L., Jordan, A., *et al.* (1993) Detection of parvovirus B19 in donated blood: a model system for screening by polymerase chain reaction. *J Clin Microbiol*, **31**, 323–8.

Miller, E., Fairley, C. K., Cohen, B. J., *et al.* (1998) Immediate and long-term outcome of human parvovirus B19 infection in pregnancy. *British J Obstet Gynaecol*, **105**, 174–8.

Miyagawa, E., Yoshida, T., Takahashi, H., *et al.* (1999) Infection of the erythroid cell line, KU812Ep6 with human parvovirus B19 and its application to titration of B19 infectivity. *J Virol Methods*, **83**, 45–54.

Moffatt, S., Yaegashi, N., Tada, K., *et al.* (1998) Human parvovirus B19 non-structural (NS1) protein induces apoptosis in erythroid lineage cells. *J Virol*, **72**, 3018–28.

Morita, E., Tada, K., Chisaka, H., *et al.* (2001) Human parvovirus B19 induces cell cycle arrest at G(2) phase with accumulation of mitotic cyclins. *J Virol*, **75**, 7555–63.

Mortimer, P. P., Humphries, R. K., Moore, J. G., *et al.* (1983a) A human parvovirus-like virus inhibits haematopoietic colony formation in vitro. *Nature*, **302**, 426–9.

Mortimer, P. P., Luban, N. L., Kelleher, J. F., *et al.* (1983b) Transmission of serum parvovirus-like virus by clotting-factor concentrates. *Lancet*, **ii**, 482–4.

Musiani, M., Zerbini, M., Gentilomi, G., *et al.* (1995) Parvovirus B19 clearance from peripheral blood after acute infection. *J Infect Dis*, **172**, 1360–3.

Nguyen, Q. T., Sifer, C., Schneider, V., *et al.* (1999) Novel human erythrovirus associated with transient aplastic anemia. *J Clin Microbiol*, **37**, 2483–7.

Nguyen, Q. T., Wong, S., Heegaard, E. D., *et al.* (2002) Identification and characterization of a second novel human erythrovirus variant, A6. *Virology*, **301**, 374–80.

Nubling, C. M., Daas, A. and Buchheit, K. H. (2004) Collaborative study for establishment of a European Pharmacopoei Biological Reference Preparation (BRP) for B19 virus DNA testing of plasma pools by nucleic acid amplification technique. *Pharmeuropa Bio*, **2003**(2), 27–34.

O'Neill, H. J. and Coyle, P. V. (1992) Two anti-parvovirus B19 IgM capture assays incorporating a mouse monoclonal antibody specific for B19 viral capsid proteins VP 1 and VP 2. *Arch Virol*, **123**, 125–34.

Ozawa, K., Kurtzman, G. and Young, N. (1986) Replication of the B19 parvovirus in human bone marrow cell cultures. *Science*, **233**, 883–6.

Patou, G., Pillay, D., Myint, S., *et al.* (1993) Characterization of a nested polymerase chain reaction assay for detection of parvovirus B19. *J Clin Microbiol*, **31**, 540–6.

Prikhod'ko, G. G., Vasilyeva, I., Reyes, H., *et al.* (2005) Evaluation of a new LightCycler reverse transcription-polymerase chain reaction infectivity assay for detection of human parvovirus B19 in dry-heat inactivation studies. *Transfusion*, **45**, 1011–19.

Public Health Laboratory Service Working Party on Fifth Disease (1990) Prospective study of human parvovirus (B19) infection in pregnancy. *BMJ*, **300**, 1166–70.

Saikawa, T., Anderson, S., Momoeda, M., *et al.* (1993) Neutralizing linear epitopes of B19 parvovirus cluster in the VP1 unique and VP1-VP2 junction regions. *J Virol*, **67**, 3004–9.

Sakata, H., Ihara, H., Sato, S., *et al.* (1999) Efficiency of donor screening for human parvovirus B19 by the receptor-mediated hemagglutination assay method. *Vox Sang*, **77**, 197–203.

Saldanha, J. and Minor, P. (1996) Detection of human parvovirus B19 DNA in plasma pools and blood products derived from these pools: implications for efficiency and consistency of removal of B19 DNA during manufacture. *Br J Haematol*, **93**, 714–9.

Sayers, M. H. (1994) Transfusion-transmitted viral infections other than hepatitis and human immunodeficiency virus infection. Cytomegalovirus, Epstein-Barr virus, human herpes virus 6, and human parvovirus B19. *Arch Pathol Lab Med*, **118**, (4), 346–9.

Schneider, B., Becker, M., Brackmann, H. H., *et al.* (2004) Contamination of coagulation factor concentrates with human parvovirus B19 genotype 1 and 2. *Thromb Haemost*, **92**, 838–45.

Schwarz, T. F., Serke, S., von Brunn, A., *et al.* (1992) Heat stability of parvovirus B19: kinetics of inactivation. *Int J Med Microbiol Virol Parasitol Infect Dis*, **277**, 219–23.

Servant, A., Laperche, S., Lallemand, F., *et al.* (2002) Genetic diversity within human erythroviruses: identification of three genotypes. *J Virol*, **76**, 9124–34.

Shimomura, S., Komatsu, N., Frickhofen, N., *et al.* (1992) First continuous propagation of B19 parvovirus in a cell line. *Blood*, **79**, 18–24.

Smith-Whitley, K., Zhao, H., Hodinka, R. L., *et al.* (2004) Epidemiology of human parvovirus B19 in children with sickle cell disease. *Blood*, **103**, 422–7.

Soderlund, M., von Essen, R., Haapasaari, J., *et al.* (1997) Persistence of parvovirus B19 DNA in synovial membranes of young patients with and without chronic arthropathy. *Lancet*, **349**, 1063–5.

Solheim, B. G., Rollag, H., Svennevig, J. L., *et al.* (2000) Viral safety of solvent/detergent-treated plasma. *Transfusion*, **40**, 84–90.

Speyer, I., Breedveld, F. C. and Dijkmans, B. A. (1998) Human parvovirus B19 infection is not followed by inflammatory joint disease during long term follow-up. A retrospective study of 54 patients. *Clin Exp Rheumatol*, **16**, 576–8.

Tabor, E. and Epstein, J. S. (2002) NAT screening of blood and plasma donations: evolution of technology and regulatory policy. *Transfusion*, **42**(9), 1230–7.

Takahashi, Y., Murai, C., Shibata, S., *et al.* (1998) Human parvovirus B19 as a causative agent for rheumatoid arthritis. *Proceedings of the National Academy of Science USA*, **95**, 8227–32.

Török, T. J. (1997). Unusual clinical manifestations reported in patients with parvovirus B19 infection. L. J. Anderson and N. S. Young Human parvovirus B19. 1(20), 61–92. Basel, Karger. Monographs in Virology. Parks, W. P. 1997. Ref Type: Serial (Book, Monograph).

Tsujimura, M., Matsushita, K., Shiraki, H., *et al.* (1995) Human parvovirus B19 infection in blood donors. *Vox Sang*, **69**, 206–12.

Wakamatsu, C., Takakura, F., Kojima, E., *et al.* (1999) Screening of blood donors for human parvovirus B19 and characterization of the results. *Vox Sang*, **76**, 14–21.

Weiland, H. T., Vermey-Keers, C., Salimans, M. M., *et al.* (1987) Parvovirus B19 associated with fetal abnormality (letter). *Lancet*, **i**, 682–3.

White, D. G., Woolf, A. D., Mortimer, P. P., *et al.* (1985) Human parvovirus arthropathy. *Lancet*, **i**, 419–21.

Woolf, A. D. (1990) Human parvovirus B19 and arthritis. *Behring Inst Mitt*, 64–8.

Wu, C. G., Mason, B., Jong, J., *et al.* (2005) Parvovirus B19 transmission by a high-purity factor VIII concentrate. *Transfusion*, **45**, 1003–10.

Yaegashi, N., Shiraishi, H., Takeshita, T., *et al.* (1989) Propagation of human parvovirus B19 in primary culture of erythroid lineage cells derived from fetal liver. *J Virol*, **63**, 2422–26.

Yoto, Y., Kudoh, T., Haseyama, K., *et al.* (1995) Incidence of human parvovirus B19 DNA detection in blood donors. *Br J Haematol*, **91**, 1017–18.

Young, N. (1988) Hematologic and hematopoietic consequences of B19 parvovirus infection. *Semin Hematol*, **25**, 159–72.

Young, N. S. and Brown, K. E. (2004) Parvovirus B19. *N Eng J Med*, **350**, 586–97.

Yunoki, M., Tsujikawa, M., Urayama, T., *et al.* (2003) Heat sensitivity of human parvovirus B19. *Vox Sang*, **85**(1), 67–8.

Zadori, Z., Szelei, J., Lacoste, M. C., *et al.* (2001) A viral phospholipase A2 is required for parvovirus infectivity. *Dev Cell*, **1**, 291–302.

Zanella, A., Rossi, F., Cesana, C., *et al.* (1995) Transfusion-transmitted human parvovirus B19 infection in a thalassemic patient. *Transfusion*, **35**, 769–72.

6 EMERGING VIRUSES IN TRANSFUSION

Jean-Pierre Allain

Introduction

The availability of a broad range of molecular biological techniques following the development of polymerase chain reaction (PCR) had a major impact on the discovery of new viruses, often outside the classical context of a clinical disease. Conversely, the same techniques were used to examine diseases of unknown aetiology where a viral involvement was suspected and a virus was identified, long, controversial, and often inconclusive data were assembled by investigators to demonstrate the connection between this viral agent and the original disease such as human herpes virus 8 (HHV-8) in multiple myeloma. Besides the virological issues, in such circumstances, relevance to transfusion was invariably examined, irrespective of pathogenicity (Allain, 2000).

In the past ten years, several extra- and intra-cellular viruses have been discovered or re-discovered and only one, West Nile virus (WNV), led to blood screening, the other viruses are at the present time considered not worthy of screening due to lack of pathogenicity (GBV-C/HGV, TTV, SEN-V) and/or high prevalence (TTV, SEN-V), or lack of evidence of transfusion-transmissibility despite clear pathogenicity, for example HHV-8. Another issue explaining the reluctance to screen was that most viruses needed genomic amplification methods for detection (please refer to Chapter 14) and this added substantially to the complication and costs of current procedures for blood testing (Allain *et al.*, 2002).

Despite these limitations of scope and practicality, it is important in the context of transfusion microbiology to be aware of these viruses whose features and pathogenicity can be better understood in the future, and this may influence future policy.

GB virus C/hepatitis G virus

Virology

GB virus C/hepatitis G virus is an enveloped RNA virus member of the Flaviviridae family (that includes HCV) which was discovered simultaneously by two groups in 1995. The virus genome organization is similar to that of HCV with which GBV-C/HGV has 25% homology at the nucleotide level (Karayiannis and Thomas, 1997). The two prototype viruses have 86% and 95% homology at the nucleotide and amino acid levels, respectively. The single strand of RNA contains a single open reading frame encoding for a polyprotein enzymatically cleaved by endogenous and cellular enzymes into three structural and several non-structural proteins including a helicase and a protease. At the 5′ and 3′ ends of the viral RNA are two non-coding regions critical for the virus replication. They are relatively more conserved than the regions coding for the three structural and other non-structural viral proteins. There is no defined region corresponding to the core protein. GB virus C/hepatitis G virus envelope glycoprotein does not seem to contain an equivalent of the hypervariable region of HCV which might explain the high frequency of recovery from infection after the development of neutralizing antibodies. Phylogenetic analysis carried out in various regions of the viral genome revealed a considerable diversity (Muerhoff *et al.*, 1996). Five genotypes have been described: genotype 1 – mostly prevalent in Africa, genotype 2 – in Europe and North America, genotypes 3 and 4 – in South-east Asia and genotype 5 in South Africa (see Table 6.1). The relative geographical specificity of these subtypes is found with 5′ NCR-based sequences but tends to erode when using other, less conserved, regions such as NS3 or NS5 (Muerhoff *et al.*, 1996).

Similar to other flavivirus, GBV-C circulates as a quasispecies of related variants despite the absence of hypervariable regions (George *et al.*, 2003). Two studies reported evidence of recombination between strains of different genotypes (Worobey and Holmes, 2001) and one case of superinfection in an immunosuppressed organ recipient was described (Fan *et al.*, 2002).

Recent studies attempting to identify the HGV target cell suggested hepatocytes and peripheral mononuclear cells. The virus appears to replicate in both cell types although no cytopathic effect was found in hepatocytes. Several studies identified HGV RNA in purified peripheral blood mononuclear cells (PBMC) but it is not known whether peripheral lymphocytes are a major or a minor target, as they are for HCV (Sheng *et al.*, 1997). Interference of GBV-C with HIV replication suggests that CD4 T-cells are a target common to both viruses.

Natural history

Limited data on the natural history of GBV-C/HGV infection is available. In HCV and HGV coinfection, occurrence of viraemia is simultaneous at approximately two weeks post-transfusion. Subsequently, GBV-C/HGV viraemia increases progressively reaching 10^5 to 10^6 copies/ml (see Figure 6.1). A period of viraemia of three months to several years follows before the development of neutralizing antibodies leading to infection recovery (Alter *et al.*, 1997). In a few cases of dual HCV and HGV infection by transfusion or in IV drug abusers, it was shown that the pre-seroconversion window period was approximately three months, similar to HCV. Following the development of specific neutralizing antibodies to the major envelope E2 protein, GBV-C/HGV RNA becomes undetectable. In immunocompetent infected individuals, such as recipients of blood

Transfusion Microbiology, eds John A. J. Barbara, Fiona A. M. Regan and Marcela C. Contreras. Published by Cambridge University Press. © Cambridge University Press 2008.

Table 6.1 Geographical distribution of GBV-C/HGV prevalence and genotypes in blood donors.

Geographic area	HGV-C/HGV RNA % prevalence in blood donors	Anti-E2 prevalence % in blood donors	Genotypes
Western Europe	1.2–3.2	3.2–15.3	2a, 2b
North America	1.7–2.7	7–10	2a, 2b
South America	5.5	19.5	2a, 2b, 3
Africa	10.3–19	20–59	1, 2a, new variant
Asia	0.8–6.6	3–6	3, 4
Australia	2.5–3	10–11	2a, 2b

Distribution of HCV and GBV-C RNA load

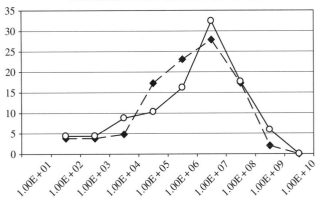

Figure 6.1 Distribution of viral load of HCV (solid line) and GBV-C (dashed line) expressed in copies/ml. HCV data are from 104 UK and Ghanian samples from our laboratory. GBV-C data are from Saito et al., (1998); *J Virol Methods*, **74**, 185–91.

for surgery or haemophiliacs who were not infected with HIV, approximately 80% recover and develop anti-E2 (Heuft et al., 1998). This proportion is compatible with the 3:1 ratio between anti-E2 and GBV-C/HGV RNA carriers observed in blood donors (see Table 6.1). An exception to this pattern has been observed in multitransfused patients with chronic congenital anaemia, such as thalassaemia major or sickle cell disease. The proportion of chronic carriers was approximately 75%, suggesting that chronic transfusion induces some degree of immunodeficiency (Lefrere et al., 1997). GB virus C/hepatitis G virus infection by transfusion of immunocompromised recipients under immunosuppressive drugs becomes significantly more often chronic (Heuft et al., 1998). Another feature of the infection is the relatively low level and the transitory nature of the antibody response. In multitransfused thalassaemics or patients with acute lymphoblastic leukaemia, nearly half of antibody positive patients became anti-E2 negative after 5–6 years of follow up. Some infected individuals may recover without the development of detectable anti-E2. It is therefore likely that, in the various populations studied, the proportion of exposed individuals might be higher than the simple sum of

RNA and anti-E2 carriers. This might explain in part the apparently lower transmission rate of GBV-C/HGV than HCV by non-virally inactivated plasma derivatives in haemophiliacs.

Transmission

The transmission features of GBV-C/HGV are remarkably similar to HCV. GB virus C has been shown to be primarily transmissible parenterally, including by transfusion, IV drug abuse and haemodialysis. Vertical transmission from infected mother to fetus or newborn seems to occur at a lower frequency than HCV transmission, although the levels of viraemia are approximately the same (see Figure 6.1). As in HCV infection, vertical transmission is related to viral load (Ohto et al., 2000). Preliminary reports suggest that nosocomial transmission, an important factor in HCV epidemiology, might be involved for GBV-C/HGV transmission (Lunel et al., 1998). Indirect evidence of homosexual or heterosexual transmission has been reported (Lefrere et al., 1999a). A progressive increase in prevalence with age suggests either nosocomial or horizontal transmission. Except in the context of parenteral transmission, GBV-C/HGV transmission appears independent of HCV epidemiology. In GBV-C marker carrier blood donors, an association was found with sexually transmitted diseases and sexual promiscuity as well as endoscopic procedures (Bjorkman et al., 2001).

GB virus C/hepatitis G virus in transfusion

Whole blood and blood components can transmit HGV but so do pooled plasma derivatives not submitted to virucidal procedures. In a recent study, 64% of recipients transfused with GBV-C RNA containing components became infected, suggesting that, compared to HCV, the threshold of infectivity is higher or that, as discussed above, some recipients have lost detectable specific antibodies but kept memory of the infection (Sentjens et al., 2003). In haemophiliacs treated with products not submitted to virucidal treatment, the rate of infection (40–50%) appears less than HCV and only 7 to 15% remain chronically viraemic. In plasma derivatives, the difference with HCV might be related to the presence of GBV-C/HGV neutralizing antibodies in plasma pools and in the IgG contaminated intermediate purity concentrates available prior to 1985. The former hypothesis is supported by the low GBV-C/HGV infection rate (despite nearly 100% detection of HGV RNA) in recipients of HCV-transmitting intravenous immunoglobulin to agammaglobulinaemic recipients. Virus inactivated products do not seem to transmit GBV-C/HGV but the rate of infection in recipients of these products remains substantial while no HCV infection is observed. This surprising observation might reflect the transmission of GBV-C/HGV through routes other than blood products in haemophiliacs.

The prevalence of GBV-C/HGV in blood donor populations in developed countries ranges between 1% and 5%, but these numbers correspond to HGV RNA positive, persistent infections (Lefrere et al., 1997; 1999a). Anti-E2 is present in three to four times more donors, indicating past infection and recovery from the infection (see Table 6.1) (Lefrere et al., 1997). In classical high-risk groups (IV drug abusers, chronic haemodialysis, recipients of multiple transfusions), the prevalence of HGV RNA ranges between 7 and 57% and anti-E2 between 25 and 62%. Transfusion recipients and other patients who are immunocompromised by immunosuppressive drugs, HIV infection, or genetically, are at higher risk of persistent infection (Heringlake *et al.*, 1996).

Pathogenicity

The main debate regarding HGV has been its pathogenicity. Having been discovered in patients with post-transfusion non-A–E hepatitis, the assumption and the initial name of the virus suggested a causal relation to hepatitis. However, many subsequent epidemiological investigations concluded that GBV-C/HGV was not a cause of viral hepatitis (Lefrere *et al.*, 1999a). In individuals persistently infected by transfusion and other routes, there is no correlation with elevation of liver enzymes. Although hepatocytes can be a target for HGV, no cytopathic effect has been found (Halasz *et al.*, 2000). However, some investigators have described the association of HGV with cases of fulminant hepatitis. One of them described an HGV genotype with specific mutations in the NS3 region in all patients (Heringlake *et al.*, 1996). These associations have not been confirmed by other groups and remain controversial (Munoz *et al.*, 1999). Similarly, the role of HGV in cases of aplastic anaemia and non-Hodgkin lymphomas has been suggested by some and denied by other investigators. To date, no definite pathogenic role can be attributed to GBV-C/HGV. At present, the pathogenicity of GBV-C/HGV remains unknown.

A new chapter of GBV-C pathogenicity was opened with the finding that HIV infected patients coinfected with GBV-C had a significantly better clinical outcome (Lefrere *et al.*, 1999b). This surprising observation was later confirmed by several groups (Tillman *et al.*, 2001 and Xiang *et al.*, 2001). The interference is clear only when both viruses actively replicate, and much less in anti-E2 carriers. There were suggestions that the mechanism of such viral interference was the competition between the two T-cell tropic viruses for the same receptors or the same cytokines. The clinical importance of this was such that there was speculation about the potential use of GBV-C infection in preventing HIV clinical progression. However, the interference lasts only whilst the virus replicates and not once antibody production occurs.

Diagnosis of GB virus C/hepatitis G virus

Although the virus clearly meets the criteria for transfusion-transmission of low prevalence of viraemia and persistence in a sizeable number of individuals, it lacks demonstrable pathogenicity and the only appropriate means of detection is genomic amplification (Lefrere *et al.*, 1997). To date, no commercial assay has been developed that could be applied to testing a large number of samples. Although not relevant to transfusion, diagnosis of GBV-C infection can also be made by detection of anti-E2 using research EIA kits prepared by diagnostic companies. As previously mentioned, antibodies are short-lived and some individuals, negative for both RNA and anti-E2, might have been infected.

Kaposi's sarcoma associated herpes virus (KSHV) or human herpes virus 8 (HHV-8)

Virology

Kaposi's sarcoma associated herpes virus or human herpes virus 8 is a gamma herpes virus whose initial sequence has been discovered by Representational Difference Analysis (RDA) in the lesion of HIV infected patients with Kaposi's sarcoma (KS) in 1994. Human herpes virus 8 has also been found in classical (non-HIV infected) KS and other tumours such as multicentre Castleman's disease (MCD) and body cavity based lymphoma (BCBL). Human herpes virus 8 also seems associated with polyneuropathy, organomegaly, endocrinopathy, M protein and skin changes (POEMS), a rare syndrome often associated with MCD (Belec *et al.*, 1999).

The genomic organization of this 140 Kb double-stranded DNA virus appears similar to other gamma-herpes virinae such as EBV or herpes virus Saimiri with which HHV-8 shares 39 and 51% amino acid identity, respectively. Like CMV and EBV, HHV-8 seems to cause a persistent infection, the viral genome remaining mostly latent in host cells when contained by the host immune system. Latent virus can be re-activated in immunocompromised hosts after HIV infection or immunosuppressive treatment.

One domain of HHV-8 (K1) is highly variable, particularly in an extra-cellular loop. Sequencing this domain revealed four different genotypes with some geographic specificity (Meng, 1999). Human herpes virus 8 seems to have two main target cells (Boschoff and Weiss, 1998). A substantial proportion of endothelial cells in KS lesions and in non-lesion tissue in KS patients contain HHV-8 genome, often in a latent state. Tumour cells of MCD and BCBL are transformed B-lymphocytes; some of them have been established as HHV-8 infected cell lines. Several cell lines harbour both HHV-8 and EBV; other cell lines permanently replicate HHV-8 only. In apparently healthy HHV-8 infected individuals, the viral genome is preferentially detected in B-cells, although there is some evidence that monocytes may also harbour the virus. While HHV-8 is detectable in virtually 100% of KS lesions, it is detected in 50–100% of patients' peripheral blood mononuclear cells (PBMC), particularly in CD19 purified B-cell fractions (see Table 6.2). The level of detectable virus seems higher in HIV infected KS, possibly in relation to an enhancing effect of the HIV Tat protein. Human herpes virus 8 has also been

Table 6.2 Serology and PCR for HHV-8 detection.

Source of samples	Per cent positive		
	Anti-HHV-8 lytic	Anti-HHV-8 latent	PCR PBMC
Patients with			
KS	80–97	83	45
Before KS	54–100	77	31
No KS	16–64	20	8
Blood donors	0–10	10	0

(Spira *et al.*, 2000)

found in PBMCs of individuals who are HIV positive or negative without KS or other lymphoid tumours.

Although not formally demonstrated, a number of converging observations suggest that HHV-8 is causal for KS (Boschoff and Weiss, 1998). In HIV infected patients, HHV-8 infection always precedes the occurrence of KS by several months. Human herpes virus 8 genome encodes and expresses the G-protein-coupled receptor (GPCR), which has been shown to act as an oncogene, inducing an angiogenic switch in cultured endothelial cells. One of the main features of HHV-8, shared in part with some other human herpes viruses, is the presence in the viral genome of sequences encoding proteins possibly involved in the monoclonal cell proliferation leading to KS and other tumours. Some of these genes have been borrowed from human cellular genes with which they have the highest homology (Boschoff and Weiss, 1998). Viral gene products essentially interfere with the normal cell cycle, which tends, upon viral aggression, to react by undergoing apoptosis. Viral Bcl2 and a product of ORF 71 can prevent apoptosis. Other viral gene products, such as cyclin 2, IL-6, IL-8-like G-coupled protein and Interferon Regulatory Factor, induce or contribute to cell proliferation. Transformed cells seem to be accompanied by secretion of vascular endothelial growth factor (VEGF) that is known to be over-expressed in KS cells, although the direct link between GPCR and induction of VEGF has not been formally demonstrated. Human primary endothelial cells infected with free HHV-8 can be immortalized. Cells acquire telomerase activity and anchorage-independent growth, all characteristics of cancer cells. In addition, infected cells produce (VEGF) that enhances the survival of uninfected cells.

Similarly to EBV, HHV-8 expresses different antigens in the latent state (latent antigens) than in the stimulated, cytolytic form (lytic antigens) (see Table 6.2). Preliminary evidence suggests that induction from latent to cytolytic stage, requiring several levels of massive stimulation, does not occur easily in cell culture and that HHV-8 infected tumours do not appear in immunocompetent individuals. In the presence of latent HHV-8 infection that has been found in a small percentage of apparently healthy individuals, a severe state of immunodepression such as caused by HIV infection or immunosuppressive drugs seems necessary for tumour induction. Conversely, KS spectacularly regresses after discontinuation of immunosuppressive regimes.

Methods of detection

The epidemiology of HHV-8 had been studied initially with genomic amplification by direct or nested PCR on PBMCs and, more than one year later, by various antibody detection assays. Peripheral blood monocyte cells do not seem the optimal sample to detect HHV-8 genome since not all KS patients are positive (see Table 6.2). Similarly, HHV-8 sequences are detected in virtually all cases of BCBL, but only in a majority of MCD or POEMS. Even when using nested PCR, sensitivity is low, particularly in HIV negative individuals. It improves when CD19 cells are used as a source of DNA but this is not very practical. Human herpes virus 8 genome has also been detected using whole blood as a source of DNA. In patients doubly infected with HIV and HHV-8, the latter

genome has been quantified by real-time PCR and found to correlate with KS clinical progression (Malnati et al., 2002). The detectability of HHV-8 is greatly dependent on the sensitivity of the genomic amplification method used, particularly nested PCR (see Chapter 14). It is recommended that several primer pairs are tested and a result is accepted as positive only when several parts of the genome can be amplified (Meng et al., 1999; Tisdale et al., 1998). The uncertainty of HHV-8 genomic detection has been to a large extent the source of the controversy with regard to the potential role of HHV-8 in multiple myeloma (MM). Great variation in the amount of virus was observed in association with tumours, ranging between 8–9 logs in KS lesions to 1–2 logs in MCD and POEMS (Lefrere et al., 1999b). In peripheral blood or PBMCs, viraemia was found in some serologically positive individuals. Patients with acquired or induced immunosuppression tend to have higher numbers of infected cells. This was suggested in kidney transplant recipients who were HHV-8 seropositive but DNA negative prior to transplant and became positive soon after the induction of immunosuppressive treatment. The simultaneous presence of HHV-8 DNA in PBMC and plasma in two patients with KS followed by the disappearance of DNA when the tumour regressed, suggests that low levels of viraemia are present but below the limit of detection in many seropositive individuals.

Antibodies to HHV-8 antigens have been detected by Western blot, immunofluorescence assay (IFA), using whole cells or isolated nuclei from HHV-8 infected cells as the antigen source (Blackbourn et al., 1997; Gao et al., 1996). At least one IFA kit is commercially available. Recombinant proteins were obtained from part of the ORF 73 or the capsid antigen from ORF 65 (Simpson et al., 1996). Enzyme linked immunosorbent assays have been developed in several laboratories but no commercial EIA is currently available. As observed with molecular detection, discrepancies between methods of antibody detection using various antigens or different cell lines have been observed (see Table 6.2). To avoid false reactions, it is recommended that multiple assay types or antigens are used and confirmation is performed, preferably by Western blot. With all assays, higher positivity rates with serological assays than with genomic amplification methods were found in patients with KS. The two types of antigens provide similar prevalence, ranging from 81 to 100% in KS patients. In seropositive, apparently healthy individuals, HHV-8 DNA is usually not detected in the peripheral cells or plasma. However, occasional blood donors were HHV-8 DNA positive in PBMC but 3 to 27% of HIV infected homosexual males without KS were positive.

Epidemiology

The epidemiology of HHV-8 appears radically different in areas where the infection is endemic and those where it is rare. In endemic areas such as Africa, tropical South America and southern Italy, the mode of transmission is essentially horizontal from mother to child or other household member and child, probably through saliva (Brayfield et al., 2003; Gao et al., 1996; Gessain et al., 1999; Mantina et al., 2001; Mbulaiteye et al., 2003).

Table 6.3 Risk of HHV-8 infection and KS post-kidney transplant.

Sero + recipients pre-transplant are at risk of KS	
Parravicini *et al.*, 1997	77% at 2 yrs
Farge *et al.*, 1999	30% at 1 yr
Frances *et al.*, 2000	28% at 3 yrs
Sero + kidney donors often transmit HHV-8	
Regamey *et al.*, 1998	83%
Seroconverting recipients are at risk of KS	
Parravicini *et al.*, 1997	25% (1/4)
Regamey *et al.*, 1998	8% (2/25)

However, there is some evidence of vertical transmission, in part related to maternal viral load (Mantina *et al.*, 2001). This explains the rapidly increasing prevalence with children's age. After age 15, there is evidence of sexual transmission between spouses or with commercial sex (Lavreys *et al.*, 2002; Mbulaiteye *et al.*, 2003). The infection rate ranges between 35 and 75% in African populations and blood donors, irrespective of the HIV status. Human herpes virus 8 DNA is found in 10–50% of PBMC from African individuals, depending on HIV status. In HIV seronegative populations, 10–20% of anti-HHV-8 positive individuals carry detectable levels of HHV-8 DNA.

In Western countries, HHV-8 seems to be sexually transmitted, particularly homosexually. In the USA and Europe, HHV-8 seropositivity has been found frequently in cohorts of homosexual men and directly related to the frequency of KS when HIV infected. Other groups at high risk of HIV infection such as intravenous drug users (IVDU) and haemophiliacs, have both a low incidence of KS and low prevalence of HHV-8 infection (Renwick *et al.*, 2002). However, there is evidence of HHV-8 transmission by IV drug use although the efficacy of transmission is considerably lower than for other viruses such as HBV, HIV or HCV (Cannon *et al.*, 2001).

A high prevalence of HHV-8 antibodies was found in 12 to 30% of homosexual males; in 6% of heterosexual males or females attending STD clinics; and in 3% of IVDU. In blood donors, seroprevalence ranged between 0 and 5% in most studies, but one study found a 20% prevalence in the USA (Blackbourn *et al.*, 1997; Lennette, 1996).

At present, the transmissibility of HHV-8 by blood and cellular blood products has not been demonstrated in studies, including a small study targeting immunosuppressed kidney transplant recipients (Blackbourn *et al.*, 1997; Cattani *et al.*, 2000; Farge *et al.*, 1999). However, transmissibility by IVDU suggests that transfusion may be infectious (Cannon *et al.*, 2001).

Human herpes virus 8 and transplantation

Kaposi's sarcoma has been described with relatively high frequency within two years after renal transplantation (1–3%). Kaposi's sarcoma after transplantation of other organs such as heart or lungs has been described (Jones *et al.*, 1998). Kidney transplant recipients HHV-8 infected prior to transplantation or infected post-transplantation, essentially by HHV-8 infected

organs, are at high risk of KS within two years after transplantation (see Table 6.3).

Reactivation of a latent HHV-8 infection by immunosuppression rather than new infection by transfusion, was observed (Parravicini *et al.*, 1997; Regamey *et al.*, 1998) and may explain HHV-8 infection in recipients who did not receive an infected organ (Jenkins *et al.*, 2002; Regamey *et al.*, 1998). Human herpes virus 8 infection or KS post-transplantation can occur either as a result of recipient occult HHV-8 infection or transmission by an organ taken from an HHV-8 infected donor (Farge *et al.*, 1999; Regamey *et al.*, 1998). Several studies have observed an increase in anti-HHV-8 prevalence after organ transplantation and an increase in antibody titres in patients seropositive pre-transplantation (Rettig *et al.*, 1997). These apparently new infections might be related to increased susceptibility to community infection or reactivation in individuals with undetectable antibody level. The only risk factors associated with post-transplantation KS are HHV-8 infection, the use of anti-lymphocyte antibodies in the immunosuppressive cocktail, and, indirectly, the patients' geographical origin, as individuals from higher HHV-8 prevalence countries are at higher risk (Farge *et al.*, 1999).

This data strongly suggests that HHV-8 infection should be systematically screened for in candidates for organ transplantation. Organ donors, particularly kidney donors, should also be tested for the presence of HHV-8 antibody in serum and HHV-8 DNA in PBMCs. Organs from HHV-8 seropositive donors should not be used. Although no evidence of HHV-8 transfusion-transmission in immunocompetent or immunocompromised recipients is available, universal leucodepletion as practised in several countries may provide an additional security by removing HHV-8 infected mononuclear cells.

Pathogenicity of human herpes virus 8 other than Kaposi's sarcoma, body cavity based lymphoma, multi centre Castleman's disease and poly neuropathy, organomegaly, endocrinopathy, M protein and skin changes

Recently, a major controversy developed regarding the potential association between HHV-8 and multiple myeloma (MM) (Farge *et al.*, 1999). Human herpes virus 8 related sequences were found in 15/15 bone marrow stromal cells in culture but not in bone marrow mononuclear cells. The same group confirmed their findings by in situ hybridization in bone marrow biopsy. A causal role of HHV-8 in MM was suggested but could not be confirmed by other investigators (Tisdale *et al.*, 1998). Besides the fact that four separate groups studying either cultured stromal cells or biopsies failed to demonstrate the presence of HHV-8 genome, several other lines of evidence do not seem to support the claim.

(1) Epidemiological data does not find any correlation between the incidences of KS and MM or of other cancer. Patients with MM do not carry antibody to HHV-8 at prevalence above the background population.

(2) Six groups studied peripheral blood dendritic cells before and after mobilization and either did not find the HHV-8 genome

or found a moderate increase in frequency corresponding to an improvement in testing sensitivity.

(3) Several investigators failed to detect the HHV-8 genome in BM by single PCR but found a weak signal with a nested method (Tisdale et al., 1998). Such a highly sensitive method also found a high frequency of positive results in the controls. Others observed a discrepancy between results obtained with different primer pairs. Not unlike an earlier controversy on the role of HTLV-I in multiple sclerosis, it appears unlikely that HHV-8 is the cause of multiple myeloma.

Several recent reports indicated that HHV-8 was involved in bone marrow failures in immunodeficient individuals receiving either organ or bone marrow transplantation (Luppi et al., 2000a; 2000b). Evidence was given that HHV-8 could directly infect bone marrow progenitor cells.

In summary, there is evidence that HHV-8 can be transmitted by blood but is not that easily transmissible by transfusion, probably because of the very small number of infected cells in infected blood donors who are not HIV infected or otherwise immunocompromised. In addition, leucodepletion of all blood components is likely to further decrease this potential risk. Individuals already infected by HHV-8 who become HIV infected or receive major immunosuppressive treatment, such as in organ transplantation, reactivate the infection and viral production increases, leading to high risk of developing KS. In addition, HHV-8 can be transmitted by the transplantation of organs from HHV-8 infected donors. There is therefore a need to screen all potential organ recipients or HIV infected individuals for anti-HHV-8 to inform them of the risk of developing KS or other related tumours. All organ donors should also be screened for antibody to HHV-8 and, when a positive result is obtained, the organ should not be transplanted.

TT virus

In late 1997, using representational differential analysis (RDA) in the serum of a patient with post-transfusion hepatitis of unknown etiology, sequences suggestive of a novel DNA virus were identified by a Japanese group of investigators. Patient TT was one of five patients with non-A–G hepatitis who had moderately elevated transaminase levels 6 to 21 weeks post-transfusion. His initials were given to the new virus.

Virology

TT virus is a small (18–50 nm) DNA, non-enveloped, virus with a 3852 nt genome, including two open reading frames. TT virus size and circular DNA make it similar to animal circovirinae (Mushawar et al., 1999; Okamoto et al., 1999). It is closely related to simian TT viruses, particularly chimpanzees that are susceptible to human TTV. In humans, TTV is remarkably variable in the ORF1 region (up to 50%) but more conserved in the 5' non-coding regions; this probably explains the major discrepancies observed in prevalence of TTV DNA depending on the primer pairs used. Several viruses with 60% or less nucleotide homology with the TTV prototype have been described (SANBAN, TUS01) and probably represent distant variants of TTV rather than new viruses.

On the basis of the N22 section of ORF 1, at least 11 genotypes have been described. When considering the whole genome, only six genotypes emerge; a genotype being defined as >30% difference at the nucleotide level. All genotypes are found in various parts of the world, consistent with TTV being a very ubiquitous virus established in humans for over a million years (Devalle and Niel, 2004). Recent data suggests that recombinations between subtypes are frequent, potentially explaining the group diversity (Manni et al., 2002).

TT virus DNA has been found in plasma and PBMCs, in saliva, faeces, tears and semen of viraemic individuals. In addition, replicative, double-stranded forms of TTV have been identified in bone marrow cells and hepatocytes. Although the level of viraemia is consistently low (median 10^4 geq/ml), even in immunocompromised individuals, TTV tends to persist for several years post infection (Lefrere et al., 2000; Pistello et al., 2001). Ultimately, viral DNA becomes undetectable either by infection recovery through an immune response or a decrease of viral production. There is indirect evidence of the second mechanism since TTV DNA negative individuals undergoing organ transplantation become viraemic days after the induction of the immunosuppressive regime, suggesting a reactivation of viral production.

Relatively little is known about the host immune response to TTV. The presence of antibodies was initially shown by an insensitive immunoprecipitation method (Tsuda et al., 1999) that found some cases where viral DNA appeared cleared by the occurrence of antibodies but some others where DNA and antibodies co-existed. Antibodies to a recombinant part of ORF1 revealed 99% positivity while 76% carried viral DNA (Ott et al., 2000). An assay detecting specific IgM was developed that showed this class of antibodies were detectable only during a few weeks after primary infection (Tsuda et al., 2001). The lower IgG prevalence found in another study might have been related to the choice of a rare antigen cross-reacting poorly with ubiquitous strains (Kakkola et al., 2004). This data seems to indicate that a neutralizing response does not occur or is not effective.

Epidemiology

Multiple routes of transmission of TTV are likely as viral DNA is found in most body fluids. In line with the low level of viraemia, vertical transmission does not seem to occur frequently. Infants are rapidly infected during the first year of life, reaching 50% prevalence of viraemia by one year of age. There is evidence that the aerosol route is the most likely to explain horizontal transmission (Lin et al., 2002; Ohto et al., 2002). Intravenous drug use does not appear a frequent route of transmission. Clear evidence of transmission by transfusion and patients in chronic dialysis has been provided. Acquired or induced immunodeficiency, including by frequent transfusions, seems to increase the rate of persistence of TTV. Transmission studies are strictly based on genomic detection of TTV, without testing for serological markers. It is therefore difficult to distinguish between reactivation, superinfection and genuine infection. Several investigators have described the simultaneous presence of multiple genotypes in humans or chimpanzees, suggesting that super-infection does occur.

Prevalence of TT virus infection

The prevalence of TTV DNA ranges between 2% and 60% in blood donors when screened with N22/ORF1 primers. It ranges between 1.5 and 27% in Europe (Kakkola *et al.*, 2004), 1 and 8% in the USA, 29 and 83% in Africa, 11 and 43% in Asia. Using NCR primers, the prevalence of TTV DNA in blood donors rises to 40 to 82% (Okamoto *et al.*, 1999; Simmonds *et al.*, 1998). This data is consistent with TTV being an extremely ubiquitous and harmless infection whose prevalence was initially underestimated because of the restriction imposed by the extreme variability of the N22 region from which the first primers were derived (Sugiyama *et al.*, 1999). It is likely that non-viraemic blood donors have recovered from the infection or that the detection methods are not sensitive enough. The relevance of TTV in the transfusion setting is therefore limited, since most blood recipients have been in contact with TTV prior to transfusion. In addition, clear cases of transfusion-transmission are not accompanied by any clinical symptoms; in particular, the ALT level remains unchanged (Lefrere *et al.*, 2000). This interpretation of available data is supported by the similar prevalence of TTV viraemia observed in multitransfused haemophiliacs, whether or not they have received virally inactivated plasma derivatives. No clear evidence of TTV inactivation with the current inactivation procedures has been provided.

Pathogenicity

To date, no specific pathogenicity has been attributed to TTV. In young children, the TTV load in nasal secretions is extremely high and might be correlated with some acute respiratory syndrome (Maggi *et al.*, 2003). It is not associated with non-A–E hepatitis and chronic carriers have normal liver function (Lefrere *et al.*, 2000). No co-factor role in the development of AIDS in HIV infected patients or of chronic liver disease in HCV infected patients has been demonstrated. The potential causal or co-factor role of TTV infection in hepatocellular carcinoma has been denied.

In summary, TTV is a ubiquitous, apparently harmless virus infecting the majority of the human population at a young age. Although transmissible by transfusion, the high prevalence in both donors and recipients make its detection by genomic amplification irrelevant to blood transfusion. The lack of solid immunity to TTV explains the apparent frequency of infection with multiple strains and recombination.

SEN virus

A novel DNA virus designated SEN virus (SEN-V) was discovered in the serum of an intravenous drug user coinfected with HIV (Alter *et al.*, 1997; Umemura *et al.*, 2001). Like HCV or GBV-C/HGV, a commercial company (DiaSorin), in collaboration with an American research group identified the new virus and performed

Table 6.4 Prevalence of active SEN-V infection.

Area	Population tested	N	SEN-V DNA + (%)
USA	Volunteer donors	436	8 (1.8)
Japan	General population	194	118 (61)
China	Volunteer donors	—	15.1%
Japan	Volunteer donors	49	14 (28.6)
Japan	Volunteer donors	277	27 (10)

Rettig *et al.* (1997) and Sheng *et al.* (1997).

the preliminary studies on its molecular biology, prevalence and clinical relevance.

SEN virus is a single-stranded DNA virus of approximately 3800 nucleotides. Phylogenetic analysis of SEN-V has demonstrated the existence of eight strains or genotypes, designated from A to H (Alter *et al.*, 1997). Though structurally similar to TTV, SEN-V has less than 55% sequence homology and less than 37% amino acid homology with the TTV prototype. Like TTV, SEN-V has been classified into the human Circoviridae family.

Active infection is frequent in healthy blood donors and general populations (see Table 6.4). Some SEN-V strains are of particularly high prevalence, especially SENV-B. SEN virus A and SENV-E are less frequently found among blood donors and do not appear to be related to non-A–E hepatitis. In contrast, genotypes D and H have been found in only 1% of blood donors but in more than 50% of non-A–E hepatitis cases. These two subtypes seem more implicated in transfusion-transmission. Chronic infection is detected in patients with various hepatic diseases. Despite the favourable ratio donors/acute hepatitis for SEN-V D and H and the fact that preliminary data suggest that SEN-V can replicate in the liver, no true association between SEN-V and liver damage has been proved so far in multiple studies conducted in Japan, Thailand, China, Canada and the USA (Mikuni *et al.*, 2002; Umemura *et al.*, 2001; 2003; Wong *et al.*, 2002; Yoshida *et al.*, 2002). As discussed with TTV, recovery and elimination of viraemia does not appear frequent and patients can be infected with multiple strains and subtypes (Kojima *et al.*, 2003). In addition, in cases of HCV/SEN-V genotype C or D coinfections, anti-viral treatment did not affect levels of SEN-V viraemia (Rigas *et al.*, 2001).

Little is known on the natural history of the infection. Chronic infections over ten years have been observed in retrospectively tested samples of infected individuals, but most patients clear viraemia during the first months of exposure. Therefore, true exposure to virus is difficult to assess, as no serological test for SEN-V antibodies is currently available. Vertical transmission occurs infrequently, probably because of relatively low viral load (Pirovano *et al.*, 2002). Most infections occur at a young age and horizontally, as for TTV. Similar to TTV, SEN-V DNA can only be detected by NAT using primers from conserved, genotype-independent regions. Qualitative PCR with primers specific to genotypes D and H, and a quantitative PCR assay based on micro-well hybridization of PCR products have also been described (Umemura *et al.*, 2001). Design of quantitative NAT for SEN-V can be complicated by the variability of the viral genome.

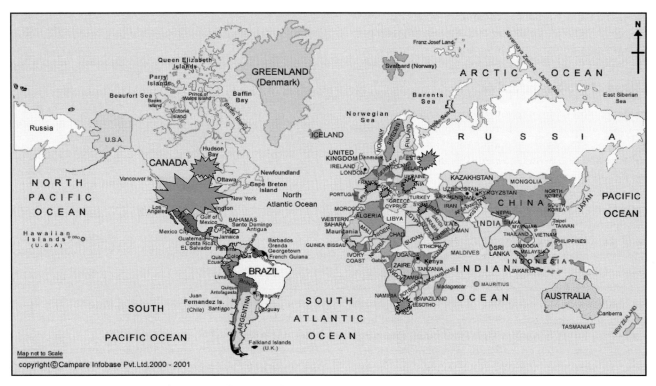

Figure 6.2 Location of recent WNV outbreaks reported in the world. Yellow stars indicate an outbreak.

A mutation rate close to that found in RNA viruses and higher than in other DNA viruses has been observed in serial samples of infected individuals (Umemura *et al.*, 2002).

SEN virus is transmitted by blood as demonstrated by comparing sequence homology between donor and recipient (Mikuni *et al.*, 2002). Moreover, transfused patients are at higher risk of acquiring SEN-V than non-transfused patients (30% SEN-V positive vs. 3.1%, p > 0.001, respectively) (see Table 6.4). The risk of infection in transfused patients increased proportionally to the number of units of blood transfused. It must be expected that, like HCV or TTV, individuals at risk of repeated parenteral exposures are coinfected with more than one SEN-V genotype (Simmonds *et al.*, 1998). No data has yet been published on SEN-V epidemiology in Europe.

There is no specific pathogenicity so far attributed to SEN-V. Contrary to initial indications, a potential association with post-transfusion hepatitis was not confirmed. No association with hepatocellular carcinoma was found in Thailand (Tangkijvanich *et al.*, 2003).

West Nile virus

West Nile virus (WNV) is a mosquito-borne flavivirus that naturally infects birds but occasionally infects other hosts such as horses or humans in limited epidemics (Brinton, 2002; Campbell *et al.*, 2002). West Nile virus was discovered in Uganda in 1937 and is endemic in Africa, the Middle East and Europe, where human outbreaks have been reported in Romania, Russia, Israel and France. It was not considered a transfusion threat until the virus was introduced in the USA in 1999, where

in three years it spread from the initial foci of New York City and Miami to cover the entire North American continent (Nash *et al.*, 2001) (please see Figure 6.2). The spread of the infection was preceded by massive numbers of bird deaths and occasional infection in humans. In 80% of cases, the infection is asymptomatic; in 20% a febrile episode called WNV fever occurs and in 1 in 150 contacts, neurological disease, particularly meningoencephalitis was reported (Anonymous, 2002a). The median age of infected individuals presenting with symptoms is 59 years and the neurological symptoms tend to occur in immunocompromised individuals such as the elderly or organ or bone marrow transplant recipients. In the USA in 2002, 3389 cases of WNV-related illnesses were reported, of whom 69% had meningoencephalitis. In this last group, 199 (9%) died and only 0.3% of those with WN fever died. The median age of deceased people was 78 years, but it ranged between 24 and 99 years (Chowers *et al.*, 2000).

Infections are reported between June and November, the mosquito season. These epidemiological features appear similar in the Middle Eastern, Eastern European and North American outbreaks (Campbell *et al.*, 2001; Chowers *et al.*, 2000).

The virus

West Nile virus is a 11 Kb single stranded positive polarity enveloped RNA virus with structural similarity with HCV and GBV-C, two other flaviviruses relevant to transfusion. Between the 5' (100 nucleotides) and 3' (600 nucleotides) non-coding regions, a single frame codes for three structural (core, membrane and envelope) proteins and seven non-structural proteins called NS1, NS2A, NS2B, NS3, NS4A, NS4B and NS5. As in HCV, NS3 is the viral protease and NS5 the viral polymerase (Brinton, 2002). No hypervariable region of the envelope protein has been described, consistent with the development of neutralizing antibodies leading to recovery from the infection. The incubation period lasts 3 to 14 days, the viral RNA being detectable at three days and the viraemic period lasting 1 to 11 days. The level of viraemia is relatively low, with a median of 10^4 copies/ml compared to 10^6 found in HCV and GBV-C infections (Anonymous, 2003). This low level of viraemia has bearing on the detection of the short infectious period relevant to transfusion. Towards the end of the viraemic period, IgM antibodies are detectable for a few weeks while an IgG response develops.

West Nile virus and transfusion

While previous limited epidemics did not draw attention to transfusion-transmission of WNV, the American outbreak was quickly marked by the transmission of the infection to four recipients of organs from an infected donor. All recipients developed severe neurological symptoms and one of them died. Subsequently, suspected and confirmed cases of WNV transmission by transfusion were described. In 2002, 33 cases were suspected and six of them were confirmed by the identification of viral RNA in the donations (Anonymous, 2002b). As a result, the health authorities in the USA and Canada mandated nucleic acid testing for WNV RNA in all blood donations from July 2003. In the first million donations screened, 329 (0.03%) were NAT reactive and 163 (0.015%) were confirmed to contain WNV RNA (Anonymous, 2003).

Detection of West Nile virus RNA

Currently, two commercial NAT assays are available. One is based on the transcription mediated amplification method and is specific for WNV (Chiron-GenProbe). The second method is by real-time RT-PCR using primers enabling co-detection of Japanese encephalitis virus, Saint Louis encephalitis virus and Murray valley virus in addition to WNV (please refer to Chapter 14). Owing to the relatively low level of viraemia during the acute phase of infection, testing is performed in pools of 6 or 16 plasma samples instead of 16, 24 or 48 plasmas as currently used for HCV and HIV RNA NAT. As approximately 50% of the reactive samples remain unconfirmed by alternative molecular assays, serological tests detecting IgM to WNV are also part of the confirmatory process.

Protection of the blood supply in countries other than North America

The WNV epidemics in the USA raised concerns about the possibility of transmission to recipients of blood components from donors who had stayed in North America. A ban of one to two months has been implemented in several European countries (Lefrere *et al.*, 2003). Several studies are currently ongoing to determine the risk of WNV transmission by blood components collected from European donors.

Conclusion

New or emerging viruses are an ongoing problem in transfusion. More research will be conducted to determine the pathogenicity of the viruses described in this chapter. Others will come. In addition, viruses prevalent in remote and circumscribed areas of the world may at any time be dispersed to the whole planet very rapidly as the SARS virus epidemic demonstrated. In most cases, these viruses are likely to be detected only with NAT, and screening for each new virus will be expensive and add to the complexity of blood screening, increasing the risk of errors. One solution to this problem has already been proposed although not widely implemented: pathogen inactivation (please refer to Chapter 19.). The viral burden already considerably reduced by the current serology and NAT could be usefully complemented by a last step that would inactivate known low prevalence, low pathogenicity, viruses and those still unknown. Despite the considerable amount of data (including in the clinical field) accumulated on several inactivating agents, more needs to be done to ensure the safety and efficacy of blood components submitted to these procedures.

Annexe

John A. J. Barbara

Respiratory infections: SARS and influenza

Classically, persistent virus infections have been recognized as the main microbial threat to transfusion safety. More recently, acute infections with transient viraemia but occurring with high incidence in a previously unexposed population (e.g. WNV, see Chapter 15) have posed different threats. With such new challenges, detection of antibodies to these infections cannot be used to identify infectious units. This is in contrast to the situation with persistent infections. The timing of the development and introduction of genomic amplification testing in a routine donation screening context has therefore proved to be very fortuitous. Although WNV provides a clear example of a significant TTI which is acute rather than persistent, it has been a problem largely restricted to North America (other than for visitors). In contrast, the appearance of new acutely infectious agents with the potential to spread globally and rapidly to the majority of the world's population must pose a potential threat to blood supplies irrespective of the brevity of any viraemia that might occur.

It is perhaps noteworthy that almost exclusively these 'new' agents posing threats to human health, by gaining the ability to spread from their original animal hosts, are RNA containing viruses. RNA viruses lack the 'molecular proof-reading' mechanisms of DNA viruses. Therefore, their mutation rates during multiplication are higher, leading to populations of 'quasispecies' which may well aid survival of the virus under evolutionary selection pressure. Indeed, evidence for this has steadily accrued. One elegant demonstration examined the 'reverse' situation. Poliovirus with a mutation in the viral polymerase replicates with increased fidelity because the mutation confers resistance to mutagenic nucleotide analogues. The mutant virus was less pathogenic than wild-type virus on poliovirus-receptor transgenic mice, even though only slight growth defects were noted in tissue culture. Extensive experiments showed that this 'high fidelity' mutant reduced viral fitness under a defined selective pressure, indicating that the reverse is also true (Pfeiffer *et al.*, 2005).

In this context consideration will be given to some of the changing characteristics of the severe acute respiratory syndrome (SARS) coronavirus and the avian influenza virus (H_5N_1), both of which are RNA viruses.

Severe acute respiratory syndrome (SARS)

Severe acute respiratory syndrome is caused by a coronavirus (hence the abbreviation SARS CoV). Early in 2003, a severe outbreak of atypical pneumonia was reported in the Guandong province of the People's Republic of China which spread from the mainland to Hong Kong in March 2003 and by June of that year 1750 cases of what became identified as SARS had occurred there. There were 286 (16%) deaths from this disease, indicating the severity of the epidemic. International air travel allowed rapid spread to several other countries, resulting in approximately 8500 cases around the world. The overall case fatality rate was 11%. Fortunately, by early July 2003 it was announced that all known chains of person-to-person transmission had been broken. To have successfully contained this epidemic in less than four months from recognition of the virus as a potential global threat represents a remarkable international public health achievement in disease control. Nevertheless, the resurgence of the disease remains a continuing possibility. Continuing monitoring and surveillance is therefore essential.

Unlike other respiratory viral infections, SARS CoV is relatively stable in the environment and also in faeces. Although respiratory droplets are likely to be a primary source of person-to-person transmission, detection of high concentrations of (stable) virus in faeces suggests that faecal contamination may, in part, be responsible for large community outbreaks such as occurred in Hong Kong.

This novel coronavirus, likely to have originated as a zoonosis, causes acute infections with outcomes ranging from the asymptomatic to fatal disease. Virus could be detected in the kidney of deceased patients and also in the blood of symptomatic patients, using nucleic acid amplification technologies. Assuming this reflects 'viable' viraemia, and if infectious virus is present in the blood prior to the onset of any symptoms, albeit only for a short period, then the potential for transfusion-transmission (especially in an epidemic situation) arises. Fortunately, no transfusion-transmitted cases were associated with the 2003 epidemic and exclusion of SARS patients, their contacts, and travellers to 'high-risk' areas as blood donors is likely to provide adequate protection for the blood supply. Nevertheless, coronaviruses such as SARS have much bigger genomes than other RNA viruses. Although they are therefore likely to evolve more slowly, their larger genome affords them greater adaptability. Vigilant surveillance remains essential.

Influenza viruses

Influenza viruses also contain RNA but can mutate and evolve more rapidly than coronaviruses. Influenza A viruses are currently attracting considerable attention, in particular the H_5N_1 strain of avian influenza commonly known as 'bird flu'. As the name implies, this is an infection of avian species thought to originate in the intestines of waterfowl such as ducks. The virus is excreted in the faeces and can be transmitted to poultry (chicken and turkeys) with a small risk of subsequent transmission to humans. However, very close contact with infected birds is necessary before the H_5N_1 strain can be transmitted to humans. By early 2007, approximately 165 people worldwide had died following infection with this virus despite it being widely epidemic in birds, especially in South-east Asia. Perhaps not surprisingly therefore, the cases in humans are mainly confined to South-east Asia, but careful international surveillance is in place because of the concern that an influenza pandemic in humans, potentially similar in scale to the devastating 1918 pandemic, might occur if the avian virus becomes 'humanized'. This might occur either by mutation or by 'reassortment' of human and avian influenza virus RNA if a person were to be simultaneously infected with the H_5N_1 strain and a currently circulating human strain. The further concern of the possibility of transmission by blood transfusion arises because, although there is no carrier state associated with influenza infection, viraemia has been reported. If an individual were to donate blood in a presymptomatic viraemic condition (and the chance of this obviously increases in an epidemic, with a high attack rate) a transfusion risk is theoretically possible.

Although unusual, the observation of live influenza virus in human serum or plasma has been occasionally reported. In 1963, low titres of virus were isolated from the blood of a patient on the fourth day of illness (Naficy, 1963). Also, in 1970, virus was recovered from blood in two patients (Lehmann and Gust, 1971). More recently H_5N_1 virus was detected in the plasma of a symptomatic five-year-old boy living near Bangkok. He subsequently died of the infection. The influenza virus was detected by reverse transcription polymerase chain reaction at a relatively low titre of 3000 copies/ml. Plasma was also inoculated into an embryonated egg. The infected embryo died within 48 hours and the allontoic fluid contained 2048 haemagglutination units (Chutinimiktul *et al.*, 2006).

However, these instances of reported viraemia relate to symptomatic infections; it is believed that viraemia may occur up to 24 hours prior to the development of symptoms. Should a human H_5N_1 epidemic occur, with a recombinant or mutated virus, symptomatic and recently convalescent potential donors would naturally be excluded but a small risk might remain from presymptomatic viraemia. The extent of this risk would relate to the incidence of infection and the length of the incubation period, as would the feasibility of exclusion of 'relevant' (however defined) contacts of infected individuals. Furthermore, if the titre of virus in the blood is likely to be low, the sensitivity of any nucleic acid testing options would be a significant issue.

ANNEXE REFERENCES

Chutinimiktul, A., Bhattarakosol, P., Srisuratanon, S., *et al.* (2006) H5N1 influenza A virus and infected human plasma. *Emerging Infectious Diseases*, **12**, 1041–3.

Lehmann, N. I. and Gust, D. (1971 Viraemia in influenza. A report of two cases. *Med J Aust*, **2**; 1166–9).

Naficy, K. (1963) Human influenza infection with proved viremia: report of a case. *N Engl J Med*, **269**, 964–6.

Pfeiffer, J. K. and Kirkegaard K. (2005) Increased fidelity reduces poliovirus fitness and virulence under selective pressure in mice. PLoS Pathog, **1**(2): e11.

REFERENCES

Allain, J.-P. (2000) Emerging viral infections relevant to transfusion medicine. *Blood Rev*, **14**, 173–81.

Allain, J.-P., Thomas, I. and Sauleda, S. (2002) Nucleic acid testing for emerging viral infections. *Transfusion Medicine*, **12**, 275–83.

Alter, H. J., Nakatsuji, Y., Melpolder, J., *et al.* (1997) The incidence of transfusion-associated hepatitis G virus infection and its relation to liver disease. *N Eng J Med*, **336**, 747–54.

Anonymous (2002a) Provisional surveillance summary of the West Nile virus epidemic – United States, January–November 2002. *MMWR*, **51**, 1129–33.

Anonymous (2002b) Public health dispatch: investigation of West Nile virus infection in recipients of blood transfusion. *MMWR*, **51**, 973–4.

Anonymous (2003) Detection of West Nile virus in blood donations – United States, 2003. *MMWR*, **52**, 769–72.

Belec, L., Si Mohammed, A., Authier F.J., *et al.* (1999) Human herpes virus 8 infection with POEMS syndrome-associated multicentric Castleman's disease. *Blood*, **93**, 3643–53.

Bjorkman, P., Naucler, A., Winqvist, N., *et al.* (2001) A case-control study of transmission routes for GB virus C/hepatitis G virus in Swedish blood donors lacking markers for hepatitis C virus infection. *Vox Sang*, **81**, 148–53.

Blackbourn, D.J., Ambroziak, J., Lennette, E., *et al.* (1997) Infectious human herpes virus 8 in a healthy North American blood donor. *Lancet*, **349**, 609–11.

Boschoff, C. and Weiss, R.A. (1998) Kaposi's sarcoma-associated herpes virus. *Adv Cancer Res*, **75**, 57–86.

Brayfield, B.P., Phiri, S., Kankasa, C., *et al.* (2003) Postnatal human herpes virus 8 and human immunodeficiency virus type 1 infection in mothers and infants from Zambia. *J Inf Dis*, **187**, 559–68.

Brinton, M.A. (2002) The molecular biology of West Nile virus: a new invader of the Western hemisphere. *Ann Rev Microbiol*, **56**, 371–402.

Campbell, G.L., Ceianu C.S. and Savage, H.M. (2001) Epidemic West Nile encephalitis in Romania: waiting for history to repeat itself. *Ann NY Acad Sci*, **951**, 94–101.

Campbell, G. L., Martin, A. A., Lanciotti, R. S., *et al.* (2002) West Nile virus. *Lancet Infect Dis*, **2**, 519–29.

Cannon, M. J., Dollard, S. C., Smith, D. K., *et al.* (2001) Blood-borne and sexual transmission of human herpes virus 8 in women with or at risk for human immunodeficiency virus infection. *N Eng J Med*, **344**, 637–43.

Cattani, P., Nanni, G., Graffeo, R., *et al.* (2000) Pretransplantation human herpes virus 8 seropositivity as a risk factor for Kaposi's sarcoma in kidney transplant recipients. *Transplant Proc*, **32**, 526–7.

Chowers, M.Y., Lang, R., Nassar, F., *et al.* (2000) Clinical characteristics of the West Nile fever outbreak, Israel, 2000. *Emerg Infec Dis*, **7**, 1–9.

Devalle, S. and Niel, C. (2004) Distribution of TT virus genomic groups 1–5 in Brazilian blood donors, HBV carriers, and HIV-1-infected patients. *J Med Virol*, **72**, 166–73.

Fan, X., Xu, Y., Detre, K, *et al.* (2002) Direct evidence for GB virus C/hepatitis G virus (GBV-C/HGV) superinfection: elimination of resident viral strain by donor strain in a patient undergoing liver transplantation. *J Med Virol*, **68**, 76–81.

Farge, D., Lebbe, C., Marjanovic, Z., *et al.* (1999) Human herpes virus-8 and other risk factors for Kaposi's sarcoma in kidney transplant recipients. *Transplantation*, **67**, 1236–42.

Frances, C., Monguet, C., Marcelin, A. G., *et al.* (2000) Outcome of kidney transplant recipients with previous human herpes virus 8 infection. *Transplantation*, **69** (9), 1776–9.

Gao, S. J., Kingsley, L., Li, M., *et al.* (1996) KSHV antibodies among Americans, Italians and Ugandans with and without Kaposi's sarcoma. *Nat Med*, **2**, 925–8.

George, S. L., Xiang, J. and Stapleton, J. T. (2003) Clinical isolates of GB virus type C vary in their ability to persist and replicate in peripheral blood mononuclear cell cultures. *Virology*, **316**, 191–201.

Gessain, A., Mauclere, P., van Beveren, M., *et al.* (1999) Human herpes virus 8 primary infection occurs during childhood in Cameroon, Central Africa. *Int J Cancer*, **81**, 189–92.

Halasz, R., Sallberg, M., Lundholm, S., *et al.* (2002) The GB virus C/hepatitis G virus replicates in hepatocytes without causing liver disease in healthy blood donors. *J Infect Dis*, **182**, 1756–60.

Heringlake, S., Osterkamp, S. and Trautwein, C. (1996) Association between fulminant hepatitis failure and a strain of GB virus C. *Lancet*, **348**, 1626–9.

Heuft, H. G., Berg, T., Schreier, E., *et al.* (1998) Epidemiological and clinical aspects of hepatitis G virus infection in blood donors and immunocompromised recipients of HGV-contaminated blood. *Vox Sang*, **74**, 161–7.

Jenkins, F. J., Hoffman, L. J. and Liegey-Dougall, A. (2002) Reactivation of and primary infection with human herpes virus 8 among solid-organ transplant recipients. *J Inf Dis*, **185**, 1238–43.

Jones, D., Ballestas, M. E., Kaye, K. M., *et al.* (1998) Primary-effusion lymphoma and Kaposi's sarcoma in a cardiac-transplant recipient. *N Eng J Med*, **339**, 444–8.

Kakkola, L., Hedman, K., Vanrobaeys, H., *et al.* (2004) Cloning and sequencing of TT virus genotype 6 and expression of antigenic open reading frame 2 proteins. *J Gen Virol*, **83**, 979–90.

Karayiannis, P. and Thomas, H.C. (1997) Current status of hepatitis G virus (GBV-C) in transfusion: is it relevant? *Vox Sang*, **73**, 63–9.

Kojima, H., Kaita, K. D., Zhang, M., *et al.* (2003) Genomic analysis of a recently identified virus (SEN virus) and genotypes D and H by polymerase chain reaction. *Antiviral Res*, **60**, 27–33.

Lavreys, L., Chohan, B., Ashley, R., *et al.* (2002) Human herpes virus 8: seroprevalence and correlates in prostitutes in Mombasa, Kenya. *J Inf Dis*, **187**, 359–63.

Lefrere, J. J., Allain, J.-P., Prati, D., *et al.* (2003) West Nile virus and blood donors. *Lancet*, **361**, 2083–4.

Lefrere, J. J., Loiseau, P., Maury, J., *et al.* (1997) Natural history of GBV-C/ hepatitis G virus infection through the follow-up of GBV-C/hepatitis G virus-infected blood donors and recipients studied by RNA polymerase chain reaction and anti-E2 serology. *Blood*, **90**, 3776–80.

Lefrere, J. J., Roudot-Thoraval, F., Lefrere, F., *et al.* (2000) Natural history of the TT virus infection through follow-up of TTV DNA-positive multiple-transfused patients. *Blood*, **95**, 347–51.

Lefrere, J. J., Roudot-Thoraval, F., Morand-Joubert, L., *et al.* (1999a) Prevalence of GB virus type C/hepatitis G virus RNA and anti-E2 in individuals at high or low risk for blood-borne or sexually transmitted viruses: evidence of sexual and parenteral transmission. *Transfusion*, **39**, 83–94.

Lefrere, J. J., Roudot-Thoraval, F., Morand-Joubert, L., *et al.* (1999b) Carriage of GBV-C/hepatitis G virus RNA is associated with slower immunologic, virologic, and clinical progression of human immunodeficiency virus disease in coinfected persons. *J Inf Dis*, **179**, 783–9.

Lennette, E. T., Blackbourn, D. J. and Levy, J. A. (1996) Antibodies to human herpes virus type 8 in the general population and in Kaposi's sarcoma patients. *Lancet*, **348**, 858–61.

Lin, H. H., Kao, J. H., Lee, P. I., *et al.* (2002) Early acquisition of TT virus in infants: possible minor role of maternal transmission. *J Med Virol*, **66**, 285–90.

Lunel, F., Frangeul, L., Chuteau, C., *et al.* (1998) Transfusion-associated nosocomial hepatitis G virus infection in patients undergoing surgery. *Transfusion*, **38**, 1097–103.

Luppi, M., Barozzi, P., Schultz, T. F., *et al.* (2002a) Bone marrow failure associated with human herpes virus 8 infection after transplantation. *N Eng J Med*, **343**, 1378–85.

Luppi, M., Barozzi, P., Schultz, T. F., *et al.* (2002b) Nonmalignant disease associated with human herpes virus 8 reactivation in patients who have undergone autologous peripheral blood stem cell transplantation. *Blood*, **96**, 2355–7.

Maggi, F., Pifferi, M., Fornai, C., *et al.* (2003) TT virus in the nasal secretions of children with acute respiratory diseases: relations to viremia and disease severity. *J Virol*, **77**, 2418–25.

Malnati, M., Broccolo, F., Nozza, S., *et al.* (2002) Retrospective analysis of HHV-8 viremia and cellular viral load in HIV-seropositive patients receiving interleukin 2 in combination with antiretroviral therapy. *Blood*, **100**, 1575–8.

Manni, F., Rotola, A., Caselli, E., *et al.* (2002) Detecting recombination in TT virus: a phylogenetic approach. *J Mol Evol*, **55**, 563–72.

Mantina, H., Kankasa, C., Klaskala, W., *et al.* (2001) Vertical transmission of Kaposi's sarcoma-associated herpes virus. *Int J Cancer*, **94**, 749–52.

Mbulaiteye, S. M., Pfeiffer, R. M., Whitby, D., *et al.* (2003) Human herpes virus 8 infection within families in rural Tanzania. *J Inf Dis*, **187**, 1780–5.

Meng, Y. X., Spira, T. J. and Bhat, G. J. (1999) Individuals from North America, Australasia, and Africa are infected with four different genotypes of human herpes virus 8. *Virology*, **261**, 106–19.

Mikuni, M., Moriyama, M., Tanaka, N., *et al.* (2002) SEN virus infection does not affect the progression of non-A to E liver disease. *J Med Virol*, **67**, 624–9.

Muerhoff, A. S., Simons, J. N., Leary, T. P., *et al.* (1996) Sequence heterogeneity within the 5-terminal region of the hepatitis GB virus C genome and evidence for genotypes. *J Hepatol*, **25**, 379–84.

Munoz, S. J., Alter, H. J., Nakatsuji, Y., *et al.* (1999) The significance of hepatitis G virus in serum of patients with sporadic fulminant and subfulminant hepatitis of unknown etiology. *Blood*, **94**, 1460–4.

Mushawar, I. K., Erker, J. C., Muerhoff, A. S., *et al.* (1999) Molecular and biophysical characterization of TT virus: evidence for a new virus family infecting humans. *Proc Ntl Acad Scie USA*, **96**, 3177–82.

Nash, D., Mostashari, F., Fine, A., *et al.* (2001) The outbreak of West Nile virus infection in the New York City area in 1999. *N Engl J Med*, **344**, 1807–14.

Ohto, H., Ujiie, N., Sato, A., *et al.* (2000) Mother-to-infant transmission of GB virus type C/HGV. *Transfusion*, **40**, 725–30.

Ohto, H., Ujiie, N., Takeuchi, C., *et al.* (2002) TT virus infection during childhood. *Transfusion*, **42**, 892–8.

Okamoto, H., Takahashi, M., Nishizawa, T., *et al.* (1999) Marked genomic heterogeneity and frequent mixed infection of TT virus demonstrated by PCR primers from coding and noncoding regions. *Virology*, **259**, 428–36.

Ott, C., Duret, L., Chemin, I., *et al.* (2000) Use of TT virus ORF1 recombinant protein to detect anti-TT virus antibodies in human sera. *J Gen Virol*, **81**, 2949–58.

Parravicini, C., Olsen, S. J., Capra, M., *et al.* (1997) Risk of Kaposi's sarcoma-associated herpes virus transmission from donor allografts among Italian post-transplant Kaposi's sarcoma. *Blood*, **90**, 2826–9.

Pirovano, S., Bellinzoni, M., Ballerini, C., *et al.* (2002) Transmission of SEN virus from mothers to their babies. *J Med Virol*, **66**, 421–7.

Pistello, M., Morrica, A., Maggi, F., *et al.* (2001) TT virus levels in the plasma of infected individuals with different hepatic and extrahepatic pathology. *J Med Virol*, **63**, 189–95.

Regamey, N., Tamm, M., Wernli, M., *et al.* (1998) Transmission of human herpes virus 8 infection from renal transplant donors to recipients. *N Engl J Med*, **339**, 1358–63.

Renwick, N., Dukers, N. H. T. M., Weverling, G. J., *et al.* (2002) Risk factors for human herpes virus 8 infection in a cohort of drug users in the Netherlands, 1985–1996. *J Inf Dis*, **185**, 1808–12.

Rettig, M. B., Ma, H. J., Vescio, R. A., *et al.* (1997) Kaposi's sarcoma-associated herpes virus infection of bone marrow dendritic cells from multiple myeloma patients. *Science*, **276**, 1851–4.

Rigas, B., Hasan, I., Rehman, R., *et al.* (2001) Effect of treatment outcome of coinfection with SEN viruses in patients with hepatitis C. *Lancet*, **358**, 1961–2.

Saito, T., Matsumoto, S., Nojiri, O., *et al.* (1998) Multicyclic reverse transcription-polymerase chain reaction assay system for quantitation of GB virus-C/hepatitis G virus RNA in serum. *J Virol Methods*, **74**, 185–91.

Sentjens, R., Basaras, M., Simmonds, P., *et al.* (2003) HGV/GB virus C transmission by blood components in patients undergoing open-heart surgery. *Transfusion*, **43**, 1558–62.

Sheng, L., Soumillion, A., Peerlinck, K., *et al.* (1997) Hepatitis G viral RNA in serum and in peripheral blood mononuclear cells and its relation to HCV-RNA in patients with clotting disorders. *Thromb Haemost*, **77**, 868–72.

Simmonds, P., Davidson, F., Lycet, C., *et al.* (1998) Detection of a novel DNA virus (TTV) in blood donors and blood products. *Lancet*, **352**, 191–5.

Simpson, G. R., Schulz, T. F., Whitby, D., *et al.* (1996) Prevalence of Kaposi's sarcoma associated herpes virus infection measured by antibodies to recombinant capsid protein and latent immunofluorescence antigen. *Lancet*, **349**, 1133–8.

Spira, T. J., Lam, L., Dollard, S. C., *et al.* (2000) Comparison of serologic assays and PCR for diagnosis of human herpes virus 8 infection. *J Clin Microbiol*, **38**, 2174–80.

Sugiyama, K., Goto, K., Ando, T., *et al.* (1999) Route of TT virus infection in children. *J Med Virol*, **59**, 204–7.

Tangkijvanich, P., Theamboonlers, A., Sriponthong, M., *et al.* (2003) SEN virus infection and the risk of hepatocellular carcinoma: a case-control study. *Am J Gastroenterol*, **98**, 2500–4.

Tillmann, H. L., Heiken, H., Knapik-Botor, A., *et al.* (2001) Infection with GB virus C and reduced mortality among HIV infected patients. *N Engl J Med*, **345**, 715–24.

Tisdale, J. F., Stewart, A. K., Dickstein, B., *et al.* (1998) Molecular and serological examination of the relationship of human herpes virus 8 to multiple myeloma: orf 26 sequences in bone marrow stroma are not restricted to myeloma patients and other regions of the genome are not detected. *Blood*, **92**, 2681–7.

Tsuda, F., Okamoto, H., Ukita, M., *et al.* (1999) Determination of antibodies to TT virus (TTV) and application to blood donors and patients with post-transfusion non-A to G hepatitis in Japan. *J Virol Methods*, **77**, 199–206.

Tsuda, F., Takahashi, M., Nishizawa, T., *et al.* (2001) IgM-class antibodies to TT virus (TTV) in patients with acute TTV infection. *Hepatology Research*, **19**, 1–11.

Umemura, T., Tanaka, Y., Kiyosawa, K., *et al.* (2002) Observation of positive selection within hypervariable regions of a newly identified DNA virus. *FEBS Let*, **510**, 171–4.

Umemura, T., Tanaka, E., Ostapowicz, G., *et al.* (2003) Investigation of SEN virus infection in patients with cryptogenic acute liver failure, hepatitis-associated aplastic anemia, or acute and chronic non-A–E hepatitis. *J Infect Dis*, **188**, 1545–52.

Umemura, T., Yeo, A. E. T., Sottini, A., *et al.* (2001) SEN virus infection and its relationship to transfusion-associated hepatitis. *Hepatology*, **33**, 1303–11.

Wong, S. G., Primi, D., Kojima, H., *et al.* (2002) Insights into SEN virus prevalence, transmission, and treatment in community-based persons and patients with liver disease referred to a liver disease unit. *Clin Infect Dis*, **35**, 789–95.

Worobey, M. and Holmes, E. C. (2001) Homologous recombination in GB virus C/hepatitis G virus. *Mol Biol Evol*, **18**, 254–61.

Xiang, J., Wunchmann, S., Diekema, D. J., *et al.* (2001) Effect of coinfection with GB virus C on survival among patients with HIV infection. *N Engl J Med*, **345**, 707–14.

Yoshida, H., Kato, N., Shiratori, Y., *et al.* (2002) Weak association between SEN virus viremia and liver disease. *J Clin Microbiol*, **40**, 3140–5.

7 BACTERIAL CONTAMINATION IN BLOOD AND BLOOD COMPONENTS

Carl P. McDonald and M. A. Blajchman

Introduction

Bacterial transmission remains a significant problem in transfusion medicine. This issue is not a new problem and was first identified more than 60 years ago with the first report of a bacterial transfusion-transmission from a blood component in 1941 (Novak, 1939; Strumia and McGraw, 1941). Since the 1970s remarkable progress has been made in increasing the safety of the blood supply with regard to viruses. Unfortunately, this has not been the case with bacterial contamination. Moreover, the continued emphasis in striving for 'zero risk' with regard to blood-borne viruses and in measures to prevent the 'potential' problem of prion transmission has possibly been to the detriment of resolving the issue of bacterial contamination. The current risk of receiving bacterially contaminated platelet concentrates, however, may be 1000 times higher than the combined risk of transfusion-transmitted infection with the human immunodeficiency virus (HIV), hepatitis C virus, hepatitis B virus and human T-cell lymphotropic virus (HTLV) (Blajchman, 2002).

In the USA, from 1985 to 1999, bacterial contamination was the most frequently reported cause of mortality after haemolytic reactions, accounting for over 10% (77/694) of transfusion fatalities (Centre for Biologics Evaluation and Research, 1999). From 1986 to 1991, 29 out of 182 (16%) transfusion-associated fatalities reported to the USA Food and Drug Administration (FDA) were caused by bacterial contamination of blood components (Hoppe, 1992).

From 1994 to 1998, the French Haemovigilance system attributed 18 deaths (four occurring in 1997) to blood components contaminated with bacteria (Debeir et al., 1999; Morel, 1999a). In France, between 1994 and 1999, bacterial transmissions comprised 22% of total transfusion-associated fatalities (Morel, 1999b). Bacterial transfusion-transmission was reported to the Haemovigilance surveillance system as the most frequently identified cause of death (Debeir et al., 1999).

The UK Serious Hazards of Transfusion (SHOT) surveillance system reported that between 1995 and 2003, bacterial transmissions accounted for 58% (29/50) of microbial transmissions (Stainsby et al., 2003). In this period in the UK, 77% (7/9) of microbial fatalities reported to SHOT were due to bacterial transfusion-transmission (Stainsby et al., 2003).

Sources of contamination

The source of bacterial contamination in blood and blood components cannot always be easily identified due to the ubiquitous nature of bacteria in the environment. Table 7.1 lists the major reported causes of bacterial contamination.

Donor arm derived

The major source of bacterial contamination is the donor arm (Goldman and Blajchman et al., 2001; Puckett et al., 1992). In the SHOT reports, potentially 80% of bacterial transmissions in which the source was defined were derived from the donor's arm (Stainsby et al., 2003). Donor arm disinfection reduces the bacterial load on the donor's arm, but does not sterilize the arm. Whilst it has been shown that 'best practice' donor arm disinfection techniques can substantially reduce the bioburden on the upper layers of the skin, it is virtually impossible to disinfect the lower layers (Goldman et al., 1997; Lee et al., 2002; McDonald et al., 2001a). During blood collection, the actual act of the phlebotomy needle passing through the skin may result in a 'skin biopsy' to allow a small core of skin containing viable bacteria to enter the collection bag (Gibson and Norris, 1958; Kojima et al., 1998). This idea was first proposed by Goldman and Blajchman in 1991 (Goldman and Blajchman, 1991), based on the findings of Gibson and Norris (Gibson and Norris, 1958).

Dimpled phlebotomy sites have been shown to be a problem with regard to disinfection. Anderson reported that four positive blood cultures of coagulase negative Staphylococci species were obtained out of 17 platelet apheresis donations from one donor (Anderson et al., 1986). The donor's antecubital fossa was heavily dimpled. Transfusion of these units resulted in two cases of sepsis. Phlebotomy from the non-dimpled left antecubital fossa gave negative blood cultures. Similar results were obtained in three of four other apheresis donors with scarred phlebotomy sites.

An interesting case of donor arm derived fatal transmission with *Clostridium perfringens* from a pooled platelet concentrate was reported in 1994 (McDonald et al., 1998). *Clostridium perfringens* is found in the soil, as well as the gut of man and other animals. This Gram-positive organism grows best anaerobically, but can also grow under aerobic conditions. *C. perfringens* produces powerful exotoxins. On investigation it was found that one of the donors who had contributed towards the platelet pool had a lower arm heavily contaminated with faecal flora. Amongst the faecal flora was *Clostridium perfringens* of the same serotype (PSG8, PS80) as that isolated from the platelet bag. The cause of the lower arm faecal contamination was probably associated with nappy changing, as the donor at the time had two young children. On interview, the donor stated that he meticulously washed his hands after nappy changing, but not his lower arm. Inadequate donor arm disinfection was the most probable cause, as after this incident the donor's arm was swabbed and cultured pre-disinfection and again faecal flora was isolated. After disinfection no bacteria were isolated, indicating that the disinfection procedure was usually effective.

Transfusion Microbiology, eds John A. J. Barbara, Fiona A. M. Regan and Marcela C. Contreras. Published by Cambridge University Press. © Cambridge University Press 2008.

Table 7.1 Possible sources of the bacterial contamination of blood components.

Sources	Cause
Donor arm derived	• Inadequate donor arm disinfection • Dimpled phlebotomy sites • Skin coring
Donor bacteraemia	• Asymptomatic donor due to a low grade infection or recovery from a recent bacterial illness • Chronic low grade bacterial infection
Contaminated collection equipment	• Transient bacteraemia • Specimen collection tubes • Blood bags
Blood processing	• Defective blood bags • Defective welds from sterile connection device • Poor hygiene in processing areas

Donor bacteraemia

The majority of bacteraemic individuals are symptomatic and would be excluded from donation. However, donors may be asymptomatic due to a low grade infection or recovery from a bacterial illness, a chronic low-grade infection or a transient bacteraemia.

Asymptomatic donors due to a low grade infection or recovery from a bacterial illness

Yersinia enterocolitica is one of the most frequently implicated organisms in red blood cell (RBC) bacterial transmissions (Jones *et al.*, 1993). This organism is a Gram-negative coccobacillus that is normally associated with a self-limiting gastrointestinal illness. Infection is spread by the ingestion of food or water contaminated with the faeces of infected humans or animals. Its optimal growth temperature is 25 °C. *Y. enterocolitica* is one of the few human pathogens that can multiply at 4 °C. It uses citrate as an energy source and growth occurs better in the presence of abundant iron; red cell concentrates are therefore an ideal culture medium. *Y. enterocolitca* proliferates in RBCs after a lag phase of 10–20 days. Transmission via transfusion of red cells is probably always due to donor bacteraemia at the time of donation, which is asymptomatic in about half of the infections (Tipple *et al.*, 2004). Transmission of contaminated RBC units can result in septicaemia and endotoxin-mediated shock. In the USA, from 1986 to 1992, 13 cases, 7 (54%) of which were fatal, were reported to the Food and Drug Administration (Centres for Disease Control, 1991). At least six cases, four of them fatal, have occurred in the UK since 1988 (Prentice, 1992). In New Zealand, from 1991 to 1997, nine units infected with Yersinia contributed to six deaths of patients and to morbidity in three other recipients (Kendrick *et al.*, 2001). The incidence of 1 case per 104 000 RBC units transfused in New Zealand is over 90 times higher than that reported in the USA (Theakston *et al.*, 1997). *Yersinia* gastrointestinal infection in New Zealand is high by international standards. This probably reflects the rural lifestyle that frequently exposes humans to animal carriers. (Fenwick, 1992; 1995).

Donor bacteraemia may be a particular issue for autologous blood donations. Exclusion criteria may be less stringent than with routine allogeneic blood donation and storage time may sometimes be longer than for allogeneic donation, allowing additional opportunity for bacterial proliferation. In Austria, a 64-year-old patient undergoing a total hip replacement was transfused with his own RBCs. After transfusion of 150 ml of RBCs. He developed symptoms of endotoxin-mediated shock and fever up to 40 °C (Haditsch *et al.*, 1994). The implicated organism was *Y. enterocolitica*. In the USA, a 13-year-old girl developed septic shock after transfusion of an autologous RBC donation. She required a bilateral amputation below the knee and developed seizures; all these complications were attributed to the Yersinia transmission (Benavides *et al.*, 2003). Autologous transfusion bacterial transmissions highlight the fact that unlike viruses, bacteria can proliferate in blood components. Autologous blood donation has potential benefit with regard to viral safety, but this is not the case with bacterial contamination.

Transmission of the enteric organisms *Campylobacter jejuni*, *Salmonella heidelberg* and *Escherichia coli* are most likely to be due to bacteraemic donors (Heal *et al.*, 1987; Pepersack *et al.*, 1979; Stainsby *et al.*, 2003). A recent case of bacterial transmission of *Salmonella enterica* to two patients (one of whom died) from a split apheresis platelet donation was shown to be due to asymptomatic infection of the donor with this organism, probably derived from his pet boa constrictor (Jarfari *et al.*, 2002).

Chronic low grade infection

Donors with low-grade chronic infections have been cited as the cause of bacterial transmissions. An extremely well cited case of *Salmonella choleraesuis* (now re-named *Salmonella enterica*) from one donor with a low grade infection of the tibia resulted in seven cases of sepsis, two of which were fatal (Rhame *et al.*, 1973). A *Serratia liquiefaciens* contamination of an autologous unit was linked to the donor's infected ischaemic toe ulcer (Duncan *et al.*, 1994).

Transient bacteraemia

Dental treatment (even tooth brushing) and medical procedures may induce transient bacteraemia. A case of *Staphylococcus aureus* platelet contamination may have been due to bacteraemia in the donor who had undergone a tooth repair two hours prior to donation (Goldman and Blajchman, 1991). Interestingly, the use of electric toothbrushes, which is now common in the Western world, has been shown to significantly increase the rate of bacteraemia, in comparison with manual brushing (Bhanji *et al.*, 2002).

Contaminated collection equipment

In 1999 in the Scandinavian countries of Denmark and Sweden, an outbreak of *Serratia marcescens* was reported (Heltberg *et al.*, 1993; Högman *et al.*, 1993). Six patients developed septicaemia after the transfusion of RBCs and platelets. The source of contamination was the heavy contamination with *S. marcescens* of the exterior of the collection bags. This contamination originated from the bag production site in Belgium. The same ribotype was isolated from the recipients, the blood bags and at the production site. Investigation of 1515 blood bags from the same lot revealed that 11 (0.73%) were contaminated with *S. marcescens*. *S. marcescens* is a ubiquitous organism in the environment, capable of growth at 4 °C and 22 °C that is also able to grow under poor nutritional conditions. All Serratia species are capable of deriving nutrients from the water-soluble plasticizer that is used to make plastic bags flexible and which leeches into the aqueous contents of blood bags during storage (Boulton *et al.*, 1998).

Contaminated vacuum tubes used for specimen collection after donation were attributed as a source of three incidents of *S. marcescens* transmission following platelet transfusion (Blajchman *et al.*, 1979). Non-sterile intravenous solutions used in apheresis collection have also been implicated as a source of blood component contamination (Kosmin, 1980).

Blood processing

Defects or damage to blood bags during processing may provide a portal of entry for bacteria. The major critical points in the process are when bags are placed under stress due to pressing or centrifugation. Minute lesions in the bag may increase in size and be more amenable to the entry of bacteria. Another 'potential' critical point is the extensive use of sterile connection device technology. Sterile connection devices connect blood bags together by welding tubing lines, allowing the aseptic transfer of the contents from one bag to the other under closed environmental conditions. At the point in the process when the system is open to the environment, microbial contamination is prevented due to the high temperature achieved; however, the incorrect functioning of these devices could possibly lead to bacterial contamination. These devices have been extensively validated for use (AuBuchon *et al.*, 1995; Kothe and PlatenKamp, 1994). In Germany, inspection of all sterile connection device welds is mandatory to prevent this theoretical risk (Thomas Montag-Lessing, personal communication).

Contaminated water baths have also been a source of blood product contamination, particularly with *Pseudomonas cepacia* (now renamed *Burkholderia cepacia*) and *P. aeruginosa* (Casewell *et al.*, 1981; Rhame and McCullough, 1979a; 1979b). Improvements in hygiene standards, facilities, greater awareness of the critical points at which bacterial contamination can occur, changes in processing techniques, quality systems, improved bag quality, audit and implementation of environmental monitoring systems have shown a marked reduction in Pseudomonas transmissions in the UK. No pseudomonad species has been reported in any bacterial transfusion-transmission to SHOT since its inception in 1995 (Stainsby *et al.*, 2003).

Prevalence of bacterial contamination

Screening and monitoring studies indicate the prevalence of bacterial contamination in pooled platelet concentrates ranges from

0.14% to 1.41% with a mean of 0.43% (see Table 7.2). In apheresis platelet concentrates the bacterial contamination rate from published data ranged from 0% to 0.89%, with a mean of 0.09% (see Table 7.2). The apheresis rate is consistently lower than that for pooled platelet concentrates, presumably due to the number of venepunctures involved, as skin contaminants are the major source of bacterial contamination. In red cell units the bacterial contamination rates from study data range from 0.01% to 0.27% with a mean of 0.10% (see Table 7.2). In general, the bacterial contamination rate of RBC units is lower than that for platelet concentrates due to the 4 °C storage temperature. The majority of bacteria are unable to proliferate at this temperature and the opposite applies to platelet concentrates which are stored at 22 °C. Care is needed, however, when comparing bacterial contamination rates between countries and even blood centres. There may be differences in testing techniques, classification of a positive reaction, donor arm disinfection techniques, use of diversion, or non use, processing methods and many other variables that might affect the bacterial contamination rate.

Organisms implicated in clinically apparent bacterial transfusion-reactions

Table 7.3 lists the organisms cited in the US study on Bacterial Contamination of Blood (BaCon), French Haemovigilance (BACTHEM) and SHOT reports, responsible for causing clinically apparent bacterial transfusions reactions and fatalities associated with contaminated platelet concentrates. Gram-positive organisms accounted for 68% (49 cases) of the transfusion reactions and Gram-negative organisms accounted for 32% (23 cases). *Staphylococcus epidermidis*, a skin commensal (20 cases), was the most frequently transmitted organism, indicating the importance of donor arm disinfection. *Escherchia coli* (nine cases) was the second most commonly transmitted organism, followed by *Staphylococcus aureus* and *Bacillus cereus*. In terms of transfusion reactions resulting in fatalities, Gram-positive organisms accounted for 37% (six cases) and Gram-negative organisms 63% (10 cases). Overall, 16 deaths (22%) resulted from 72 transfusion reactions.

The RBC data from BaCon, BACTHEM and SHOT indicate that Gram-positive organisms accounted for 47% (14 cases) of clinically apparent transfusion reactions and Gram-negative 53% (16 cases) (see Table 7.4). Gram-positive coagulase negative Staphylococci (six cases), including *Staphylococcus epidermidis*, were the most frequently transmitted organisms overall. *Acinetobacter* (four cases) and *Serratia* sp. (four cases) were the most frequently transmitted Gram-negative organisms. Gram-positive organisms were responsible for 14% (one case) and Gram-negative for 86% (six cases) of fatal RBC-associated cases.

In BaCon, BACTHEM and SHOT reports, RBCs accounted for 29% (30 cases) of transmissions compared with 71% (72 cases) associated with platelet concentrates. Overall transmissions with RBCs accounted for 30% of fatalities, compared with 70% with platelet concentrates. Platelet concentrates are the major cause of morbidity and mortality with regard to transfusion-associated bacterial transmission. The 22 °C-storage

Table 7.2 Prevalence of bacterial contamination of cellular blood components.

Blood product type	Country	Number of units tested/transfused	Positives	Reference
Pooled platelets	Australia	1517	13 (0.86%)[a]	(Cummings *et al.*, 2001)
	Belgium	17675	93 (0.52%)[a]	(Claeys and Verhaeghe, 2000)
	Belgium	12968	152 (1.2%)	(Schelstraete *et al.*, 2000)
	Brazil	13454	21 (0.16%)[a]	(Wendel *et al.*, 2000)
	Croatia	71	1 (1.41%)[a]	(Vuk *et al.*, 2003)
	England	6730	34 (0.5%)[a]	(McDonald *et al.*, 2002a)
	Hong Kong	21503[b]	10 (0.3%)[a]	(Chiu *et al.*, 1994)
	Netherlands	2123	14 (0.65%)[a]	(Laport *et al.*, 1999)
	Netherlands	3033	27 (0.9%)[a]	(Van der Meer *et al.*, 2002)
	USA	4995	4 (0.08%)[a]	(Leiby *et al.*, 1997)
	USA	3141	6 (0.2%)[a]	(Yomtovian, 1993)
	USA	712[b]	1 (0.14%)[a]	(Barrett *et al.*, 1993)
TOTAL		87922	376 (0.43%)	
Apheresis platelets	Brazil	3553	16 (0.45%)[a]	(Wendel *et al.*, 2000)
	Croatia	273	2 (0.89%)[a]	(Vuk *et al.*, 2003)
	England	3017	6 (0.2%)[a]	(McDonald *et al.*, 2002a)
	USA	2678	1 (0.04%)[a]	(AuBuchon *et al.*, 2002b)
	USA	17928[b]	5 (0.03%)[a]	(Barrett *et al.*, 1993)
	USA	2476	0 (0.00%)[a]	(Yomtovian, 1993)
	USA	5197[b]	1 (0.02%)[a]	(Dzieczkowski *et al.*, 1995)
TOTAL		35122	31 (0.09%)	
Red blood cells	Brazil	20206	55 (0.27%)[a]	(Wendel *et al.*, 2000)
	Croatia	2465	3 (0.12%)[a]	(Vuk, 2003)
	England	4183	3 (0.1%)	(McDonald *et al.*, 2002a)
	USA	31385[b]	1 (0.003%)[a]	(Barrett *et al.*, 1993)
	USA	7080	1 (0.01%)	(Dzieczkowski *et al.*, 1995)
TOTAL		61136	60 (0.1%)	

[a] Confirmed positive
[b] Number of units transfused

temperature of platelet concentrates allows for the growth of a wide range of bacteria. These organisms are capable of proliferation to levels of 10^6 to 10^{11} cfu/ml in this environment and at this storage temperature (Brecher *et al.*, 2000a; McDonald *et al.*, 2001b; Punsalang, 1989; Wagner *et al.*, 1995a; Wenz, 1993). Not unexpectedly with growth to these levels, contaminated units can lead to morbidity and mortality. The minimal bacterial level which is specifically associated with a transfusion reaction is, however, as yet unknown. Moreover, platelet concentrates are invariably given to patients with an impaired immune system and who are granulocytopenic; they will be more susceptible than normal individuals to bacterial infections.

Incidence of bacterial transfusion reactions

The rate reported for bacterial contamination of blood components clearly exceeds the incidence of bacterial reactions

following transfusion. A contaminated blood component has the potential to cause a transfusion reaction but this depends on a range of factors. These include the health of the patient, the type of antibiotic therapy being administered, the bacterial inoculum level transfused, as well as the nature of the particular organism (or even strain) transfused. At present there is scant data on the true rate of bacterial transfusion reactions. The current available data on the possible rate of bacterial transfusion reactions is summarized in Table 7.5. In general, only the most severe transfusion reactions are likely to be reported and under-reporting undoubtedly occurs. This is particularly relevant for platelet concentrates as these are invariably given to immunocompromised patients who frequently succumb to infection from other sources and the platelet concentrate may not be considered as the source of the bacterial infection. Also, the organisms transmitted from the blood component may, to a clinical microbiologist, not be considered inherently pathogenic.

Table 7.3 Summary of organisms implicated in bacterial transmission from platelet concentrates.

Organism	Total transmissions	Fatalities
Staphylococcus epidermidis	20	1
Staphylococcus aureus	7	1
Bacillus cereus	7	3
Coagulase negative staphylococcus	4	0
Streptococcus species	4	0
Group B streptococcus	3	1
Propionibacterium acnes	3	0
Enterococcus faecalis	1	0
Total Gram-positive organisms	49 (68%)	6 (37%)
Escherichia coli	9	3
Serratia species	4	3
Enterobacter species	4	1
Klebsiella species	2	1
Yersinia enterocolitica	1	0
Morganella morganii	1	1
Acinetobacter species	1	0
Proteus species	1	1
Total Gram-negative organisms	23 (32%)	10 (63%)
Total	**72**	**16**

Data from BaCon; BACTHEM; SHOT; Kuehnert *et al.*, 2001; Perez *et al.*, 2001; Stainsby *et al.*, 2003.

Table 7.4 Summary of organisms implicated in bacterial transmission from RBC concentrates.

Organism	Total transmissions	Fatalities
Coagulase negative staphylococcus	4	0
Staphylococcus aureus	2	0
Bacillus cereus	2	0
Staphylococcus epidermidis	2	1
Streptococcus species	2	0
Enterococcus faecalis	1	0
Propionibacterium acnes	1	0
Total Gram-positive organisms	14 (47%)	1 (14%)
Acinetobacter species	4	1
Serratia species	4	2
Yersinia enterocolitica	2	1
Pseudomonas species	2	1
Escherichia coli	1	0
Enterobacter species	1	1
Klebsiella species	1	0
Proteus species	1	0
Total Gram-negative organisms	16 (53%)	6 (86%)
Total	**30**	**7**

Data from BaCon; BACTHEM; SHOT; Kuehnert *et al.*, 2001; Perez *et al.*, 2001; Stainsby *et al.*, 2003.

Strategies to reduce bacterial transfusion-transmission (see Table 7.6)

Reducing the risk of blood component contamination

Improved donor selection

Donor selection/screening is intended to exclude blood donations from individuals with clinically inapparent bacteraemia. Screening is usually based on either questioning the donor with regard to symptoms of infection or the determination of the donor's temperature. As previously stated, *Y. enterocolitica* is one of the organisms most frequently transmitted by RBC transfusions. Questioning and deferral of donors with regard to a history of gastrointestinal illness has been suggested as a measure to prevent *Y. enterocolitica* transmission. It has been reported that history taking would prevent 50% of *Y. enterocolitica* transmissions, but at a cost of 11% of donors (Prentice, 1992). This measure, therefore, would have only a limited effect in preventing bacterial transmission, but could have a very serious effect on the blood supply.

Improved donor arm disinfection

Skin disinfection prior to venepuncture remains a vital first line of defence in preventing the bacterial contamination of blood components with coagulase-negative Staphylococci, *Staphylococcus aureus*, *Corynebacterium* sp., *Propionibacterium acnes* and

Table 7.5 Rate of bacterial transfusion reactions and fatalities per million units transfused.

Study	Apheresis platelets	Whole-blood-derived platelets	Red blood cells	Case fatality rate (%)
Perez *et al.*, 2001.	31.8	71.8	5.8	16.0
Kuehnert *et al.*, 2001.	9.9	10.6	0.2	26.5
Ness *et al.*, 2001.	74.5	67.0	not determined	17.4

Bacillus sp. These skin flora are the most commonly detected bacteria in screening and monitoring studies (de Korte *et al.*, 2001; 2002; McDonald *et al.*, 2004c; Soeterboek *et al.*, 1997). In the BaCon, SHOT and Haemovigilance surveillance system studies, resident skin flora potentially account for 57% of platelet concentrate and 37% of RBC-associated bacterial transmissions (Kuehnert *et al.*, 2001; Perez *et al.*, 2001; Stainsby *et al.*, 2003). Skin derived organisms would appear to be the major source of bacterial contamination of blood components and transient skin flora have been cited frequently in bacterial transmissions (McDonald *et al.*, 1998). Taking resident and transient skin derived organisms together, they account for over 90% of platelet

Table 7.6 Strategies to reduce bacterial transmission by transfusion.

Reducing the risk of product contamination	(1) Improving donor screening
	(2) Improved donor arm disinfection
	(3) Diversion
Improving blood component processing and storage	(1) Optimize storage temperature
	(2) Limit storage time
	(3) Leucodepletion
	(4) Overnight hold
Reducing recipient exposures to blood donors	(1) Reduce transfusion triggers
	(2) Optimize transfusion indications
	(3) Increase use of apheresis-derived platelet products
Bacterial screening	(1) Visual inspection
	(2) Microscopic examination
	(3) Molecular techniques
	(4) Endotoxin detection
	(5) Culture techniques
	(6) Rapid techniques
Pathogen reduction	Platelet concentrates:
	(1) Intercept system (amotosalen/UVA)
	(2) Mirasol (riboflavin/UVA)
	Red cells:
	(1) Inactine
	(2) FRALE

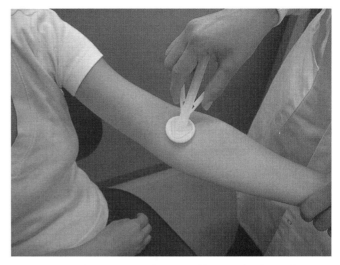

Figure 7.1 Skin disinfection procedure using chloraprep disinfection device.

In Australia, single use chlorhexidine alcohol was shown to be an acceptable method of disinfection (Wong *et al.*, 2004). Lee has shown that povidine-iodine and isopropyl alcohol is more effective than cetrimide/chlorhexidine and isopropyl alcohol. The bacterial contamination rate in platelet concentrates was reduced from 0.072% to 0.042% (Lee *et al.*, 2002). Critical factors affecting the extent of skin disinfection efficiency are the type of disinfectant or disinfectants used, concentration of the disinfectant, quantity of disinfectant applied, drying time, the type of application device and the application method. Also, an essential factor for efficacy is that the phlebotomy team is motivated, trained and educated in the importance of donor arm disinfection. In England, the performance of donor arm cleansing is monitored on a regular basis (McDonald *et al.*, 2004b).

Donor arm cleansing is a disinfection procedure and not a sterilization step. There is a limit to the amount of time the disinfectant can be applied and the type of chemical that can be applied to the human skin. Bacterial bioburden may be considerable at the antecubital fossa, and a recent study has indicated that over 50% of donors have 10^5 organisms/cm^2 at the venepuncture site pre-disinfection (McDonald *et al.*, 2001a). Therefore, improved donor arm disinfection is not a panacea for preventing bacterial transmission, but needs to be combined with other preventive measures.

Diversion

Diversion is based on the principle that contaminants from the donor's skin will be carried in the initial flow of blood. Redirection of the initial flow of blood from the collection bag into a pouch or side arm will thus reduce the bacterial contamination in the donation bag. Diversion will not result in blood wastage, as the contents of the pouch can be utilized for microbial and blood group serology purposes. As previously stated, the majority of bacterial contamination in blood components is skin derived. Diversion studies have shown a substantial reduction in bacterial contamination rates in the number of blood components found on monitoring to contain bacteria (see Table 7.7). Diversion, together with improved donor arm disinfection, has been shown

concentrate and 70% of RBC transmissions cited in the BaCon, SHOT and Haemovigilance reports (Kuehnert *et al.*, 2001; Perez *et al.*, 2001; Stainsby *et al.*, 2003).

Many blood services are now introducing 'best practice' donor arm disinfection techniques. Three separate studies have shown an application of 70% isopropyl alcohol followed by tincture of iodine to be a 'best practice' procedure (Goldman *et al.*, 1997; McDonald *et al.*, 2001a; Pleasant *et al.*, 1994). Indeed, this technique has been widely used throughout Canada for over five years. In England, the same technique was trialled with apheresis donors and shown to reduce the bacterial contamination observed in outdated platelet concentrates by 57% (McDonald unpublished data). A commercial two-minute, two-stage disinfection procedure (Donor Prep Kit (DPK), Mediflex, Kansas, USA), was deemed by the National Blood Service of England, after field trial evaluation, to take too long and potentially to lead to long waiting times for donors. Therefore an alternative rapid method was sought (see Figure 7.1). The Chloraprep disinfection device (Mediflex, Kansas, USA), a one-stage procedure consisting of a 30-second application of 70% isopropyl alcohol and 2% chlorhexidine gluconate with a 30-second drying time was shown to have equivalent disinfection efficiency to the DPK (99.8% reduction with both techniques) (McDonald *et al.*, 2002c).

Table 7.7 Reduction in bacterial contamination achieved with diversion of initial aliquot.

Study	Component cultured	% Reduction achieved
Olthuis *et al.*, 1995	Apheresis	88%
Bruneau *et al.*, 2001	Whole blood	72%
McDonald *et al.*, 2004c	Whole blood	47%
De Korte *et al.*, 2002	Whole blood	40%
Bos *et al.*, 2002	Pooled platelet concentrates	53%
Schneider *et al.*, 2002	Pooled platelet concentrates	58%

Table 7.8 Age of products causing bacterial transfusion reactions SHOT 1995–2003 (N = 29).

	Platelets Age (in days) at use							RBCs
	1	2	3	4	5	NK	**ALL**	
All species	0	2	3	6	10	4	**25**	4
Bacillus cereus				3(1[a])		1	**4**	
Coagulas negative staphylococci				1			**1**	1 (23 days)
Enterobacter aerogenes			1[a]				**1**	
Escherichia coli	1[a]	1[a]				1	**3**	
Group B streptococcus			1	1		1	**3**	
Morganella morganii				1			**1**	
Serratia liquifaciens								1
Staphylococcus aureus					2	1[a]	**3**	
Staphylococcus epidermidis		1[a]		2	6		**9**	1 (32 days)
Yersinia entercolitica								1[a] (33 days)

[a] Infection was implicated in the death of a recipient

NK – Not known

to improve the reduction achieved to 77% (McDonald *et al.*, 2004c). Improved donor arm disinfection and diversion, although substantially reducing contamination from skin derived organisms, cannot prevent transmission from bacteraemic blood donors.

Improving blood component processing and storage

Optimizing storage temperature

Storage temperature of blood components is a significant factor influencing bacterial proliferation. Red blood cells are stored at 4 °C and platelet concentrates at 22 °C. The majority of bacteria are unable to proliferate at the RBC storage temperature and it has been suggested that a decrease to 0 °C will reduce bacterial proliferation of those psychrophilic organisms that are able to grow at 4 °C (Bradley *et al.*, 1997)

Platelet concentrate storage at 22 °C provides a temperature at which most types of bacteria are able to proliferate. Reduction of the platelet concentrate storage temperature to 4 °C will prevent bacterial proliferation from the majority of organisms cited in platelet transfusion-transmissions (Currie *et al.*, 1997). However, it has been shown that platelet concentrates stored at 4 °C rapidly leave the circulation post-transfusion (Vostal and Mondoro, 1997). Hoffmeister has recently described a mechanism elucidating the rapid clearance of 'chilled' (4 °C) platelet concentrates in experimental animals and its prevention. Such observations could lead to a potential resolution of this issue, if applicable to humans (Hoffmeister *et al.*, 2003a; 2003b; Snyder *et al.*, 2003).

Limit storage time

Theoretically, the longer the storage period of a bacterially contaminated blood product unit, the greater the likelihood that the bacteria present would multiply to sufficient numbers to cause a transfusion reaction in a recipient. In the SHOT reports, of the cases where the age of the implicated blood component was known, 75% of platelet concentrate transfusion reactions occurred when the product was 4–5 days old (Stainsby *et al.*, 2003) (see Table 7.8). Therefore, reducing the shelf life to three days might have prevented these transmissions. However, such an approach would result in supply problems. Interestingly,

SHOT reported that 50% of the transmissions that resulted in a fatality were from platelet concentrates aged 2–3 days. Therefore, reduction in shelf life would not have prevented some of these fatal cases.

In some European centres (Scandinavia and the Netherlands) the introduction of the bacterial screening of platelet concentrates using automated blood culture systems enabled the shelf life to be extended to seven days (McDonald *et al.*, 2000; Munksgaard *et al.*, 2004). In the USA, in 1983, the platelet concentrate shelf life was extended from five to seven days (Simon *et al.*, 1983). In 1983 alone, four fatal bacterial transfusion reactions were reported to the Food and Drug Administration (FDA) (Heal *et al.*, 1987). In response, apparently solely due to the increased risk of bacterial contamination, the FDA returned the shelf life to five days (Heal *et al.*, 1987; Punsalang *et al.*, 1989).

It has been suggested that a reduction in RBC storage time to 25 days could prevent Yersinia transmission, which proliferates after a lag phase of 10 to 20 days. However, an FDA study reports that reduction in storage time to 25 days would significantly reduce the blood supply (by 20%) (Hoppe, 1992). In the UK, a fatality was reported in a patient receiving a *Y. enterocolitica* contaminated RBC unit that had only been stored for 16 days (Jones *et al.*, 1993).

In the SHOT reports, all cases of bacterial transmission from RBCs in which the shelf life was known, were from units stored for more than 22 days (Stainsby *et al.*, 2003) (see Table 7.8).

Leucodepletion filters

Leucodepletion of blood and blood components has been introduced by many blood services, but invariably for reasons other than to address the issue of bacterial contamination. Filtration reduces the level of bacterial contamination but is not 100% effective, nor is it effective for all bacterial species (Dzik, 1995; Holden et al., 2000; Stainsby et al., 2003; Vasconcelos, 2001). The potential mechanisms of reduction of bacterial contamination by leucodepletion filters can be either physical retention of bacteria in the filtration process, physical injury resulting in cell death, and/or removal of macrophages which have phagocytosed bacteria. Bacterial growth kinetics have been shown to be the same in leucodepleted and non-leucodepleted platelet concentrates (McDonald et al., 2001b).

Overnight hold

Many blood services hold whole blood at 18–22 °C overnight prior to component preparation. It has been shown that storage at 22 °C does not adversely affect the properties of blood components (Pietersz et al., 1989). Overnight hold has logistical benefits for blood services, allowing flexibility in component preparation and the potential availability of microbiological test results prior to processing. Bacteriologically, overnight hold may promote a reduction in bacterial contamination by allowing time for natural anti-bacterial activities, such as activation of the complement cascade and macrophage bacterial engulfment to have their effect. Högman et al. have shown that hold at 22 °C for several hours and then leucodepletion resulted in the removal of certain bacterial species (Högman et al., 1991). Wagner et al. reported that the overnight hold of bacterially spiked whole blood units for 24 hours without leucodepletion resulted in a significant increase in bacterial number in RBCs, but not in platelet concentrates and plasma (Wagner et al., 1995b). In units that were leucodepleted, where 7/8 bacterial species were tested, there was no significant difference between units held for 8 hours (routine practice) and 24 hours. In platelet concentrates prepared from units held for 24 hours, a significant reduction in bacterial number was observed for 7/10 bacterial species, for two species no difference was found and for one species a small, but significant increase was observed compared to the units held for 8 hours. In another study, it was concluded that a hold for 16 hours at 22 °C before component preparation delays bacterial growth and that the effect appeared to be white cell mediated (Sanz et al., 1997). A comparison of the bacterial contamination rate in whole blood within two hours of collection and after overnight hold at 20 °C, using an automated blood culture system, showed no significant difference between the two groups (de Korte et al., 2001). This study did not take into account the effect of leucodepletion.

Other studies have suggested that an overnight hold at 20–22 °C appears to have no adverse effect regarding bacterial contamination and may even be beneficial, particularly if leucodepletion is performed. In-depth studies are required to determine whether the effects of variations in individual processing methods may be of significance.

Reducing recipient exposures to blood donors

Reduce transfusion triggers

Reducing the number of allogeneic transfusions to recipients would reduce the risk from the whole gamut of microbial agents. Publications recommending reduced transfusion triggers appear to suggest that this approach would reduce patient risk without detriment to the patient (Hebert et al., 1999; Schiffer et al., 2001).

Optimizing transfusion indications

Clinical audit of the usage of blood components has frequently indicated that blood components are often transfused to patients inappropriately. A reduction in inappropriate usage would, therefore, reduce patient exposure. A vigorous system of audit and education of health care workers would be appropriate to encourage a reduction in inappropriate transfusions.

Increased use of apheresis-derived platelet concentrates

Reports have consistently indicated that the bacterial contamination rates in pooled platelets are greater than that for apheresis platelets. For example, the increased use of apheresis platelet concentrates from 51.7% to 99.4% over a 12-year period was shown to result in a decrease in septic transfusion reactions to platelets from 1 in 4818 to 1 in 15 098 (Ness et al., 2001). Exclusive use of apheresis platelet concentrates would reduce patient donor exposure by a factor of 4 to 6, but this would only represent a partial risk reduction of transfusion-associated sepsis.

Bacterial screening

The challenge of bacterial screening

Viral screening for specific blood-borne viruses has been implemented for over 30 years by blood services throughout the world. In countries with high Human Development Indexes (HDI's) the blood supply is now extremely safe regarding viral risks, due to the development of exquisitely sensitive and specific assays. In comparison, bacterial screening can be said to be in its 'infancy'. Numerous countries have now implemented screening programmes for platelet concentrates (see Table 7.9). In comparison with viral screening, bacterial screening poses a unique challenge for the following reasons:

(1) Unlike viruses, bacteria can multiply during the storage of blood components.
(2) The initial inoculum may be extremely low and be undetectable early in the shelf life.
(3) A broad spectrum of bacteria contaminate blood components, unlike viruses in which only a limited range are transfusion-transmitted.
(4) Most bacterial transmission is due to exogenous contamination. Unlike with viruses, antibody response, which could then be conveniently screened for, is therefore not pertinent.
(5) Rapid, sensitive, simple and specific tests are not yet available.
(6) Testing may not be appropriate 'immediately' post-collection in contrast with viral screening.

Table 7.9 Overview: worldwide bacterial screening of platelet concentrates.

Country	Percentage screened (date commenced)	Screening system
• Belgium (Flanders)	100% (1998)	BacT/ALERT
• Netherlands	100% (2001)	BacT/ALERT
• Wales	100% (2003)	BacT/ALERT
• USA	100% (2004)	Mixed
• Canada	100% (2004)	Mixed
• Republic of Ireland	100% (2004)	BacT/ALERT
• Northern Ireland	90% (2000)	BacT/ALERT
• Scotland	75% (2000)	BacT/ALERT
• Sweden/Denmark/ Norway	60% (1996)	BacT/ALERT
• China	Limited	BacT/ALERT
• Brazil	Limited	BacT/ALERT
• England	Limited	BacT/ALERT

(7) Screening at more than one time point may be required during the shelf life of the product to 'guarantee' negativity at the point of transfusion. The virology test results are valid for the donation regardless of the storage time period.

(8) Individual components from each donation may require bacterial screening. A single screening test suffices for all components with regard to viral testing.

(9) Donor exclusion has limited benefit with regard to preventing bacterial contamination, but is highly effective for viruses.

Bacterial growth kinetics

Figure 7.2 illustrates bacterial growth kinetics in a contaminated blood component. Initially, at the point of contamination, there is a lag phase in bacterial growth in which the bacteria are metabolizing, but not multiplying. The lag phase can be hours or even days, and is dependent on various factors such as environment, temperature, species and whether the organism has been damaged or 'shocked'. At this early point, bacterial numbers may be low. It has been stated that bacterially contaminated units at the time of collection typically contain less than 10 cfu/ml and there may be only 1–10 colonies present per bag (Goodnough *et al.*, 2003; Wagner, 1997; Wagners *et al.*, 1996). Therefore, screening during the lag phase of growth may not detect bacterial contamination due to few or no bacteria present in the sample taken. Bacteria then enter an exponential growth phase during which rapid multiplication occurs. If only one organism is present in a particular unit and that organism had a doubling time (time taken for one round of multiplication) of 20 minutes (a typical time period), approximately 2.6×10^5 would be present per bag after six hours. Spiking experiments have shown that platelet concentrates are an excellent growth medium for bacteria and levels of 10^8–10^{12} cfu/ml have regularly been obtained (Brecher *et al.*, 2000a; McDonald *et al.*, 2001b; Punsalang *et al.*,

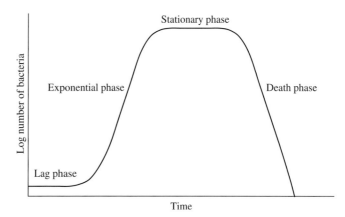

Figure 7.2 Bacterial growth kinetics. The time course for each phase varies for each bacterial species.

1989; Wagner *et al.*, 1995a; Wenz *et al.*, 1993). The exponential phase ends due to the exhaustion of available nutrients or because of the accumulation of the toxic products of bacterial metabolism. The bacteria then enter the stationary phase in which, as in the lag phase, metabolism is occurring without multiplication. Bacteria in the stationary phase eventually die, the death phase, which is also exponential in nature. The death phase occurs because of a number of factors, the most important one being the depletion of cellular reserves. It must be noted that when bacteria multiply to sufficient numbers, the toxins produced can be sufficient to cause morbidity and mortality in the recipient, even though these bacteria may not be viable at the time of transfusion.

Bacterial contamination of blood components will not always result in bacterial multiplication. The organisms may not be able to survive the storage conditions and so die. Autosterilization due to the presence of natural bactericidal agents in the blood component (e.g. complement), may result in death of the organism (McDonald *et al.*, 2005a). Also, bacteria may survive in the unit in low numbers, but not multiply.

Screening issues

The key screening issues are:
(1) When to test.
(2) What volume to test.
(3) Which assay to use.

In the majority of cases, screening near the time of collection will usually be associated with a low bacterial number and therefore an extremely sensitive assay will be required under such circumstances. A large sample volume will need to be taken from the component to be tested in order to enhance the probability of detection of the bacteria present. Screening at this time parallels that of virological screening and therefore is operationally 'friendly' (see Figure 7.3a). Culture assays which are extremely sensitive would be the most appropriate to use, although with extremely sensitive tests, 18–24 hours is required to obtain a positive test result (Brecher *et al.*, 2005; McDonald *et al.*, 2002b; Ortolano *et al.*, 2003; Pall Corporation, 2003). Paradoxically, screening at this time would often detect bacteria that may not

(a)

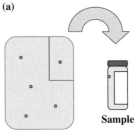

Platelet bag

Sample

For:
    Operationally 'friendly'

Against:
    Sampling probability
    Requirement for a large sample volume?

Current options:
    Culture (i.e. BacT/ALERT, PALL eBDS)

(b)

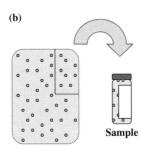

Platelet bag

Sample

For:
    Increased detection probability
    Possibility of reduction in sample volume
    Possibility of pooling (cost reduction)

Against:
    Operational difficulties

Current options:
    Culture (i.e. BacT/ALERT, PALL eBDS)
    Rapid tests (i.e. Scansystem)

Figure 7.3 Testing strategies: (a) Testing on day 1 (immediately after preparation/collection); (b) testing on day 2 (or later in shelf life).

be able to survive in the product or organisms that do not enter into an exponential growth phase (i.e. surviving but not multiplying).

Screening at 24 hours or later post-donation will have the benefit that the bacteria present are able to grow in the blood component and will potentially have entered the exponential phase of growth. Under such circumstances bacterial numbers may be sufficient to allow the use of less sensitive, but rapid, tests (1–2 hours) compared with culture (see Figure 7.3b). Culture would also be appropriate for screening. At present there are no rapid and highly sensitive assays readily available. Reduction in sample volume and the possibility of pooling to reduce the cost of bacterial testing may be achievable with bacterial screening at 24 hours or later. In Hong Kong, five samples at day 2 of shelf life are pooled into one culture bottle for the bacterial screening of whole blood derived platelet concentrates (Liu *et al.*, 1999). Operationally, this strategy provides challenges and may require the holding of a product and its release until screening results are obtained. Indeed, a major policy change may be required in transfusion medicine with regard to the period of time a product can be classed as bacterially negative, the number of tests that will need to be performed and the testing time or times. More than one test may be required on a product and theoretically the daily screening of the inventory may be required. An alternative strategy would be to screen early in the product's shelf life using a sensitive assay such as culture and then using a rapid, less sensitive test, later in the shelf life. Obviously, the most appropriate point to screen for bacteria would be at the point of transfusion, but with current technology this would appear not to be operationally feasible.

An ideal bacterial assay needs to be rapid (less than two hours), sensitive (approximately 1 cfu/ml), specific, inexpensive, simple and be associated with low labour costs. At present the ideal assay has yet to be produced, but considerable development is now underway and, as previously stated, some screening programmes (sometimes of low sensitivity) have been put in place by numerous blood services.

Bacterial detection methods

Visual inspection

It has been noted that in some cases of an RBC-associated transfusion-transmission of bacteria, distinct colour changes (darkening of the unit) had been observed in the contaminated unit (Franzin and Gioannini, 1992; Goldman and Blajchman, 1991; Hoppe, 1992). Kim *et al.* thus proposed examination of the unit, comparing the colour of the bag with the distal segment, which would tend not be contaminated if the inoculum level were low (Hoppe, 1992; Kim *et al.*, 1992). This colour change has been attributed to bacterial oxygen consumption, leading to desaturation as well as the marked haemolysis of red cells. In a study, visual inspection could detect units as potentially contaminated when the initial bacterial contamination content was in the range 1.8×10^4 to 1.6×10^9 cfu/ml (Pickard *et al.*, 1998). The colour change due to bacterially contaminated RBC units responsible for patient morbidity has not always been noted (McDonald *et al.*, 1996). In platelet concentrates, visual inspection to try and detect a decrease in platelet 'swirling', has been suggested as a possible method to detect bacterial contamination. Platelets with good viability have a discoid morphology and reflect light, producing a 'swirling' visual effect. Non-discoid (poor viability), spherical platelets do not show this swirling. A decrease in swirling will occur at lower pH, which potentially will be caused by bacterial metabolism. Several studies have shown that platelets ceased to swirl at levels of 10^7 to 10^9 bacterial cfu/ml; however, as many as 18% of day five platelets do not swirl, which means the majority of non-swirling units will not be bacterially contaminated (Bertolini and Murphy, 1994; Wagner and Robinette, 1996).

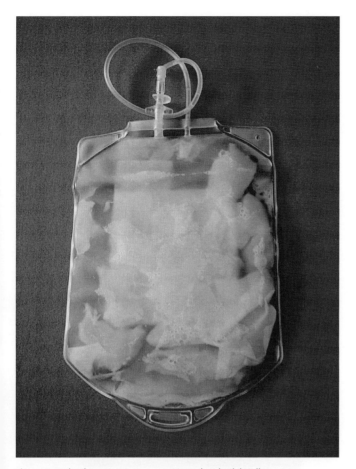

Figure 7.4 Platelet concentrate contaminated with *Klebsiella oxytoca*.

Visual inspection of blood components at the time of issue and transfusion is a prudent, cost-efficient, quality control measure, but it is not specific and only sensitive enough to detect highly contaminated units. Figure 7.4 shows a four-day old apheresis contaminated platelet unit that was about to be transfused. The health care worker visually inspected the unit and deemed it to be 'abnormal' for transfusion. The large white amorphous mass in the unit is likely to be a platelet clot caused by *Klebsiella oxytoca*, a Gram-negative organism which was found to be present in the unit at a concentration of 10^6 cfu/ml. Visual inspection prevented the transfusion of this unit, which would undoubtedly have caused a severe if not fatal transfusion-associated reaction (unpublished data).

Microscopic examination

Gram and acridine orange staining have been investigated as a possible pre-transfusion approach for the detection of bacteria in platelet concentrates (Barrett *et al.*, 1993; McCarthy and Senne, 1980; Mitchell and Brecher, 1999; Reik and Rubin, 1981; Yomtovian, 1993). Both assays do not determine viability, are quite insensitive and will only detect heavily contaminated units. The sensitivity of Gram and acridine orange staining is in the order of 10^6 cfu/ml and 10^5 cfu/ml. These tests are inexpensive and easy to perform, but do require skilled personnel to interpret the results (McCarthy and Senne, 1980; Reik and Rubin, 1981). Acridine

orange requires a fluorescent microscope and both methods involve the use of potentially mutagenic compounds. The most appropriate time to employ these assays would be at the point of transfusion or for the screening of units later in shelf life, when bacterial numbers may be sufficiently high for detection (i.e. $>10^6$ cfu/ml). The sensitivity of these assays is inappropriate for use as a routine screening assay in a blood centre.

Molecular techniques

Molecular techniques have been deemed by some investigators to be the panacea for microbial detection and have been continually cited as specific and sensitive. This is the case for certain viral agents and for the identification of specific bacteria, but for the broad spectrum detection of bacteria this has not been the case. Chaney *et al.*, using a universal ribosomal RNA sequence, obtained a detection level of 10^5–10^9 cfu/ml (Chaney *et al.*, 1999). A 16 S ribosomal RNA assay has been developed, which in screening 2146 samples in parallel with the BacT/ALERT system detected all culture assay positives (Mohammadi *et al.*, 2005). Sensitivity of the assay is in the order of 10–100 cfu/ml (Mohammadi *et al.*, 2003). GeneProbe (San Diego, CA), using a ribosomal RNA sequence obtained a sensitivity of 1–5×10^5 cfu/ml (Mimms, 2002). Using a similar approach, contamination was detected at levels of 10^2–10^5 cfu/ml (Chongokolwatana *et al.*, 1993). Brecher *et al.* (1993; 1994) designed a non-amplified chemiluminescence-linked universal bacterial ribosomal RNA gene probe detecting bacteria at levels of 10^5 cfu/ml or greater. Sen (2000) and Sen *et al.* (2001) designed a multiplex 5′-nuclease PCR assay for the detection of *Enterobacteriaceae* with a security of 1–8 cfu/ml.

Problems have been encountered with molecular assays because the reagents themselves are prone to contamination with bacterial nucleic acid. Bacterial contamination of reagents, especially the polymerase enzymes, causes false-positive results. As yet, no commercial molecular technique is available.

Endotoxin detection

Lipopolysaccharides, cell wall components of Gram-negative bacteria, are responsible for the endotoxin mediated septic shock syndrome. Detection of this Gram-negative component has been suggested as a method for the detection of Gram-negative bacteria, particularly *Yersinia enterocolitica*. The Limulus amoebocyte lysate (LAL) test using the LAL reagent prepared from horseshoe crab haemolymph has been shown to be the most sensitive and specific (Bang, 1953; Hochstei, 1987; Levin and Bang, 1964a; 1964b; 1968).

The endotoxin asssay was discovered by accident when an American horseshoe crab *Limulus polyphemus* died from intravascular blood coagulation after contact with bacterial endotoxin during marine research. The enzyme mediating this coagulation was subsquently isolated from the crab's circulating blood cells (amoebocytes). The in vitro test developed using the *Limulus* amoebocyte lysate (LAL) reagent that spectrophotometrically monitors the reaction between a test sample and the purified enzyme lysate. The test is sensitive, quantitative and rapid (Cooper, 2001). Because of this it has become the test of choice for endotoxin detection. Nevertheless, due to natural fluctuations in the source material, stability and sensitivity of the assay depends on an individual manufacturer's formulation (Lane, 2004). This problem and the requirement to bleed live animals stimulated the development of recombinant LAL reagents that do not depend on the use of horseshoe crabs. These reagents have recently become commercially available (Lane, 2006).

Studies using the LAL assay for the detection of bacteria in RBC have shown a sensitivity range from 10^1 to 10^5 cfu/ml, but 100% detection was not always obtained (Arduino et al., 1989). More importantly, a test based on endotoxin detection will not detect Gram-positive bacteria, which comprise a substantial proportion of the septic transfusion episodes, particularly those associated with platelet concentrates.

Culture techniques

Culture systems offer the most sensitive assays at present, but to achieve adequate sensitivity, incubation periods of 8–24 hours are required for bacterial detection (Brecher, 2005; McDonald et al., 2005a; Ortolano et al., 2003; Pall Corporation, 2003). Nonetheless, these systems are now extensively utilized for the screening of platelet concentrates to detect bacterial contamination.

Automated blood culture systems

These systems were originally designed for clinical microbiology laboratory usage and accordingly have a proven track record for performing patient derived blood cultures in the hospital environment. The majority of hospital microbiology departments possess a system and could offer this resource to hospital based blood centres (AuBuchon et al., 2002a). These systems have been adapted for the screening of blood components. A sample is inoculated into a culture bottle containing bacterial growth media. The culture bottle is then loaded into an incubator associated with the system. Specific sample identification is maintained through barcoding. At this point the process is fully automated and the system can alert the operator to a positive result. At the end of the incubation period these systems indicate that non-reactive bottles need to be unloaded. The presence of bacteria in a culture tube is determined by the detection of carbon dioxide, which is a by-product of bacterial metabolism. Transfer of results can be direct to the main computer system, obviating transcription errors. Aerobic and anaerobic culture can be performed with these systems by using culture bottles that have the appropriate atmosphere. Automated blood culture systems which have been evaluated for the screening of blood components include BacT/ALERT, BACTEC (Becton Dickinson) and ESP (TREK) (Gonzales et al., 2004; Kahwash et al., 2004; Macauley et al., 2003). These systems allow for a large number of samples to be screened, with low labour costs, specific sample identification, and they are sensitive and specific.

BacT/ALERT

BacT/ALERT is by far the most widely utilized instrument for the screening and monitoring of blood components (see Figure 7.5).

BacT/ALERT has been used in Scandinavia for the routine screening of blood components since the 1980s (Bjork and Johnson, 1998; Gong et al., 1994; Högman and Gong, 1994). The product has a CE mark and is FDA approved for the screening of platelet concentrates for quality control purposes. BacT/ALERT is a modular system and consists of an incubator unit (housing 240 culture bottles), controller module (for loading, unloading and positive/negative indication) and an optional database management system (BacT/VIEW) (see Figure 7.5). Six incubation modules can be linked to each controller module with a maximum capacity for

BacT/ALERT System

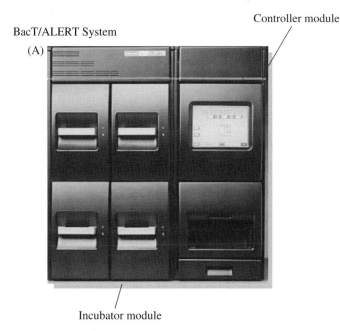

Incubator module

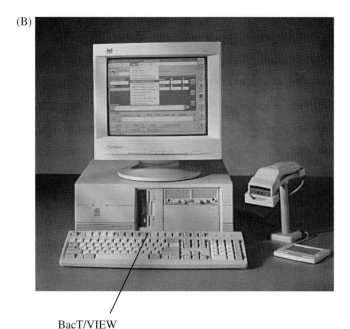

BacT/VIEW
Data management system

Figure 7.5 BacT/ALERT System showing the incubator module, controller module (A) and the data management system (B).

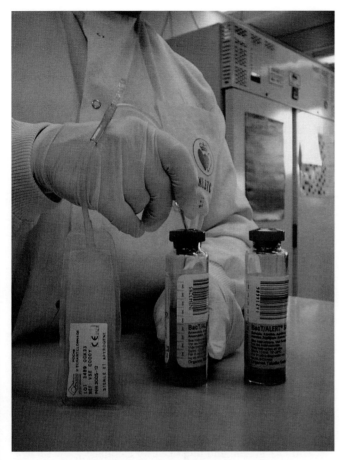

Figure 7.6 BacT/ALERT culture bottle inoculation using a sample pouch.

1440 bottles. A sample of a blood component is required to be taken from the unit under test. Normally sampling of units to be tested is performed by using a sample pouch (see Figure 7.6) which has a needle present for the easy inoculation of the BacT/ALERT bottles. These can be attached to the primary pack using a sterile connection device to maintain a closed system or can be integral to the blood product pack to be tested. The sample pouch is then filled under gravity until the requisite volume is obtained. It is essential that the unit to be sampled is thoroughly mixed prior to filling the pouch. The pouch is then removed from the platelet bag using a heat sealer to maintain a closed system throughout the process. Inoculation of BacT/ALERT bottles is performed by the penetration of the rubber septum with the needle attached to the sample pouch. The BacT/ALERT bottles are at negative pressure and draw the contents of the pouch into the culture bottles. The bottles are graduated so the fill volume can be determined. Inoculation of the BacT/ALERT culture bottles is best performed in a laminar flow cabinet to reduce exogenous contamination. Disinfection of the septum of the BacT/ALERT culture bottles, using 70% alcohol, needs to be performed prior to inoculation.

BioMérieux (Basingstoke, Hants., UK) manufacture a range of culture bottles. Extensive evaluation has been performed on the performance of the various culture bottles for the detection of bacteria associated with bacterial transfusion-transmission

(Brecher *et al.*, 2001; 2005). Standard BacT/ALERT culture bottles contain tryptic soya broth and BioMérieux manufacture a blood product bottle which is the standard bottle, but which has undergone additional quality control. The paediatric bottle (only aerobic version available) and FAN bottles contain peptone enriched tryptic soya broth, supplemented with brain heart infusion medium and activated charcoal for the removal of antibiotics for testing clinical patients. The maximum fill volume for all bottles is 10 ml with the exception of the paediatric bottle (4 ml). Detection of low level contamination is enhanced by increased fill volume (Brecher *et al.*, 2001; 2004; 2005; McDonald *et al.*, 2001b; 2002b). Standard and paediatric bottles are generally used for the screening of blood products (AuBuchon *et al.*, 2002a; Claeys & Verhaeghe, 2000; McDonald *et al.*, 2000; Macauley *et al.*, 2003; Pearce *et al.*, 2004; Wendel *et al.*, 2000).

Specific sample identification is maintained throughout the entire process by barcoding. The unique identification number on each BacT/ALERT bottle can be linked to the unit number by entry of these details into the BacT/VIEW information system or an in-house system.

Inoculated bottles are loaded onto the system by first scanning them on the controller module, which reads the unique BioMérieux barcode label on the bottles. Bottles are then placed in the incubator module, generally set at 35 °C, which is an adequate growth temperature for the majority of bacteria. The system maintains specific sample identification throughout the process and will detect, for example, if a bottle has been removed before the end of the established incubation period. At this point the system requires no operator intervention until a positive has been detected or until the end of the established incubation period.

In the base of each BacT/ALERT bottle is a sensory device, which consists of a semi-permeable membrane containing water and a pH sensitive dye. As bacteria grow in the nutrient broth present in the BacT/ALERT bottles, they produce carbon dioxide. This diffuses through the membrane in the base of the bottle, reacting with the water present to produce carbonic acid, which causes a change in pH. This causes the pH sensitive dye to change from green to yellow (see Figure 7.7). The BacT/ALERT system scans each bottle with a beam of light every ten minutes and light is reflected back from the base of the bottle to a detector measuring reflectance, that is, a colour change (see Figure 7.8). Three algorithms are present within the system (see Figure 7.9):

(1) Substantial acceleration: two hours of exponential growth.
(2) Rate: in which carbon dioxide is produced at a rate only likely as a result of microbial respiration, not the respiration of cellular blood components.
(3) Initial threshold: for those specimens already positive when loaded.

Positive bottles will be indicated by the system and a prompt to unload negative bottles will be provided by the system. Scanning out of negative and positive bottles on the system is recommended, as this acts as an additional reconciliation step.

BioMérieux have now developed a software system for the direct notification of results of bacterial cultures to hospitals and blood centres. BacT/Notify allows the automatic notification

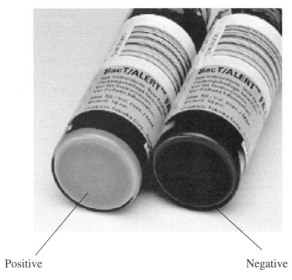

Figure 7.7 BacT/ALERT positive (yellow) and negative (green) bottles.

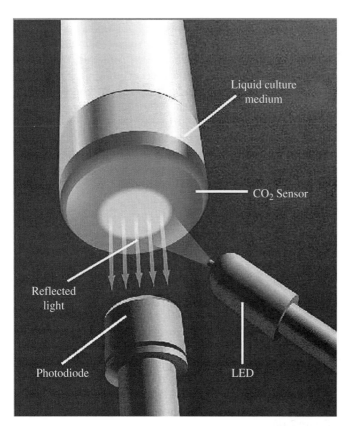

Figure 7.8 BacT/ALERT culture bottle reading mechanism.

of results by fax, email or pager and also allows access to the most recent culture results via a secure web source (Hay *et al.*, 2004). This is particularly relevant when cultures are maintained on the system even after the release of the product from the blood centre. This will be beneficial in the recall and timely reporting of positive results. Many BacT/ALERT users culture for the duration of the whole shelf life of platelet concentrates.

Theoretically, BacT/ALERT will detect one viable bacterial cell inoculated into the BacT/ALERT culture bottle with the

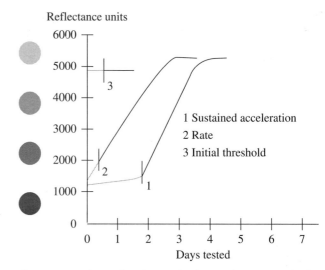

Figure 7.9 BacT/ALERT algorithms used in the BacT/ALERT system for the detection of bacteria.

appropriate atmosphere and media for growth of that organism. This applies to all current culture systems. BacT/ALERT has been shown to detect in the order of 1 cfu/ml (McDonald *et al.*, 2005a). Table 7.10 presents data of initially reactive and confirmed positive rates using the BacT/ALERT system for the screening of platelet concentrates. In these studies the definition of a confirmed positive is one in which the reactive unit is retested again using the BacT/ALERT system and the organism identified is the same as that from the initial reactive bottle. Caution is needed when analysing data for initially reactive and confirmed positive results as these are not always so rigorously defined.

In general, the initially reactive rate is considerably higher than the confirmed positive rate (see Table 7.10). This might be due either to exogenous contamination of the incubation bottle during sampling, autosterilization of bacteria due to bactericidal factors present in the platelet concentrate (i.e. complement), low sample number, non-proliferating bacteria, or death of the bacteria.

Exogenous contamination in testing with BacT/ALERT can be minimized with dedicated, trained staff using good aseptic techniques and the use of a laminar flow or safety cabinet for bottle inoculation (Macauley *et al.*, 2003).

Pall eBDS

The Pall eBDS is a second-generation culture assay, superseding the Pall BDS (McDonald *et al.*, 2004a; 2005a; Ortolano *et al.*, 2003; Rock *et al.*, 2004). Sensitivity of the Pall eBDS has been considerably improved compared with the BDS (McDonald *et al.*, 2005a). BacT/ALERT uses carbon dioxide as a marker for the detection of bacterial growth. In contrast, Pall eBDS uses oxygen consumption as the marker for detecting bacterial growth (Ortolano *et al.*, 2003). As aerobic bacteria grow, they consume oxygen and the decrease in oxygen concentration is detected in the system's culture pouch.

Table 7.10 Worldwide data from bacterial screening of platelet concentrates using the BacT/ALERT system.

Country	No. tested				Initial reactive	Confirmed reactive	Shelf life at time of sampling	Reference
	Pooled	Apheresis	Single	Unspecified				
Belgium	75 829				1.05%	0.82%	Day 0	(Blajchman et al., 2005)
		31 998			0.74%	0.57%		
Brazil	13 454				0.26%	0.16%	Day 1	(Wendel et al., 2000)
		3553			0.59%	0.45%		
Denmark	22 165				0.22%	0.15%	Day 0	(Blajchman et al., 2005)
Netherlands	17 675				1.7%	1.1%	Not stated	(Claeys and Verhaeghe, 2000)
			6885		1.4%	0.8%		
Northern Ireland	3285				0.72%	0.36%	Day 2/3	(Macauley et al., 2003)
		1600			0.25%	0.06%		
UK	296				1.0%	0.3%	Day 3	(McDonald, 2000)
US		2678			0.6%	0.0%	Day 2	(AuBuchon et al., 2002a)
Wales				8927	0.48%	0.05%	Day 1	(Pearce et al., 2004)

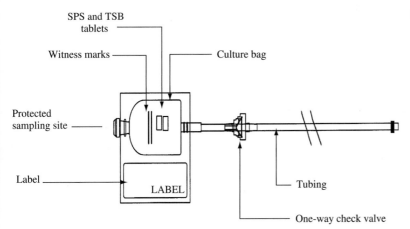

SPS and TSB tablets

Witness marks

Culture bag

Protected sampling site

Label

LABEL

Tubing

One-way check valve

Figure 7.10 The Pall eBDS system shown schematically.

The system consists of a culture pouch, which can be attached to the unit to be tested using a sterile connection device (see Figures 7.10 and 7.11). Alternatively, the device can be integral to the primary platelet pack. A 4 ml sample of the unit to be tested is passed into the aliquot culture pouch under gravity (see Figure 7.12). The system is therefore 'closed' and exogenous contamination is theoretically not an issue. Pall eBDS has a non-return valve to prevent back-flow from the culture pouch into the primary pack. The culture pouch contains two tablets; each of these contain trypticase soya broth (TSB) to promote bacterial proliferation and sodium polyanethol sulphonate (SPS). The SPS inhibits bactericidal activity in plasma and aggregates any platelets present to reduce any confounding platelet oxygen metabolism. After sampling, the culture pouch is disconnected from the primary pack and the tubing section containing the non-return valve discarded (see Figure 7.13). The culture pouch is then placed in a horizontal platelet agitator at 35°C and incubated for a minimum period of 24 hours (see Figure 7.14). At the end of the incubation period, the oxygen content of the culture pouch is read using an oxygen analyser (see Figure 7.15).

Specific sample identification is maintained throughout the process by the use of barcode labels and electronic data transmission obviates transcription errors. The cut-off level for a positive reaction for platelet concentrates containing plasma and platelet additive solution (PAS) is less than or equal to 9.4% (plasma) and 16.2% (PAS) oxygen content respectively. There are concerns about the cut-off level which may require redefining when more field data is available (Nguyen et al., 2004). The system has FDA approval for quality control purposes and has a CE mark (see Figure 7.16).

At present, the Pall eBDS has been implemented at 30 sites (23 USA, 4 Europe, 3 Middle East). Sensitivity of the system is comparable to that of the BacT/ALERT system. This is not surprising as both systems use tryptic soya broth as a growth medium, incubation is at 35°C, and both the BacT/ALERT bottles and the Pall eBDS pouches are agitated (McDonald et al., 2005a).

In screening 118 067 platelet concentrates from March to November 2004 with the Pall eBDS system in 23 US blood centres, the initial reactive rate was 0.1 (1 in 1001) (Stein Holme, Pall

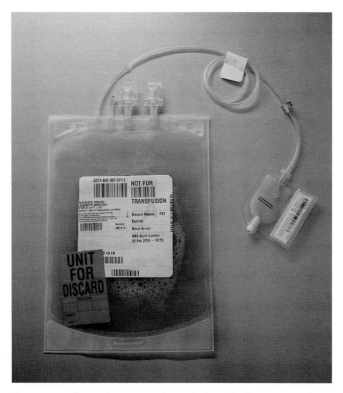

Figure 7.11 Pall eBDS detection pouch attached to a platelet concentrate bag.

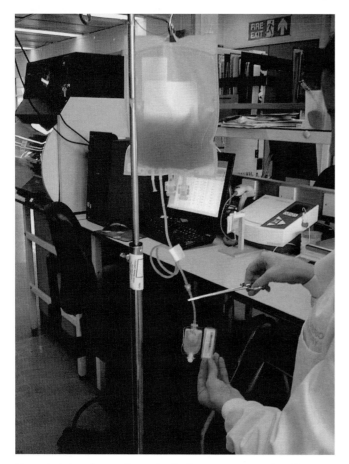

Figure 7.12 Sampling an aliquot of a platelet concentrate into the Pall eBDS system pouch.

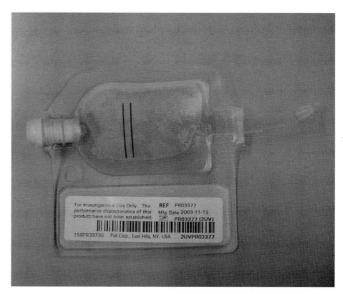

Figure 7.13 The Pall eBDS sample pouch.

Corporation, personal communication). It is difficult to analyse repeat reactives, confirmed positives and false-positives because of the lack in standardized definition in these terms. Evaluation of the system is in progress for the screening of red cell concentrates (Yu *et al.*, 2004).

Pall eBDS provides a simple, easy-to-use, closed sampling system. In contrast, exogenous contamination is possible with the BacT/ALERT as this has an open sampling system. A greater sample volume can be taken for BacT/ALERT, which potentially can increase sensitivity, although a balance is required between the volume taken for bacterial screening and that required for patient use. BacT/ALERT continually reads and reports every ten minutes. BacT/ALERT bottles can be incubated until the end of the shelf life of the product. Pall eBDS gives a single 'one-off' result at the end of the incubation period, which must be incubated for a minimum of 24 hours. The space required for both systems is comparable and implementation of either system depends on the logistics of individual blood centres or hospital blood banks.

Rapid techniques

Scansystem

The Scansystem (Hemosystems, Marseilles, France) is one of the first generation of commercial rapid detection systems (under 90 minutes) to be made available for the detection of bacteria in platelet concentrates (Morel *et al.*, 2002; Ribault *et al.*, 2004a). The Scansystem has a CE mark and has FDA approval for quality control use in the USA. At present, the system is under evaluation by several blood services (Jacobs *et al.*, 2005).

An initial sample preparation stage is required with the Scansystem. This consists of pooling three 3 ml samples, from different platelet concentrates under test, into a pooling bag of the Scansystem platelet kit (see Figure 7.17a). Luer connections are present in the device for the separation of each stage of the

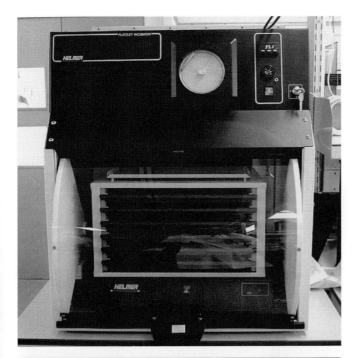

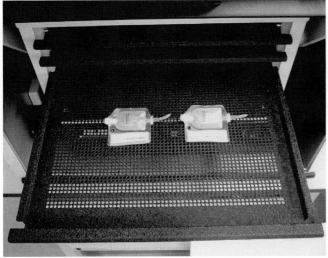

Figure 7.14 The Pall eBDS incubator.

process. The pool is mixed and 3 ml of pooled sample together with 6 ml of air are taken into the system's syringe (see Figure 7.17b). The Scansystem platelet kit is then agitated on a flat bed shaker for 40 minutes at room temperature. The syringe contains a specific fluorescent double-stranded DNA label for uptake by any bacteria present, and a monoclonal antibody to aggregate any platelets present. After the 40-minute agitation stage the syringe's contents are forced through a 5 µm filter into the lysis bag. The 5 µm filter retains the platelet aggregates, but allows the passage of bacteria into the lysis bag (see Figure 7.17c). Residual platelets are destroyed by the lysis solution present in the bag. The lysis solution renders the membranes of any bacteria present permeable, increasing the uptake of the fluorescent label. Contents of the platelet kit are then mixed by inversion and suspended vertically for 20 minutes at room

temperature. After incubation the contents of the lysis bag are filtered through a 0.4 µm membrane (see Figure 7.17d). Any bacteria present will be retained on the membrane. The 0.4 µ black membrane is then removed from the sample preparation kit (see Figure 7.18) and placed in the Scansystem analyser (see Figure 7.19), which has been moistened with phosphate buffered saline (PBS) on a sub-membrane. The membrane is then taken into the Scansystem analyser and a 488 nm argon laser causes fluorescence of any fluorchrome present. Automatic computer analysis is part of the system. The entire scanning procedure lasts approximately three minutes. An image of any fluorescent particles present on the membrane is then displayed by the Scansystem. Currently, manual microscopic verification is required for each test performed. The membrane is removed from the analyser drawer and placed on an attached fluorescent microscope stage. Bacteria present on the membrane are then verified microscopically (see Figure 7.20). A confirmed positive result is one in which 10 or more fluorescent signals out of 50 are identified as bacteria, corresponding to a ratio of ≥ 0.20.

The Scansystem provides rapid testing (less than 90 minutes) but is labour intensive and requires a skilled operator. Sensitivity is in the order of 10^3 cfu/ml and is species dependent (McDonald et al., 2005b). Schneider et al. screened 813 platelet concentrates using the Scansystem and BacT/ALERT and detected four initial reactives using the BacT/ALERT system (Schneider et al., 2003). None of the BacT/ALERT initial reactives were confirmed by standard microbiological methods or by the Scansystem.

The assay has now been developed for the screening of RBC with a pool size of 20 units and a sensitivity of approximately 1 cfu/ml (Ribault, 2004b; 2004c).

Dielectrophoresis

A rapid detection system Bac-Detect (Blood Analysis, Slough, UK) has been developed for the screening of platelet concentrates, based on the principle of dielectrophoresis (Betts et al., 1999) (see Figure 7.21). Dielectrophoresis occurs when cells are placed in non-uniform electric fields. The cells move towards, and accumulate on electrodes (regardless of the direction of the applied field), as determined by their dielectric properties (conductivity and permittivity) rather than by their charges (as would occur in electrophoresis). There is an initial sample preparation step using 1 ml of the platelet concentrate to be tested. Platelets are removed from the sample using a lysis solution and any residual platelet or platelet debris is removed by centrifugation. The sample preparation stage takes approximately 30 minutes. Sample is then pipetted into a microelectrode well and electrophoresized for 30 minutes; bacteria present are then collected onto electrodes (see Figure 7.21). The detection is accomplished by the measurement of impedance. With the current system 24 samples can be tested per hour. Initial evaluation of a prototype system has shown a detection level of 10^4 cfu/ml for *Escherichia coli*, *Bacillus cereus* and *Clostridium perfringens* and a level of 10^5 cfu/ml for group *B* Streptococcus (McDonald, 2005c). The system detects both live and dead bacteria. Bac-Detect may potentially offer a rapid, easy to use and low labour

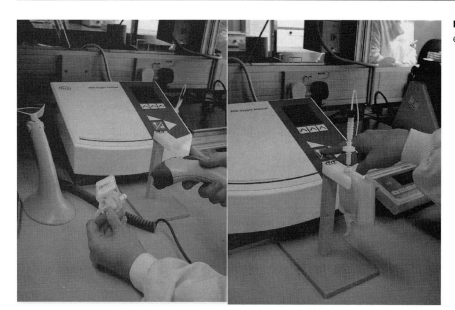

Figure 7.15 Reading the oxygen content in the Pall eBDS pouch.

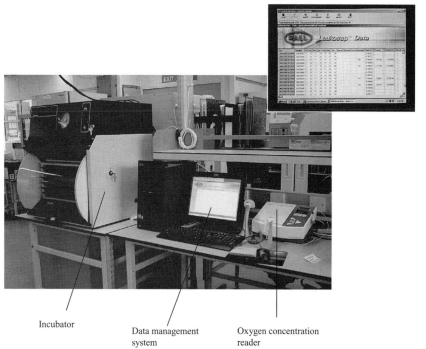

Figure 7.16 The Pall eBDS equipment showing the various components of the system.

Incubator

Data management system

Oxygen concentration reader

cost system for screening platelet concentrates. Further evaluation of the system is necessary.

Metabolic changes (pH and glucose)

The majority of proliferating bacteria will metabolize glucose and produce acid, lowering the pH. Measurement of glucose and pH has been evaluated and, indeed, utilized in the USA for the detection of bacteria in platelet concentrates (Burstain *et al.*, 1997; Choo *et al.*, 2004; Cocco *et al.*, 2004; Hahn *et al.*, 2004; Werch *et al.*, 2002). An advantage of this system is that it is extremely rapid if using multi-reagent dipsticks (glucose 30 seconds and pH

60 seconds). Sensitivity is species specific but is in the range 10^5–10^8 cfu/ml. In general, only high bacterial levels are detected and specificity is questionable (Amorim *et al.*, 2004; Nguyen *et al.*, 2004; Puca *et al.*, 2004).

Microvolume fluorimetry

An assay using antibiotic labelled probes which bind to bacteria and are detected by microvolume fluorimetry has been developed (Adams *et al.* 1997; Brecher *et al.* 2000b; Dietz *et al.*, 1996; Dzik, 1997; Lee *et al.*, 2002). A sensitivity of 10^5 cfu/ml was obtained with *S. epidermidis* (Brecher *et al.*, 2000b). However, since the initial

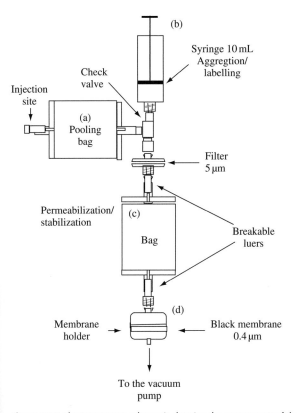

Figure 7.17 The Scansystem schematic showing the components of the system.

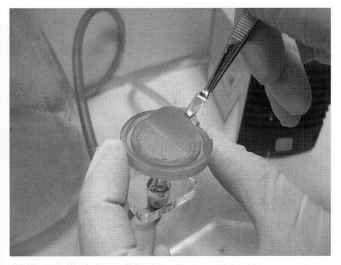

Figure 7.18 Membrane filter of the Scansystem.

publication in 2000 there appears to have been no further development using this technology. The sensitivity reported would indicate the ability to detect only heavily contaminated units.

Flow cytometry

An assay has been developed by the German Red Cross in Springe, in conjunction with Becton Dickinson. The fluorescent dye thiazole orange is used to stain bacterial nucleic acid for the detection of bacteria in platelet concentrates (Mohr *et al.*, 2003).

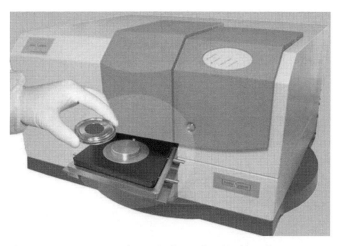

Figure 7.19 Scansystem analyser, membrane placed in the analyser.

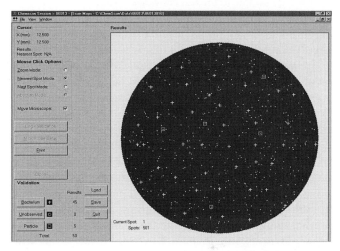

Figure 7.20 Scansystem visual display of fluorescent particles from the Scansystem analyser.

The stained bacteria are detected by flow cytometry, a technique available in many blood centres. A 50 µl sample from the platelet concentrate is lysed and stained (five minutes). The sample is then analysed in a flow cytometer using a 488 nm argon laser (10 to 30 seconds) (Mohr *et al.*, 2003). Sensitivity of the assay is reported to be in the order of 10^4 cells/ml. The assay will detect both live and dead bacteria and is extremely rapid, low cost, easy to perform, with the potential for automation. Current sensitivity will only allow detection of a relatively high bacterial load, so the assay is only of potential value later in the shelf life of the product. Development work using this approach is still in progress.

Bacterial cell wall detection

Assays that detect the bacterial cell wall are currently under development. The Pan Genera Detection (PGD) assay detects conserved class-specific cell wall bacterial antigens; lipoteichoic acid on Gram-positives and lipopolysaccharides on Gram-negative bacteria (Hall & Lejoie, 2004). There are potentially 200 000–2 000 000 targets per bacterium. Gram-positive and Gram-negative antibodies are configured in a double antibody (a)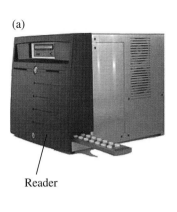

Reader

(b)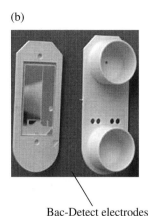

Bac-Detect electrodes

(c)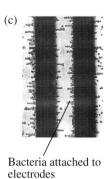

Bacteria attached to electrodes

Figure 7.21 The Bac-Detect system (dielectrophoresis) showing (a) analyser; (b) electrodes in which sample is placed; (c) view of bacteria attached to electrodes.

assay format. The test involves application of 500 µl of platelet concentrate sample to the test cartridge. The sample reacts with antibody-coated gold colloid via capillary action. The presence of bacteria is detected when immobilized Gram-positive and Gram-negative antibodies capture gold tagged bacterial antigens and a visible red line is formed on the test line of the assay cartridge. The test time is approximately 20–30 minutes. Sensitivity of the assay is approximately 10^3 cfu/ml (http://www.veraxbiomedical.com).

Another assay in development is based on the binding of specific proteins and derived peptides to the peptidoglycan component of the bacterial cell wall (Immunetics Inc., Boston, USA) (Beausang *et al.*, 2004; Kagan and Levin, 2001). The assay can be performed in a single tube or in a microplate and read visually or using an enzyme immunoassay (EIA) microplate reader at 450 nm. Colour development is directly proportional to the amount of peptidoglycan present (Beausang *et al.*, 2004). Two peptide markers have enabled the detection of 11 bacterial species (three Gram-positive and eight Gram-negative) (Kagan and Levin, 2001) The assay time is 25 minutes and the sensitivity for the detection of *Serratia marcescens* and *Staphylococcus epidermidis* was 10^2 cfu/ml (Beausang *et al.*, 2004). Both assays may potentially allow 'point of transfusion' screening. Further evaluation of this system is warranted.

Pathogen reduction

Please refer to Chapter 19.

Pathogen reduction technologies are under development for the inactivation of viral, bacterial and parasitic microbial agents. The majority of these systems involve the addition of a chemical, which binds to DNA. Binding to DNA or RNA prevents the organism transcribing DNA and RNA, so replication is blocked. This will ultimately interfere with metabolic function, resulting in cell death. Nucleic acid is an ideal target as this is not present in plasma, RBCs and platelets. These processes have the additional benefit that leucocytes contain DNA and these will also be inactivated. Leucocyte inactivation will potentially prevent graft-versus-host disease as well as cytokine-induced transfusion reactions.

There is sometimes an incorrect assumption that gamma irradiation will solve the problem of bacterial contamination. Doses

Psoralen

Amotosalen

Figure 7.22 Chemical structures of psoralen and amotosalen.

of 75 Gy do not effectively prevent the growth of bacteria (Huston, 1998). Dose levels of 25–30 Gy are generally applied to blood components to prevent graft versus host disease. This dose level has been shown to inactivate T lymphocytes, but levels as high as 4–12 kGy are required to inactivate bacteria, and this may compromise platelet function (Block, 2001). Therefore, gamma irradiated components are just as likely to cause a bacterial transfusion reaction as are non-irradiated units.

Platelet concentrate pathogen reduction systems

The intercept system

Cereus (Concord, California, USA) in collaboration with Baxter (Deerfield, Illinois, USA), have developed the Intercept system for the pathogen reduction of platelet concentrates (http://www.cerus.com). The psoralen based compound amotosalen hydrochloride is used (see Figure 7.22). Amotosalen-HCl intercalates with nucleic acids and each amotosalen molecule has two reactive sites. In the presence of long wavelength ultraviolet light (UVA), reversibly intercalated amotosalen-HCl reacts with pyrimidine bases to form permanent covalent bonds, cross-linking strands of nucleic acid (see Figure 7.23). This cross-linking prevents transcription and blocks replication (see Figure 7.24). At the end of the process residual amotosalen-HCl and photodegradation products are removed by a compound absorption device (CAD) (see Figure 7.25). The system requires product standardization with regard to total volume and

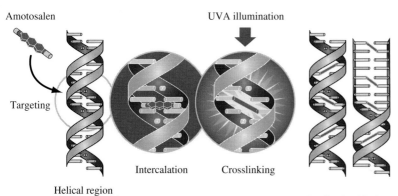

Figure 7.23 Amotosalen: mechanism of action.

Amotosalen

UVA illumination

Targeting

Intercalation   Crosslinking

Helical region
of DNA and RNA

Replication blocked

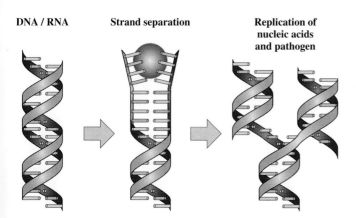

DNA / RNA   **Strand separation**   **Replication of nucleic acids and pathogen**

Figure 7.24 Nucleic acids must 'Unzip' during replication of pathogens.

platelet concentration. Currently, Baxter (Deerfield, Illinois, USA) platelet additive solution (Intersol) must be utilized in the process in the ratio 65% Intersol to 35% plasma. Illumination of the platelet concentrates is performed at 3J/cm² for 3–6 minutes. Removal of residual psoralen then takes a minimum of 4–6 hours depending on product type. Standardization of the product may pose logistical problems. An 11% loss of platelets and volume has been reported with the process (Picker *et al.*, 2004). There are still residual concerns with regard to the possible long-term adverse genotoxic and mutagenic effects of the transfusion of psoralen and psoralen derivatives into patients. However, successful clinical trials have been performed with no evidence of such problems as yet.

In spiking experiments, the bacterial reduction achieved ranges from >5.6 to >7.0 $\log_{10}$ (see Table 7.11). It appears that spores cannot be inactivated by this (Knutson *et al.*, 2000), unless inspissation of the spore to a vegetative phase has occurred.

The system is CE marked and is awaiting FDA approval in the USA. At present it is in routine use in 12 sites in Europe (three in Scandinavia, four in Spain, three in Italy and two in Belgium) and under evaluation in others (Janetzko *et al.*, 2004; Picker *et al.*, 2004). The system is being adapted for plasma treatment, but is not suitable for RBCs as the UVA light is absorbed by haemaglobin, reducing intercalation with nucleic acid.

Mirasol system

The Mirasol system is under development by Navigant Biotechnologies (Lakewood, Colorado, USA) in conjunction with Gambro (Lakewood, Colorado, USA). Mirasol uses the naturally occurring vitamin riboflavin (B_2) (see Figure 7.26). At present, the system is primarily under development for the pathogen reduction of platelet concentrates, but it is potentially adaptable for plasma and RBC units. Riboflavin in the presence of light can act as a photosensitizer producing nucleic acid reactive oxygen mediated damage (Ito *et al.*, 1993; Joshi, 1985). Illuminated riboflavin can also form new compounds (Olsen *et al.*, 1996; Piper *et al.*, 2001) (adducts) with thiamine and adenine (Ennever and Speck, 1983). Either process interferes with DNA and RNA replication.

In the current Mirasol process, riboflavin is added to the platelet concentrate bag. The bag is illuminated with broad spectrum light (6.2 J/ml) for ten minutes and then made available for transfusion (see Figure 7.27). No removal step is required as the residual riboflavin and photo by-products are considered to be non-toxic.

Riboflavin and light treatment can produce membrane and protein damage as well as nucleic acid damage. Haemolysis of RBCs has been reported when using this process. Platelet concentrate function and quality studies have shown that riboflavin and light treated units are within acceptable limits (Corbin, 2002; Goodrich *et al.*, 2001; Li *et al.*, 2004).

In a bacterial spiking experiment logarithmic reductions ranging from 3.1–5.5 were observed (see Table 7.12). The low reduction achieved with *Bacillus cereus* may be because this system is also unable to inactivate spore forming bacteria. Further assessment of bacterial inactivation as well as clinical trials is needed. Launch of the Mirasol system was planned for 2008.

Red cell inactivation system

Inactine (Pen 110)

The Inactine system is under development by Vitex (Watertown, MA, USA) for pathogen reduction of RBCs. Inactine (Pen 110) is chemically related to ethylenimine (see Figure 7.28). Inactine electrostatically binds to nucleic acid, by which it is activated to a reactive form, enabling a covalent bonding with nucleic acids (Budowsky *et al.*, 1996; Hemminki, 1984). Binding of the inactine to the nucleic acid prevents replication (O'Connor *et al.*, 1988). No illumination is required in this process, an obvious advantage given the density of RBCs in a red cell unit.

In this process, inactine is added to RBC units for 6–24 hours at 22–24 °C. At the end of this period any residual inactine is removed by multiple saline washes using a cell washer (AuBuchon *et al.*, 2002b; Zavizion *et al.*, 2003). Sodium thiosulphate can be used as an inactine quencher (AuBuchon *et al.*, 2002b). Spiking of RBC units at a concentration of 10–100 cfu/ml of the psychrophillic bacteria, *Yersinia enterocolitica*, *Pseudomonas fluorescens* and *Pseudomonas putida* and treatment with 0.1% (v/v) inactine for 24 hours resulted in no bacterial growth after 42 days' storage (Zavizion *et al.*, 2003). With an increase in inoculum level to 10^4 cfu/ml, growth was obtained with *Yersinia enterocolitica* and *Pseudomonas fluorescens* in two of the three RBC units studied, by day 14 of storage (Zavizion *et al.*, 2001). Therefore inactine may not be able to inactivate higher bacterial loads.

At present, Phase III clinical trials of inactine treated RBCs have been voluntarily suspended because one patient in the study developed an unanticipated immune response (http://www.vitechnologies.com). Vitex are currently modifying their RBC inactivation process to reduce the possibility of unexpected immunological responses.

FRALE

Cerus (Concord, California, USA) are developing a system for pathogen reduction of RBCs. A Frangible Anchor Linker Effector (FRALE) compound is used (S-303) based on the structure of quinacrine, which is similar to the toxic agent mustard gas (used to such devastating effect in World War I) (see Figure 7.29) (Cook *et al.*, and Wollowitz, 1997; Greenman *et al.*, 1998). FRALE bonds with nucleic acid preventing replication. A frangible (breakable/fragile) ester bond is present in FRALE compounds. This bond is broken down at a rate slower than that of bonding of the FRALE compound with nucleic acid. Therefore, it allows breakdown of the unreacted FRALE compound. No illumination is required with FRALE treatment.

Treatment of RBCs with 150 µ S-303 and a two-hour incubation was associated with a bacterial reduction that ranged from 4.8–7.4 $\log_{10}$ (see Table 7.13). Data are not yet available for the effect on spore forming bacteria.

In September 2003, all S-303 phase III clinical trials were suspended because two treated patients developed antibodies to red cells (http://cerus.com). Cerus, however, continue to develop this system and are in the process of developing changes that may greatly diminish the likelihood of antibody reaction in red cells.

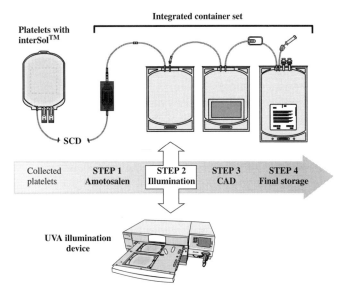

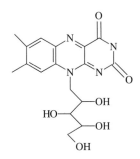

Figure 7.26 Riboflavin structure

Figure 7.25 Steps in the use of INTERCEPT platelet system using Helinx™ Technology.

Table 7.11 Bacterial reduction achieved with amotosalen-HCl And UV light.	
Bacteria	Logarithmic reduction ($\log_{10}$)
Staphylococcus epidermidis	>6.6
Escherichia coli	>6.4
Treponema pallidum	>7.0
Klebsiella pneumoniae	>5.6
Lactobacillus	>6.9
Bifidabacterium adolescentis	>6.5
Propionibacterium acnes	>6.7

Lin, 1997; Savoor, 2002; Zuckerman, 2003.

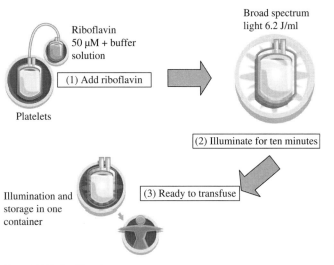

Figure 7.27 The Mirasol process.

Table 7.12 Bacterial reduction observed with riboflavin and light.

Bacteria	Logarithmic reduction ($\log_{10}$)
Staphylococcus epidermidis	5.1
Escherichia coli	4.7
Staphylococcus aureus	4.5
Bacillus cereus	3.1
Klebsiella pneumoniae	5.5

Goodrich et al., 2002.

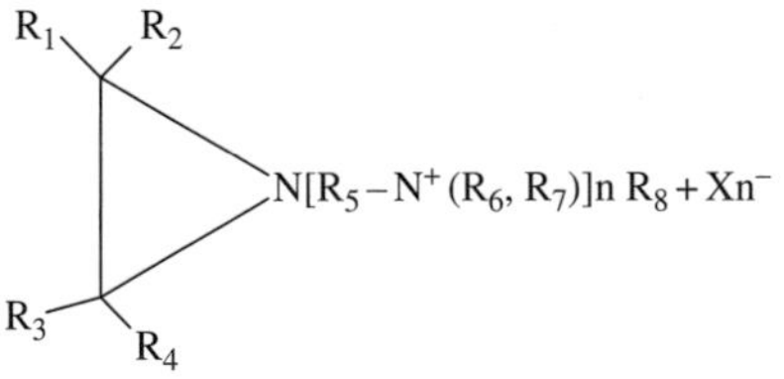

Figure 7.28 Structure of inactine (Pen 110).

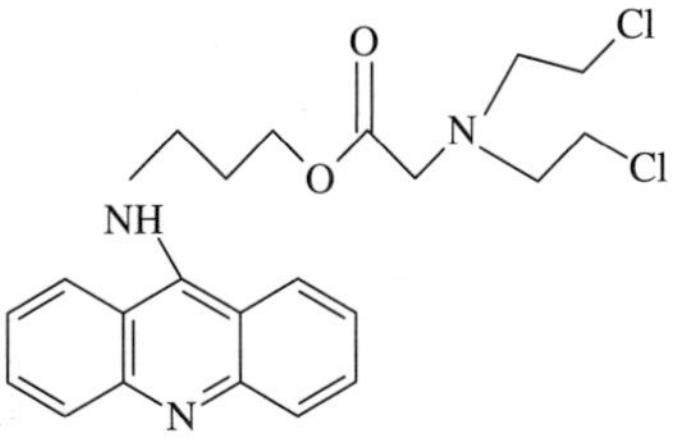

Figure 7.29. FRALE structure (S-303).

Table 7.13 Bacterial reduction achieved with S-303 (FRALE).

Organism	Reduction ($\log_{10}$) achieved
Yersinia enterocolitica	> 7.0
Salmonella typhimurium	4.8
Escherichia coli	> 7.4
Listeria monocytogenes	> 7.0
Staphylococcus epidermidis	5.2
Desinococcus radiodurans	> 6.0

Stassinopoulos, et al., 2000.

Conclusion

The bacterial contamination of blood components has been (and for the foreseeable future will continue to be) a serious threat to transfusion safety. Septic transfusion reactions associated with the transfusion of blood components contaminated with bacteria can potentially result in very serious transfusion-associated consequences. In fact, the presence of bacteria in blood components has been associated with more transfusion-associated adverse events than that caused by all the other microbiological agents that affect the blood supply combined.

It is important to recognize that many transfusion-associated septic events go unrecognized and undiagnosed because health care workers do not always think of blood components as the potential source of the bacterial infections in their patients. Moreover, many of the recipients of bacterially contaminated blood components are often granulocytopenic, and/or immunosuppressed. They may therefore be particularly susceptible to transfusion-associated bacterial infection and its consequences.

As outlined in this chapter, a large array of strategies (summarized in Table 7.6) have evolved to try and reduce the risk of transfusion-associated bacterial transmission. Many of these strategies have been implemented in many countries; we believe that the bacterial detection systems designed to screen out bacterially contaminated blood components play an important role in this regard (Fang et al., 2005). However, bacterial testing has been shown to be of somewhat limited efficacy (Benjamin and Mintz, 2005; Blajchman et al., 2005). As many as 50% of contaminated blood components may be undetected by culturing; particularly if sampled early in storage (Blajchman et al., 2005) ('false-negative' culture). The clinical risk of false-negative bacterial cultures, however, has not yet been clearly defined (Benjamin and Mintz, 2005). In addition, many of the other interventions proposed have both theoretical and practical limitations. Despite such limitations, it has become clear that cases of transfusion-associated sepsis could be prevented by the application of bacterial screening and/or other interventions listed in Table 7.6. (Benjamin & Mintz 2005; Fang et al., 2005).

In relation to the limitations of many of the current approaches to reducing the risk of transfusion-associated bacterial transmission, it appears that the 'ideal' strategy for the prevention of transfusion-associated bacterial sepsis would be the implementation of effective and safe methods for completely inactivating bacteria (as well as other microbiological agents). If manufacturers continue to invest in their development (despite the less than enthusiastic response from the majority of professionals, because of high cost for the small additional gain and implications for the throughput of component production), such methods are likely to become readily available over the next decade, particularly those that can be applied to platelet preparations. In addition to being safe, the systems would need to be highly effective in inactivating a wide range of bacterial species, including those that are spore forming. Finally, and most importantly, pathogen inactivated blood components should be free of potential toxicological problems (short and long term) for the recipient.

Pathogen inactivation systems for blood components are actively being developed and some 'first-generation' systems are now clinically available in Europe. Given all these developments, the reduction (and even the possible elimination) of transfusion-associated septic reactions is a realistic possibility in the foreseeable future (Benjamin and Mintz, 2005; Fang et al., 2005).

Acknowledgements

The authors would like to thank Julia Colvin, Siobhan McGuane and Mary Fielder for their assistance in preparation of this document.

Annexe

Brian C. Dow

Syphilis

Definition and characteristics of the agent

There are four main human treponemes that are known to be pathogenic:

(1) *Treponema pallidum* subspecies *pallidum* (syphilis)
(2) *Treponema pallidum* subspecies *endemicum* (bejel)
(3) *Treponema pallidum* subspecies *pertenue* (yaws)
(4) *Treponema carateum* (pinta).

Bejel, yaws and pinta are normally transmitted by non-sexual skin contact, mainly between children living in poor hygiene conditions.

Syphilis, caused by infection with *Treponema pallidum*, is, however, sexually transmitted and can be classified into several clinical stages. Primary syphilis is characterized by a painless genital ulcer (chancre) that appears around three weeks from infection. Around one-third of untreated primary infections will progress to secondary infections six to eight weeks later. Secondary syphilis is recognized by a symmetrical maculopapular rash involving the palms of hands and soles of feet. Around one-third of untreated secondary infections will develop latent infection. Latent syphilis infection is by definition asymptomatic and one-third of untreated cases will progress to tertiary syphilis. Tertiary syphilis may occur up to 40 years after the primary infection and usually involves central nervous and cardiovascular systems with lesions occurring in bones, skin, viscera, eyes and elsewhere in the body.

Transmission

Syphilis is normally transmitted through sexual contact with an infected individual. Congenital transmission can also occur. Although rare, transfusion-transmission can occur, particularly where blood is unscreened (as in poorer regions of the world). The incubation period for primary syphilis is usually around three weeks (9 to 90 days). The first transfusion-transmitted syphilis case was reported in 1915, but by 1941 138 cases were known (De Schryver and Meheus, 1990). The advent and gradual improvement of routine blood screening tests led to very few cases occurring (probably around one every 20 years).

Testing

Serological blood screening tests for syphilis have been in use for more than 60 years. Originally non-treponemal based tests such as the Venereal Diseases Research Laboratory (VDRL) and rapid plasma reagin (RPR) tests were used. These non-specific tests used a combination of cardiolipin antigen bound to charcoal to detect antilipin antibody produced in early syphilis infection. Such non-specific tests were capable of detecting between 50 and 70% of early primary syphilis infections but antibody levels waned after the secondary phase of infection (after three months

to one year) in either treated or untreated individuals (Young, 1992). Persistent reactivity suggested either continued infection or, alternatively, false-positive results. Confirmatory testing using treponema-based antigen systems was necessary to determine if this reactivity was true or false (Egglestone and Turner, 2000). Because cardiolipin (which mimics treponemal antigens) was used, approximately two-thirds of 'reactive' samples in testing were cross-reacting 'biological false-positives'.

A further complication is that infections of all four major types of pathogenic treponemes (syphilis, bejel, yaws and pinta) will produce antibodies that are reactive and indistinguishable by all specific syphilis assays. Epidemiological investigation on counselling a positive donor is necessary to help ascertain the type of treponeme infection.

During the 1990s, most blood services took the World Health Organization's advice and replaced the reagin tests with specific treponema based haemagglutination assays (TPHA). When used on the Olympus blood grouping machine, the TPHA assays do not have any of the subjectiveness associated with manual TPHA test reading.

More recently, both Northern Ireland and the Irish blood services have replaced their manual TPHA assays with syphilis EIAs. It should be noted that both TPHA and syphilis EIAs are extremely sensitive, such that remote past syphilis infections (as long ago as 50 or 60 years) will usually be reactive. In recent years manufacturers have utilized recombinant materials rather than purified and sonicated treponemes as source antigenic materials in various TPHA-based assays and EIAs. This has helped to provide more stable kits with little, if any, batch to batch variation. For some years gelatin particle agglutination assays (TPPA) have been available as an alternative to TPHA.

Confirmation of syphilis reactive screening tests is normally carried out using a confirmatory algorithm utilizing sensitive alternative EIA tests. If an alternative EIA is reactive then an immunoblot (see Figure 7.1) (please refer to Figure 12.7 in colour plate section) is performed together with a specific IgM EIA.

Window period

Levels of the organism in blood are variable and any bacteraemia may be short-lived. There is a general paucity of data regarding the possibility that blood taken early in the window period of early syphilis infection may cause infection in recipients, although it must be theoretically possible. The availability of polymerase chain reaction (PCR) tests for syphilis may assist in investigating the rare instance of a reported transfusion-transmitted syphilis infection or alternatively re-bleeding and testing implicated donors may prove easier (Orton, 2001). Nevertheless, until such time as such a case is investigated, then it is unlikely that our scientific knowledge will be augmented.

Risk factors

The main risk factors associated with syphilis infection are obviously those donors who are sexually promiscuous, for example men who have had sex with men (MSM).

Estimated risk of transfusion-transmission

The UK has not had a reported case of syphilis transfusion-transmission for some time. Indeed, the USA claims a period of over 30 years with no reported case (Orton, 2001). This apparent low incidence may have many explanations:

(1) The treponemes are comparatively fragile, such that storage for 72 hours at 4 °C will irretrievably damage the organism.

(2) Syphilis serological donor testing removes most infective donations.

(3) Those 'window-period' infective donations that elude detection may be transfused to recipients who are also receiving antibiotic therapy; infection is therefore avoided.

(4) Alternatively, syphilis infection may be occurring but symptoms are not recognized as transfusion-transmitted syphilis.

Conclusion

There has been much debate whether to retain or cease syphilis donor testing. The US American Association of Blood Banks (AABB) dropped the requirement in 1985 but the FDA did not support the proposal because syphilis testing was a potential surrogate for high risk behaviour for HIV infection. Even in 2000, it was felt that there was insufficient scientific data to warrant discontinuation of syphilis donor testing in the USA. To cease testing would provide minimal cost savings when compared to the current commercial NAT assays. Moreover, in 2000–2005 there has been a resurgence in syphilis infection in the UK general population (initially amongst MSMs) and this has been reflected by an increased number of blood donors with evidence of early primary syphilis infection (as demonstrated by the presence of IgM antibodies) (L. J. Brant personal communication). This recent increase in recently acquired syphilis is suggestive that more blood donors are practising high-risk sexual behaviours. This obviously has significant implications regarding the safety of the blood supply from agents that are normally sexually transmitted but may also be unknowingly transfusion-transmitted. Most would therefore favour retention of syphilis donor testing.

ANNEXE REFERENCES

De Schryver, A. and Meheus, A. (1990) Syphilis and blood transfusion: a global perspective. *Transfusion*, **30**, 844–7.

Egglestone, S. I. and Turner, A. J. L. for the PHLS Syphilis Serology Working Group (2000) Serological diagnosis of syphilis. *Commun Dis Public Health*, **3**, 158–62.

Orton, S. (2001) Syphilis and blood donors: what we know, what we do not know, and what we need to know. *Transfus Med Rev*, **15**, 282–92.

Young, H. (1992) Syphilis: new diagnostic directions. *Int J STD AIDS*, **3**, 391–413.

REFERENCES

Adams, M. R., Johnson, D. K. and Busch, M. P. (1997) Automatic volumetric capillary cytometry for counting white cells in white cell-reduced platelet-pheresis components. *Transfusion*, **37**, 29–37.

Amorim, L., Lopes, M., Oliveira, J. F., *et al*. (2004) Bacterial detection in platelet concentrates: a comparison between urine strips and culture. *Transfusion*, **44** (Supplement), 48A.

Anderson, K. C., Lew, M. A. and Gorgone, B. C. (1986) Transfusion-related sepsis after prolonged platelet storage. *Am J Med*, **81**, 405–11.

Arduino, A. M., Bland, L. A. and Tipple, M. A. (1989) Growth and endotoxin productions of *Yersinia enterocolitica* and *Enterobacter agglomerans* in packed erythrocytes. *J Clin Microbiol*, **27**, 1483–5.

AuBuchon, J. P., Cooper, L. K., Leach, M. F., *et al*. (2002a) Experience with universal bacterial culturing to detect contamination of apheresis platelet units in a hospital transfusion service. *Transfusion*, **42**, 855–61.

AuBuchon, J. P., Pickard, C. and Herschel, L. (1995) Sterility of plastic tubing welds in components stored at room temperature. *Transfusion*, **35**, 303–7.

AuBuchon, J. P., Pickard, C. A., Herschel, L. H., *et al*. (2002b) Production of pathogen-inactivated RBC concentrates using PEN 110 chemistry: a phase I clinical study. *Transfusion*, **42**, 146–52.

Bang, F. B. (1953) The toxic effect of a marine bacterium on Limulus and the formation of blood clots. *Bio Bull*, **105**, 361–2.

Barrett, B. B., Andersen, J. W. and Anderson, K. C. (1993) Strategies for the avoidance of bacterial contamination of blood components. *Transfusion*, **33**, 228–33.

Beausang, L. A., Levin, A. and Kovalenko, V. (2004) A rapid assay for the detection of bacteria in platelet units. *Transfusion*, **44** (Supplement), 47A.

Benavides, S., Nicol, K., Koranyi, K., *et al*. (2003) Yersinia septic shock following an autologous transfusion in a pediatric patient. *Transfus Apheresis, Sci*, **28**, 19–23.

Benjamin, R. J. and Mintz, P. D. (2005) Bacterial detection and extended platelet storage: the next step forward. *Transfusion*, **45**, 1832–5.

Bertolini, F. and Murphy, S. (1994) A multicenter evaluation of reproducibility of swirling in platelet concentrates. *Transfusion*, **34**, 796–801.

Betts, W. B. and Brown, A. P. (1999) Dielectrophoretic analysis of microbes in water. *Journal of Applied Microbiology Symposium Supplement*, **85**, 201S–13S.

Bhanji, S., Williams, B., Sheller, B., *et al*. (2002) Transient bacteremia induced by toothbrushing: a comparison of the Sonicare toothbrush with a conventional toothbrush. *Pediatr Dent*, **24**, 295–9.

Bjork, P. and Johnson, U. (1998) Detection of bacterial growth in platelet concentrates (Abstract). *Vox Sang*, **74** (Suppl.), 1267.

Blajchman, M. A. (2002) Incidence and significance of the bacterial contamination of blood components. *Dev Bio*, **108**, 59–67.

Blajchman, M. A., Beckers, E. A., Dickmeiss, E., *et al*. (2005) Bacterial detection of platelets: current problems and possible resolutions. *Transfus Med Rev*, **19**, 259–72.

Blajchman, M. A., Thornley, J. H., and Richardson, H. (1979) Platelet transfusion-induced *Serratia marcescens* sepsis due to vacuum tube contamination. *Transfusion*, **19**, 39–44.

Block, S. S., ed. (2001) *Disinfection, Sterilization, and Preservation*. 5th edn. Lippincott Williams & Wilkins, Philadelphia.

Bos, H., Yedema, T. H. and Luten, M. (2002) Reduction of the incidence of bacterial contamination by pre-donation drawing blood for safety tests. *Vox Sang*, **83** (Suppl.2), 14.

Boulton, F. E., Chapman, S. T. and Walsh, T. H. (1998) Fatal reaction to transfusion of red-cell concentrate contaminated with *Serratia liquefaciens*. *Transfus Med*, **8**, 15–8.

Bradley, R. M., Gander, R. M. and Patel, S. K. (1997) Inhibitory effect of 0°C storage on the proliferation of *Yersinia enterocolitica* in donated blood. *Transfusion*, **37**, 691–5.

Brecher, M. E., Hay, S. N., and Rothenberg, S. J. (2004) Validation of BacT/ALERT plastic culture bottles for use in testing of whole-blood-derived leukoreduced platelet-rich-plasma-derived platelets. *Transfusion*, **44**, 1174–8.

Brecher, M. E., Heath, D. and Hay, S. (2005) Evaluation of a new generation culture bottle using the BacT/ALERT 3D microbial detection system on 9 common contaminating organisms found in platelet components. *Transfusion*, **42**, 774–9.

Brecher, M. E., Hogan, J. J. and Boothe, G. (1993) The use of a chemiluminescence-linked universal bacterial ribosomal RNA gene probe and blood gas analysis for the rapid detection of bacterial contamination in white cell reduced and non-reduced platelets. *Transfusion*, **33**, 450–7.

Brecher, M. E., Hogan, J. J. and Boothe, G. (1994) Platelet bacterial contamination and the use of a chemiluminescence-linked universal bacterial ribosomal RNA gene probe. *Transfusion*, **34**, 750–5.

Brecher, M. E., Holland, P. V., Pineda, A. A., *et al.* (2000a) Growth of bacteria in inoculated platelets: implications for bacteria detection and the extension of platelet storage. *Transfusion*, **40**, 1308–12.

Brecher, M. E., Means, N. and Jere, C. S. (2001) Evaluation of the BacT/ALERT 3D microbial detection system for platelet bacterial contamination: an analysis of 15 contaminating organisms. *Transfusion*, **41**, 477–82.

Brecher, M. E., Wong, E. C. C., Chen, S. E., *et al.* (2000b) Antibiotic-labeled probes and microvolume fluorimetry for the rapid detection of bacterial contamination in platelet components: a preliminary report. *Transfusion*, **40**, 411–3.

Bruneau, C., Perez, P., Chassaigne, M., *et al.* (2001) Efficacy of a new collection procedure for preventing bacterial contamination of whole-blood donations. *Transfusion*, **41**, 74–81.

Budowsky, E. I., Zalesskaya, M. A., Nepomnyashchaya, N. M., *et al.* (1996) Principles of selective inactivation of the viral genome: dependence for the rate of viral RNA modification on the number of protonizable groups in ethyleneimine. *Vaccine Res*, **5**, 29–39.

Burstain, J. M., Brecher, M. E., Workman, K., *et al.* (1997) Rapid identification of bacterially contaminated platelets using reagent strips: glucose and pH analysis as markers of bacterial metabolism. *Transfusion*, **37**, 255–8.

Casewell, M. W., Slater, N. and Cooper, J. E. (1981) Operating theatre water-baths as a cause of Pseudomonas septicaemia. *J Hosp Infect*, **2**, 237–40.

Center for Biologics Evaluation and Research (1999) Workshop on bacterial contamination of platelets, Bethesda. www.fda.gov.cber/minutes/bact092499.pdf.

Centers for Disease Control. (1991) *Yersinia enterocolitica* bacteremia and endotoxin shock associated with red blood cell transfusion – United States. *Morbidity and Mortality Weekly Report*, **40**, 176–8.

Chaney, R., Rider, J. and Pamphilon, D. (1999) Direct detection of bacteria in cellular blood products using bacterial ribosomal RNA-directed probes coupled to electrochemiluminescence. *Transfus Med*, **9**, 177–88.

Chiu, E. K., Yuen, K. Y., Lie, A. K., *et al.* (1994) A prospective study of symptomatic bacteremia following platelet transfusion and of its management. *Transfusion*, **34**, 950–4.

Chongokolwatana, V., Morgan, M. and Feagin, J. C. (1993) Comparison of microscopy and a bacterial DNA probe for detecting bacterially contaminated platelets (Abstract). *Transfusion*, **33**(Suppl.), 50S.

Choo, Y., Rudon, L., Czajkowska, Z., *et al.* (2004) Bacterial screening of platelet concentrates using dipstick measurements of glucose and pH: validation in a tertiary care hospital. *Transfusion*, **44** (Suppl.), 51A.

Claeys, H. and Verhaeghe, B. (2000) Bacterial screening of platelets (abstract). *Vox Sang*, **78** (Suppl. 1), 374.

Cocco, A. E., Yomtovian, R. A., Jacobs, M. R., *et al.* (2004) Platelet bacterial contamination masquerading as a RBC febrile non-hemolytic transfusion reaction (FNHTR): a case report. *Transfusion*, **44** (Suppl.), 134A.

Cook, D. and Wollowitz, D. (1997) Method for inactivating pathogens in red cell compositions using quinacrine mustard. [5691132], USA Patent.

Cooper, J. F. (2001) The bacterial endotoxins test: past, present and future. *European Journal of Parenteral Sciences*, **6**, 89–93.

Corbin, F., III. (2002) Pathogen inactivation of blood components: current status and introduction of an approach using riboflavin as a photosensitizer. *Int J Hematol*, **76** Suppl. 2, 253–7.

Cummings, B., Colville, V., Hudson, N., *et al.* (2001) Routine surveillance is a sensitive and practical way to detect bacterial contamination of platelet units (abstract). *Transfusion Clinique et Biologique*, **8** (Suppl. 1), 23S.

Currie, L. M., Harper, J. R. and Allan, H. (1997) Inhibition of cytokine accumulation and bacterial growth during storage of platelet concentrates of 4 °C with retention of in vitro functional activity. *Transfusion*, **37**, 18–24.

Debeir, J., Noel, L., Allen, J.-P., *et al.* (1999) The French hemovigilance system. *Vox Sang*, **77**, 77–81.

Dietz, L., Debrow, R. S. and Manian, B. S. (1996) Volumetric capillary cytometry – a new method for absolute cell enumeration. *Cytometry*, **23**, 177–86.

Duncan, K. L., Ransley, J. and Elterman, M. (1994) Transfusion-transmitted *Serratia liquifaciens* from an autologous blood unit (letter). *Transfusion* **34**, 738–9.

Dzieczkowski, J. S., Barrett, B. B., Nester, D., *et al.* (1995) Characterization of reactions after exclusive transfusion of white cell-reduced cellular blood components. *Transfusion*, **35**, 20–5.

Dzik, W. (1995) Use of leukodepletion filters for the removal of bacteria. *Immunol Invest*, **24**, 95–115.

Dzik, W. H. (1997) A general method for concentrating blood samples in preparation for counting very low numbers of white cells. *Transfusion*, **37**, 277–83.

Ennever, J. F. and Speck, W. T. (1983) Photochemical reactions to riboflavin: covalent binding to DNA and to poly (dA). poly (dT) (short communication). *Pediatr Res*, **17**, 234–6.

Fang, C. T., Chambers, L. A., Kennedy, J., *et al.* (2005) Detection of bacterial contamination in apheresis platelet products: American Red Cross experience, 2004, *Transfusion*, **45**, 1845–52.

Fenwick, S. G. (1992) Pharyngitis and infections with *Yersinia enterocolitica* (letter). *NZ Med J*, **105**, 112.

Fenwick, S. G. and McCarthy, M. D. (1995) *Yersinia enterocolitica* is a common cause of gastroenteritis in Auckland. *N Z Med J*, **108** (1003), 269–71.

Franzin, L. and Gioannini, P. (1992) Growth of Yersinia species in artificially contaminated blood bags. *Transfusion*, **32**, 673–6.

Gibson, T. and Norris, W. (1958) Skin fragments removed by injection needles. *Lancet*, **2**, 983–5.

Goldman, M. and Blajchman, M. A. (1991) Blood product-associated bacterial sepsis. *Transfusion Med Rev*, **5**, 73–83.

Goldman, M. and Blajchman, M. A. (2001) Bacterial contamination. In *Transfusion Reaction*, ed. M. Popovsky, 2nd edn, pp. 133–59. Bethesda, MD, American Association of Blood Banks

Goldman, M., Roy, G., Frechette, N., *et al.* (1997) Evaluation of donor skin disinfection methods. *Transfusion*, **37**, 309–12.

Gong, J., Högman, C. F. and Lundholm, M. (1994) Novel automated microbial screening of platelet concentrates. *APMIS*, **102**, 72–8.

Gonzales, R., Durham, L. and Mark, O. (2004) Validation of the versatrek blood detection system for detection of bacterial contamination of platelets (abstract). *Transfusion*, **44**, 47A.

Goodnough, L. T., Shander, A. and Brecher, M. E. (2003) Transfusion medicine: looking to the future. *Lancet*, **361**, 161–9.

Goodrich, L., Douglas, I. and Urioste, M. (2002) Riboflavin photoinactivation procedure inactivates significant levels of bacteria and produces a culture negative product (abstract). *Transfusion*, **42** (Suppl.), 16S.

Goodrich, L. L., Hasen, E. T. and Gampp, D. (2001) Riboflavin pathogen inactivation process yields good platelet cell quality and expedient viral kill (abstract). *Blood*, **98** (Suppl.), 540a.

Greenman, W. M., Grass, J. A., Talib, S. *et al.* (1998) Method of treating leukocytes, leukocyte compositions and methods of use thereof. Cerus Corp (US) EP1005531. www.freepatentsonline.com/EP1005531A2.html.

Haditsch, M., Binder, L., Gabriel, C., et al. (1994) *Yersinia enterocolitica* septicemia in autologous blood transfusion. *Transfusion*, **34**, 907–9.

Hahn, L. F., Casciola, T. M., Triulzi, D. J., *et al.* (2004) Validation of pH determination on random donor platelets for the detection of bacteria. *Transfusion*, **44** (Suppl.), 48A.

Hall, J. and Lajoie, C. (2004) Correlation of PGD test result and pH of platelet concentrates inoculated with bacteria. *Transfusion*, **44** (Suppl.), 49A.

Hay, S. N., Brecher, M. E., Rothenberg, S. J., *et al.* (2004) Validation of the BacT/Notify remote notification software system. *Transfusion*, **44** (Suppl.), 53A.

Heal, J. M., Jones, M. E., Forey, J., *et al.* (1987) Fatal *salmonella septicemia* after platelet transfusion. *Transfusion*, **27**, 2–5.

Hebert, P. C., Wells, G. and Blajchman, M. A. (1999) A multicenter, randomized controlled clinical trial of transfusion requirements in critical care. *N Engl J Med*, **340**, 409–17.

Heltberg, O., Skov, F., Gerner-Smidt, P., *et al.* (1993) Nosocomial epidemic of *Serratia marcescens* septicemia ascribed to contaminated blood transfusion bags. *Transfusion*, **33**, 221–7.

Hemminki, K. (1984) Reactions of ethyleneimine with guanosine and deoxyguanosine. *Chem Biol Interact*, **48**, 249–60.

Hochstei, H. D. (1987) The LAL test versus the rabbit pyrogen test for endotoxin detection: Update 87. *Pharm Technol*, **11**(6), 124–9.

Hoffmeister, K. M., Felbinger, T. W., Falet, H., *et al.* (2003b) The clearance mechanism of chilled blood platelets. *Cell*, **112**, 87–97.

Hoffmeister, K. M., Josefsson, E. C., Isaac, N. A., *et al.* (2003a) Glycosylation restores survival of chilled blood platelets. *Science*, **301**, 1531–4.

Högman, C. F., Fritz, H. and Sandberg, L. (1993) Post-transfusion *Serratia marcescens* septicemia. *Transfusion*, **33**, 189–91.

Högman, C. F., Gong, J. and Eriksson, L. (1991) White cells protect donor blood against bacterial contamination. *Transfusion*, **31**, 620–6.

Högman, C. F. and Gong, J. (1994) Studies of one invasive and two non-invasive methods for detection of bacterial contamination of platelet concentrates. *Vox Sang*, **67**, 351–5.

Holden, F., Foley, M. and Devin, G. (2000) Coagulase-negative staphylococcal contamination of whole blood and its components: the effect of WBC reduction. *Transfusion*, **40**, 1508–13.

Hoppe, P. A. (1992) Interim measures for detection of bacterially contaminated red cell components. *Transfusion*, **32**, 199–201.

http://www.cerus.com

http://www.veraxbiomedical.com

http://www.vitechnologies.com

Huston, B. M., Brecher, M. E. and Bandarenko, N. (1998) Lack of efficacy for conventional gamma irradiation of platelet concentrates to abrogate bacterial growth. *Am J Clin Pathol*, **109**, 734–47.

Ito, K., Inoue, S., Yamamoto, K., *et al.* (1993) 8-hydroxyguanosine formation at the 5′ site of 5′-GG-3′ sequences in double-stranded DNA by UV radiation with riboflavin. *J Bio Chem*, **268**, 13221–7.

Jacobs, M. R., Bajaksouzian, S., Windau, A., *et al.* (2005) Evaluation of the Scansystem method for detection of bacterially contaminated platelets. *Transfusion*, **45**, 265–9.

Janetzko, K., Lin, L., Eichler, H., *et al.* (2004) Implementation of the INTERCEPT blood system for platelets into routine blood bank manufacturing procedures: evaluation of apheresis platelets. *Vox Sang*, **86**, 239–45.

Jarfari, M., Forsberg, J., Gilcher, R. O., *et al.* (2002) *Salmonella sepsis* caused by a platelet transfusion from a donor with a pet snake. *N Engl J Med*, **347**, 1075.

Jones, B. L., Saw, M. H., Hanson, M. F., *et al.* (1993) *Yersinia enterocolitica* septicaemia from transfusion of red cell concentrate stored for 16 days. *J Clin Pathol*, **46**, 477–8.

Joshi, P. C. (1985) Comparison for the DNA-damaging property of photosensitised riboflavin via singlet oxygen (^{1}O$_2$) and superoxide radical O$_2$ mechanisms. *Toxicol Lett*, **26**, 211–7.

Kagan, D. and Levin, A. E. (2001) Rapid assay for bacterial contamination of platelets. *Transfusion*, **41** (Suppl.), 34S.

Kahwash, E. B., Leonard, J. and Redmon, M. (2004) BACTEC detection of bacteria in platelet pools (abstract). *Transfusion*, **44**, 47A.

Kendrick, C. J., Baker, B., Morris, A. J., *et al.* (2001) Identification of Yersinia-infected blood donors by anti Yop IgA immunoassay. *Transfusion*, **41**, 1365–72.

Kim, D. M., Brecher, M. E. and Bland, L. A. (1992) Visual identification of bacterially contaminated red cells. *Transfusion*, **32**, 221–5.

Knutson, F., Alfonso, R. and Dupuis, K. (2000) Photochemical inactivation of bacteria and HIV in buffy-coat-derived platelet concentrates under conditions that preserve in vitro platelet function. *Vox Sang*, **78**, 209–16.

Kojima, K., Togashi, T., Hasegawa, K., *et al.* (1998) Subcutaneous fatty tissue can stray into a blood bag. *Vox Sang*, **74**(Suppl. 1), Abstract 1205.

Korte, D. de, Marcelis, J. H. and Soeterboek, A. M. (2001) Determination of the degree of bacterial contamination of whole-blood collections using an automated microbe-detection system. *Transfusion*, **41**, 815–8.

Korte, D. de, Marcelis, J. H., Verhoeven, A. J., *et al.* (2002) Diversion of first blood volume results in a reduction of bacterial contamination for whole-blood collections. *Vox Sang*, **83**, 13–6.

Kosmin, M. (1980) Bacteremia during leukapheresis (letter). *Transfusion*, **20**, 115.

Kothe, F. C. and Platenkamp, G. J. (1994) The use of the sterile connection device in transfusion medicine. *Transfus Med Rev*, **VIII**, 117–22.

Kuehnert, M. J., Roth, V. R., Haley, N. R., *et al.* (2001) Transfusion-transmitted bacterial infection in the United States, 1998 through 2000. *Transfusion*, **41**, 1493–9.

Lane, S. R., Nicholls, P. J. & Sewell, R. D. E. (2004) The measurement and health impact of Endotoxin contamination in organic dusts from multiple sources: focus on the cotton industry. *Inhalation Toxicology*. **16**, 217–29.

Lane, S. R., Sewell, R. D. E. (2006) Endotoxins and glucans: Environmental trouble makers. *Biologist*, **53**, 129–34.

Laport, R., Bakker, M., Van Schayk, A., *et al.* (1999) Detection of bacterial contamination of platelet concentrates (abstract). *VI Regional European Congress of the International Society of Blood Transfusion*, **66**.

Lee, C. K., Ho, P. L., Chan, N. K., *et al.* (2002) Impact of donor arm skin disinfection on the bacterial contamination rate of platelet concentrates. *Vox Sang*, **83**, 204–8.

Leiby, D. A., Kerr, K. L., Campos, J. M., *et al.* (1997) A retrospective analysis of microbial contaminants in outdated random-donor platelets from multiple sites. *Transfusion*, **37**, 259–63.

Levin, J. and Bang, F. B. (1964a) A description of cellular coagulation in the Limulus. *Bull John Hopkins Hospital*, **115**, 337–45.

Levin, J. and Bang, F. B. (1964b) The role of endotoxin in the extracellular coagulation of Limulus blood. *Bull Johns Hopkins Hosp*, **115**, 265–74.

Levin, J. and Bang, F. B. (1968) Clottable protein in Limulus: its localization and kinetics of its coagulation by endotoxin. *Thromb Diath Haemorrh*, **19**, 186–97.

Li, J., de Korte, D. and Woolum, M. D. (2004) Pathogen reduction of buffy coat platelet concentrates using riboflavin and light: comparisons with pathogen-reduction technology-treated apheresis platelet products. *Vox Sang*, **87**, 82–90.

Lin, L. (1997) Photochemical inactivation of viruses and bacteria in platelet concentrates by use of a novel psoralen and long-wavelength ultraviolet light. *Transfusion*, **37**, 423–35.

Liu, H. W., Yuen, K. Y., Cheng, T. S., *et al.* (1999) Reduction of platelet transfusion-associated sepsis by short-term bacterial culture. *Vox Sang*, **77**(1), 1–5.

Macauley, A., Chandrasekar, A., Geddis, G., *et al.* (2003) Operational feasibility of routine bacterial monitoring of platelets. *Transfus Med*, **13**, 189–95.

McCarthy, L. R. and Senne, J. E. (1980) Evaluation of acridine orange stain for detection of micro-organisms in blood cultures. *J Clin Microbiol*, **11**, 281–5.

McDonald, C. P., Barbara, J. A. and Hewitt, P. E. (1996) *Yersinia enterocolitica* transmission from a red cell unit 34 days old. *Transfus Med*, **6**, 61–3.

McDonald, C. P., Colvin, J., Mahajan, P., *et al.* (2002a) National monitoring of the bacterial contamination rate of blood products using the BacT/ALERT system (abstract). *Clin Microbiol Infec*, **8** (Suppl. 1), 152.

McDonald, C. P., Colvin, J., Robbins, S., *et al.* (2005b) The use of a solid phase fluorescent cytometric technique for the detection of bacteria in platelet concentrates. *Transfus Med*, **15**, 175–83.

McDonald, C. P., Colvin, J. and Smith, R. (2004a) A novel method for the detection of bacteria in platelet concentrates utilising oxygen consumption as a marker for bacterial growth. *Transfus Med*, **14**, 391–8.

McDonald, C. P., Hartley, S., Orchard, K., *et al.* (1998) Fatal *Clostridium perfringens* sepsis from a pooled platelet transfusion. *Transfus Med*, **8**, 19–22.

McDonald, C. P., Lowe, P., Robbins, S., *et al.* (2001a) Evaluation of donor arm disinfection techniques. *Vox Sang*, **80**, 135–41.

McDonald, C. P., Pearce, S., Wilkins, K., *et al.* (2005a) Pall eBDS an enhanced bacterial detection system for screening platelet concentrates. *Transfus Med*, **15**, 259–68.

McDonald, C. P., Robbins, S. and Shahram, M. (2004b) Monitoring donor arm disinfection: essential for blood safety? (abstract). *Vox Sang*, **87**, S6.

McDonald, C. P., Rogers, A., Cox, M., *et al.* (2002b) Evaluation of the 3D BacT/ALERT automated culture system for the detection of microbial contamination of platelet concentrates. *Transfus Med*, **12**, 303–9.

McDonald, C. P., Roy, A., Lowe, P., *et al.* (2000) The first experience in the United Kingdom of the bacteriological screening of platelets to increase shelf life to seven days. (abstract). *Vox Sang*, **78** (Suppl. 1), 375.

McDonald, C. P., Roy, A., Lowe, P., *et al.* (2001b) Evaluation of the BacT/Alert automated blood culture system for detecting bacteria and measuring their growth kinetics in leucodepleted and non-leucodepleted platelet concentrates. *Vox Sang*, **81**, 154–60.

McDonald, C. P., Roy, A., Mahajan, P., *et al.* (2004c) Relative values of the interventions of diversion and improved donor-arm disinfection to reduce the bacterial risk from blood transfusion. *Vox Sang*, **86**, 178–82.

McDonald, C. P., Roy, A., Mahajan, P., *et al.* (2002c) Evaluation of the Chloroprep disinfection system (abstract). *Vox Sang*, **83** (Suppl. 2), 5.

McDonald, C. P., Smith, R. and Colvin, J. (2005c) Evaluation of a novel dielectrophoresis system for the rapid detection of bacteria in platelet concentrates (abstract). *Transfusion*, **41** (Suppl.), 34S.

Mimms, L. (2002) Bacterial contamination of blood products – measures toward risk reduction, 2002. 6th Scientific Symposium German Red Cross, Dresden.

Mitchell, K. M. T. and Brecher, M. E. (1999) Approaches to the detection of bacterial contamination in cellular blood products. *Transfus Med Rev*, **13**, 132–44.

Mohammadi, T., Pietersz, R. N. I., Vandenbroucke-Grauls, C. M. J. E., *et al.* (2005) Detection of bacteria in platelet concentrates: comparison of broad-range real-time 16 S rDNA polymerase chain reaction and automated culturing. *Transfusion*, **45**, 731–6.

Mohammadi, T., Reesink, H. W., Vandenbroucke-Grauls, M. J. E., *et al.* (2003) Optimization of real-time PCR assay for rapid and sensitive detection of eubacterial 16S ribosomal DNA in platelet concentrates. *J Clin Microbiol*, **41**, 4796–8.

Mohr, H., Spengler, H.-P., Lambrecht, B., *et al.* (2003) Flow cytometric sterility testing of platelet concentrates. *VIII European Congress of the International Society of Blood Transfusion*, p85.

Morel, P. (1999b) Bacterial contamination of platelets workshop, Bethseda. fda gov/cber/minutes/bact092499 pdf 1999. 13–10–2005

Morel, P., Deschaseaux, M., Bertrand, X., *et al.* (2002) Detection of bacterial contamination in platelet concentrates using Scansystem: first results (abstract). *Transfusion*, **42** (Suppl.).

Morel, P. C. (1999a) *The French Experience in the Prevention of Transfusion Incidents Due to Bacterial Contamination.* Bacterial Contamination of Platelets Workshop, FDA, Washington.

Munksgaard, L., Albjerg, L., Lillevang, S. T., *et al.* (2004) Detection of bacterial contamination of platelet components: six years' experience with the BacT/ALERT system. *Transfusion*, **44**, 1166–73.

Ness, P., Braine, H. and King, K. (2001) Single-donor platelets reduce the risk of septic platelet transfusion reactions. *Transfusion*, **41**, 857–61.

Nguyen K.-A., Yamamoto, T. and Sandhu, H. (2004) Performance evaluation of the Pall eBDS bacterial detection method and direct comparison with BacT/Alert, pH and swirling. *Transfusion*, **44** (Suppl.), 25A.

Novak, M. (1939) Preservation of stored blood with sulfanilamide. *JAMA*, **113**, 2227–9.

O'Connor, T. R., Boiteux, S. and Laval, J. (1988) Ring-opened 7-methylguanine residues in DNA are a block to in vitro DNA synthesis. *Nucl Acid Res*, **16**, 5879–94.

Olsen, J. H., Hertz, H. and Kjaer, S. K. (1996) Childhood leukemia following phototherapy for neonatal hyperbilirubinemia (Denmark). *Cancer Causes Control*, **7**, 411–4.

Olthuis, H., Puylaert, C., Verhagen, C., *et al.* (1995) Method for removal of contamination bacteria during venepuncture. Presented at the Fifth International Society of Blood Transfusion Regional Congress, Venice, Italy 2–5 July 1995 (abstract).

Ortolano, G. A., Freundlich, L. F. and Holme, S. (2003) Detection of bacteria in WBC-reduced PLT concentrates using percent oxygen as a marker for bacteria growth. *Transfusion*, **43**, 1276–84.

Pall Corporation (2003) Bacteria detection system for leukocyte-reduced platelet transfusion products-sample set. Pall BDS package insert. East Hills, NY.

Pearce, S., Hayward, M., Rowe, G., *et al.* (2004) Routine bacterial monitoring of platelets (abstract). *Vox Sang*, **87**(Suppl. 3), 27.

Pepersack, F., Prigogyne, T. and Butzler, J. P. (1979) *Campylobacter jejuni* post-transfusion septicemia (letter). *Lancet*, 2, 911.

Perez, P., Salmi, L. R., Follea, G., *et al.* (2001) Determinants of transfusion-associated bacterial contamination: results of the French BACTHEM Case-Control Study. *Transfusion*, **41**, 862–72.

Pickard, C., Herschel, L. and Seery, P. (1998) Visual identification of bacterially contaminated red blood cells (abstract). *Transfusion*, **38** (Suppl.), 12S.

Picker, S. M., Speer, R. and Gathof, B. S. (2004) Evaluation of processing characteristics of photochemically treated pooled platelets: target requirements for the INTERCEPT blood system comply with routine use after process optimization. *Transfus Med*, **14**, 217–23.

Pietersz, R. N., de Korte, D. and Reesink, H. W. (1989) Storage of whole blood for up to 24 hours at ambient temperature prior to component preparation. *Vox Sang*, **56**, 145–50.

Piper, J. T., Murphy, S. E. and Schuyler, R. (2001) Evaluation of acute toxicity and genotoxicity risks associated with the riboflavin photoproduct lumichrome (abstract). *Transfusion*, **41** (Suppl.), 90S.

Pleasant, H., Marini, J. and Stehling, L. (1994) Evaluation of three skin preps for use prior to phlebotomy (abstract). *Transfusion*, **34** (Suppl.), 14S.

Prentice, M. (1992) Transfusing *Yersinia enterocolitica. BMJ*, **305**, 663–4.

Puca, K. E., Boyer, T. C., Grygny, C.-J., *et al.* (2004) A blood center experience using pH paper for detection of bacterial contamination of whole blood-derived platelets. *Transfusion*, **44** (Suppl.), 51A.

Puckett, A., Davison, G., Entwistle, C. C., *et al.* (1992) Post-transfusion septicaemia 1980–1989: importance of donor arm cleansing. *J Clin Pathol*, **45**, 155–7.

Punsalang, A., Heal, J. M. and Murphy, P. J. (1989) Growth of Gram-positive and Gram-negative bacteria in platelet concentrates. *Transfusion*, **29**, 596–9.

Reik, H. and Rubin, S. J. (1981) Evaluation for the buffy-coat smear for rapid detection of bacteremia. *JAMA* 245, 357–9.

Rhame, F. S. and McCullough, J. (1979a) Follow-up on nosocomial *Pseudomonas cepacia* infection. *MMWR*, **28**, 409.

Rhame, F. S., McCullough, J. J. and Cameron, S. (1979b) *Pseudomonas cepacia* infections caused by thawing cryoprecipitate in a contaminated water bath (abstract). *Transfusion*, **19**, 653–4.

Rhame, F. S., Root, R. K., MacLowry, J. D., *et al.* (1973) *Salmonella septicemia* from platelet transfusions. Study of an outbreak traced to a hematogenous carrier of *Salmonella cholerae-suis. Ann Intern Med*, **78**, 633–41.

Ribault, S., Faucon, A. and Faure, I. (2004a) Bacterial detection in red blood cell concentrates using Scansystem (abstract). *Transfusion*, **44**, 50A.

Ribault, S., Grave, L. and Faucon, A. (2004b) Detection of bacterial growth in contaminated red blood cell concentrates using Scansystem (abstract). *Transfusion*, **44**, 50A.

Ribault, S., Harper, K., Grave, L., *et al.* (2004c) Rapid screening method for the detection of bacteria in platelet concentrates. *J Clin Microbiol*, **42**(5), 1903–8.

Rock, G., Neurath, D., Toye, B. *et al.* (2004) The use of a bacteria detection system to evaluate bacterial contamination in PLT concentrates. *Transfusion*, **44**, 337–42.

Sanz, C., Pereira, A. and Vila, J. (1997) Growth of bacteria in platelet concentrates obtained from whole blood stored for 16 hours at 22 °C before component preparation. *Transfusion*, **37**, 251–4.

Savoor, A. R., Mababangloob, R., Kinsey, J., *et al.* (2002) The intercept blood system for platelets inactivities anaerobic bacteria (abstract). *Transfusion*, **42** (Suppl), 925.

Schelstraete, B., Bijens, B. and Wuyts, G. (2000) Prevalence of bacteria in leuco-depleted pooled platelet concentrates and apheresis platelets: current status in the Flemish blood service (abstract). *Vox Sang*, **78** (Suppl. 1), 372.

Schiffer, C. A., Anderson, K. C. and Bennett, C. L. (2001) Platelet transfusion for patients with cancer: clinical practice guidelines of the American Society of Clinical Oncology. *J Clin Oncol*, **19**, 1519–38.

Schneider, T., Tunez, V. and Fontaine, O. (2002) Benefits of the pre-donation sampling pouch in order to reduce bacterial contamination of pooled platelet concentrates (abstract). *Vox Sang*, **83**(Suppl. 2), 162.

Schneider, T., Tunez, V., Vens, T., *et al.* (2003) A comparative study of the Scansystem and the BacT/ALERT (abstract). *Transfusion*, **43**, 9S.

Sen, K. (2000) Rapid identification of *Yersinia enterocolitica* in blood by the 5' nuclease PCR assay. *J Clin Microbiol*, **38**, 1953–8.

Sen, K. and Asher, D. M. (2001) Multiplex PCR for detection of Enterobacteriaceae in blood. *Transfusion*, **41**, 1356–64.

Simon, T. L., Nelson, E. J., Carmen, R., *et al.* (1983) Extension of platelet concentrate storage. *Transfusion*, **23**, 207–12.

Snyder, E. L. and Rinder, H. M. (2003) Platelet storage – time to come in from the cold? *N Eng J Med*, **348**(20), 2032–3.

Soeterboek, A. M., Wells, F. H. W. and Marcelis, J. H. (1997) Sterility testing of blood products in 1994/1995 by three cooperating blood banks in the Netherlands. *Vox Sang*, **72**, 61–2.

Stainsby, D., Cohen, H., Jones, H., *et al.* (2003) Serious Hazards of Transfusion (SHOT). *SHOT Annual Report*, 1–88.

Stassinopoulos, A., Mababangloob, R. S., Dupuis, K. W., *et al.* (2000) Bacterial inactivation in leukoreduced PRBC treated with Helinx (abstract). *Transfusion*, **40** (Suppl.), 38S.

Strumia M. M. and McGraw J. J. (1941) Frozen and dried plasma for civil and military use. *JAMA*, **116**, 2378–82.

Theakston, E. P., Morris, A. J., and Streat, S. J. (1997) Transfusion transmitted *Yersinia enterocolitica* infection in New Zealand. *Aust NZ J Med*, **27**, 62–7.

Tipple, M. A., Bland, L. A., Murphy, J. J., *et al.* (2004) Sepsis associated with transfusion of red cells contaminated with *Yersinia enterocolitica*. *Transfusion*, **30**, 207–13.

Van der Meer, P. F., Dekker, W. J. A., Pietersz, R. N. I., *et al.* (2002) Bacterial screening of platelet concentrates in routine (abstract). *Vox Sang*, **83** (Suppl. 2), 16.

Vasconcelos E. (2001) Leucodepletion, bacterial contamination and virus inactivation: a Portuguese blood centre experience. *Transfus Apher Sci*, **25**, 215–6.

Vostal, J. G., and Mondoro, T. H. (1997) Liquid storage of platelets: a revitalized possible alternative for limiting bacterial contamination of platelet products. *Transfus Med Rev*, **11**, 286–95.

Vuk, T., Balija, M. and Jukic, I. (2003) Bacterial contamination of blood products 1998–2001 (abstract). *VIII European Congress of International Society of Blood Transfusion*, p. 272.

Wagner, S. (1997) Transfusion related bacterial sepsis. *Curr Opin Hematol*, **4**, 464–9.

Wagner, S. J. and Robinette, D. (1996) Evaluation of swirling, pH and glucose tests for the detection of bacterial contamination in platelet concentrates. *Transfusion* **36**, 989–93.

Wagner, S. J., Moroff, G., Katz, A. J., *et al.* (1995a) Comparison of bacterial growth in single and pooled platelet concentrates after deliberate inoculation and storage. *Transfusion* **35**, 298–302.

Wagner, S. J., Robinette, D. and Nazario, M. (1995b) Bacteria levels in components prepared from deliberately inoculated whole blood held for 8 or 24 hours at 20 to 24 °C. *Transfusion*, **35**, 911–6.

Wendel, S., Fontao-Wendel, R., Germano, S., *et al.* (2000) Screening of bacterial contamination in a routine scale for blood component production in a Brazilian blood bank (abstract). *Vox Sang*, **78** (Suppl.), p. 376.

Wenz, B., Ciavarella, D. and Freundlich L. (1993) Effect of prestorage white cell reduction on bacterial growth in platelet concentrates. *Transfusion*, **33**, 520–3.

Werch, J. B., Mhawech, P., Stager, C. E., *et al.* (2002) Detecting bacteria in platelet concentrates by use of reagent strips. *Transfusion*, **42**, 1027–31.

Wong, P. Y., Colville, V. and White, V. L. (2004) Appraisal of a proprietary preparation for pre-donation donor arm disinfection (abstract). *Transfusion*, **44**, 50A.

Yomtovian, R. (1993) A prospective microbiologic surveillance program to detect and prevent the transfusion of bacterially contaminated platelets. *Transfusion*, **33**, 902–9.

Yu, J. C., Chong, C., Cortus, M. A., *et al.* (2004) Bacteria growth in leukoreduced AS-3 red cell concentrates (RCC)a and detection with PALL eBDS. *Transfusion*, **44** (Suppl.), 45A.

Zavizion, B., Serebryanik, D. and Purmal, A. (2001) Collection system equivalency using the INACTINE process for pathogen inactivation: bacterial inactivation assessment (abstract). *Transfusion*, **41** (Suppl.), 89S.

Zavizion, B., Serebryanik, D., Serebryanik, I., *et al.* (2003) Prevention of *Yersinia enterocolitica*, *Pseudomonas fluorescens* and *Pseudomonas putida* outgrowth in deliberately inoculated blood by a novel pathogen-reduction process. *Transfusion*, **43**, 135–42.

Zuckerman, A. J. (2003) Intercept blood system: crosslinks under the spotlight. *Pathol. Pract*, November, 2–3.

8 THE PROTOZOAN PARASITES

David A. Leiby and Silvano Wendel

Transmission of infectious agents by blood transfusion has been an ongoing concern of transfusion medicine for decades. For years, the focus of concern has appropriately been on a variety of viral agents (e.g. HIV, hepatitis viruses, West Nile virus) that are known to pose blood safety risks. However, in recent years, infections resulting from protozoan parasites have received more prominent attention largely due to two factors. First, the success in controlling transfusion-transmitted viral agents has resulted in those infections caused by parasitic agents being more visible. Second, changing donor demographics and the norm of worldwide travel have introduced many parasitic agents, which were once thought to be exotic, to non-endemic developed countries. With the increased interest in preventing the transmission of protozoan parasites, new interventions, not based on viral models, are required. In this chapter we have attempted to explore these and other transfusion issues surrounding those protozoan parasites that pose blood safety risks (see Table 8.1).

Plasmodium spp. – malaria

Malaria is a life-threatening parasitic disease transmitted by mosquitoes (Warrell *et al.*, 2002). Human malaria is transmitted by four different species: *Plasmodium falciparum, Plasmodium vivax, Plasmodium ovale* and *Plasmodium malariae*, which require two different hosts to complete their life cycle – an *Anopheles* mosquito (sexual stage) and humans (asexual stage).

When infected female mosquitoes bite humans (see Figure 8.1), they release small asexual sporozoites through their salivary gland into the bloodstream. These are amotile, spindle shaped, 10–15 μm long organisms. They circulate for a very short time (less than 60 minutes), until they invade hepatocytes (exoerythrocytic stage), where they undergo a schizogonic step (repeated nuclear division) lasting 5 to 31 days, ending with the rupture of mature schizonts and release of merozoites (from 2000 for *P. malariae*, up to 40 000 for *P. falciparum*) into the bloodstream. They invade circulating red blood cells (erythrocytic stage), with some differences in the invasive capacity observed among the four species, given that *P. falciparum* is able to invade erythrocytes of all ages, whereas *P. vivax* and *P. ovale* prefer younger red cells or reticulocytes, and *P. malariae* prefers senescent red cells. Another schizogony occurs in red cells, with generation of schizonts (ring forms) and subsequent release of additional merozoites (4 to 24 according to the *Plasmodium* species), which infect other red cells, continuing this asexual stage (see Figure 8.2). This schizogonic process is rather regular, lasting 48 hours for *P. falciparum, P. vivax* and *P. ovale* (tertian fever), and 72 hours for *P. malariae* (quartan fever).

Merozoites released from liver cells cannot subsequently reinvade other hepatocytes and perpetuate the process. However, some *P. vivax* and *P. ovale* sporozoites give rise to hypnozoites (a very latent exoerythrocytic form), which remain dormant inside the hepatic parenchyma for approximately five years before starting the exoerythrocytic schizogonic stage, inducing late relapses if proper treatment is not applied.

In parallel, after several divisions, some erythrocytic parasites undergo another cyclical step and differentiate into sexual gametocytes. Once released, instead of invading red cells, they are ingested by another mosquito during a blood meal, beginning the sexual reproduction (fertilization) in the insect stomach, leading to development of oocysts under the basal membrane, where after a reduction division (sporogony), thousands of free sporozoites are released in the insect's haemocoel. They migrate towards the mosquito salivary gland, thereby completing their life cycle (López-Antuñano and Schmunis, 1990; Tabor, 1982; WHO, 1987). In addition to the classical, vectorial transmission, induced malaria can also be transmitted by blood transfusion (Wendel, 2003), organ transplantation (Salutari *et al.*, 1996; Talabiska *et al.*, 1996; Tran *et al.*, 1997), sharing of intravenous drugs or needles, accidental laboratory exposure, congenitally, or rarely in persons living close to or working at airports (Thellier *et al.*, 2001). The latter are presumed to be caused by infected insects travelling in the plane and evading the routine insecticidal spraying in the craft.

The first case of transfusion-transmitted malaria (TTM)[1] was reported in 1911 by Woolsey (Woolsey, 1911), and more than 3000 cases have been described so far (Turc, 1990), though these numbers may represent less than 50% of the actual cases (International Forum, 2004). Although malaria has been eradicated in almost all European countries (Rouger, 1999), the USA (Shah *et al.*, 2004), Australia (Farrugia, 2004) and Japan (Kano and Kimura, 2004), it was still present in 106 countries of the world in 2001 (available at: http://www.who.int/GlobalAtlas/DataQuery/browse.asp?catID=012802000000&lev=4). In this same year, WHO reported that more than 1200 million people were infected in 72 countries, but these estimates include 350 to 515 million new cases annually, with 270 to 400 million due to *P. falciparum* (70% in Africa and 20% in South-east Asia), nearly 1 million deaths, with 90% in Africa south of Sahara, mostly in children (http://mosquito.who.int/malariacontrol). Quite recently, a study claimed that the real number is almost two-fold greater than the

---

[1] According to WHO terminology (WHO, 1963), transfusion malaria is also defined as *induced malaria* (transmitted by mechanical means, such as transfusions, organ transplantation, deliberate infection for malaria therapy, contaminated needles or injection equipment).

Transfusion Microbiology, eds John A. J. Barbara, Fiona A. M. Regan and Marcela C. Contreras. Published by Cambridge University Press. © Cambridge University Press 2008.

Table 8.1 Protozoan parasitic agents transmissible by blood transfusion.

Agent	Disease
Plasmodium spp.	Malaria
P. falciparum	
P. vivax	
P. malariae	
P. ovale	
Babesia spp.	Babesiosis
B. microti	
WA-1	
Toxoplasma gondii	Toxoplasmosis
Leishmania spp.	Leishmaniasis
L. donavani	
Trypanosoma cruzi	Chagas' disease
	American trypanosomiasis

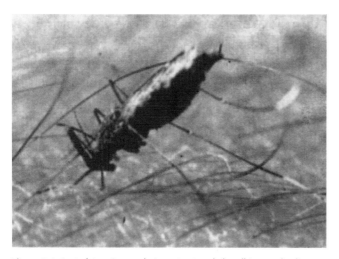

Figure 8.1 Central American malaria vector *Anopheles albimanus* feeding on a person.

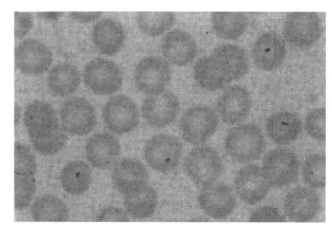

Figure 8.2 Ring forms of *Plasmodium falciparum* within red blood cells.

Chataing, 1988; Frey-Wettstein *et al.*, 2001; International Forum, 1987; Rouger, 1999; Tabor, 1982; Warrell *et al.*, 2002; WHO 1992a; 1992b). In the UK, there is a trend for continuous increases of imported malaria in the last two decades, mainly arising from *P. falciparum* cases (Bradley *et al.*, 1998).

The annual incidence of TTM ranges from 0.25–0.67 cases/million units in the USA (Nahlen *et al.*, 1991) and Canada (Shehata *et al.*, 2004), respectively, to more than 50 cases/million units in endemic regions (Bruce-Chwatt, 1972; 1974; 1982). Even in non-endemic countries, where complete eradication has been accomplished, the ever increasing migration flow has played a greater role in the last three decades, as observed in France in the 1980s, with more than 100 cases described (Chataing, 1988).

Infected blood donors may harbour parasites for many years, especially those from endemic regions who are partially immune and demonstrate an absence of symptoms, or those donors who have received chemoprophylaxis. Different periods of infection are seen for each species; it is widely known that *P. falciparum* can be cleared within one year, although longer periods (8–13 years) have been described (Bruce-Chwatt, 1982; Kitchen *et al.*, 2005; Mungai *et al.*, 2001; Turc, 1990). *Plasmodium vivax* and *P. ovale* usually do not persist for more than 3–4 years, but infections after 6–8 years or even more have also been described (Frey-Wettstein *et al.*, 2001). Longer periods of persistence, ranging from 10 to 50 years for *P. malariae* were reported in the former USSR (Bruce-Chwatt, 1982; Duhanina and Žukova, 1965) and in the USA (Bruce-Chwatt, 1972; 1974; 1982). Despite the atypical instances of prolonged periods for *P. falciparum*, *P. ovale* and *P. vivax*, it seems unlikely that a donor will remain infective after five years of infection, which is the basis for questioning blood donors in some countries.

Transfusion-transmitted malaria is transmitted either by asexual forms present in the red blood cells, usually from asymptomatic donors who carry a low level parasitaemia or rarely in the period between the sub-clinical parasitaemia and the onset of symptoms (usually associated with previous chemoprophylaxis). Gametocytes are not infective, and free merozoites are present in the bloodstream for a very short period, and do not maintain viability in stored blood. The chances of infection by circulating sporozoites immediately after the mosquito bite,

one predicted by WHO (Snow *et al.*, 2005), with 515 million people affected by *P. falciparum* alone. In addition, nearly 40% of the world population (or 2 billion people in 2005) still remain exposed to varying degrees of risk of malarial infection (Snow *et al.*, 2005; WHO, 1992a; 1992b). Comprehensive compilations from annually reported cases in Europe can be found in the European Network on Imported Infectious Disease Surveillance (www.tropnet.net).

Transmission by blood components is either a consequence of the sanitary conditions of a country or region, when complete eradication has not yet been achieved (e.g. tropical Africa, India, Sri Lanka, Brazilian Amazon basin, etc.), or is due to cases imported to either developed, non-endemic places by immigrants or travellers from endemic areas within countries where both endemic and non-endemic regions are geographically quite distinct (Alves *et al.*, 2000), or to non-endemic countries, where vectorial malaria has been completely controlled (Bellmann *et al.*, 2000; Bradley *et al.*, 1998; Bruce-Chwatt, 1972; 1974; 1982;

though theoretically possible within a 60-minute period (Fairley, 1947), has not been associated with transfusion cases. Transmission from symptomatic donors is very unlikely and when noted, usually occurs in endemic regions.

The minimum level of parasitaemia that leads to infection is not known. For *P. vivax* a total of ten parasites/ml were successful in inducing experimental transmission (Bruce-Chwatt, 1982). In addition, an infection rate of 1–2 parasites/ml equates to nearly half a million parasites in a single whole blood unit, a number far above the minimum necessary to induce an active infection in the recipient (International Forum, 1987). Even if the real value is unknown, one can assume that one infected unit of blood transfused to a naive recipient results in transmission of infection. (Shehata *et al.*, 2004).

Blood components

Though transmission occurs mainly through red cell components (whole blood or packed red cells), all other blood components (liquid or frozen, untreated fresh plasma, platelets and granulocyte concentrates) cannot be regarded as cell-free and thus devoid of viable infective parasites (Council of Europe, 2005). Infectivity is retained even in glycerolized units preserved at −70 °C and then thawed. Red cell preservatives containing adenine seem to enhance parasite viability. No infection has been associated with freeze-dried plasma or industrialized derivatives (albumin, immunoglobulin, etc.), even if derived from potentially infected donors; these donations can be regarded as safe if used exclusively as plasma for fractionation. Though viability at 4–6 °C storage is less than five days for *P. malariae* and up to ten days for *P. falciparum*, holding units for 7–10 days in order to achieve relative protection is not justified.

A survey covering the period 1950–1972 showed that *P. malariae* was responsible for 48% of cases, *P. vivax* for 19%, *P. falciparum* for 5%, *P. ovale* for very rare cases and 30% could not be determined. During the period 1973–1980, the distribution was 38% for *P. malariae*, 42% for *P. vivax* and *P. ovale* and 20% for *P. falciparum* (Bruce-Chwatt, 1982). Another survey conducted in the USA covering the period 1963–1999, when 93 TTM were reported in 28 states, showed that the distribution was 35% for *P. falciparum*, 27% for *P. vivax*, 25% for *P. malariae*, 5% for *P. ovale*, 3% mixed and 2% for unidentified species (Mungai *et al.*, 2001). This same study demonstrated that the pattern of the distribution of the causative species in the USA in the past three decades has shifted from *P. malariae* and *P. vivax* (as reported by Nahlen *et al.* (Nahlen *et al.*, 1991) to *P. falciparum*. Conversely, the distribution among different endemic regions also shows a wide variation; in Africa, *P. falciparum* is the most common agent (WHO, 1992a; 1992b), while *P. vivax* is the most common in India (Wells and Ala, 1985) and Brazil (Alves *et al.*, 2000; Andrade and Wanderley, 1991; Ferreira, 1993).

A dramatic decrease in TTM was expected after malaria was eradicated in the USA in 1951 (CDC, http://www.cdc.gov/mmwr/PDF/ss5301.pdf, 2004). Due to successive wars, American troops returning from Korea and Vietnam (and lately from Somalia) with malaria were responsible for TTM in this country, despite

appropriate preventive measures. On the other hand, migratory movements, particularly from Africa and India into Europe, and from South-east Asia and South America into North America (International Forum, 1987), were also responsible for TTM. Therefore, specific measures are now taken in order to prevent parasite transmission.

Donor questioning

The first measure is the taking of an accurate history from candidate donors, including place of birth, previous places of residence throughout their lifetime, immigration and a complete account of prior travel during the past three years. (In the UK, donors are asked about travel throughout life.) The use of specific questionnaires is aimed at excluding three types of infected donors:

- Anyone, for example non-immune travellers, who acquired malaria abroad, in order to prevent donation during relapses after specific treatment (*P. vivax* and *P. ovale*) or asymptomatic parasitaemia following inadequate chemoprophylaxis.
- Individuals, including military personnel, returning from endemic areas.
- Foreign visitors or immigrants from endemic regions who are usually immune and asymptomatic. Some individuals may be semi-immune and therefore infected but asymptomatic. Repeated exposure to malarial parasites, which is particularly common in areas of high density infection in the mosquitoes (e.g. sub-Saharan Africa/Papua New Guinea), results in a semi-immune state and these individuals remain a lifelong risk because if re-exposed and infected they remain well but could transmit malaria through their blood donations (Kitchen *et al.*, 2005).

Regulations vary in different countries (AABB, 2005; Council of Europe, 2005). In the USA, as a general policy, travellers or residents of non-malarious areas coming from malarious areas (irrespective of chemoprophylaxis) should be deferred for a one-year period, if they have been free of malaria symptoms. Immigrants from malarious areas (provided they have been asymptomatic) should be deferred from three to five years; the same period applies in some countries for those who have had a diagnosis of malaria and became asymptomatic after appropriate treatment. In the UK the ban is lifelong unless the potential donor is shown to be non-immune, that is, they have a negative test for antibodies to malaria. Though this measure has been considered effective for *P. falciparum*, *P. vivax* and *P. ovale*, a recent UK case shows the flaws of relying solely on deferral of donors for a certain time period after exposure to eliminate the risk of transmission through blood (Kitchen *et al.*, 2005). At the time, a deferral period of only five years since last exposure was in place. As a result of this case, donors in the UK who fulfil the criteria for possible semi-immunity are permanently barred unless shown to have no anti-malarial antibodies. In addition, a finite donor deferral period is not valid for *P. malariae*, for which longer periods of infectivity are recorded (Mungai, 2001; Purdy *et al.*, 2004). This led Canada to adopt a permanent deferral for donors reporting a history of diagnosis or treatment of malaria at any time in the past (Slinger *et al.*, 2001). Since the world malarial zone is so vast, an alphabetical list of countries reporting malaria transmission and a geographical malarial map (provided by Roll Back Malaria, WHO: www.mosquito.who.int/malariacontrol) should be present in every collection facility and is in use in the UK. Questionnaires are valid only for products where viable red cell components are present, but may be disregarded for donations intended exclusively for plasma fractionation. Unfortunately, screening potentially infected donors only by questionnaires brings two additional problems (Sazama, 1991):

- *Low specificity*, by rejecting a somewhat high number of healthy donors. One study in the USA (Mungai *et al.*, 2001) using a six-month interval after travel before testing, estimated that about 50 000 blood units are excluded annually (out of an estimated 14 million units collected per year). In the USA also, malaria is the most common cause of long-term donor deferral for those over 40 years of age or for first-time donors aged 16 to 24 years (Custer *et al.*, 2004). A worse scenario was observed in Australia, where up to 100 000 units (out of a total collection of 900 000 whole blood donations) were being lost annually until quite recently (Farrugia, 2004). Even despite recent changes in testing and selection algorithms, about 40 000 units of blood are still lost every year in Australia (Albert Farrugia, personal communication). Thus, validation of donor questionnaires and donor interviewers or historians (Lee *et al.*, 2003) is quite important in order to increase the specificity of current measures applied, for parasitic diseases.
- *Low sensitivity*: after careful examination of all 93 cases of TTM in the USA reported to the CDC in the period 1963–1999 (Mungai *et al.*, 2001) (with an incidence of less than 1 case/ million units of blood), the donor-questionnaire process failed in approximately two-thirds of the 93 cases. In this study, if the current guidelines were correctly applied, still a third of cases would not be prevented, mostly due to *P. malariae*. This has recently been confirmed by CDC (Shah *et al.*, 2004). Besides, the interviewer can only rely upon the accuracy of the donors' history, which may be fallible in some cases (Arafat *et al.*, 2003; Nahlen *et al.*, 1991), since many of them have been infected in childhood or do not remember the episode.

In the light of these problems, some non-endemic countries have introduced a series of specific strategies aimed at reducing the risk, such as temporary exclusion of those returning from specific WHO-defined endemic areas, temporary/permanent exclusion of candidate donors with a positive malaria history, and specific serological screening, which is applied only to selected suspected donors, such as immigrants or individuals born in endemic areas, or those who have had malaria three to five years before donation (Chataing, 1988; Chiodini *et al.*, 1997; Council of Europe, 2005; Kitchen *et al.*, 2005). With such a strategy, 5–10% of donors in France (Chataing, 1988; Soler *et al.*, 2003) who were tested by an indirect immunofluorescence assay (IFAT) were confirmed as infective. In the UK, recent work detecting antibodies by an antiglobulin EIA test (Kitchen *et al.*, 2004) with both recombinant *P. falciparum* and *P. vivax* antigens, reported saving from unnecessary rejection 94.5% of non-plasma components from donors with a malaria risk. Current estimates in the UK are that up to 30 000 donors would be lost per year in the

absence of serological testing of donors with a history of exposure. Non-immune travellers or donors who have been immigrants from malarial areas can be tested six months after their last day in a malarial area.

Other more radical positions in non-endemic regions, such as the permanent exclusion of all persons who have had malaria at any point in their lifetime have been proposed (Shah *et al.*, 2004; Shehata *et al.*, 2004), but this should be carefully analysed, since most of them actually do not carry parasites. This is particularly important in places where shortage of suitable blood is a concern. (Please refer to Chapter 28.) In countries where malaria is endemic, the exclusion of previously infected donors for three years may be unsuitable. Besides, the use of screening tests to detect *Plasmodium* antibodies may also be inadequate, since most assays denote only a previous infection and not the presence of a recent infection and/or circulating parasites. In such cases, it seems that testing for malarial antigens may be satisfactory (Choudhury *et al.*, 1988).

On the other hand, in remote endemic areas, where it is virtually impossible to rely upon uninfected donors, where neither screening tests nor adequate blood collection facilities are present, the following procedures are recommended:

- Exclude candidates who have had malaria in the previous 12 months or those with a febrile episode in the last 30 days. This procedure has been used in the highly endemic Brazilian Amazon area (Brazilian Ministry of Health, 2004), although a substantial number of donors from part of this region (who claimed no previous malaria history) were found to have malarial antibodies (Ferreira *et al.*, 1993), which may be due to an imprecise donor history or misdiagnosis of asymptomatic previous cases. Thus, purely epidemiological criteria should be regarded with caution when blood donation in endemic areas is concerned.
- In very remote endemic areas, where no organized blood services are available, one alternative is to introduce the use of chloroquine in donors 48 hours before donation or a single dose immediately before, and then accept donation. This measure is generally used in conjunction with treatment of the recipient with preventive chemoprophylaxis, particularly neonates after an exchange-transfusion (Ibhanesebor *et al.*, 1996), who must be continuously treated for a month. Unfortunately, preventive chemoprophylaxis of recipients is not advisable for pregnant or breast-feeding women, and is ineffective for drug-resistant *P. falciparum* strains, which are responsible for the worst cases (Bruce-Chwatt, 1982; Tabor, 1982). This should be regarded as a last resort, and should not be considered when recipients are from non-endemic regions (non-immune).

The use of inactivating agents might be a suitable alternative in the near future. Although past studies have proposed some activities with merocyanine 540 (MC540)(Smith *et al.*, 1991; 1992), Pc4 (a phtalocyanin) (Lustigman and Ben-Hur, 1996), and crystal violet (gentian violet) (Amato Neto *et al.*, 1987), none of these compounds have been considered for further studies in the past ten years. More recently, Inactine PEN110, an electrophilic agent chemically related to binary ethylenimine has shown considerable effect on the viability of *P. falciparum* (Zavizion *et al.*, 2004).

However, it seems that we are still a long way from pathogen inactivation agents that can be widely used for RBC components.

Screening tests

Screening tests for malaria are aimed at the detection of circulating antibodies or antigens (Bruce-Chwatt, 1982; Chataing, 1988; Wells and Ala, 1985):

- *Detection of antibodies*, based mainly on indirect immuno-fluorescence assay (IFAT) or EIA, using *P. falciparum*, non-human parasites (that show some cross-reactivity with human antibodies), purified or recombinant antigens. These tests are useful for interpreting high titred or negative sera, denoting, respectively, the presence or absence of infection. However, low titred sera must, in most cases, be supplemented by a thorough interview with the donor (International Forum, 1987). Though IgG antibody titres usually correlate with the number of past malarial attacks (Ferreira *et al.*, 1993), the presence of antibodies does not necessarily mean the presence of circulating parasites, especially among donors from endemic regions. Antibodies detected by IFAT are present in >95% of infected donors, and usually arise 7–14 days after the onset of infection by *P. falciparum* (with longer periods for other species). They persist for several years in those who are subject to continuous exposure (immune donors from endemic countries), especially when infection occurs by *P. malariae*, where long latency periods and high titres are found. After proper malaria treatment, these antibodies tend to persist for 6–12 months. Thus, this method is highly recommended for screening donors in non-endemic countries as demonstrated in France for over 20 years (Chataing, 1988; Soler *et al.*, 2003). On the other hand, it seems to be unsuitable in highly endemic regions, where a high prevalence of antibody positive donors is found, suggesting instead the adoption of antigen detection (see below). Though in the window phase the sensitivity of IFAT or EIA ranges from 50 to 80% (Assal *et al.*, 1999; Draper and Sirr, 1980), it is unlikely that donors in the acute infection period will feel well enough to donate blood, especially in non-endemic countries. An initial strategy of using combined IFAT and EIA tests for malarial antibody screening of donors with relevant histories in the UK (Chiodini *et al.*, 1997) was withdrawn in 1999, when an improved test based on three recombinant antigens for *P. falciparum* and one for *P. vivax* became available (Kitchen *et al.*, 2004). Given the wide window-period phase, detection of antibodies is fallible in early, acute cases (sensitivity is up to 85–90%). However, if a proper and valid questionnaire is applied, most of those negative, acute phase donors will be temporarily rejected: for example, in the UK, donors are deferred for six months after the last possible exposure to malaria. False-positive reactions are observed in a minority of cases; some are related to commercial kits using A_1 red blood cell cultures (which results in binding of natural anti-A mainly from group O individuals)(Soler *et al.*, 2003), or cross-reactivity to HIV antibodies, particularly in highly endemic areas (Fonseca *et al.*, 2000). More recently, a new technology, using flow-cytometry-based-multiplexed immunoassays was

proposed (Jani *et al.*, 2002), especially for developing countries. However, these assays still need to be standardized and evaluated not only in developed Western countries, but also after regional or field studies in endemic countries. Nevertheless, this method, given its low cost and multiple tests performance, might be a suitable option for some countries in the future.

- *Detection of antigens/parasites*: the method mostly used is the thick smear test; however, it lacks sensitivity, with a limit of 50 parasites/μl, or 0.001% infected RBC, which is only achieved by highly qualified technicians. In practice, detection occurs at a level of 0.01% of RBC infected (Moody, 2002), which is a far greater level than the minimum necessary for transmission of infection. It is also highly subjective, leads to lapses of concentration by technical staff (a very boring procedure) and cannot be used as a mass screening method, particularly where blood services are not fully established or developed (usually in regions where TTM is an important problem). One study in the USA showed that examination of thick smears prevented only 10% of TTM and identified only 31% (8/26) of donors implicated in TTM (Nahlen *et al.*, 1991).

The detection of parasites within erythrocytes has been achieved by IFAT in endemic countries with the use of acridine orange (Choudhury *et al.*, 1988; Kawamoto, 1991; WHO, 1987), where parasites are viewed through a capillary tube with a special lens in a fluorescent microscope. Sensitivity reaches 5–50 parasites/μl, but lower levels of parasitaemia than this may still produce up to 2.5×10^6 parasites in one unit of blood (Bruce-Chwatt, 1982).

The description of *PfHRP-2*, a water soluble, histidine-rich antigen present in immature *P. falciparum* gametocytes (Parra *et al.*, 1991; Rock *et al.*, 1987) and the production of monoclonal antibodies (MoAb) against it, have been the basis of two distinct methods for detection of circulating antigens. The first one is an EIA test (Davidson *et al.*, 1999; Namsiriponpun *et al.*, 1993; Taylor and Voller, 1993). The second one is a rapid lateral flow immunochromatographic test (dipstick or rapid diagnostic test – RDT), based on MoAb fixed onto a cellulose strip. However, given that the first RDTs that appeared on the market were specific for *P. falciparum*, most of them are no longer available and have been replaced by at least two main groups of RDTs. One uses a combination of MoAb against HRP-2 and plasmodial aldolase (Meier *et al.*, 1992) (a panspecific malarial enzyme – NOW ICT P.f/P.v – Binax, Portland, USA) and the other is based on the detection of parasite-specific lactate dehydrogenase (Piper *et al.*, 1996) (through a combination of one specific MoAb for *P. falciparum* and two other panspecific MoAb against all plasmodia LDH – OptiMAL IT, Diamed, Cressier, Switzerland), allowing detection of both *P. falciparum* and *P. vivax*. Although these methods are easy to perform, good sensitivity is achieved only when the parasite concentration is >100/μl, and specificity ranges from 40 to 93% (Moody, 2002). Since WHO recommends a sensitivity of up to 100 parasites/μl (0.002% parasitaemia) (WHO, 2003), and a high positive likelihood ratio (LR – or a high post-test probability) and a low negative LR (to rule out malaria infection in negative results), these might be suitable alternatives for regions where skilled microscopy technicians are not available or where thick or thin film examination cannot be considered as first-line methods (i.e. non-endemic countries) (De Monbrison *et al.*, 2004). Even though these results are problematic for *P. ovale* and *P. malariae*, which are both less frequent in the context of transfusion-transmission, the results are not devoid of clinical importance. More comprehensive data on rapid diagnostic tests for malaria can be found elsewhere (Bell, 2002; Craig *et al.*, 2002; Moody, 2002; Peyron *et al.*, 1994; Playford and Walker, 2002; Rubio *et al.*, 2001; Seed *et al.*, 2005; WHO, 2003). Despite the aforementioned suggestion, one has to view it with some caution; false-positive results can be observed in the presence of rheumatoid factor, and low level parasitaemia (ranging from 50 to 5000/μl) can be seen in donors who are non-immune travellers returning from endemic areas, which may not be detected by these methods, but which can still infect recipients. Thus, it is highly important that validated questionnaires should be used in combination with testing (Orton *et al.*, 2000). A combination of testing potentially infected donors for the simultaneous presence of malarial antibodies and antigens was reported in France (Silvie *et al.*, 2002), which showed increased sensitivity and shortened sero-conversion (from 11.4 ± 1.6 to 5.3 ± 1.1 days) as compared to screening by IFAT method only.

A screening procedure using PCR was published using Vietnamese blood donors (Vu *et al.*, 1995), with a sensitivity for *P. falciparum* of 1–4 parasites/50 μl, and for *P. vivax* of 40–130 parasites/50 μl which is 100 times more sensitive than that achieved by blood films. Though this test has been applied in a developing country, its high cost, particularly in regions with limited resources (where malaria is of great concern), still renders this method unsuitable. Conversely, non-reactive PCR assays are reported among donors who were allegedly implicated in induced malaria from developed countries (Shah *et al.*, 2004; Purdy *et al.*, 2004; Arafat *et al.*, 2003). Although several nested PCR tests have subsequently been developed, all entail a laborious and time-consuming procedure. More recently, a real-time PCR, which is able to discriminate all four species at a sensitivity of 30 parasites/μl was proposed (De Monbrison *et al.*, 2003) for infected travellers with low level parasitaemia, blood transfusion or transplant recipients and, possibly, for blood donors, especially in endemic areas. However, parasite densities below the level of detection should still be considered as highly infective, posing some questions on the real value of this method as the main screening procedure in blood banks. A small study in Spain adopted PCR as a strategy for testing blood donors with a potential risk for malaria (Barea *et al.*, 2001); only 4% of cases were discarded, with some 42% of donors returning for subsequent donation, and no transmission reported to recipients. A Canadian study demonstrated the cost-effectiveness of adopting PCR testing when compared with deferring donors by a standard questionnaire (Shehata *et al.*, 2004). It should, however, be noted that even a test as sensitive as PCR will not prevent transmission when parasitaemia is at very low levels, in the large inoculation of a transfusion.

A major problem is still the definition of a gold standard for screening of blood donors. Though in many countries IFAT is considered as such, one cannot expect 100% sensitivity or specificity from this method. False-positive and negative results have

always to be considered and suitable materials for preparation of this test are not readily available for many laboratories. Furthermore, they are derived only from *P. falciparum* strains; although this is the most common species, the fact that one has to rely on cross-reactions to detect the other species of *Plasmodium* renders this method far from ideal. In addition, a recent study with recombinant EIA antigens demonstrated its superiority in results obtained on proven cases (Kitchen *et al.*, 2004). In summary, it is clear that there is not a single and standard approach to prevent malaria transmission by blood components in non-endemic and endemic countries; it is up to each country to define what would be the most appropriate strategy to be applied (International Forum, 2004).

Babesia spp. – babesiosis

The *Babesia* spp. are intraerythrocytic protozoan parasites, closely related to *Plasmodium*, that are the aetiologic agents of babesiosis. The first case of human babesiosis was reported in 1957 and occurred in Yugoslavia (Skrabalo and Deanovic, 1957), while the first US case was described in 1966 on Nantucket Island, Massachusetts (Scholtens *et al.*, 1968). Following the initial recognition of *Babesia* spp. in humans, hundreds of cases of human babesiosis have been reported in the USA and more than 30 cases in Europe (Gorenflot *et al.*, 1998; Homer *et al.*, 2000; White *et al.*, 1998; Zintl *et al.*, 2003). Human babesiosis has now been identified in Mexico, Egypt, South Africa, Japan and parts of Asia. However, most cases occur in the USA and Europe, and are caused by *B. microti* and *B. divergens*, respectively (Bush *et al.*, 1990; Homer *et al.*, 2000; Meer-Scherrer *et al.*, 2004; Michael *et al.*, 1987; Osorno *et al.*, 1976; Saito-Ito *et al.*, 2000; Shih *et al.*, 1997; Zintl *et al.*, 2003). Recent accounts suggest a much wider distribution of these agents than was initially thought; *B. divergens* is apparently present in the USA and *B. microti* is endemic in Europe (Beattie *et al.*, 2002; Gray *et al.*, 2002; Herwaldt *et al.*, 2004; Meer-Scherrer *et al.*, 2004). Further complicating our understanding of the parasite's geographical distribution are several *Babesia*-like agents, which are phylogenetically distinct from *B. microti* and *B. divergens*, and have been described in the USA (WA-1, CA-1, MO-1) and Europe (EU-1) (Herwaldt *et al.*, 2003a). Thus, the recognized geographical distribution of the *Babesia* spp. and associated cases of human disease continue to expand, indicating a growing public health concern.

Babesiosis is a zoonotic disease, transmitted among animals and humans by adult and nymphal stages of *Ixodes* ticks infected with the parasite. During the course of a blood meal, ticks release thousands of infective sporozoites into dermal tissue during the latter stages of feeding (Homer *et al.*, 2000). Since most *Ixodes* ticks require 48 hours or more to reach repletion, ticks must be attached for at least this long to transmit *Babesia* infection. Vector species vary geographically: *I. scapularis*, the common deer or black legged tick acts as the vector for *B. microti* in the northeastern and upper mid-western USA. In Europe, the vector for *B. microti* is *I. trianguliceps*, but this tick is rarely thought to bite humans (Gray *et al.*, 2002), leading some to suggest that the sheep tick, *I. ricinus* may be responsible for the parasite's transmission

(Duh *et al.*, 2001; Walter and Weber, 1981). *Ixodes ricinus*, however, is primarily recognized as the European vector of *B. divergens*. In most cases, the vectors of *Babesia*-like agents (e.g. MO-1, EU-1) have not been described, but for WA-1 it is thought to be *I. pacificus*. Also critical for perpetuating the parasite's life cycle are reservoir and transport hosts. The most common reservoir host for *B. microti* is the white-footed mouse, *Peromyscus leucopus*. The reservoir host(s) for WA-1, CA-1 and MO-1, however, have yet to be established, but may also be *P. leucopus*. In Japan, the reservoir host for *B. microti* is thought to be the local field mouse, *Apodemus speciosus* (Shiota *et al.*, 1984). In most instances the white-tailed deer, a non-competent vector for *B. microti*, acts as maintenance and transport host for adult ticks of *I. scapularis*. For *B. divergens* in Europe, cattle are not only the reservoir host for human infections, but also the definitive host for the parasite.

Babesia infections in humans demonstrate a range of clinical features that vary from asymptomatic disease to severe, life-threatening illness. The severity of disease is influenced by the immune status of the host and the infecting species of *Babesia*. For example, asymptomatic infections are not uncommon in association with *B. microti* and are likely to go undetected. If symptomatic, *B. microti* infections tend to be relatively benign, with patients experiencing mild flu-like symptoms one to six weeks after exposure that self-resolve, leading to the eventual clearance of the parasite. Characteristic symptoms may include fever, headache, chills, drenching sweats, myalgia and malaise. For certain at-risk populations (e.g. infants, the asplenic, immunocompromised and elderly) *B. microti* infection can induce severe complications, including haemolytic anaemia, thrombocytopenia, haematuria, renal failure and mortality rates that approach 5% (Meldrum *et al.*, 1992). Asplenic patients are particularly susceptible to severe infections; in some cases parasitaemia levels have been reported to approach 85%, resulting in life-threatening anaemia (Homer *et al.*, 2000). These patients may require drug treatment or, in rare instances, an exchange blood transfusion designed to lower overall levels of parasitaemia. Drug treatment options include a seven-day course of quinine and clindamycin or the equally effective, but better tolerated, tandem of atovaquone and azithromycin (Krause *et al.*, 2000). In cases of severe disease or haemodynamic instability attributed to high levels of parasitaemia, an exchange transfusion may be required to rapidly decrease overall parasitaemia and related haemolysis (Dorman *et al.*, 2000; Powell and Grima, 2002).

Compared with *B. microti*, infections with *B. divergens* and WA-1 have been observed to be more severe, often producing life-threatening disease. In Europe, the approximately 30 cases of human babesiosis have been attributed to infection with *B. divergens* and almost all patients were asplenic (Gorenflot *et al.*, 1998; Zintl *et al.*, 2003). Disease onset in these patients is rapid (1–3 weeks) and symptoms include haemoglobinuria with jaundice, due to severe haemolysis, resulting in mortality rates of 42% (Homer *et al.*, 2000). Similarly, WA-1 infections in humans have been more severe than *B. microti*, even among immunocompetent patients (Quick *et al.*, 1993), an observation confirmed in animal models (Dao and Eberhard, 1996; Wozniak *et al.*, 1996).

Accurate diagnosis of babesial infections is complicated by the asymptomatic nature of many infections, particularly those caused by *B. microti*, and the limited number of reliable assays available to confirm infection. Infections with relatively high parasitaemias can be detected directly by examination of thin or thick blood smears stained with Wright or Giemsa for red cells containing *B. microti* merozoites. Unfortunately, parasitaemia levels associated with most *Babesia* infections are extremely low, falling well below the detection limits of a blood smear. Inoculation of appropriate susceptible rodent hosts, gerbils for *B. divergens* and hamsters or mice for *B. microti*, allows in vivo amplification of infection and subsequent detection by examination of rodent blood smears. However, this approach requires repeated sampling over the course of eight weeks, making it impractical for rapid diagnosis.

The 'gold standard' for *Babesia* testing remains the IFAT, which uses *Babesia* infected red cells obtained from rodents as the antigen source to detect human IgM or IgG antibodies specific for *Babesia* spp. Detection of IgM antibodies may indicate a recent infection, but confirmation requires the subsequent detection of IgG antibodies in follow-up samples (Herwaldt *et al.*, 2003b; Krause *et al.*, 1996a). Persons exposed to *B. microti* develop IgG antibody titres that persist for months to years and are readily detectable by IFAT. In contrast, infections with *B. divergens* progress too rapidly to make antibody detection useful. Although valuable for patient diagnosis in a clinical setting, IFAT is not a feasible option for screening blood since it does not lend itself to automation or large scale testing that may be required by blood banks if testing is ever considered for implementation. Alternatively, several EIA based tests using recombinant antigens have been reported that may prove promising in the future (Houghton *et al.*, 2002; Lodes *et al.*, 2000). These tests would have the advantage of being easily adapted to existing test platforms that provide required automation and throughput.

During the early acute phase of infection, *Babesia* organisms are sometimes detectable in the peripheral blood before significant antibody titres are present (i.e. window period). Thus, NAT represents an important potential adjunct to serological testing. Several papers have described highly conserved sequences of the small-subunit rRNA (ss-rDNA) gene in *Babesia* that have been employed as the target of sensitive and specific PCR assays (Krause *et al.*, 1998; Persing *et al.*, 1992). Indeed, these techniques have already been used to demonstrate parasitaemia in blood donors (Leiby *et al.*, 2005). It is not clear, however, if and when blood screening for *Babesia* is likely to be introduced, or if an intervention is even warranted. Nevertheless, as will be described below, based on recent seroprevalence estimates and the frequency with which *B. microti* is transmitted by blood transfusion, blood screening should perhaps be considered in the near future, at least in parts of the USA.

There have been relatively few studies on the prevalence of *Babesia* spp. in blood donors. An early study by Popovsky and colleagues reported that 29 of 779 (3.7%) Cape Cod (Massachusetts) blood donors were seropositive for *B. microti* (Popovsky *et al.*, 1988). A smaller study on Shelter Island (New York) observed that 5 of 115 (4.3%) blood donors had *B. microti* antibodies (Linden *et al.*, 2000). More recently, a serological study of approximately 1000 blood donors from both Wisconsin and Connecticut reported that 0.3 and 0.6 %, respectively, were *B. microti* positive (Leiby *et al.*, 2002a). A follow-up study in Connecticut reported on the seroprevalence rate for donors in *Babesia*-endemic and non-endemic areas of the state: 24 of 1745 (1.4%) for endemic and 6 of 1745 (0.3%) for non-endemic areas (Leiby *et al.*, 2005). Of particular significance, this study also tested selected seropositive donors for parasitaemia and observed that 10 of 19 (53%) had demonstrable parasitaemia.

Seroprevalence studies outside the USA and those for other species of *Babesia* are less numerous. Several studies have reported seemingly high seroprevalence rates for WA-1, including 20.1% among 124 Sacramento (California) blood donors, but questions have been raised about the specificity of the assay used in these studies (Fritz *et al.*, 1997; Homer *et al.*, 2000). Several small studies have been conducted in Germany investigating *B. divergens* and *B. microti*. The first study reported that 8 of 100 (8%) healthy blood donors had antibodies to *B. microti* (Hunfeld *et al.*, 1998). The latter study tested 120 German donors and observed two (1.7%) with *B. divergens* and one (0.8%) had *B. microti* antibodies (Hunfeld *et al.*, 2002). These studies and other case reports of babesiosis in Europe suggest that *Babesia* spp. are probably present in many parts of the continent, but comprehensive epidemiological studies to identify their geographic distribution are awaited.

Given the observed seroprevalence rates in parts of the USA and confirmation that many seropositive donors are likely to be parasitaemic, it is not surprising that transfusion-transmitted *Babesia* is a growing USA problem. To date, over 50 cases of transfusion-transmission have been reported for blood recipients ranging in age from neonatal to 79 years (Leiby and Gill, 2004). This figure, however, is likely to be an underestimate as many cases do not get reported or are asymptomatic and overlooked by physicians. All transfusion cases described to date have involved *B. microti*, except for two cases involving WA-1, one of which occurred in a premature infant and the other in a 76-year-old man (Herwaldt *et al.*, 1997; Kjemtrup *et al.*, 2002). Transfusion cases have also been reported from Japan and Canada (Jassoum *et al.*, 2000; Matsui *et al.*, 2000), but the latter case involved a donor who acquired a *B. microti* infection in the USA and subsequently donated blood in Canada six months later. Follow-up blood samples provided by this donor were positive by blood smear, IFAT (1:1024) and PCR; however, the donor was asymptomatic. The Japanese case implicated a locally acquired *B. microti* variant that demonstrated 99.2% homology with the US isolate. While no cases have been reported to date in Europe, recent seroprevalence studies identifying *B. microti* and *B. divergens* in the general population as well as in blood donors, suggest that reports of transmission by transfusion may well occur in future.

Most transmission cases have involved red cell units, but platelet units (likely to be 'contaminated' with red cells) have been implicated on several occasions. Based on empirical and case report evidence, *B. microti* survives for 21 and 35 days, respectively, in stored red cells (Eberhard *et al.*, 1995; Mintz *et al.*, 1991). In most cases, implicated donors were asymptomatic and had

no recollection of an associated tick bite. Observed incubation periods in blood recipients are generally one to nine weeks post-transfusion. While many transfusion-transmitted cases have minimal clinical impact on recipients, severe life-threatening complications can arise in those recipients at greatest risk for severe disease (e.g. elderly, asplenic, etc.). Reported symptoms among infected recipients include fever, chills, fatigue and haemolytic anaemia, which have contributed to fatal outcomes in several cases. In these patients, rapid diagnosis and treatment, coupled with exchange transfusions in severe cases, are critical to successful clinical outcomes.

Two studies conducted in Connecticut provide estimates of the risk of transmitting *B. microti* by transfusion. The first study, by Gerber and colleagues, determined the transmission risk by prospectively measuring seroconversions in cardiothoracic surgery patients who had received multiple transfusions (Gerber *et al.*, 1994). They reported the risk of transmission by red cells to be 1 in 601 (0.17%; 95% CI, 0.004–0.9%) transfused units, while the risk associated with platelets was 0 in 371 (0%; 95% CI, 0 – 0.8%). A later study estimated the risk from red cell transfusion to be 1 in 1800 based on local seroprevalence (0.3–1.4 %) and parasitaemia (56%) rates, in combination with the transmission rate (26%) identified through look-back investigations (Cable *et al.*, 2001). Taken together, these risk determinations suggest that interventions to prevent transmission of *B. microti* by transfusion should be considered. However, as already discussed, risk factor questions are unreliable and effective blood screening assays are not available at this time.

The primary risk factor for acquiring *Babesia* infection is exposure to ticks carrying the parasite. Exposure to ticks is most often associated with people involved in outdoor activities such as hiking or gardening that place them in close proximity to ticks and deer. However, as has been well documented, most people infected with a tick-borne disease (e.g. Lyme disease, babesiosis) do not recall an associated tick bite. Previous attempts to link a history of bites with higher levels of *Babesia* specific antibodies in blood donors have failed to demonstrate significant differences (Leiby *et al.*, 2002a). Indeed, blood donors reporting tick bites may actually be less likely to be infected since they routinely search for and promptly remove ticks after exposure. From the standpoint of blood centre interventions, risk-factor questions appear to lack sensitivity and are of limited value in identifying potentially infectious donors.

Another proposed intervention is to avoid collecting blood in *Babesia*-endemic areas during the height of the transmission season (i.e. June–September) when ticks are actively feeding (McQuiston *et al.*, 2000). While this approach would be effective at reducing potential transmission, it would produce detrimental effects on blood availability. This approach also does not preclude potentially infectious donors from donating blood in areas considered to be non-endemic for *Babesia*. Another drawback to seasonal blood collections are recent observations of apparent chronicity associated with *B. microti* infections. Based on PCR results, parasitaemia has been shown to persist for up to 18 months in some patients (Krause *et al.*, 1998). Recent studies in *B. microti* seropositive donors have confirmed these findings, demonstrating that parasitaemia can persist for months (Leiby et al., 2002b). This study also showed that many seropositive donors can maintain elevated antibody titres for years in the absence of measurable parasitaemia. This suggests that available PCR methods are not sufficiently sensitive to detect the parasite's presence. However, an alternative explanation is that the parasite remains sequestered in remote tissues or is present in peripheral blood intermittently, at low numbers (Krause et al., 1996b). Chronicity may also be related to the ability of some Babesia parasites to undergo antigenic variation, bind host proteins to the infected red cell surface or undergo monoallelic expression of different members of multigene families, thereby evading the host immune response (Allred, 2003).

Toxoplasma gondii – toxoplasmosis

Toxoplasma gondii is an obligate intracellular protozoan parasite that has a cosmopolitan distribution and is the aetiologic agent of toxoplasmosis. Worldwide, up to one-third of the human population is thought to be infected, with even higher rates reported in some regions (Montoya and Liesenfeld, 2004). Most infections are acquired from ingestion of oocysts passed by cats, the primary or definitive host for this parasite, or by eating raw or undercooked meat containing T. gondii cysts. Generally, exposure to T. gondii is uneventful, but for developing fetuses or immunocompromised patients, infections can be problematic.

The life cycle of T. gondii involves three separate and distinct stages; oocysts, tachyzoites and bradyzoites. In the feline host, T. gondii produces an enteroepithelial phase not seen in other hosts, resulting in the release of oocysts (10–13 μm × 9–11 μm) via the faeces. Cats may shed millions of oocysts during an acute infection with peak production during the first week. Within days oocysts undergo sporulation to contain infective sporozoites that are in turn ingested by a mammalian host, including humans. Once ingested, sporozoites of T. gondii enter a variety of host cells and begin dividing as elongate, often crescent-shaped tachyzoites (2–3 μm wide × 4–6 μm long). Rapid replication produces 8 to 16 tachyzoites that rupture the host cell, releasing the tachyzoites for dissemination and subsequent infection of new cells where replication occurs anew. Peripheral blood carries tachyzoites to distal sites including the brain, heart and skeletal muscles. In response to the host immune response, tachyzoites transform to bradyzoites during chronic infections and persist within tissues cysts. Replication dramatically slows, and the encysted parasite becomes relatively quiescent, but remains viable for years. The cyst itself may vary in size from 8 μm to 100 μm, and may contain up to 60 000 organisms.

Although cats are the only host capable of producing viable oocysts, a wide variety of mammalian species serve as intermediate hosts, including humans and domestic animals. Humans become infected through the consumption of raw or undercooked meat (often pork or lamb) that contains the encysted parasite. Similarly, water or food sources contaminated with oocysts from cat faeces also transmit the infection to humans. Several variations of this life cycle can occur, with congenitally transmitted human infections representing those with the greatest public health

significance (Dunn et al., 1999; Gavinet et al., 1998; Wong and Remington, 1994). Toxoplasma gondii transmission has also been reported from solid organ transplantation (Rynin et al., 1979; Sluiters et al., 1989). As will be discussed in greater detail later, the presence of tachyzoites in the peripheral blood, including within leucocytes, has led to rare cases of transfusion-transmission (Beauvais et al., 1976; Raisanen, 1978; Siegel et al., 1971). Lastly, recrudescence of acute infections in humans is becoming increasingly common among immunosuppressed patients (e.g. AIDS) when encysted bradyzoites become reactivated and replicate as tachyzoites (Luft and Remington, 1992).

In general, toxoplasmosis is a relatively benign, self-limiting disease that is often asymptomatic in most patients. Clinical symptoms (when present) are limited and may include malaise, fever and cervical lymphadenopathy. However, the severity of infection is influenced by the strain of T. gondii, age of the host and the host's immune status. Toxoplasmosis can have more severe implications in congenital cases or in patients with AIDS. In the former, clinical disease can occur in the unborn fetus of pregnant women who acquire the infection at or near the time of conception. While the fetus is often unaffected, severe complications, including hydrocephalus and mortality can occur at birth or later in life. In the case of AIDS patients and other immunocompromised persons (e.g. organ transplant recipients), acute infections can occur that are either newly acquired, or in most cases, arise via recrudescence of encysted bradyzoites. In cases of severe toxoplasmosis, damage to the brain, eyes, or other organs can occur. Since many blood recipients can be considered immunocompromised, the potential for more severe infections following transfusion needs to be considered.

Seroprevalence rates for T. gondii in humans vary worldwide and are influenced by the age of the population, socioeconomic conditions and geographic location. A recent US study (n = 17 658) reported that the seroprevalence rate for T. gondii among humans was 22.5% (Jones et al., 2001), but in other parts of the world seroprevalence rates are often much higher, even among blood donors (Al-Amari, 1994; Galván-Ramírez et al., 2005; Montoya and Liesenfeld, 2004; Nissapatorn et al., 2002). In most populations seroprevalence rates are observed to increase with age, which is probably attributable to increased exposure over time.

Since toxoplasmosis is generally asymptomatic, clinical diagnosis can be problematic. In suspected cases of toxoplasmosis in humans, diagnosis is accomplished by direct or indirect detection. Direct detection of the parasite can be made by histological analysis of blood smears and tissue biopsies, in vitro culture of the parasite from blood or body fluids, inoculation of mice with blood or biopsy materials (e.g. lymph node), or by PCR (Montoya and Liesenfeld, 2004; Remington et al., 2004). Direct detection is highly specific because identification is dependent upon the parasite's presence, but at the same time this limits the sensitivity of these approaches since the parasite is generally present in blood and tissues in low numbers. Enhanced sensitivity can be obtained through mouse inoculation or PCR, the former being dependent upon replication of the parasite in the mouse, while the latter amplifies gene sequences of interest. In the blood service environment, only PCR is practical, particularly for acute or 'window-period' infections. Several target sequences are routinely used in *T. gondii* nested PCR assays; the 35-fold repetitive B1 gene and the 300-fold repetitive AF146527 are the most common (Burg *et al.*, 1989; Dupouy-Camet, 1993; Filisetti *et al.*, 2003; Homan *et al.*, 2000). The recent introduction of real-time PCR provides enhanced sensitivity and a shorter turnaround time compared to traditional PCR (Costa *et al.*, 2000; 2001). In the future, advances in DNA micro-arrays may be used to identify donors infected with *T. gondii* and other protozoan parasites in multiplex systems (Duncan, 2004).

Indirect methods of diagnosis are largely dependent upon serologic assays designed to measure *T. gondii* antibodies including IFAT, EIA and Western blots (Balsari *et al.*, 1980; Remington *et al.*, in press; Walton *et al.*, 1966). These assays can be used to detect IgG, IgM and in the case of infants, IgA antibodies. However, due to the high prevalence of seroreactivity in the general population, only seroconversion or the presence of IgM antibodies would be indicative of a recent infection. Indeed, IgM antibodies arise during the first week of infection, rapidly peak and then decline, while IgG antibodies appear 1–2 weeks post-infection and persist lifelong. Alternatively, the IgG avidity test, which measures the functional affinity of IgG antibodies, can be used to differentiate between recent and past infections (Hedman *et al.*, 1989; Liesendfeld *et al.*, 2001). Antibody affinity increases with time; thus IgG affinity measurements for past *T. gondii* infections would be high, whereas recent infections would demonstrate IgG antibodies with low affinity. Taken together, the persistence of antibodies in a large portion of the general population, combined with the difficultly in differentiating a recent from past infection, makes a blood screening intervention for *T. gondii* unlikely at this time.

Interventions designed to prevent transmission of *T. gondii* may also be ill-advised given that transfusion-transmitted *T. gondii* must be considered an extremely rare event. No recent cases of transfusion-transmission have been published, but as already discussed, the literature contains several older accounts involving leucocyte transfusions for chronic myelogenous leukaemia (Beauvais *et al.*, 1976; Siegel *et al.*, 1971). However, the blood recipients in these cases were immunocompromised, which probably left them more susceptible to infection. In some respects the rarity of transfusion cases is surprising since the infection rate among the general population is relatively high and tachyzoites are demonstrable in the peripheral blood where they have been reported to persist for up to 14 months post-infection (Miller *et al.*, 1969). Tachyzoites have also been shown to remain viable in stored blood products (i.e. citrated blood) for up to 50 days at 5 °C (Talice *et al.*, 1957). Thus, while the infective form of the parasite is present in peripheral blood and it survives standard storage conditions, few transmission cases have been reported. Perhaps transmission cases are not recognized, but given the high rate of exposure among the general population, many blood recipients may be immune to reinfection unless they are naive or immunocompromised. Alternatively, with the advent of leucoreduction, *T. gondii* infected cells may be removed by the filtration process.

Leishmania spp. – leishmaniasis

The *Leishmania* spp. are obligate intracellular protozoan pathogens of human blood cells derived from the monocyte lineage. The parasite is endemic, primarily in tropical and subtropical regions worldwide, but is also present in southern Europe, where it causes leishmaniasis. Leishmaniasis is a vector-borne illness that is spectral in nature, ranging from cutaneous disease characterized by self-curing lesions to more serious visceral forms of disease associated with cells and organs of the reticuloendothelial system that is life-threatening if left untreated. Globally, 350 million people are estimated to be at risk for infection with *Leishmania* spp. and 2 million new infections are reported each year (Herwaldt 1999).

Natural infections are acquired following exposure to *Leishmania* infected phlebotomine sandflies of the genera *Phlebotomous* (Old World) or *Lutzomyia* (New World), which transmit the infective, flagellated promastigote stage (15–20 μm × 1.5–3.5 μm + 15–28 μm flagellum) to the human host during the course of a blood meal. Promastigotes initially infect localized dermal macrophages or Langerhan cells, then replicate intracellularly as ovoid, unflagellated amastigotes (2–4 μm) until the host cell ruptures. Released amastigotes are in turn phagocytosed by new monocytes/macrophages; although in the visceral syndrome the amastigotes are disseminated systemically, with a predilection for the spleen, liver and lymph nodes. Sandflies acquire the infection while feeding on an infected mammalian host that varies by species of *Leishmania* and geographic location, but can include humans, dogs and rodents. Ingested amastigote forms are passed to the midgut of the sandfly where they transform to promastigotes and undergo replication. Several days later promastigotes migrate to the oesophagus and pharynx from which they are released during subsequent blood meals. Other modes of transmission include congenital and parenteral, the latter including blood transfusion that will be discussed later (Berman, 1997; Desjeux, 1996).

Cutaneous disease is caused primarily by *L. major* and *L. tropica* in the Old World, while parasites associated with the *L. mexicana* complex (i.e. *L. mexicana, L. amazonensis, L. venezuelensis*) are the most common aetiological agents in the New World, but representatives of the *Viannia* subgenus (e.g. *L. [V.] braziliensis, L. [V.] panamensis, L. [V.] gyanensis*) have also been implicated. The incubation period for new infections ranges from a few days to weeks. Most cases of cutaneous leishmaniasis are initially characterized by a localized papule that evolves into a nodule, leading to an ulcerative lesion and months to years later, atrophic scars (Herwaldt, 1999). Manifestations of infection, however, vary widely and may include single or multiple lesions, regional adenopathy, lesion pain or secondary bacterial infections. Some infections also demonstrate latency, persistence, dissemination and reactivation (Guevara *et al.*, 1993; Nuwayri-Salti *et al.*, 1992; Rossell *et al.*, 1992; Saravia *et al.*, 1990). In the New World, mucocutaneous forms of disease (espundia) caused by the *Viannia* subgenus complex are also observed. This form of disease at first appears similar to cutaneous disease, but later develops chronic and severely necrotic lesions associated with naso-oropharyngeal mucosal tissues.

Visceral forms of leishmaniasis, also called Kala-azar, result from *L. donovani* or *L. infantum* infections in the Old World and *L. chagasi* in the New World. As for other forms, visceral disease initially starts as a localized, self-healing lesion, but with dissemination of the parasite to internal organs via the reticuloendothelial system, marked wasting, fever, malaise, pancytopenia and hepatosplenomegaly can ensue. Left untreated, visceral leishmaniasis is generally fatal within several years (Berman, 1997; Desjeux, 1996; Herwaldt, 1999).

Diagnosis of *Leishmania* infection can be accomplished directly by isolation of the parasite from infected patients. Tissue biopsies or aspirates derived from skin lesions, bone marrow, spleen or liver are used to demonstrate the unchecked proliferation of the parasite (amastigote form) by staining with Giemsa. These same tissues or blood can also be added to tissue culture media (e.g. diphasic NNN medium) supportive of the in vitro proliferation of promastigotes (Bowdre *et al.*, 1981). Observed parasites can be speciated by isoenzyme analysis or by several molecular approaches including PCR (Ravel *et al.*, 1995; Rodriguez *et al.*, 1994; Smyth *et al.*, 1992). Serological tests for detection of antibody, which can persist for years in visceral infections, are routinely employed in the research environment. Recently, an IgG antibody test for the recombinant leishmanial polypeptide K39 has been described that shows promise as a clinical assay (Badaro *et al.*, 1996; Houghton *et al.*, 1998). Unfortunately serological assays have limited application in cutaneous infections because antibody levels are extremely low. Polymerase chain reaction represents a sensitive technique for identifying *Leishmania* kinetoplast DNA (kDNA) in peripheral blood samples; however, as for serological assays, this approach probably has limited usefulness for cutaneous disease (Nuzum *et al.*, 1995; Rodriguez *et al.*, 1994; Smyth *et al.*, 1992). Treatments for leishmaniasis are available, and for years have relied upon pentavalent antimony compounds and various lipid formulations of amphotericin B (Berman, 1997; Herwaldt, 1999).

The intracellular niche of *Leishmania* and the parasite's ability to survive in stored blood components (25 days at 4°C) would predict its likely transmission by transfusion (Grogl *et al.*, 1993), but relatively few cases have been reported worldwide. The literature contains reports of at least ten cases of transmission, most occurring in young children, infants and neonates, but only one case has been reported in the last five years (André *et al.*, 1957; Cohen *et al.*, 1991; Chung *et al.*, 1948; Cummins *et al.*, 1995; Kostmann *et al.*, 1963; Mathur and Samantaray, 2004; Mauny *et al.*, 1993; Singh *et al.*, 1996). Virtually all cases implicated the visceral form of *Leishmania*, which is not surprising considering the chronic nature of these infections and the presence of infected cells in the peripheral blood. Incubation periods ranged from months to years. The most recent case (in 2004) was the first to implicate a platelet product in transmission, whereas the previous cases involved red cells or whole blood (Mathur and Samantaray, 2004). It is perhaps surprising that more transfusion cases have not been reported, but as is true for several other transmissible agents, the majority of transfusion cases may not be easily recognized. Also, infected cells may only be found in the peripheral blood intermittently, thereby decreasing the likelihood

of transmission. Thus, the likelihood of a transfusion acquired infection with *Leishmania* appears to be negligible in most parts of the world.

The potential for transfusion-transmitted *Leishmania* has been brought to the forefront in the USA, and to a lesser extent Europe, by the ongoing conflict in Iraq. During the period from January 2003 through April 2005, the US military reported nearly 850 parasitologically confirmed cases of leishmaniasis in personnel serving in and near Iraq (http://www.pdhealth.mil/downloads/leishmaniasis_information_28%20April%2005.pdf). While the large majority of cases involved cutaneous disease, four cases of the visceral form were also reported. These cases, coupled with reports of leishmaniasis in military personnel serving in Afghanistan, have led to the implementation of a one-year deferral for all military or civilian personnel who return to the USA from Iraq. Personnel serving in Afghanistan would be likely to be deferred for potential exposure to *Plasmodium* spp. While the likelihood of *Leishmania* transmission appears low, previous reports of viscerotropic forms of cutaneous leishmaniasis have led the military and US blood services to be cautious (Magill *et al.*, 1993). Indeed, a study from Natal, Brazil identified 21 asymptomatic blood donors that were seroreactive for *L. donovani*, of which five (24%) were PCR positive and nine (43%) were positive by a dot-blot hybridization assay (Otero *et al.*, 2000). Additionally, a study on *L. infantum* in a population of asymptomatic French blood donors reported that 76 of 565 (13.5%) were seropositive for the parasite (Le Fichoux *et al.*, 1999). Perhaps more importantly, this latter study confirmed the presence of the parasite in 16 seropositive donors by parasite kDNA amplification or blood culture (7 kDNA +, 7 culture +, 2 kDNA and culture +). Clearly, research studies designed to determine if cutaneous forms of *Leishmania* are also present in the peripheral blood would greatly enhance our understanding of this issue.

The limited number of transfusion cases involving *Leishmania* spp. suggests that interventions to prevent transmission may not be warranted, especially in non-endemic countries. Since leishmaniasis is a vector-borne disease, the primary risk factor for acquiring infection is exposure to a *Leishmania* infected sandfly. In general, this will restrict exposures to those areas in which *Leishmania* is endemic. For non-endemic areas such as the USA and much of Europe, the primary risk factor (much like malaria) will be travel to areas where *Leishmania* is endemic. Thus, deferrals based on travel histories could be considered, but this approach would result in the unnecessary loss of many eligible donors. Testing options are limited, but as already discussed, the recent development of a K39 based assay for visceral leishmaniasis may be useful for selective testing. Polymerase chain reaction techniques have been described indicating that NAT, at least for visceral leishmaniasis, is feasible. However, NAT may be problematical from the standpoint of assay sensitivity due to the limited number of infected cells present in peripheral blood and sample size issues. Considerations must be given to techniques that concentrate infected cells and/or testing of larger blood volumes, perhaps on repeat samples. Alternatively, given that the *Leishmania* are localized to monocytes, the potential application of leucoreduction filters to minimize transfusion-transmission warrants further study. A recent study also reported on the effectiveness of *Leishmania* inactivation by psoralen (amotosalen HCl), but this study was limited to extracellular parasites, not infected monocytes (Eastman, *et al.*, 2005).

Trypanosoma cruzi – Chagas' disease

American trypanosomiasis or Chagas' disease occurs only in the American continent, whose agent is the protozoan *Trypanosoma cruzi*. Chagas' disease was initially described in 1909 by Carlos Chagas, in the hinterlands of Brazil, who demonstrated in a series of papers the nature of the protozoan, its morphology in the bloodstream, life cycle in the digestive system of invertebrates (triatomines), cultivation in agar blood and transmission to vertebrates. He also reported in 1911 the first congenital case and raised the possibility that the human digestive system might also be affected (Chagas, 1909a; 1909b; 1909c; 1909d; 1911; 1922; Chagas Filho C., 1959).

Transmission by blood transfusion (TT) was first suggested by Mazza in Argentina, in 1936 (Mazza *et al.*, 1936). Others later supported his original concept in Brazil, Uruguay and Argentina. The first donors found to be infected were described in 1949 in Brazil (Pellegrino, 1949), later confirmed by others in 1951 (Faria, 1951). The first two cases of TT Chagas' disease were published in 1952 (Freitas *et al.*, 1952a) and at the same period, the value of chemoprophylaxis with crystal violet (gentian violet) was studied (Nussenzweig *et al.*, 1953). Though regarded as a strictly Latin American problem, Chagas' disease transmission through blood components became recognized in North America in the late 1980s (Cimo *et al.*, 1993; Galel *et al.*, 1997; Geiseler *et al.*, 1987; Grant *et al.*, 1989; Leiby *et al.*, 1996; Nickerson *et al.*, 1989).

There are about 100 million people exposed or at risk of infection in endemic areas, and from 18 to 20 million possibly infected (Leiby *et al.*, 1997a; Prata, 2001; Schmunis, 1994; Umezawa *et al.*, 2001; WHO, 2002) to less than 8 million more recently (PAHO, 2006) in 18 Latin American countries (it has not been described in Cuba and the Dominican Republic). It is estimated that 2 to 3 million individuals manifest chronic symptoms (cardiac or gastrointestinal), with nearly 45 000 annual deaths (TDR, 2007). That makes Chagas' disease a main contributor to early retirement and years lost from incapacity. Actually, when Chagas' disease is measured by DALYs (disability-adjusted life years), it shows the highest DALY in all of Latin America, whereas the remaining infectious diseases of public significance (malaria, schistosomiasis, leishmaniasis, leprosy, filariasis and onchocercosis) together represent less than 25% of Chagas' disease's economic burden (Silveira, 2002; World Bank, 1993). On a global scale, Chagas' disease represents the third tropical disease in DALYs, after malaria and schistosomiasis (Moncayo, 1993).

The Southern Cone Initiative (Resolution 04-3), launched in 1991 (Panamerican Health Organization, 1992), followed by the Andean Countries Initiative (Panamerican Health Organization, 2003), both under the auspices and support of Panamerican Health Organization (PAHO), have as a main objective the elimination of domiciliary infestation by *Triatoma infestans* (the main

reduviid bug) and complete control over transfusional transmission within a timeframe spanning ten years (Panamerican Health Organization, 1997). Thus, these countries imposed a rigid governmental control and mandatory serological screening of donated blood; in addition national blood programmes became a target to be pursued in this region. This action was also enhanced by the 51st World Health Assembly, which deemed the control of Chagas' disease as one of its main priorities (World Health Assembly, 1998).

Trypanosoma cruzi is a long and slender protozoan (order Kinetoplastida, family Trypanosomatidae), with a single nucleus, a flagellum, and a kinetoplast that is a structure unique to the order and contains the mitochondrial DNA (i.e. kinetoplast DNA or kDNA), mainly organized into a network of interlocked minicircles, with 20 000 to 25 000 copies per kinetoplast.

There are three stages in its life cycle:

(1) *Amastigotes*, round and intracellular forms (1.5–4.0 μm diameter, with no flagellum), found as clusters in infected cells of vertebrates (macrophages, muscle fibres, testis, ovaries, thyroid and adrenal glands, and in the central nervous system) or in the invertebrate triatomine stomach.

(2) *Epimastigotes*, with a juxtanuclear kinetoplast and flagellum, present in the foregut of the insect vector (rarely found in the bloodstream of vertebrates).

(3) *Trypomastigotes*, usually 'C' or 'U' shaped (12–20 μm diameter), the flagellum emerging from a post-nuclear kinetoplast, with great motility; in vertebrates, they are found in the bloodstream, lymph and cerebrospinal fluid, especially in the acute phase, while in invertebrates they can be found in the duodenum and hindgut (metacyclic trypomastigotes).

There are more than 100 different strains of *T. cruzi*, each one with a particular preference for humans, domestic or sylvatic reservoirs (Wendel *et al.*, 1992a). In the bloodstream, a polymorphism is also observed, with two different 'polar' forms (macrophagetropic and non-macrophage). In addition to the morphological differences among strains, polymorphism can also be observed according to different isoenzyme patterns (zymodemes) (Miles, 1980; 1983), kDNA cleavage by RFLP (schyzodemes)(Morel *et al.*, 1980), or molecular sequencing of several parasite genes (Avila *et al.*, 1990). Recently, the genome sequence has been characterized (El-Sayed *et al.*, 2005).

Invertebrates responsible for transmission of *T. cruzi* are haematophagus bugs (family *Reduvidae* and sub-family *Triatominae*), with over 110 different species listed worldwide. However, only 40 species are adapted to human habitats, serving as a significant vector for *T. cruzi* only in the New World, where they can be detected from latitude 42° N (northern California, Utah, Maryland) to latitude 46° S (Patagonia). They are known in English as the 'kissing bug' or 'cone-nosed bug', in Spanish as 'Vinchuca' and in Portuguese as 'Barbeiro'.

These bugs are present in nature, and transmission of *T. cruzi* occurs either under the sylvatic condition or by the peridomestic or intra-domiciliary routes. In nature, triatomines feed mainly on monkeys, marmosets, sloths, armadillos and skunks, and live on trees (bark holes); for peridomestic or intra-domiciliary transmission (cats, dogs and humans are the main reservoirs) some species are well adapted to very rudimentary human dwellings (made with wattle or bamboo and filled with mud, unplastered walls, and palm-thatched roofs). These huts are usually found in isolated poor areas of Latin America, grouped into small clusters or scattered around lowly populated villages. After a blood meal, the infected bug defaecates near the bite wound, leaving infective metacyclic trypomastigotes in faeces that enter the host through the bite wound, mucosal membranes or following localized scratching. After a 20–30 hour period, a binary division begins in the cytoplasm, generating 50 to 500 intracellular amastigotes every 12 hours, with differentiation to trypomastigotes, lysing the infected cells and subsequently releasing parasites into the bloodstream, enabling invasion of other cells, leading to the host death, or more frequently, to the development of an immune process that controls parasitaemia without parasite eradication. Thus, parasitaemia is only observed in the acute process, while in the chronic stage of Chagas' disease, only subpatent parasitaemia is present. In addition to this step in the vertebrate host, bloodstream forms can be subsequently ingested by other bugs, completing the infective cycle. There is no spontaneous cure, nor normal relapses, except when a host immunosuppressive condition ensues (e.g. organ transplant, oncological treatments or AIDS) (Nishioka et al., 1993).

Chagas' disease is also transmitted by congenital transmission, breast-feeding, accidental laboratory contamination, organ transplant (Chocair et al., 1981; Ferraz and Figueiredo, 1993), blood transfusion (Wendel et al., 1992a) or by incidental oral ingestion of contaminated food (Valente et al., 1999).

Since the American continent comprises more than 20 different countries, a wide range of infected donor rates is observed in different regions, ranging from a low of 0.01% in the USA, to 60% in certain Bolivian cities (Dias and Brener, 1984; Leiby, 1997a; Schmunis, 1991; 1994; 1997; Wendel et al., 1992a; Wendel and Gonzaga, 1993; Wendel, 1997). Ongoing surveys display a progressive decrease in the prevalence of *T. cruzi* among Latin American blood donors. There are at least three main reasons for this observation:

(1) *Efficient sanitary programmes* – a persistent effort among several countries to eradicate domiciliary bugs and improve housing over the past 20 years is supported mainly by the Southern Cone Ministerial Initiative (Panamerican Health Organization, 1992). As a result of these programmes, younger generations show lower rates of infection, as demonstrated by several studies (Aguilera et al., 1994; Andrade et al., 1992a; Martelli et al., 1992; PAHO-OPS, 1994; Segovia et al., 1993; Segura et al., 1985; Wendel and Biagini, 1995; Wendel, 2005; Zicker et al., 1990a).

(2) *Pattern of migration* – as endemic, rural areas become more developed, a decrease of emigration to urban areas is expected. Therefore, it is possible that many cities currently have more donors who were originally born in urban areas than 20 to 30 years ago (Quinteros et al., 1990).

(3) *Replacement of paid donors* – the replacement of paid donors by voluntary, altruistic donors is probably one of the most important factors contributing to the decrease in the prevalence of infected donors.

With the exception of lyophilized plasma (Amato Neto et al., 1996) and fractionated blood products, all blood components are infective. *Trypanosoma cruzi* remains viable at $4\,^{\circ}C$ for at least 18 days (Sullivan, 1944) or up to 250 days when kept at room temperature (Weinman and MacAlister, 1947). Frozen strains are infective for longer periods (Filardi and Brener, 1975; Weinman and MacAlister, 1947). The viability of the parasite is somewhat lower in frozen components (up to 24 hours), though several haemophiliacs treated only with cryoprecipitate have been infected (Cerisola et al., 1972; Lorca et al., 1988; Schlemper Jr, 1978).

In many places, blood transfusion is recognized as the second most important way of transmission of Chagas' disease; on the other hand it can be recognized as the main route in industrialized countries (e.g. Canada, USA and Spain)(Cimo et al., 1993; Geiseler et al., 1987; Grant et al., 1989; Nickerson et al., 1989; Villalba et al., 1992). The true number of reported cases is grossly underestimated, since no more than 300 cases have been published in the literature (Kirchhoff, 1989; 1993; Schmunis, 1994; Wendel, 1993). Several factors play a key role in this issue: the lack of knowledge or awareness of the disease (especially observed in industrialized, non-endemic areas), no interest or limited resources in continuing the medical evaluation of a suspected transfusion case and, finally, a reluctance to report well established cases if they might reflect badly on the standards of the given blood services. In addition, a positive factor recently observed in Latin America is that there has been a measurable decrease in observed cases associated with developed urban blood services (Schmunis and Cruz, 2005).

Although the reported cases in countries of the northern hemisphere are quite few, the recent and intense emigration to these countries is a factor of some concern. Currently, it is estimated that there are at least 12 400 000 legal Latin-American immigrants in the USA, 500 000 in Europe, 500 000 in Japan and 100 000 in Australia (Schmunis, 1994; Wendel et al., 1993). It is expected that 50 000 to 370 000 immigrants in North America are infected by *T. cruzi* (Kirchhoff & Neva 1985), and nearly 75 000 of them might involve some cardiac manifestation (Milei et al., 1992). All these factors show that Chagas' disease is slowly but gradually changing its natural geographical limits, placing other countries at risk of something unexpected only a decade ago (Wendel, 1993a).

The potential for infection by blood components depends on several factors, including the amount of transfused blood, the parasite strain, the presence of parasitaemia at the time of donation and the recipient's immune status. Additionally, the probability of infection is highly dependent on whether screening tests are performed in blood banks (Schmunis and Cruz, 2005; Wendel, 1993; 1993b). Data derived during the 1960s and 1970s demonstrated that the true infectivity rate associated with a single infected whole blood unit was around 12–25% (Cerisola et al., 1972; Coura et al., 1966; Rohwedder, 1969), though a higher value (46.7%) was observed in Bolivia (Zuna et al., 1979). Perhaps low level parasitaemia (less than 1:20 ml whole blood) and the concomitant presence of antibodies in the donor's bloodstream are partially responsible for incomplete infectivity. In addition, there are no data showing different patterns of infectivity as far as different components are concerned. Currently, there are several screening tests for *T. cruzi* antibodies in Latin America (Panamerican Health Organization, 2002). Although sensitivity is still far from what is observed for viral screening tests (97 to 99%) (Luquetti, 2000), universal screening of all blood donations has dramatically changed the transfusion risks in Latin America during the past few years. In countries where this strategy has been fully implemented, the residual risk of infection is calculated to be around 1:200 000 units (Schmunis and Cruz, 2005; Wendel *et al.*, 1992b; Wendel 2005), with clustered spatial geographic distribution.

The clinical findings observed in recipients of infected units are similar to those observed when infection occurs by insect transmission, except for the chagoma at inoculation, a typical swelling of skin, face or eyelids (representing the entry site of parasites), which is not observed. The incubation period varies from 20 to 40 days (ranging from 8 to 120 days). Fever is by far the most common and sometimes the only disease manifestation. Lymphadenopathy and hepatosplenomegaly may also be present and the association of these latter symptoms must always be suspected in recipients transfused with blood from untested donors. Cardiac arrhythmia (disturbances of atrioventricular conduction, ECG alterations or reduction of ejection fraction), leading to pericardial effusion and/or cardiac arrest can be observed. Death, though uncommon, occurs in the most severe cases, usually immunocompromised recipients. The central nervous system can also be affected (somnolence, fatigue and tremors are the most common symptoms). Myoclonus, seizures, meningitis or meningoencephalitis, though very rare, occur mainly in immunocompromised patients. The gastrointestinal system is usually spared in acute Chagas' disease. Approximately 20% of infected recipients are completely asymptomatic, raising no suspicion of diagnosis. In fact, in non-endemic areas from industrialized countries, this rate might be somewhat higher than in endemic countries.

After the acute phase, a spontaneous recovery will ensue after 6–8 weeks, but may extend up to four months. Thereafter, the disease follows its natural course to an indeterminate phase (persisting for years or decades), representing the majority of cases. In the chronic phase, cardiac, gastrointestinal or neurological symptoms are observed after several years, usually not linked to an acute phase. When the heart is affected, the myocardium becomes thin, with enlargement of the right and left chambers. Disturbances of atrioventricular conduction and Adams-Stokes syndrome (right bundle branch block) may supervene. Apical aneurysm of the left ventricle with thrombi attached to the endocardium is often found, leading to peripheral embolism. The gastrointestinal system is compromised in 8–10% of patients, with denervation of autonomic parasympathetic ganglia (Auerbach's plexus) and oesophageal or colonic hypotonia. Enlargement of the oesophagus or colon also occurs and is known as megasyndromes (e.g. megacolon or megaesophagus).

One of the key issues concerning the clinical findings among blood donors is that they are, in the vast majority of cases, asymptomatic. They can be subdivided into three main groups:

(1) *Serological Chagas' disease* – only antibodies are found, without any evidence of symptoms, comprising 60% to 80% of all infected donors.
(2) *Latent chronic phase* – donors show visceral abnormalities, as evidenced by different diagnostic tests (X-ray, CT scan, ECG), but are still asymptomatic, requiring close monitoring and follow-up, as clinical symptoms may supervene in the future.
(3) *Symptomatic donors* – representing the minority of cases; often symptoms are not persistent or specific.

Since there is an overlap between these groups, the true prevalence of each one is difficult to ascertain, although about 50% of patients with heart or gastrointestinal abnormalities show clinical symptoms. One study of 291 donors with Chagas' disease (Gontijo, 1989) revealed that 54% were in the indeterminate phase, 38% with cardiac, 18% with digestive and 10% with both cardiac and digestive symptoms. Among them, 79.5% with chronic cardiopathy and 75% with oesophagopathy were in the initial stage of clinical evolution and severe heart disease was found in only 3.1% of these cases.

Prevention of TT Chagas' disease can be accomplished by three different strategies (Wendel, 1993a):

(1) *History taking and questionnaires to the donors* – this includes exclusion of paid donations (still present in up to 2% of global donations (http://www.who.int/bloodsafety/global_database/en/)). There is a trend to find more infected donors among older donors, first-time donors or those living for longer periods in endemic areas (Wendel and Biagini, 1995; 2005; Zicker *et al.*, 1990a). Donors who live in infested dwellings or acknowledge having been bitten by the riduvid bug must be excluded from donation. Specific questionnaires have been used in parts of North America and Europe to identify high-risk donors (Appleman *et al.*, 1993; Barea *et al.*, 2004; Council Of Europe, 2005; Read *et al.*, 1994).
(2) *Serological tests* – several methods are available for screening in Latin America, and more recently, one of them has been implemented in the USA.
(3) *Chemoprophylaxis* – the first attempt to achieve parasite inactivation of whole blood was by addition of thimerosal in 1952 (Freitas *et al.*, 1952b). Subsequently, more than 1000 compounds have been tested to date; among them, only a few have shown some trypanocidal effect (Cover and Gutteridge, 1982), for example crystal violet, which totally eliminates *T. cruzi* viability within 24 hours at a concentration of 1:4000 or 200 µg/ml (0.6 mM) (Docampo *et al.*, 1983, 1993; Docampo and Moreno, 1984; Nussenzweig *et al.*, 1953). Presence of light (130 W/m^2) and reducing agents (ascorbate acid – 10 mM) enhances this reaction 17-fold (Docampo *et al.*, 1983), reducing both exposure time (20 minutes) and dye concentration (1:16 000 or 0.4 m*M*) has the same efficacy (Ramirez *et al.*, 1995; Souza, 1989).

The effect of crystal violet was extensively studied in the blood of chronic phase donors, and was shown to be effective against all parasite stages (amastigotes, epimastigotes and trypomastigotes) (Docampo *et al.*, 1983; Schlemper Jr, 1978) and several different strains (e.g. Y, FL, G, J, M, Peru and Sonya). In an experimental study with 18 recipients transfused with seropositive blood that had been treated, none developed infection (Amato Neto, 1958). Rezende *et al.* (Rezende *et al.*, 1965) reported that among a group of 774 recipients transfused with unscreened blood components, where at least 300 were likely to be derived from infected donors, none developed acute or chronic infection. The Brazilian experience, involving over 50 000 units has confirmed the efficacy of crystal violet treatment (Souza, 1989). However, this compound is not devoid of side effects on red blood cells (i.e. Rouleaux formation, slight decrease of ATP and 2,3 DPG) and platelets, due to direct action on mitochondrial calcium metabolism (Docampo *et al.*, 1993). In recipients, a slight purple colour is observed that lasts for 24 hours. In addition, crystal violet has been shown to be carcinogenic in rodents, though no effect was observed in humans (Docampo and Moreno, 1990). The maximum infusion dosage for recipients (5 to 10 mg/Kg) is still not clearly defined; this value is easily achieved with 2500 mL of treated whole blood, but its real effect in massive transfusions is still open to question. Infusion of crystal violet in infants is associated with WBC depression. The long-term effect is also unknown, though some patients transfused with over 36000 mL of treated blood during a six-month period have been reported (Rezende, 1965). In an attempt to achieve overall pathogen reduction other methods have been extensively evaluated in the past few years; among the several new agents tested, amotosalen-HCl (Van Voorhis *et al.*, 2003) and INACTINE Pen-110 (Zavizion *et al.*, 2004) have proven to be quite satisfactory. However, these products are still not widely used on a global scale.

Detection of parasites by direct examination of peripheral blood smears or indirect methods (culture systems such as xenodiagnosis or haemocultures), though still regarded as true 'gold standards' for diagnosis, are impractical for routine use. In addition, a negative result still does not preclude the presence of infection, given that the sensitivity of these methods rarely reaches 85% (Chiari, 1992; Wendel *et al.*, 1997), and both methods require up to 120 days for full and conclusive results.

Because of the relatively low sensitivity and technical problems observed by xenodiagnosis and haemoculture in chronic patients, PCR is being extensively studied for detecting Chagas' disease. The main difficulty in adopting PCR for the diagnosis of Chagas' disease in chronic patients derives from the low and intermittent parasitaemia observed in an important proportion of chronic carriers. In order to obviate this concern, investigators have focused on highly conserved DNA sequences present on the *T. cruzi* genome, mostly contained within the parasite's kDNA (Avila *et al.*, 1991; 1993; Britto *et al.*, 1995; Gomes *et al.*, 1999; Wincker *et al.*, 1994). However, the need for chaotropic agents (guanidine HCl) for better DNA extraction (Avila *et al.*, 1991), associated with variable sensitivity (45 to 100%) (Antaz *et al.*, 1999; Brenière *et al.*, 1992; Britto *et al.*, 1995; Galvão *et al.*, 2003; Lages-Silva *et al.*, 2001, Marcon *et al.*, 2002; Salomone *et al.*, 2003; Silber *et al.*, 1997; Vera-Cruz *et al.*, 2003; Virreira *et al.*, 2003; Zingales *et al.*, 1998) has precluded the adoption of this method as a gold standard thus far. Also, false-positive results may be more common than expected (Avila *et al.*, 1993; Brenière *et al.*, 1992; Castro *et al.*, 2002; Gomes *et al.*, 1999).

Thus, as a practical procedure, one has to rely on testing for antibodies to the parasite, which is easily performed with relatively low cost and high sensitivity (though with variable specificity). There are several methods commercially available in Latin America (Cura and Wendel, 1994; Ferreira, 1992), mostly based on EIA (Brashear *et al.*, 1995; Carvalho *et al.*, 1993; Ferreira *et al.*, 1991; Hoffman *et al.*, 1997; Houghton *et al.*, 1996; Voller *et al.*, 1975; Wendel *et al.*, 1993), Indirect Haemagglutination (Andrade *et al.*, 1992b; Luquetti, 1990; Zicker *et al.*, 1990b) or Indirect Immunofluorescence Assay (IFAT) (Camargo and Sawza, 1966; Fife Jr and Mushel, 1959), using whole parasites or crude lysates as antigen sources, although intense research has been carried out on the development of synthetic peptides or recombinant antigens. *Trypanosoma cruzi* antibody titres are quite variable in infected people, and usually bear no relationship to clinical symptoms; they also vary in the same individual throughout their lifetime.

The current serological methods are also prone to cross-reaction with sera containing antibodies against other infectious agents such as yeasts, *Leishmania* spp. (Kala-azar and mucocutaneous leishmaniasis), *T. rangeli* (a non-pathogenic agent found in Venezuela, Colombia, Peru, Ecuador, Panama and Costa Rica), *T. gambiensis* (the agent of the sleeping sickness or African trypanosomiasis), *H. muscarum, L. seymoury, C. fasciculata* and other trypanosomatids. In addition, non-specific IgM directed against phosphocoline (Lal and Ottesen, 1989), an antigenic fraction widely present in several mycobacteria and parasites, is also responsible for cross-reaction, rendering the serological methods for *T. cruzi* antibody detection still open to improvement. One has also to bear in mind that indefinite results are seen in approximately 3–5% of all blood donors, characterized by a reactive result in only one assay (usually with clearly negative or very low titres in a second test).

These issues pose significant problems for the counselling of reactive donors in endemic areas. For this reason, supplementary assays are also necessary to confirm the screening test results. Though several methods have been proposed as potential confirmatory assays (Almeida *et al.*, 1994; 1997; Chiller *et al.*, 1990; Costa *et al.*, 1997; Lanar and Manning, 1984; Malchiodi *et al.*, 1994; Reed *et al.*, 1987; Rosfjord *et al.*, 1990; Sabino *et al.*, 1997), cross-reactivity has also been demonstrated as a problem in many of these tests. Thus, maybe only two methods deserve some attention at this point:

(1) *Western blot* – using highly purified trypomastigote excreted-secreted antigens (TESA) (Kesper *et al.*, 2000; Silveira-Lacerda *et al.*, 2004; Umezawa *et al.*, 1996).

(2) *Radioimmunoprecipitation assay (RIPA)* – when lysed cultured epimastigotes containing a radioisotope (^{125}I) are tested against serum, displaying two major glycoprotein bands (gp 72 and gp 90)(Kirchhoff *et al.*, 1987; Leiby 1997b; Winkler *et al.*, 1995).

However, both methods have shown some flaws in a recent Brazilian survey (Wendel, 2005), suggesting that they still should be considered as 'imperfect gold standards' (Zhou *et al.*, 2002).

Conclusion

In the light of current blood safety, one has to focus on the concept of a 'Safety Tripod' (Farrugia, 2004), based on the following principles: selection of appropriate and 'low-risk' donors, usage of screening tests for the relevant marker of infection and elimination of residual pathogens. Though most aspects of this approach have been incorporated into current practice in developed countries, even greater benefits will be achieved once they are properly established in developing countries, where parasite infections are more prevalent and therefore pose a greater risk to the recipient population. Several problems remain: the geographic distribution of parasitic infections, patterns of emigration, high numbers of asymptomatic donors, lack of medical knowledge for correct diagnosis, and the need for technical refinements for laboratory screening. Therefore, some parasites remain a major threat for transfusions worldwide. Thus, every country must be aware of their particular epidemiological pattern and adopt a combination of procedures to prevent transmissions, especially those countries that were considered risk-free until very recently.

REFERENCES

AABB (2005) *Standards for Blood Banks and Transfusion Services.* 23rd edn. Bethesda, MD, USA, American Association of Blood Banks.

Aguilera, X. M., Apt, W. B., Rodriguez, J. T., *et al.* (1994) Eficacia del control del vector de la enfermedad de Chagas demonstrada a través de la infección humana. *Rev Med Chile*, **122**, 259–64.

Al-Amari, O. M. (1994) Prevalence of antibodies to *Toxoplasma gondii* among blood donors in Abha, Asir Region, south-western Saudi Arabia. *J Egypt Public Health Assoc*, **69**, 77–88.

Allred, D. R. (2003) Babesiosis: persistence in the face of adversity. *Trends Parasitol*, **19**, 51–5.

Almeida, I. C., Covas, D. T., Soussumi, L. M. T. and Travassos, L. R. (1997) A highly sensitive and specific chemiluminescent enzyme-linked immunosorbent assay for diagnosis of active *Trypanosoma cruzi* infection. *Transfusion*, **37**, 850–57.

Almeida, I. C., Ferguson, M. A. J., Schenkman, S., *et al.* (1994) Lytic anti-alpha-galactosyl antibodies from patients with chronic Chagas' disease recognise novel O-linked oligosaccharides on mucin-like GPI-anchored glycoproteins of *Trypanosoma cruzi*. *Biochem J*, **304**, 793–802.

Alves, M. J. C. P., Rangel, O. and Souza, S. S. A. P. (2000) Malária na região de Campinas, São Paulo, Brasil, 1980 a 1994. *Rev Soc Bras Med Trop*, **33**, 53–60.

Amato Neto, V. (1958) Contribuição ao conhecimento da forma aguda da Doença de Chagas – Tese: Faculdade de Medicina da Universidade de São Paulo.

Amato Neto, V., Leonhardt, H. and Souza, H. B. W. T. (1996) Liofilização do plasma: Medida capaz de evitar a transmissão da Doença de Chagas em Bancos de Sangue. *Rev Inst Med Trop São Paulo*, **8**, 122–4.

Amato Neto, V., SaníAna, E. J., Pinto, P. L. S., *et al.* (1987) Estudo experimental sobre a possibilidade de prevenção da malária pós transfusional através do uso de violeta de genciana. *Rev Saúde Publ S Paulo*, **21**, 497–500.

Andrade, A. L. S. S., Zicker, F., Luquetti, A. O., *et al.* (1992a) Surveillance of *Trypanosoma cruzi* by serological screening of school children. *Bull WHO*, **70**, 625–9.

Andrade, A. L. S. S., Martelli, C. M. T., Luquetti, A. O., *et al.* (1992b) Serologic screening for *Trypanosoma cruzi* among blood donors in central Brazil. *Bull Pan Am Health Organ*, **26**, 157–64.

Andrade, J. C. R. and Wanderley, D. M. V. (1991) Malária induzida no Estado de São Paulo, Brasil. *Rev Soc Bras Med Trop*, **24**, 157–61.

André, R., Brumpt, L., Dreyfus, B., *et al.* (1957) Cutaneous leishmaniasis, cutaneous-glandular leishmaniasis and transfusional kala-azar. *Bull Mém Soc Méd Hôpit Paris*, **25/26**, 854–60.

Antaz, P. R. Z., Medrano-Mercado, N., Torrico, F., *et al.* (1999) Early, intermediate, and late acute stages in Chagas' disease: a study combining anti-galactose IgG, specific serodiagnosis, and polymerase chain reaction analysis. *Am J Trop Med Hyg*, **61**, 308–14.

Appleman, M. D., Shulman, I. A., Saxena, S., *et al.* (1993) Use of a questionnaire to identify potential blood donors at risk for infection with *Trypanosoma cruzi*. *Transfusion*, **33**, 61–4.

Arafat, R., Long, S., Perry, M., *et al.* (2003) Probable transfusion-transmitted malaria – Houston, Texas, 2003. *MMWR*, **52**, 1076.

Assal, A., Kauffmann-Lacroix, C., Rodier, M. H., *et al.* (1999) Comparison de deux techniques de détection des anticorps anti-*Plasmodium falciparum*: Falciparum-spot IF® (BioMérieux) et Malaria IgG Celisa® (BMD). Résultats préliminaires. *Transf Clin Biol*, **6**, 119–23.

Avila, H., Gonçalves, A. M., Nehme, N. C., *et al.* (1990) Schizodeme analysis of *Trypanosoma cruzi* stocks from South and Central America by analysis of PCR-amplified minicircle variable region sequences. *Molec Biochem Parasitol*, **42**, 175–88.

Avila, H., Pereira, J. B., Thiemann, O., *et al.* (1993) Detection of *Trypanosoma cruzi* in blood specimens of chronic chagasic patients by polymerase chain reaction amplification of kinetoplast minicircle DNA: comparison with serology and xenodiagnosis. *J Clin Microbiol*, **31**, 2421–6.

Avila, H. A., Sigman, D. S., Cohen, L. M., *et al.* (1991) Polymerase chain reaction of *Tripanosoma cruzi* kinetoplast minicircle DNA isolated from whole blood lysates: diagnosis of chronic Chagas' disease. *Mol Biochem Parasitol*, **48**, 211–22.

Badaro, R., Benson, D., Eulalio, M. C., *et al.* (1996) rK39: a cloned antigen of *Leishmania chagasi* that predicts active visceral leishmaniasis. *J Infect Dis*, **173**, 758–61.

Balsari, A., Poli, G., Molina, V., *et al.* (1980) ELISA for toxoplasma antibody detection: a comparison with other serodiagnostic tests. *J Clin Pathol*, **33**, 640–3.

Barea, L., Cañavate, C., Flores, M., *et al.* (2004) Seroprevalence of anti-*Trypanosoma cruzi* in blood donors coming from Chagas' diasease endemic countries. *Vox Sang*, **87** (Suppl. 3), Abstract W 01.03.

Barea, L., Gonzalez, R., Bueno, J. L., *et al.* (2001) Strategy for the acceptance of blood donors coming from malaria areas. *Transfusion*, **41**(Suppl.), 75S.

Beattie, J. F., Michelson, M. L. and Holman, P. J. (2002) Acute babesiosis caused by *Babesia divergens* in a resident of Kentucky. *N Eng J Med*, **347**, 697–8.

Beauvais, B., Garin, J. F., Lariviere, M., *et al.* (1976) Toxoplasmose et transfusion. *Ann Parasitol Hum Comp*, **51**, 625–35.

Bell, D. (2002) Malaria rapid diagnostic tests: one size may not fit all (letter). *Clin Microbiol Rev*, **15**, 771–2.

Bellmann, R., Sturm, W., Pechlaner, C., *et al.* (2000) Imported malaria: six cases of severe *Plasmodium falciparum* infection in Innsbruck, Austria, within a period of five weeks (February/March 1999). *Wien Klin Wochenschr*, **112**, 453–8.

Berman, J. D. (1997) Human leishmaniasis: clinical, diagnostic and chemotherapeutic developments in the last ten years. *Clin Infect Dis*, **24**, 684–703.

Bowdre, J. H., Campbell, J. L., Walker, D. H., *et al.* (1981) American mucocutaneous leishmaniasis. Culture of a *Leishmania* species from peripheral blood leukocytes. *Am J Clin Pathol*, **75**, 435–8.

Bradley, D. J., Warhurst, D. C., Blaze, M., *et al.* (1998) Malaria imported into the United Kingdom in 1996. *Euro Surveill*, **3**, 40–2.

Brashear, R. J., Winkler, M. A., Schur, J. D., *et al.*, (1995) Detection of antibodies to *Trypanosoma cruzi* among blood donors in the south-western and western United States. 1 Evaluation of the sensitivity and specificity of an enzyme immunoassay for detecting antibodies to *T. cruzi*. *Transfusion*, **35**, 213–8.

Brazilian Ministry of Health, Resolution 153 (2004). www.anvisa.gov.br.

Brenière, S. F., Bosseno, M. F., Revollo, S., *et al.* (1992) Direct identification of *Trypanosoma cruzi* natural clones in vectors and mammalian hosts by polymerase chain reaction amplification. *Am J Trop Med Hyg*, **46**, 335–41.

Britto, C., Cardoso, M. A., Ravel, C., *et al.* (1995) *Trypanosoma cruzi*: parasite detection and strain discrimination in chronic chagasic patients from north-eastern Brazil using PCR amplification of kinetoplast DNA and non-radioactive hybridization. *Exp Parasitol*, **81**, 462–71.

Bruce-Chwatt, L. J. (1972) Blood transfusion and tropical disease. *Trop Dis Bull*, **69**, 825–62.

Bruce-Chwatt, L. J. (1974) Transfusion malaria. *Bull WHO*, **50**, 337–46.

Bruce-Chwatt, L. J. (1982) Transfusion malaria revisited. *Trop Dis Bull*, **79**, 827–40.

Burg J. L., Grover, C. M., Pouletty P., *et al.* (1989) Direct and sensitive detection of a pathogenic protozoan, *Toxoplasma gondii*, by polymerase chain reaction. *J Clin Microbiol*, **27**, 1787–92.

Bush, J. B., Isaäcson, M., Mohamed, A. S., *et al.* (1990) Human babesiosis – a preliminary report of two suspected cases in southern Africa. *S Afr Med J*, **78**, 699.

Cable, R. G., Badon, S., Trouern-Trend, J., *et al.* (2001) Evidence for transmission of *Babesia microti* from Connecticut blood donors to recipients. *Transfusion*, **41**(Suppl.), 12S–13S.

Camargo, M. E. and Souza, S. L. (1966) The use of filter paper blood smears in a practical fluorescent test for American trypanosomiasis serodiagnosis. *Rev Inst Med Trop S Paulo*, **8**, 255–8.

Carvalho, M. R., Krieger, M. A., Almeida, E., *et al.* (1993) Chagas' disease diagnosis: evaluation of several tests in blood bank screening. *Transfusion*, **33**, 830–4.

Castro, A. M., Luquetti, A. O., Rassi, A., *et al.* (2002) Blood culture and polymerase chain reaction for the diagnosis of the chronic phase of human infection with *Trypanosoma cruzi*. *Parasitol Res*, **88**, 894–900.

Cerisola, J. A., Rabinovich, A., Alvarez, M., *et al.* (1972) Enfermedad de Chagas' y la transfusion de sangre. *Bol Of Sanit Panam*, **63**, 203–21.

Chagas Filho, C. (1959) Carlos Chagas – Oficina Gráfica da Universidade do Brazil.

Chagas, C. (1909a) Nova espécie morbida do homem, produzida por um *Trypanosoma* (*Trypanosoma cruzi*): Nota prévia. *Brasil Médico*, **23**, 161.

Chagas, C. (1909b) Neue Trypanosomen. *Arch Schiffs Tropenhyg*, **13**, 120–2.

Chagas, C. (1909c) Uber eine neue Trypanosomiasis des Menschen. *Arch Schiffs Tropenhyg*, **13**, 351–3.

Chagas, C. (1909d) Nova tripanozomiase humana. Estudos sobre a morfolojia e o ciclo evolutivo do *Schizotrypanum cruzi* n.g., n.s.p., ajente etiolójico de nova entidade mórbida no homem. *Mem Inst Oswaldo Cruz*, **1**, 159–218.

Chagas, C. (1911) Nova entidade mórbida do homem. Resumo geral de estudos etiolójicos e clínicos. *Mem Inst Oswaldo Cruz*, **3**, 219–75.

Chagas, C. (1922) The discovery of *Trypanosoma cruzi* and of American Trypanosomiasis. *Mem Inst Oswaldo Cruz*, **15**, 1–11.

Chataing, B. (1988) Prevention du paludisme transfusionel. *Rev Franc Transf Immunohematol*, **31**, 81–8.

Chiari, E. (1992) Diagnostic tests for Chagas' disease. In *Chagas' Disease (American Trypanosomiasis): Its Impact on Transfusion and Clinical Medicine*, eds S. Wendel, Z. Brener, M. E. Camargo, A. Rassi, pp. 153–164. São Paulo, ISBT Brazil 92.

Chiller, T. M., Samudio, M. A. and Zoulek, G. (1990) IgG antibody reactivity with *Trypanosoma cruzi* and *Leishmania* antigens in sera of patients with Chagas' disease and leishmaniasis. *Am J Trop Med Hyg*, **43**, 650–6.

Chiodini, P. L., Hartley, S., Hewitt, P. E., *et al.* (1997) Evaluation of a malaria antibody ELISA and its value in reducing potential wastage of red cell donations from blood donors exposed to malaria, with a note on a case of transfusion-transmitted malaria. *Vox Sang*, **73**, 143–8.

Chocair, P. R., Sabbaga, E., Amato Neto, V., *et al.* (1981) Transplante de rim: nova modalidade de transmissão da doença de Chagas'. *Rev Med Trop S Paulo*, **23**, 282.

Choudhury, N., Jolly, J. G., Mahajan, R. C., *et al.* (1988) Selection of blood donors in malaria endemic countries. *Lancet*, **ii**, 972–3.

Chung, H. L., Chow, H. K. and Lu, J. P. (1948) The first two cases of transfusion kala-azar. *Chinese Med J*, **66**, 325–6.

Cimo, P. L., Luper, W. E. and Scouros, M. A. (1993) Transfusion-associated Chagas' disease in Texas: report of a case. *Tex Med*, **89**, 48–50.

Cohen, C., Corazza, F., De Mol, P., *et al.* (1991) Leishmaniasis acquired in Belgium. *Lancet*, **338**, 128.

Costa, G. C. V., Teixeira, M. G. M., Borges-Pereira, J., *et al.* (1997) A recombinant antigen and peptide line immunoassay (LIA) as an alternative diagnostic test for Chagas' disease. *Mem Inst Oswaldo Cruz*, **92** (Suppl. 1), 267.

Costa, J. M., Ernault, P., Gautier, E., *et al.* (2001) Prenatal diagnosis of congenital toxoplasmosis by duplex real-time PCR using fluorescence resonance energy transfer hybridization probes. *Prenat Diagn*, **21**, 85–8.

Costa, J. M., Pautas, C., Ernault, P., *et al.* (2000) Real-time PCR for diagnosis and follow-up of toxoplasma reactivation after allogeneic stem cell transplantation using fluorescence resonance energy transfer hybridization probes. *J Clin Microbiol*, **38**, 2929–32.

Council of Europe (2005) *Guide to the Preparation, Use and Quality Assurance of Blood Components* (11th edn) (available at www.coe.int).

Coura, J. R., Nogueira, E. S. and Silva, J. R. (1966) Índices de transmissão da doença de Chagas por transfusão de sangue de doadores na fase crônica da doença. *O Hospital*, **69**, 115–22.

Cover, B. and Gutteridge, W. E. (1982) A primary screen for drugs to prevent transmission of Chagas' disease during blood transfusion. *Trans Roy Soc Trop Med Hyg*, **76**, 633–5.

Craig, M. H., Bredekamp, B. L., Vaughan Williams, C. H., *et al.* (2002) Field and laboratory comparative evaluation of ten rapid malaria diagnostic tests. *Trans R Soc Trop Med Hyg*, **96**, 258–65.

Cummins, D., Amin, S., Ozay, H., *et al.* (1995) Visceral leishmaniasis after cardiac surgery. *Arch Dis Child*, **72**, 235–6.

Cura, E. and Wendel, S. (eds) (1994) *Manual de Procedimientos de Control de Calidad para los Laboratorios de Serologia de los Bancos de Sangre*. PAHO/HPC/HPT/94.21, Washington DC, USA.

Custer, B., Johnson, E. S., Sullivan, S. D., *et al.* (2004) Quantifying losses to donated blood supply due to deferral and miscollection. *Transfusion*, **44**, 1417–26.

Dao, A. H. and Eberhard, H. L. (1996) Pathology of acute fatal babesiosis in hamsters experimentally infected with the WA-1 strain of *Babesia*. *Lab Invest*, **74**, 853–9.

Davidson, N., Woodfield, G. and Henry, S. (1999) Malarial antibodies in Auckland blood donors. *N Z Med Journal*, **112**, 181–3.

De Monbrison, F., Angei, C., Staal, A., *et al.* (2003) Simultaneous identification of the four human *Plasmodium* species and quantification of *Plasmodium* DNA load in humans by real-time polymerase chain reaction. *Trans Royal Soc Trop Med Hyg*, **97**, 387–90.

De Monbrison, F., Gérome, P., Chaulet, J. F., *et al.* (2004) Comparative diagnostic performance of two commercial rapid tests for malaria in a non-endemic area. *Eur J Clin Microbiol Infect Dis*, **23**, 784–6.

Desjeux, P. (1996) Leishmaniasis: public health aspects and control. *Clin Dermatol*, **14**, 417–23.

Dias, J. C. P. and Brener, Z. (1984) Chagas' disease and blood transfusion. *Mem Inst Oswaldo Cruz*, **79**, l39–47.

Docampo, R. and Moreno, S. N. J. (1984) Free radicals metabolites in the mode of action of chemotherapeutic agents and phagocytic cells on *Trypanosoma cruzi*. *Rev Inf Dis*, **6**, 223–38.

Docampo, R. and Moreno, S. N. J. (1990) The metabolism and mode of action of gentian violet. *Drug Met Rev*, **22**, 161–78.

Docampo, R., Gadelha, F. R., Moreno, S. N. J., *et al.* (1993) Disruption of Ca^{+2} homeostasis in *Trypanosoma cruzi* by crystal violet. *J Eur Microbiol*, **40**, 311–6.

Docampo, R., Moreno, S. N. J., Muniz, R. P., *et al.* (1983) Light-enhanced free radical formation and trypanocidal action of gentian violet (crystal violet). *Science*, **220**, 1292–5.

Dorman, S. E., Cannon, M. E., Telford, S. R., *et al.* (2000) Fulminant babesiosis treated with clindamycin, quinine, and whole-blood exchange transfusion. *Transfusion*, **40**, 375–80.

Draper, C. C. and Sirr, S. S. (1980) Serological investigation in retrospective diagnosis of malaria. *Br. J Med*, **2**, 1575–6.

Duh, D., Petrovec, M. and Avsic-Zupanc, T. (2001) Diversity of *Babesia* infecting European sheep ticks (*Ixodes ricinus*). *J Clin Microbiol*, **39**, 3395–7.

Duhanina, N. N. and Žukova, T. A. (1965) Transmission of malaria through blood transfusion: an epidemiological study in the USSR. World Health Organization, WHO/Mal/503.65 (available at: whqlibdoc.who.int/malaria/WHO_Mal_503.65.pdf).

Duncan, R. (2004) DNA microarray analysis of protozoan parasite gene expression: outcomes correlate with mechanisms of regulation. *Trends Parasitol*, **20**, 211–5.

Dunn, D., Wallon, M., Peyron, F., *et al.* (1999) Mother-to-child transmission of toxoplasmosis: risk estimates for clinical counselling. *Lancet*, **353**, 1829–33.

Dupouy-Camet, J., de Souza, S. L., Maslo, C., *et al.* (1993) Detection of *Toxoplasma gondii* in venous blood from AIDS patients by polymerase chain reaction. *J Clin Microbiol*, **31**, 1866–9.

Eastman, R. T., Barrett, L. K., Dupuis, K., *et al.* (2005) *Leishmania* inactivation in human pheresis platelets by a psoralen (amotosalen HCl) and long-wavelength ultraviolet irradiation. *Transfusion*, **45**, 1459–63.

Eberhard, M. L., Walker, E. M. and Steurer, F. J. (1995) Survival and infectivity of *Babesia* in blood maintained at 25 °C and 2–4 °C. *J Parasitol*, **81**, 790–2.

El-Sayed, N. M., Myler, P. J., Bartholomeu, D. C., *et al.* (2005) The genome sequence of *Trypanosoma cruzi*, etiologic agent of Chagas' disease. *Science* **309**, 409–15.

Fairley, N. H. (1947) Sidelights on malaria in man obtained by subinoculation experiments. *Trans R Soc Trop Med Hyg*, **40**, 621–76.

Faria, P. (1951) Sífilis, Maleita, Doença de Chagas e Transfusão. *Folia Clin Biol*, **17**, 113–7.

Farrugia, A. (2004) The mantra of blood safety: time for a new tune? *Vox Sang*, **86**, 1–7.

Ferraz, A. S. and Figueiredo, J. F. C. (1993) Transmission of Chagas' disease through transplanted kidney: occurrence of the acute form of the disease in two recipients from the same donor. *Rev Inst Med Trop S Paulo*, **35**, 461–3.

Ferreira, A. W. (1992) Serological diagnosis – tests for Chagas' disease serodiagnosis: a review. In *Chagas' Disease (American Trypanosomiasis): Its Impact on Transfusion and Clinical Medicine*, eds S. Wendel, Z. Brener, M. E. Camargo and A. Rassi, pp. 179–93. São Paulo, ISBT Brazil 92.

Ferreira, A. W., Belem, Z. R., Moura, M. E. G., *et al.* (1991) Aspectos da padronização de testes sorológicos para a Doença de Chagas': Um teste imunoenzimático para a triagem de doadores de sangue. *Rev Inst Med Trop S Paulo*, **33**, 123–8.

Ferreira, M. V., Camargo, L. M. A., Carvalho, M. E., *et al.* (1993) Prevalence and levels of IgG and IgM antibodies against *Plasmodium falciparum* and *P. vivax* in blood donors from Rondonia, Brazilian Amazon. *Mem Inst Oswaldo Cruz*, **88**, 263–9.

Fife, E. H. Jr. and Mushel, L. H. (1959) Fluorescent antibody technique for serodiagnosis of *Trypanosoma cruzi* infection. *Proc Soc Exp Biol (NY)*, **101**, 540–3.

Filardi, L. S. and Brener, Z. (1975) Cryopreservation of *Trypanosoma cruzi* bloodstream forms. *J Protozool*, **22**, 398–401.

Filisetti, D., Gorcii, M., Pernot-Marine, E., *et al.* (2003) Diagnosis of congenital toxoplasmosis: comparison of targets for detection of *Toxoplasma gondii* by PCR. *J Clin Microbiol*, **41**, 4826–8.

Fonseca, M. O., Pang, L., Ávila, S. L. M., *et al.* (2000) Cross-reactivity of anti-*Plasmodium falciparum* antibodies and HIV tests. *Trans Roy Soc Trop Med Hyg*, **94**, 171–2.

Freitas, J. L. P., Amato Neto, V., Sonntag, R., *et al.* (1952a) Primeiras verificacões de transmissão acidental da molestia de Chagas ao homem por transfusão de sangue. *Rev Paul Med*, **40**, 36–40.

Freitas, J. L. P., Biancalana, A., Amato Neto, V., *et al.* (1952b) Moléstia de Chagas em bancos de sangue na capital de S. Paulo. *O Hospital*, **41**, 99–106.

Frey-Wettstein, M., Maier, A., Markwalder, K., *et al.* (2001) A case of transfusion transmitted malaria in Switzerland. *Swiss Med Wkly*, **131**, 320.

Fritz, C. L., Kjemtrup, A. M., Conrad, P. A., *et al.* (1997) Seroepidemiology of emerging tick-borne infectious diseases in a northern California community. *J Infect Dis*, **175**, 1432–9.

Galel, S., Wolles, S. and Stumpf, R. (1997) Evaluation of a selective donor testing strategy. *Transfusion*, **37**, Suppl. 9S, S296.

Galván-Ramírez, M. L., Covarrubias, X., Rodríguez, R., *et al.* (2005) *Toxoplasma gondii* antibodies in Mexican blood donors. *Transfusion*, **45**, 281–2.

Galvão, L. M. C., Chiari, E., Macedo, A. M., *et al.* (2003) PCR assay for monitoring *Trypanosoma cruzi* parasitemia in childhood after specific chemotherapy. *J Clin Microbiol*, **41**, 5066–70.

Gavinet, M. F., Robert, F., Firtion, G., *et al.* (1998) Congenital toxoplasmosis due to maternal reinfection during pregnancy. *J Clin Microbiol*, **35**, 1276–7.

Geiseler, P. J., Ito J. I., Tegtemeier, B. R., *et al.* (1987) Fulminant Chagas' disease in bone marrow transplantation. 27th Intersc Conf on Antimicro Agents and Chemoter, Washington. *Am Soc for Microbiol*, (Abstract), **418**.

Gerber, M. A., Shapiro, E. D., Krause, P. J., *et al.* (1994) The risk of acquiring Lyme disease or babesiosis from a blood transfusion. *J Inf Dis*, **170**, 231–4.

Gomes, M. L., Galvão, L. M. C., Macedo, A. M., *et al.* (1999) Chagas' disease diagnosis: comparative analysis of parasitologic, molecular and serologic methods. *Am J Trop Med Hyg*, **60**, 205–10.

Gontijo, E. C. D. (1989) Doença de Chagas Transfusional na Região Metropolitana de Belo Horizonte: aspectos clínico-epidemiológicos e a questão institucional. Thesis. Belo Horizonte, Universidade Federal de Minas Gerais, 1–179.

Gorenflot, A., Moubri, K., Precigout, E., *et al.* (1998) Human babesiosis. *Ann Trop Med Parasitol*, **92**, 489–501.

Grant, I., Gold, J. W. H., Wittnee, M., *et al.* (1989) Transfusion associated acute Chagas' disease acquired in the United States. *Ann Intern Med*, **111**, 849–51.

Gray, J., von Stedingk, L. V., Gürtelschmid, M., *et al.* (2002) Transmission studies of *Babesia microti* in *Ixodes ricinus* ticks and gerbils. *J Clin Microbiol*, **40**, 1259–63.

Grogl, M., Daugirda, J. L., Hoover, D. L., *et al.* (1993) Survivability and infectivity of viscerotropic *Leishmania tropica* from Operation Desert Storm participants in human blood products maintained under blood bank conditions. *Am J Trop Med Hyg*, **49**, 308–15.

Guevara, P., Ramírez, J. L., Rojas, E., *et al.* (1993) *Leishmania braziliensis* in blood 30 years after cure. *Lancet*, **341**, 1341.

Hedman, K., Lappalainen, M., Seppala, I., *et al.* (1989) Recent primary toxoplasma infection indicated by a low avidity of specific IgG. *J Infect Dis*, **159**, 736–9.

Herwaldt, B. L. (1999) Leishmaniasis. *Lancet*, **354**, 1191–9.

Herwaldt, B. L., Bruyn, G., Pieniazek, N. J., *et al.* (2004) *Babesia divergens*-like infection, Washington State. *Emerg Infect Dis*, **10**, 622–9.

Herwaldt, B. L., Cacciò, S., Gherlinzoni, F., *et al.* (2003a) Molecular characterization of a non-*Babesia divergens* organism causing zoonotic babesiosis in Europe. *Emerg Infect Dis*, **9**, 942–8.

Herwaldt, B. L., Kjemtrup, A. M., Conrad, P. A., *et al.* (1997) Transfusion-transmitted babesiosis in Washington State: first reported case caused by a WA1-type parasite. *J Infect Dis*, **175**, 1259–62.

Herwaldt, B. L., McGovern, P. C., Gerwel, M. P., *et al.* (2003b) Endemic babesiosis in another eastern state: New Jersey. *Emerg Infect Dis*, **9**, 184–8.

Hoffman, A., Jaczko, B., Jones, J., *et al.* (1997) Evaluation of a prototype screening ELISA and supplemental analysis for the serological identification of Chagas' disease. *Transfusion*, **37** (Suppl.), S181.

Homan, W. L., Vercammen, M., De Braekeleer, J., *et al.* (2000) Identification of a 200- to 300-fold repetitive 529 bp DNA fragment in *Toxoplasma gondii*, and its use for diagnostic and quantitative PCR. *Int J Parasitol*, **30**, 69–75.

Homer, M. J., Aguilar-Delfin, I., Telford, S. R., *et al.* (2000) Babesiosis. *Clin Microbiol Rev*, **13**, 451–69.

Houghton, R. L., Benson, D., Skeiky, Y., *et al.* (1996) Multi-epitope peptide ELISA for detection of serum antibodies to *Trypanosoma cruzi* in patients with treated and untreated Chagas' disease. *Transfusion*, **36** (Suppl.), S137.

Houghton, R. L., Homer, M. J., Reynolds, L. D., *et al.* (2002) Identification of *Babesia microti*-specific immunodominant epitopes and development of a peptide EIA for detection of antibodies in serum. *Transfusion*, **42**, 1488–96.

Houghton, R. L., Petrescu, M., Benson, D. R., *et al.* (1998) A cloned antigen (recombinant K39) of *Leishmania chagasi* diagnostic for visceral leishmaniasis in human immunodeficiency virus type 1 patients and a prognostic indicator for monitoring patients undergoing drug therapy. *J Infect Dis*, **177**, 1339–44.

Hunfeld, K. P., Allwinn, R., Peters, S., *et al.* (1998) Serologic evidence for tick-borne pathogens other than *Borrelia burgdorferi* (TOBB) in Lyme borreliosis patients from mid-western Germany. *Wien Klin Wochenschr* **119**, 901–8.

Hunfeld, K. P., Lambert, A., Kampen, H., *et al.* (2002) Seroprevalence of *Babesia* infections in humans exposed to ticks in mid-western Germany. *J Clin Microbiol*, **40**, 2431–6.

Ibhanesebor, S. E., Otobo, E. S. and Ladipo, O. A. (1996) Prevalence of malaria parasitemia in transfused donor blood in Benin City, Nigeria. *Ann Trop Ped*, **16**, 93–5.

International Forum (1987) Which are the appropriate modifications of existing regulations designed to prevent the transmission of malaria by blood transfusion, in view of the increasing frequency of travel to endemic areas? *Vox Sang*, **52**, 138–48.

International Forum (2004) Are current measures to prevent transfusion-associated protozoal infections sufficient? *Vox Sang*, **87**, 125–38.

Jani, I. V., Janossy, G., Brown, D. W. G., *et al.* (2002) Multiplexed immunoassays by flow cytometry for diagnosis and surveillance of infectious diseases in resource-poor settings. *Lancet Infect Dis*, **2**, 243–50.

Jassoum, S. B., Fong, I. W., Hannach, B., *et al.* (2000) Transfusion-transmitted babesiosis in Ontario: first reported case in Canada. *Can Commun Dis Rep*, **26**, 9–13.

Jones, J. L., Kruszon-Moran, D., Wilson, M., *et al.* (2001) *Toxoplasma gondii* infection in the United States: seroprevalence and risk factors. *Am J Epidemiol*, **154**, 357–65.

Kano, S. and Kimura, M. (2004) Trends in malaria cases in Japan. *Acta Tropica*, **89**, 271–8.

Kawamoto, F. (1991) Rapid diagnosis of malaria by fluorescence microscopy with light microscopy and interference filters. *Lancet*, **i**, 200–2.

Kesper, N., Almeida, K. A., Stolf, M. S., *et al.* (2000) Immunoblot analysis of trypomastigote excreted-secreted antigens as a tool for characterization of *T. cruzi* strains and isolates. *J Parasitol*, **86**, 862–7.

Kirchhoff, L. V. (1989) *Trypanosoma cruzi*: a new threat to our blood transfusion supply (Editorial). *Ann Intern Med*, **111**, 773–5.

Kirchhoff, L. V. (1993) American trypanosomiasis (Chagas' disease) a tropical disease now in the United States. *N Engl J Med*, **329**, 639–44.

Kirchhoff, L. V. and Neva, F. A. (1985) Chagas' disease in Latin American immigrants. *JAMA*, **254**, 3058–60.

Kirchhoff, L. V., Gam, A. A., Gusmão, R. A., *et al.* (1987) Increased specificity of serodiagnosis of Chagas' disease by detection of antibody to the 72- and 90-kilodalton glycoproteins of *Trypanosoma cruzi*. *J Infect Dis*, **155**, 561–4.

Kitchen, A., Mijovic, A. and Hewitt, P. (2005) Transfusion-transmitted malaria: current donor selection guidelines are not sufficient. *Vox Sang*, **88**, 200–1.

Kitchen, A. D., Lowe, P. H. J., Lalloo, K., *et al.* (2004) Evaluation of a malarial antibody assay for use in the screening of blood and tissue products for clinical use. *Vox Sang*, **87**, 150–5.

Kjemtrup, A. M., Lee, B., Fritz, C. L., *et al.* (2002) Investigation of transfusion transmission of a WA1-type babesial parasite to a premature infant in California. *Transfusion*, **42**, 1482–7.

Kostmann, R., Barr, M., Bengtsson, E., *et al.* (1963) Kala-azar transfered by exchange blood tranfusions in two Swedish infants. *Proceedings of the Seventh International Congress of Tropical Medicine and Malaria*, **2**, 384.

Krause, P. J., Lepore, T., Sikand, V. K., *et al.* (2000) Atovaquone and azithromycin for treatment of babesiosis. *N Engl J Med*, **343**, 1454–8.

Krause, P. J., Ryan, R., Telford, S., *et al.* (1996a) Efficacy of immunoglobulin M serodiagnositic test for rapid diagnosis of acute babesiosis. *J Clin Microbiol*, **34**, 2014–6.

Krause, P. J., Spielman, A., Telford, S. R., *et al.* (1998) Persistent parasitemia acute babesiosis. *N Engl J Med*, **339**, 160–4.

Krause, P. J., Telford, S., Spielman, A., *et al.* (1996b) Comparison of PCR with blood smear and inoculation of small animals for diagnosis of *Babesia microti* parasitemia. *J Clin Microbiol*, **34**, 2971–4.

Lages-Silva, E., Crema, E., Ramirez, L. E., *et al.* (2001) Relationship between *Trypanosoma cruzi* and human chagasic megaesophagus: blood and tissue parasitism. *Am J Trop Med Hyg*, **65**, 435–41.

Lal, R. B. and Ottesen, E. A. (1989) Phosphocoline epitopes on helminth and protozoal parasites and their presence in the circulation of infected human patients. *Trans Roy Soc Trop Med Hug*, **83**, 652–5.

Lanar, D. E. and Manning, J. E. (1984) Major surface proteins and antigens on the different in vivo and in vitro forms of Trypanosoma cruzi. *Mol Biochem Paras*, **11**, 119–31.

Le Fichoux, Y., Quaranta, J. F., Aufeuvre, J. P., *et al.* (1999) Occurrence of *Leishmania infantum* parasitemia in asymptomatic blood donors living in an area of endemicity in southern France. *J Clin Microbiol*, **37**, 1953–7.

Lee, S. J., Wilkinson, S. L., Battles, J. B., *et al.* (2003) An objective structured clinical examination to evaluate health historian competencies. *Transfusion*, **43**, 34–41.

Leiby, D., Gill, J., Johnson, S. T., *et al.* (2002b) Lessons learned from a natural history study of *Babesia microti* infection in Connecticut blood donors. *Transfusion*, **42**(Suppl.), 30S.

Leiby, D. A. and Gill, J. E. (2004) Transfusion-transmitted tick-borne infections: a cornucopia of threats. *Transfusion Med Rev*, **18**, 293–306.

Leiby, D. A., Chung, A. P., Cable, R. G., *et al.* (2002a) Relationship between tick bites and the seroprevalence of *Babesia microti* and *Anaplasma phagocytophila* (previously *Ehrlichia* sp.) in blood donors. *Transfusion*, **42**, 1585–91.

Leiby, D. A., Chung, A. P. S., Gill, J. E., *et al.* (2005) Demonstrable parasitemia among Connecticut blood donors with antibodies to *Babesia microti*. *Transfusion*, **45**: 1804–10.

Leiby, D. A., Jensen, N. C., Fucci, M. C., *et al.* (1997a) Prevalence of *Trypanosoma cruzi* antibodies in a blood donor population at low risk. *Transfusion*, **37** (Suppl. 9S), S297.

Leiby, D. A. Wendel, S., Takaoka, D. T., *et al.* (1997b) Confirmatory testing for *Trypanosoma cruzi* antibodies: validation of radioimmunoprecipitation (RIPA) testing. *Transfusion*, **37** (Suppl. 9S), S301.

Leiby, D. A., Yund, J., Read, E. J., *et al.* (1996) Risk factors for *Trypanosoma cruzi* infection in seropositive blood donors. *Transfusion* **36**, (Suppl. 9S) S228.

Liesendfeld, O., Montoya, J. G., Kinney, S., *et al.* (2001) Effect of testing for IgG avidity in the diagnosis of *Toxoplasma gondii* infection in pregnant women: experience in a US reference laboratory. *J Infect Dis*, **183**, 1248–53.

Linden, J. V., Wong, S. J., Chu, F. K., *et al.* (2000) Transfusion-associated transmission of babesiosis in New York State. *Transfusion*, **40**, 285–9.

Lodes, M. J., Houghton, R. L., Bruinsma, E. S. *et al.* (2000) Serologic expression cloning of novel immunoreactive antigens of *Babesia microti*. *Infect Immun*, **68**, 2783–90.

López-Antuñano, F. J. and Schmunis, G. (eds) (1990) *Diagnosis of malaria*. Scientific Publication No. 512. Washington DC, USA, Pan American Health Organization.

Lorca, M., Lorca, J., Child, R., *et al.* (1988) Prevalencia de la infección por *Trypanosoma cruzi* en pacientes politransfundidos. *Rev Med Chile*, **116**, 112–6.

Luft, B. J. and Remington, J. S. (1992) Toxoplasmic encephalitis in AIDS. *Clin Infect Dis*, **15**, 211–22.

Luquetti, A. O. (1990) Use of *Trypanosoma cruzi* defined proteins for diagnosis – multicentre trial, serological and technical aspects. *Mem Inst Oswaldo Cruz*, **85**, 497–505.

Luquetti, A. O. (2000) Diagnóstico etiológico da doença de Chagas. *Rev Pat Trop*, **29** (Suppl.), 145–9.

Lustigman, S. and Ben-Hur, E. (1996) Photosensitized inactivation of *Plasmodium falciparum* in human red cells by phthalocyanines. *Transfusion*, **36**, 543–6.

Magill, A. J., Grogl, M., Gasser, R. A., *et al.* (1993) Visceral infection caused by *Leishmania tropica* in veterans of Operation Desert Storm. *N Engl J Med*, **328**, 1383–7.

Malchiodi, E. L., Chiaramonte, M. G., Taranto, N. J., *et al.* (1994) Cross reactivity studies and differential serodiagnosis of human infections caused by *Trypanososma cruzi* and *Leishmania* spp; use of immunoblotting and ELISA with purified antigen (Ag 163B6). *Clin Exp Immunol*, **97**, 417–23.

Marcon, G. E. B., Andrade, P. D., Albuquerque, D. M., *et al.* (2002) Use of a nested polymerase chain reaction (N-PCR) to detect *Trypanosoma cruzi* in blood samples from chronic chagasic patients and patients with doubtful serologies. *Diagn Microbiol Infect Dis*, **43**, 39–43.

Martelli, C. M. T., Andrade, A. L. S. S., Silva, A. S., *et al.* (1992) Risk factor for *Trypanosoma cruzi* infection among blood donors in Central Brazil. *Mem Inst Oswaldo Cruz*, **87**, 339–43.

Mathur, P. and Samantaray, J. C. (2004) The first probable case of platelet transfusion-transmitted visceral leishmaniasis. *Transfusion Med*, **14**, 319–21.

Matsui, T., Inoue, R., Kajimoto, K., *et al.* (2000) First documentation of transfusion-associated babesiosis in Japan (article in Japanese with English summary). *Rinsho Ketsueki*, **41**, 628–34.

Mauny, I., Blanchot, I., Degeilh, B., *et al.* (1993) Leishmaniose viscérale chez un nourrisson en Bretagne: discussion sur les modes de transmission hors des zones endémiques. *Pédiatrie*, **48**, 237–9.

Mazza, S., Montana, A., Benitez, C., *et al.* (1936) Transmisión de '*Schizotrypanum cruzi*' al niño por leche de la madre con enfermedad de Chagas. *Publ MEPRA*, **28**, 41–6.

McQuiston, J. H., Childs, J. E., Chamberland, M. E., *et al.* (2000) Transmission of tick-borne agents of disease by blood transfusion: a review of known and potential risks in the United States. *Transfusion*, **40**, 274–84.

Meer-Scherrer, L., Adelson, M., Mordechai, E., *et al.* (2004) *Babesia microti* infection in Europe. *Curr Microbiol*, **48**, 435–7.

Meier, B., Dobeli, H. and Certa, U. (1992) Stage-specific expression of aldolase isoenzymes in the rodent malaria parasite *Plasmodium bergei*. *Mol Biochem Parasitol*, **52**, 15–27.

Meldrum, S. C., Birkhead, G. S., White, D. J., *et al.* (1992) Human babesiosis in New York State: an epidemiological description of 136 cases. *Clin Infect Dis*, **15**, 1019–23.

Michael, S. A., Morsy, T. A. and Montasser, M. F. (1987) A case of human babesiosis (preliminary case report in Egypt). *J Egypt Soc Parasitol*, **17**, 409–10.

Milei, J., Mautner, B., Storino, R., *et al.* (1992) Does Chagas' disease exist as an undiagnosed form of cardiomyopathy in the United States? (Editorial) *Am H Journ*, **123**, 1732–5.

Miles, M. A. (1980) Further enzymic characters of *Trypanosoma cruzi* and their evaluation for strain identification. *Trans Roy Sci Trop Med Hyg*, **74**, 221–37.

Miles, M. A. (1983) The epidemiology of South American trypanosomiasis – biochemical and immunological approaches and their relevance to control. *Trans Roy Soc Trop Med Hyg*, **77**, 5–23.

Miller, M. J., Aronson, W. J. and Remington, J. S. (1969) Late parasitemia in asymptomatic acquired toxoplasmosis. *Ann Intern Med*, **71**, 139–45.

Mintz, E. D., Anderson, J. F., Cable, R. G., *et al.* (1991) Transfusion-transmitted babesiosis: a case report from a new endemic area. *Transfusion*, **31**, 365–8.

Moncayo, A. (1993) Chagas' disease. Tropical disease research. Progress 1991–92. *Eleventh Programme Report of the UNDP/World Bank/WHO Special Programme for Research and Training in Tropical Diseases (TDR)*, pp. 67–75. Geneva, World Health Organization.

Montoya, J. G. and Liesenfeld, O. (2004) Toxoplasmosis. *Lancet*, **363**, 1965–76.

Moody, A. (2002) Rapid diagnostic tests for malaria parasites. *Clin Microbiol Rev*, **15**, 66–78.

Morel, C., Chiari, E., Plessman-Camargo, E., *et al.* (1980) Strains and clones of *Trypanosoma cruzi* can be characterized by pattern of restriction endonuclease products of kinetoplast DNA minicircles. *Proc Natl Acad Sci USA*, **77**, 6810–14.

Mungai, M., Tegtmeier, G., Chamberland, M., *et al.* (2001) Transfusion-transmitted malaria in the United States from 1963 through 1999. *N Engl J Med*, **344**, 1973–8.

Nahlen, B. L., Lobel, H. O., Cannon, S. E., *et al.* (1991) Reassessment of blood donor selection criteria for the United States travellers to malarious areas. *Transfusion*, **31**, 798–804.

Namsiriponpun, V., Wilde, H., Pamsandang, P., *et al.* (1993) Field study of an antigen-detection ELISA specific for *Plasmodium falciparum* malaria. *Trans R Soc Trop Med Hyg*, **87**, 32–4.

Nickerson, P., Orr, P., Schoeder, M. C., *et al.* (1989) Transfusion associated *Trypanosoma cruzi* infection in a non-endemic area. *Ann Inter Med*, **111**, 851–3.

Nishioka, A. S., Ferreira, M. S., Rocha, A., *et al.* (1993) Reactivation of Chagas' disease successfully treated with benznidazole in a patient with acquired immunodeficiency syndrome. *Mem Inst Oswaldo Cruz*, **88**, 493–6.

Nissapatorn, V., Kamarulzaman, A., Init, I., *et al.* (2002) Seroepidemiology of toxoplasmosis among HIV-infected patients and healthy blood donors. *Med J Malaysia*, **57**, 304–10.

Nussenzweig, V., Sonntag, R., Biancalana, A., *et al.* (1953) Ação de corantes trifenil-metanicos sobre o *Trypanosoma cruzi* 'in vitro'. Emprego da Violeta de Genciana na profilaxia da transmissão da Moléstia de Chagas por transfusão de sangue. *O Hospital*, **44**, 731–44.

Nuwayri-Salti, N., Mu'Atassem, D., Salman, S., *et al.* (1992) Chronic cutaneous leishmaniasis: leishmania parasites in blood. *Int J Dermatol*, **31**, 562–4.

Nuzum, E., White, F., Thakur, C., *et al.* (1995) Diagnosis of symptomatic visceral leishmaniasis by use of the polymerase chain reaction on patient blood. *J Infect Dis*, **171**, 751–4.

Orton, S. L., Virvos, V. J. and Williams, A. E. (2000) Validation of selected donor-screening questions: structure, content, and comprehension. *Transfusion*, **40**, 1407–13.

Osorno, B. M., Vega, C., Ristic, M., *et al.* (1976) Isolation of *Babesia* spp. from asymptomatic human beings. *Vet Parasitol*, **2**, 111–20.

Otero, A. C. S., da Silva, V. O., Luz, K. G., *et al.* (2000) Short report: occurrence of *Leishmania donovani* DNA in donated blood from seroreactive Brazilian blood donors. *Am J Trop Med Hyg*, **62**, 128–31.

PAHO-OPS (1994) III Reunión de la Comisión Intergubernamental para la Eliminación del Triatoma infestans y la interrupción de la tripanosomiasis Americana Transfusional. OPS/HPC/HCT/94–37 1–21, Montevideo, Uruguay.

Panamerican Health Organization (1992) I Reunión de la Comisión Intergubernamental del Cono Sur para la Eliminación de T. infestans y la Interrupción de la Transmision de la Tripanosomiasis Americana Transfusional, OPS, OPS/HCP/HCT/PNSP/92.18.

Panamerican Health Organization (1997) Iniciativa del Cono Sur. VI Reunión Intergubernamental para la eliminación de Triatoma infestans y la interrupción de la tripanosomiasis americana por transfusión. Documento OPS/HPC/HCT 98/102, 83pp.

Panamerican Health Organization (2002) Southern Cone Initiative to Control/Eliminate Chagas (INCOSUR) PAHO, 2002 (available at: http://www.paho.org/English/HCP/HCT/DCH/incosur.htm).

Panamerican Health Organization (2003) Va. Reunión de la Comisión Intergubernamental (CI) de la Iniciativa Andina de Control de la Transmisión Vectorial y Transfusional de Chagas – Guyaquil, Ecuador, Mayo 2003 – OPS, 2003 (available at: http://www.paho.org/Spanish/AD/DPC/CD/dch-v-inicandina.htm).

Panamercial Health Organization (2006) Estimación Cuantitativa de la Enfermedad de Chagas en las Américas-OPS/HDM/CD/425-06.

Parra, M. E., Evans, C. B. and Taylor, D. W. (1991) Identification of *Plasmodium falciparum* histidine-rich protein 2 in the plasma of humans with malaria *J Clin Microbiol*, **29**, 1629–34.

Pellegrino, J. (1949) Transmissão da doença de Chagas pela transfusão de sangue. Primeiras comprovações sorológicas em doadores e candidatos a doadores de sangue. *Rev Bras Méd*, **6**, 297–301.

Persing, D. H., Mathiesen, D., Marshall, W. F. (1992) Detection of *Babesia microti* by polymerase chain reaction. *J Clin Micro*, **30**, 2097–103.

Peyron, F., Martet, G. and Vigier, J. P. (1994) Dipstick antigen-capture assay for malaria detection. *Lancet*, **343**, 1502–3.

Piper, R. C., Vanderjagt, D. L., Holbrook, J. J., *et al.* (1996) Malaria lactate dehydrogenase: target for diagnosis and drug development. *Ann Trop Med Parasitol*, **90**, 433.

Playford, E. G. and Walker, J. (2002) Evaluation of the ICT malaria P.f./P.v. and the OptiMal rapid diagnostic tests for malaria in febrile returned travelers. *J Clin Microbiol*, **40**, 4166–71.

Popovsky, M. A., Lindberg, L. E., Syrek, A. L., *et al.* (1988) Prevalence of *Babesia* antibody in a selected blood donor population. *Transfusion*, **28**, 59–61.

Powell, V. I. and Grima, K. (2002) Exchange transfusion for malaria and *Babesia* infection. *Transfusion Med Rev*, **16**, 239–50.

Prata, A. (2001) Clinical and epidemiological aspects of Chagas' disease. *Lancet Infect Dis*, **1**, 92–100.

Purdy, E., Perry, E., Gorlin, J., *et al.* (2004) Transfusion-transmitted malaria: unpreventable by current donor exclusion guidelines? *Transfusion*, **44**, 464.

Quick, R. E., Herwaldt, B. L., Thomford, J. W., *et al.* (1993) Babesiosis in Washington State: a new species of *Babesia*? *Ann Intern Med*, **119**, 284–90.

Quinteros, Z. T., Troncoso, M. C., Arnesi, N., *et al.* (1990) Comportamientos migratórios en donantes de sangre y su relación com infección chagásica. *Cuad Med Soc*, **54**, 3–14.

Raisanen, S. (1978) Toxoplasmosis transmitted by blood transfusions. *Transfusion*, **18**, 329–32.

Ramirez, L. E., Lages-Silva, E., Painetti, G. M., *et al.* (1995) Prevention of transfusion-associated Chagas' disease by sterilization of *Trypanosoma cruzi*-infected blood with gentian violet, ascorbic acid, and light. *Transfusion*, **35**, 226–30.

Ravel, S., Cuny, G., Reynes, J., *et al.* (1995) A highly sensitive and rapid procedure for direct PCR detection of *Leishmania infantum* within human peripheral blood mononuclear cells. *Acta Trop*, **59**, 187–96.

Read, E. J., Leiby, D. A. and Dodd, R. Y. (1994) Seroprevalence of *Trypanosoma cruzi* (*T. cruzi*) in blood donors with and without risk infection. *Blood*, **84** (Suppl. 1), Abstract 1853.

Reed, S. G., Badaró, R. and Lloyd, R. M. C. (1987) Identification of specific and cross-reactive antigens of *Leishmania donovani chagasi* by human infection sera. *J Immunol*, **138**, 1598–1601.

Remington, J. S., Araujo, F. G. and Desmonts, G. (in press) Recognition of different toxoplasma antigens by IgM and IgG antibodies in mothers and their congenitally infected newborns. *J Infect Dis*, **152**, 1020–4.

Remington, J. S., Thulliez, P. and Montoya, J. G. (2004) Recent developments for diagnosis of toxoplasmosis. *J Clin Microbiol*, **42**, 941–5.

Rezende, J. M., Zupelli, W. and Bafutto, M. (1965) O problema da transmissão da doença de Chagas por transfusão de sangue. Emprego da Violeta de Genciana como medida profilática. *Rev Goiana Méd*, **11**, 35–47.

Rock, E. P., Marsh, K., Saul, S. J., *et al.* (1987) Comparative analysis of the *Plasmodium falciparum* histidine-rich proteins HRP1, HRP2, and HRP3 in malaria diagnosis of diverse origin. *Parasitology*, **95**, 209–27.

Rodriguez, N., Guzman, B., Rodas, A., *et al.* (1994) Diagnosis of cutaneous leishmaniasis and species discrimination of parasites by PCR and hybridization. *J Clin Microbiol*, **32**, 2246–52.

Rohwedder, R. W. (1969) Infección chagásica en doadores de sangre y las probabilidades de transmitirla por medio de la transfusion. *Bol Chile Parasitol*, **24**, 88–93.

Rosfjord, E. C., Mikhael, K. S., Rowland, E. C., *et al.* (1990) Analysis of antibody cross-reactivity in experimental American trypanosomiasis. *J Parasitol*, **76**, 698–702.

Rossell, R. A. de, de Duran, R. J., Rossell, O., *et al.* (1992) Is leishmaniasis ever cured? *Trans R Soc Trop Med Hyg*, **86**, 251–3.

Rouger P. (1999) Du paludisme au paludisme post-transfusionnel. *Transf Clin Biol*, **6**, 72–4.

Rubio, J. M., Buhigas, I., Subirats, M., *et al.* (2001) Limited level of accuracy provided by available rapid diagnosis tests for malaria enhances the need for PCR-based reference laboratories. *J Clin Microbiol*, **39**, 2736–7.

Rynin, F. W., McLeod, R., Maddox, J. C., *et al.* (1979) Probable transmission of *Toxoplasma gondii* by organ transplantation. *Ann Intern Med*, **90**, 47–9.

Sabino, E. C., Salles, N., Stoops, E., *et al.* (1997) Evaluation of Chagas' Innolia assay as a confirmatory test for Chagas' disease. *Mem Inst Oswaldo Cruz*, **92**, (Suppl. 1), 266.

Saito-Ito, A., Tsuji, M., Wei, Q., *et al.* (2000) Transfusion-acquired, autochthonous human babesiosis in Japan: isolation of *Babesia microti*-like parasite with hu-RBC-SCID mice. *J Clin Microbiol*, **38**, 4511–16.

Salomone, O. A., Basquiera, A. L., Sembaj, A., *et al.* (2003) *Trypanosoma cruzi* in persons without serologic evidence of disease, Argentina. *Emerg Infect Dis*, **9**, 1558–62.

Salutari, P., Sica, S., Chiusolo, P., *et al.* (1996) *Plasmodium vivax* malaria after autologous bone marrow transplantation: an unusual complication. *Bone M Transpl*, **18**, 805–6.

Saravia, N. G., Weigle, K., Segura, I., *et al.* (1990) Recurrent lesions in human *Leishmania braziliensis* infection – reactivation or reinfection? *Lancet*, **336**, 398–402.

Sazama, K. (1991) Prevention of transfusional-transmitted malaria: is it time to revisit the standards (Editorial). *Transfusion*, **31**, 786–8.

Schlemper, B. R. Jr. (1978) Estudos experimentais de Quimio-profilaxia de transmissão da doença de Chagas por transfusão sangüínea. *Rev Pat trop*, **7**, 55–111.

Schmunis, G. A. (1991) *Trypanosoma cruzi*, the etiologic agent of Chagas' disease: status in the blood supply in endemic and non-endemic countries. *Transfusion*, **31**, 547–57.

Schmunis G. A. (1994) *American Trypanosomiasis as a Public Health Problem, in Chagas' disease and the nervous system*. PAHO Scientific Publication 994, No. 547, pp. 3–29, Washington DC, USA.

Schmunis, G. A. (1997) Tripanosomíase Americana: seu impacto nas Américas e perspectivas de eliminação. In *Clínica e terapêutica da Doença de Chagas*, eds J. C. P. Dias and J. R. Coura, pp 11–23, Rio de Janeiro, Brazil, Editora Fiocruz.

Schmunis, G. A. and Cruz, J. R. (2005) Safety of the blood supply in Latin America. *Clin Microbiol Rev*, **18**, 12–29.

Scholtens, R. G., Braff, E. H., Healy, G. R., *et al.* (1968) A case of babesiosis in man in the United States. *Am J Trop Med Hyg*, **17**, 810–13.

Seed, C. R., Kitchen, A. and Davis, T. M. E. (2005) The current status and potential role of laboratory testing to prevent transfusion-transmitted malaria. *Transfus Med Rev*, **19**, 229–40.

Segovia, A. M. and López Dias, M. (1993) Infección Chagásica en varones de 18 años de edad en província de Salta durante los años 1985–1992. *Medicina (Buenos Aires)*, **53** (Suppl. 1), 87–8.

Segura, E. L., Pérez, A. C., Yanovsky, J. F., *et al.* (1985) Decrease in the prevalence of infection by *Trypanosoma cruzi* (Chagas' disease) in young men of Argentina. *PAHO Bull*, **19**, 252–66.

Shah, S., Filler, S., Causer, L. M., *et al.* (2004) Malaria surveillance – United States. *MMWR*, **53** (SS01), 21–34. Also available at: www.cdc.gov/mmwr/PDF/ss/ss5301.pdf.

Shehata, N., Kohli, M. and Detsky, A. (2004) The cost-effectiveness of screening blood donors for malaria by PCR. *Transfusion*, **44**, 217–28.

Shih, C. M., Liu, L. P., Chung, W. C., *et al.* (1997) Human babesiosis in Taiwan: asymptomatic infection with a *Babesia microti*-like organism in a Taiwanese women. *J Clin Microbiol*, **35**, 450–4.

Shiota, T., Kurimoto, H., Haguma, N., *et al.* (1984) Studies on *Babesia* first found in murine in Japan: epidemiology, morphology and experimental infection. *Zentralbl Bakteriol Mikrobiol Hyg [A]*, **256**, 347–55.

Siegel, S. E., Lunde, M. N., Gelderman, A. H., *et al.* (1971) Transmission of toxoplasmosis by leukocyte transfusion. *Blood*, **37**, 388–94.

Silber, A. M., Búa, J., Porcel, B. M., *et al.* (1997) *Trypanosoma cruzi*: specific detection of parasites by PCR in infected humans and vectors using a set of primers (BP1/BP2) targeted to a nuclear DNA sequence. *Exp Parasitol*, **85**, 225–32.

Silveira, A. C. (2002) Introdução – in O controle da doença de Chagas nos países do Cone Sul da América – História de uma Iniciativa Internacional 1991/2001, pp. 16–41. *OPS*.

Silveira-Lacerda, E. P., Silva, A. G., Junior, S. F., *et al.* (2004) Chagas' disease: application of TESA-blot in inconclusive sera from a Brazilian blood bank. *Vox Sang*, **87**, 204–7.

Silvie, O., Thellier, M., Rosenheim, M., *et al.* (2002) Potential value of *Plasmodium falciparum*-associated antigen and antibody detection for screening of blood donors to prevent transfusion-transmitted malaria. *Transfusion*, **42**, 357–62.

Singh, S., Chaudhry, V. P. and Wali, J. P. (1996) Transfusion-transmitted kala-azar in India. *Transfusion*, **36**, 848–9.

Skrabalo, Z. and Deanovic, Z. (1957) Piroplasmosis in man: report of a case. *Doc Med Geogr Trop*, **9**, 11–6.

Slinger, R., Giulivi, A., Bodie-Collins, M., *et al.* (2001) Transfusion-transmitted malaria in Canada. *Can Med Assoc J*, **164**, 377–9.

Sluiters, J. F., Balk, A. H. M. M., Essed, C. E., *et al.* (1989) Indirect enzyme-linked immunosorbent assay for immunoglobulin G and four immunoassays for immunoglobulin M to *Toxoplasma gondii* in a series of heart transplant recipients. *J Clin Microbiol*, **27**, 529–35.

Smith, O. M., Dolan, A. S. and Dvorak, J. A.. (1992) Merocyanine 540-sensitized photoinactivation of human erythrocytes parasitized by *Plasmodium falciparum*. *Blood*, **80**, 21–4.

Smith, O. M., Traul, D. L., McOlash, L., *et al.* (1991) Evaluation of merocyanine 540 – sensitized photoirradiation as a method for purging malarially infected red cells from blood. *J Inf Dis*, **163**, 1312–7.

Smyth, A. J., Ghosh, A., Hassan, M. Q., *et al.* (1992) Rapid and sensitive detection of *Leishmania* kinetoplast DNA from spleen and blood samples of kala-azar patients. *Parasitology*, **105**, 183–92.

Snow, R. W., Guerra, C. A., Noor, A. M., *et al.* (2005) The global distribution of clinical episodes of *Plasmodium falciparum* malaria. *Nature*, **434**, 214–7.

Soler, C. P., Gerome, P., Soullié, B., *et al.* (2003) Comparaison de techniques de depistage des anticorps anti-paludiques utilisées en transfusion. *Med Trop*, **63**, 587–9.

Souza, H. M. (1989) The present state of chemoprophylaxis in transfusional Chagas' disease (Editorial) *Rev Soc Bras Med Trop*, **22**, 1–3.

Sullivan, T. S. (1944) Viability of *Trypanosoma cruzi* in citrated blood stored at room temperature. *J Parasitol*, **30**, 200.

Tabor, E. (1982) *Infectious Complications of Blood Transfusion*. New York, Academic Press.

Talabiska, D. G., Komar, M. J., Wytock, D. H., *et al.* (1996) Post-transfusion acquired malaria complicating orthotopic liver transplantation. *Am J Gastroenterol*, **91**, 376–9.

Talice, R. V., Gurri, J., Royol, J., *et al.* (1957) Findings on toxoplasmosis in Uruguay; survival of *Toxoplasma gondii* in human blood in vitro (Article in Spanish). *Ann Fac Med Repub Montev Urug*, **42**, 143–7.

Taylor, D. W. and Voller, A. (1993) The development of a simple antigen detection ELISA for *Plasmodium falciparum* malaria. *Trans R Soc Trop Med Hyg*, **87**, 29–31.

Thellier, M., Lusina, D., Guiguen, C., *et al.* (2001) Is airport malaria a transfusion-transmitted malaria risk? *Transfusion*, **41**, 301–2.

Tran, V. B., Tran, V. B. and Lin, K. H. (1997) Malaria infection after allogeneic bone marrow transplantation in a child with thalassemia. *Bone M Transpl*, **19**, 1259–60.

Turc, J. M. (1990) Malaria and blood transfusion. In *Emerging Global Patterns in Transfusion-transmitted Infections*, eds R. G. Westphal, K. B. Carlson and J. M. Turc, pp. 31–43. Arlington, VA, USA, American Association of Blood Banks.

Umezawa, E., Nascimento, N. S., Kasper, N. J. R., *et al.* (1996) Immunoblot assay using excreted-secreted antigen of *Trypanosoma cruzi* in serodiagnosis of congenital, acute, and chronic Chagas' disease. *J Clin Microbiol*, **34**, 2143–7.

Umezawa, E. S., Stolf, A. M. S., Corbett, C. E. P., *et al.* (2001) Chagas' disease. *Lancet*, **357**, 797–9.

Valente, S. A. S., Valente, V. C. and Fraiha Neto, H. (1999) Considerations on the epidemiology and transmission of Chagas' disease in the Brazilian Amazon. *Mem Inst Oswaldo Cruz*, **94** (Suppl. 1), 395–8.

Van Voorhis, W. C., Barrett, L. K., Eastman, R. T., *et al.* (2003) *Trypanosoma cruzi* inactivation in human platelet concentrates and plasma by a psoralen (amotosalen HCl) and long-wavelength UV. *Antimicrob Agents Chemother*, **47**, 475–9.

Vera-Cruz, J. M., Magallón-Gastelum, E., Grijalva, G., *et al.* (2003) Molecular diagnosis of Chagas' disease and use of an animal model to study parasite tropism. *Parasitol Res*, **89**, 480–6.

Villalba, R., Fornés, G., Alvarez, M. A., *et al.* (1992) Acute Chagas' disease in a recipient of a bone marrow transplant in Spain: case report. *Clin Inf Dis*, **14**, 594–5.

Virreira, M., Torrico, F., Truyens, C., *et al.* (2003) Comparison of polymerase chain reaction methods for reliable and easy detection of congenital *Trypanosoma cruzi* infection. *Am J Trop Med Hyg*, **68**, 574–82.

Voller, A., Draper, C., Bidwell, D. E., *et al.* (1975) A micro-plate enzyme-linked immunosorbent assay (ELISA) for Chagas' disease. *Lancet*, **1**, 426–9.

Vu T. T., Phan, N. T., Le, T. T., *et al.* (1995) Screening donor blood for malaria by polymerase chain reaction. *Trans R Soc Trop Med Hyg*, **89**, 44–7.

Walter, G. and Weber, G. (1981) A study on the transmission (transstadial, transovarial) of *Babesia microti*, strain 'Hannover i,' in its tick vector, *Ixodes ricinus*. *Tropenmed Parasitol*, **32**, 228–30.

Walton, B. C., Benchoff, B. M. and Brooks, W. H.. (1966) Comparison of the indirect fluorescent antibody test and methylene blue dye test for detection of antibodies to *Toxoplasma gondii*. *Am J Trop Med Hyg*, **15**, 149–52.

Warrell, D. A., Gilles, H. A. and Gilles, H. M. (2002) *Bruce-Chwatt's Essential Malariology*, 4th edn. London, Edward Arnold.

Weinman, D. and MacAlister, J. (1947) Prolonged storage of human pathogenic protozoa with conservation of virulence. *Am J Hyg*, **45**, 102–21.

Wells, L. and Ala, F. A. (1985) Malaria and blood transfusion. *Lancet*, **i**, 1317–8.

Wendel, S. (1993a) Blood banking preventive approaches for Chagas' disease. *Mem Inst Oswaldo Cruz*, **88** (Suppl.), 59–60.

Wendel, S. (1993b) Chagas' disease: an old entity in new places (Editorial). *Int J Art Organs*, **16**, 117–9.

Wendel, S. (1997) Doença de Chagas Transfusional. In *Clínica e Terapêutica da Doença de Chagas*, eds J. C. P. Dias and J. R. Coura, pp. 411–27. Rio de Janeiro, Brazil, Editora Fiocruz.

Wendel, S. (2003) The protozoal parasites – malaria and Chagas' disease. In *Blood Safety and Surveillance*, eds J. V. Linden and C. Bianco, pp. 355–98. New York, Marcel Dekker, Inc.

Wendel, S. (2005) Risco residual da transmissão da infecção por *Trypanosoma cruzi* por via transfusional no Brasil. PhD Thesis. Faculdade de Medicina da Universidade de São Paulo, Brazil, USP/FM/SBD-20/05.

Wendel, S. and Biagini, S. (1995) Absence of serological surrogate markers for *Trypanosoma cruzi* infected blood donors. *Vox Sang*, **69**, 44–9.

Wendel, S. and Gonzaga, A. L. (1993) Chagas' disease and blood transfusion: a new world problem? *Vox Sang*, **64**, 1–12.

Wendel, S., Brener, Z., Camargo, M., *et al.* (eds), (1992a) *Chagas' Disease (American Trypanosomiasis): Its Impact on Transfusion and Clinical Medicine*. ISBT, Brasil '92, SBHH.

Wendel, S., Lopes, V. H. G., Batemarchi, M. V., *et al.* (1993) High levels of false positive reaction for *Trypanosoma cruzi* antibodies tests used for blood donor screening. *Transfusion*, **33** (Suppl.) Abstract S155, 41S.

Wendel, S., Siqueira, R. V., Lopes, V. H. G., *et al.* (1992b) Assessing the performance of *Trypanosoma cruzi* antibody detection currently in use in Brazilian blood centres: a few answers from a large prevalence study. *Rev Paul Med*, **110**(5), Abstract TTD 16.

Wendel, S., Takaoka, D. T., Fachini, R., *et al.* (1997) Serological screening tests for *Trypanosoma cruzi* antibodies: the role of supplemental methods. *Transfusion*, **37** (Suppl.), S298.

White, D. J., Talarico, J., Chang, H. G., *et al.* (1998) Human babesiosis in New York State. Review of 139 hospitalized cases and analysis of prognostic factors. *Arch Intern Med*, **158**, 2149–54.

Wincker, P., Britto, C., Pereira, J. B., *et al.* (1994) Use of a simplified polymerase chain reaction procedure to detect *Trypanosoma cruzi* in blood samples from chronic chagasic patients in a rural endemic area. *Am J Trop Med Hyg*, **51**, 771–7.

Winkler, M. A., Brashear, R. J., Hall, H. J., *et al.* (1995) Detection of antibodies to *Trypanosoma cruzi* among blood donors in the southwestern and western United States. II – Evaluation of a supplemental enzyme immunoassay and radioimmuneprecipitation assay for confirmation of seroreactivity. *Transfusion*, **35**, 219–25.

Wong, S. Y. and Remington, J. S. (1994) Toxoplasmosis in pregnancy. *Clin Infect Dis*, **18**, 853–61.

Woolsey, G. (1911) Transfusion for pernicious anaemia: two cases. *Ann Surg*, **53**, 132–5.

World Bank (1993) The World Bank Development Report 1993. Investing in Health. World development indicators. Washington, University Press.

World Bank (2007) WHO Special Programme for Research and Training in Tropical Diseases – TDR. Available at http://www.who.int/tdr/diseases/chagas/diseaseinfo.htm.

World Health Assembly (1998) Resolution WHA.51.14, Geneva, World Health Assembly.

World Health Organization (1963) Terminology of malaria and of malaria eradication: report of a drafting committee. Geneva, Switzerland, World Health Organization; 32.

World Health Organization (1987) The biology of malaria parasites – *Technical Report Series* 743, World Health Organization, Geneva, Switzerland.

World Health Organization (1992a) World malaria situation in 1990. *Weekly Ep Record*, **67**, 161–8 (Part I).

World Health Organization (1992b) World malaria situation in 1990. *Weekly Ep Record*, **67**, 169–76(Part II).

World Health Organization (2002) Chagas' disease – TDR strategic direction, February, 2002 (available at: http://www.who.int/tdr/diseases/chagas/direction.htm.)

World Health Organization (2003) Malaria rapid diagnosis – making it work. Meeting Report 20–23.01.2003 (RS/2003/GE/05(PHL)) (available at: http://mosquito.who.int).

World Health Organization (2004) Global database on blood Safety (available at: http://www.who.int/bloodsafety/global_database/en/).

World Health Organization (WHO) *Roll Back Malaria* (available at: http://mosquito.who.int/malariacontrol).

Wozniak, E. J., Lowenstine, L., Hemmer, R., *et al.* (1996) Comparative pathogenesis of human WA1 and *Babesia microti* isolates in a Syrian hamster model. *Lab Anim Sci*, **46**, 507–15.

Zavizion, B., Pereira, M., Jorge, M. M., *et al.* (2004) Inactivation of protozoan parasites in red blood cells using INACTINE PEN110 chemistry. *Transfusion*, **44**, 731–8.

Zhou, X. H., Obuchowski, N. A. and McClish, D. K. (2002) *Statistical Methods in Diagnostic Medicine*. New York, John Wiley & Sons.

Zicker, F., Martelli, C. M. T., Andrade, A. L. L. S., *et al.* (1990a) Trends of *T. cruzi* infection based on data from blood bank screening. *Rev Inst Med Trop S Paulo*, **39**, 132–7.

Zicker, F., Smith, P. G., Luquetti, A. O., *et al.* (1990b) Mass screening for *Trypanosoma cruzi* infections using the immunofluorescence, ELISA and hemagglutination tests on serum samples and on blood eluates from filter paper. *Bull WHO*, **68**, 465–71.

Zingales, B., Souto, R. P. and Mangia, R. H., (1998) Molecular epidemiology of American trypanosomiasis in Brazil based on dimorphisms of rRNA and mini-exon gene sequences. *Intern J Parasitol*, **28**, 105–12.

Zintl, A., Mulcahy, G., Skerrett, H. E., *et al.* (2003) *Babesia divergens*, a bovine blood parasite of veterinary and zoonotic importance. *Clin Microbiol Rev*, **16**, 622–36.

Zuna, H., Recacoechea, M., Bermudez, H., *et al.* (1979) Transmissión de la enfermedad de Chagas por via transfusional en Santa Cruz de la Sierra, Bolivia. *Bol Inf CENENTROP*, **5**, 49–56.

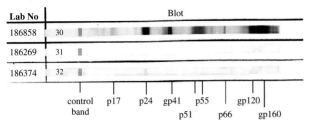

Figure 4.3 HIV Western blot (genelabs HIV 2.2) strip 30 confirmed positive, strip 31 negative, strip 32 indeterminate (p24).

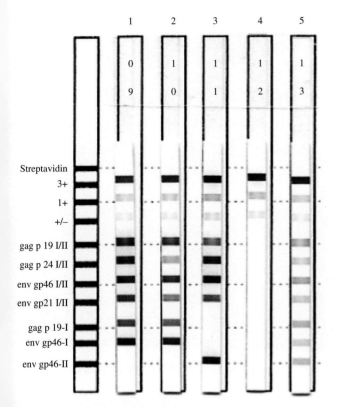

Figure 4.6 HTLV immunoblot (INNOLIA).
strips 09 and 10 confirmed anti-HTLV-I positive, strip 11 confirmed anti-HTLV-II positive, strip 12 negative, strip 13 positive control.

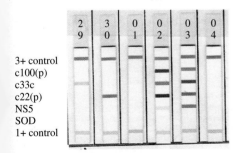

Figure 12.3 RIBA-3 HCV immunoblot.
29 indeterminate
30 indeterminate
01 negative
02 positive
03 positive control
04 negative control.

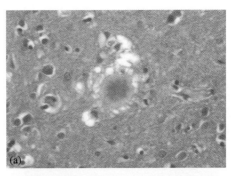

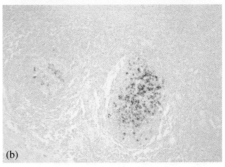

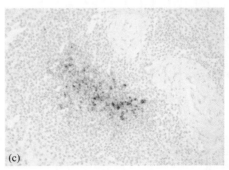

Figure 9.2 (a) PrP accumulation in the brain as florid plaques (centre) in variant CJD. Haematoxylin and eosin stain, original magnification × 400. (b) PrP accumulation within a germinal centre in the tonsil in variant CJD. KG9 anti-PrP antibody, original magnification × 200. (c) PrP accumulation within a germinal centre in the spleen in variant CJD. 3F4 anti-PrP antibody, original magnification × 200.

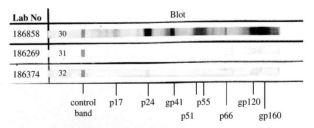

Figure 12.5 HIV Western blot (Genelabs HIV 2.2).
strip 30 confirmed positive
strip 31 negative
strip 32 indeterminate (p24).

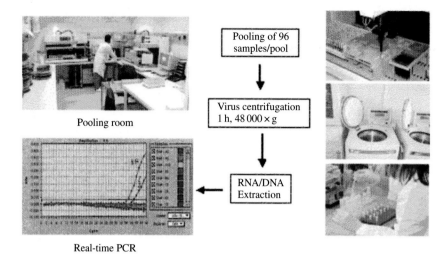

Pooling of 96 samples/pool

↓

Virus centrifugation 1 h, 48 000 × g

↓

RNA/DNA Extraction

←

Pooling room

Real-time PCR

Figure 14.2 Implementation of PCR in Frankfurt Transfusion Service.

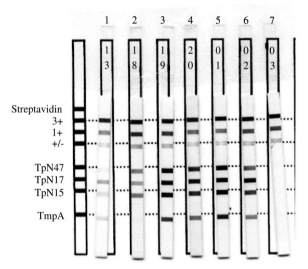

Streptavidin
3+
1+
+/-

TpN47
TpN17
TpN15

TmpA

1 2 3 4 5 6 7

Figure 12.7 Syphilis immunoblot (INNOLIA). strips 13 to 02 confirmed positive strip 03 negative.

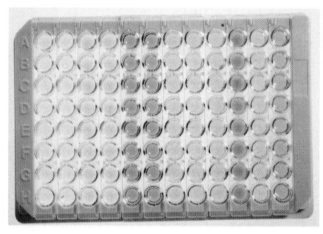

Figure 17.2 Colour monitoring of a microplate EIA using colour change and coloured reagents.

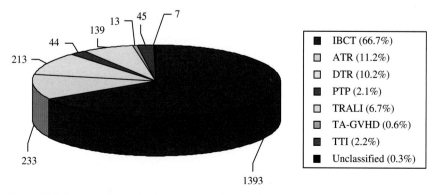

Figure 21.3 Questionnaires by incident 1996–2003 (n = 2087). IBCT: incorrect blood component transfused; ATR: acute transfusion reaction; DTR: delayed transfusion reaction; PTP: post-transfusion purpura; TRALI: transfusion-related acute lung injury; TA-GVHD: transfusion-associated graft versus host disease; TTI: transfusion-transmitted infection.

9 PRION DISEASES

Marc L. Turner, Patricia E. Hewitt, Moira Bruce
and James W. Ironside

Introduction

Prion diseases include a spectrum of disorders in animals and man (see Table 9.1). Scrapie, endemic in sheep and goat populations throughout most of the world, was first recognized over 250 years ago and was demonstrated to be experimentally transmissible in 1936. Chronic wasting disease (CWD) is endemic in Rocky Mountain elk, white-tailed deer and mule deer in several areas of the USA and is increasing in both incidence and geographic distribution. The routes by which these two endemic prion diseases are transmitted remain unclear. Transmissible mink encephalopathy was first recorded to have occurred in 1947 in farmed mink in Wisconsin and was probably transmitted through prion infected food.

Bovine spongiform encephalopathy (BSE) was first recognized in the UK in 1985/86 (Wells *et al.*, 1987). Affected cattle become apprehensive, hypersensitive, ataxic and generally difficult to handle, giving rise to the common name of mad cow disease. It remains unclear whether BSE arose spontaneously in cattle or resulted from transmission of scrapie from sheep, but onward transmission is thought to have occurred through the practice of feeding cattle ruminant-derived meat and bone meal. Over 180 000 clinical cases of BSE have been reported in the UK since 1985, though the annual incidence has now fallen to just over 100 cases per annum. Over 4500 infected cattle have been detected elsewhere, mainly in Europe, the majority associated with the export of BSE infected cattle or meat and bone meal from the UK. It is estimated that between 1 and 2 million cattle may have become infected and entered the human food chain before developing evidence of clinical disease (Donnelly *et al.*, 2002). Unlike scrapie, BSE has shown itself capable of spreading to other species, including domestic and exotic cats (feline spongiform encephalopathy) and exotic ungulates such as kudu, gemsbok and nyala in British zoos (exotic ungulate encephalopathy). Experimentally, BSE has been transmitted to rodents, primates, sheep, goats and pigs.

Several forms of prion disease have been described in man (see Table 9.1). Sporadic or classical Creutzfeldt-Jakob disease (CJD) was first described in the early 1920s (Creutzfeldt, 1920; Jakob, 1921) and occurs with an incidence of around 1/million population/annum throughout the world, with no clear relationship to the prevalence of other prion diseases such as scrapie. The disease presents at a median age of 68 years, with a rapidly progressive dementia, myoclonus, ataxia, visual abnormalities and motor dysfunction, normally leading to death in 2–6 months. Kuru was first described in the Fore people of the Papua New Guinea highlands in 1957 and takes a somewhat different clinical form with cerebellar ataxia as a prominent feature, leading to progressive neurological deterioration and death within approximately 12 months (Gajdusek and Zigas, 1957). At one time kuru was endemic in the Fore people, affecting up to 1% of the population, and is thought to have been transmitted orally through ritualistic cannibalistic funeral rites. The incubation period is between 5 and 30 years and although cannibalistic rites were discontinued in 1959/60, occasionally patients still develop clinical disease, suggesting that the upper limit of the incubation period could be 40–50 years or perhaps beyond the normal human lifespan.

Over 200 cases of CJD have been transmitted by medical intervention. Some of these events have involved inoculation into the central nervous system from inadequately sterilized neurosurgical instruments, stereotactic EEG electrodes or corneal or dura mater grafts. Others have involved peripheral transmission via cadaveric derived pituitary growth and follicular stimulating hormone (Brown *et al.*, 1992). Inoculation directly into the nervous system is associated with a relatively short incubation period (median 18 months, range 1–2 years) and a rapidly progressive dementia, whilst peripheral transmission leads to longer and more variable incubation periods (median 12 years, range 5–30 years) with cerebellar ataxia. These clinical differences are reflected in the distribution of neuropathological lesions.

Variant CJD was first described in 1996 (Will *et al.*, 1996) and differs from sporadic and other forms of CJD in a number of important respects. The disease affects a younger age group (median 28 years, range 12–74 years) and often presents with depression or anxiety, followed by dysaesthesia and cerebellar ataxia. Patients progress to generalized dementia, myoclonus and choreoathetosis over a period of 7–36 months. The epidemiological, clinical, neuropathological and experimental data all support the thesis that variant CJD is caused by the same prion strain as BSE in cattle and as BSE transmitted naturally and experimentally to other animals. Variant CJD represents a different strain of prion disease from those seen in sporadic CJD and scrapie (Bruce *et al.*, 1997). To date there have been 166 cases of variant CJD in the UK (National CJD Surveillance Unit), twenty-three in France, four in Eire, three in the USA, two in the Netherlands, and Portugal, and one each in Canada, Japan, Saudi Arabia, Spain and Italy. Two of the Irish and US cases along with the Canadian case are thought to have been infected in the UK. The other US case is thought to have been infected as a child in Saudi Arabia. The remaining cases are thought to be endogenous to the countries in which they were described. It remains unclear how many people may be currently incubating the disease. The incidence appears to be falling and recent mathematical projections have suggested an upper limit of around 70

Transfusion Microbiology, eds John A. J. Barbara, Fiona A. M. Regan and Marcela C. Contreras. Published by Cambridge University Press. © Cambridge University Press 2008.

Section 1: Agents

Table 9.1 Transmissible spongiform encephalopathies in animals and man.

Animals	Man
Scrapie (sheep, goats)	Sporadic/classical Creutzfeldt-Jakob disease (CJD)
Chronic wasting disease (CWD) (white-tailed and mule deer and Rocky Mountain elk)	Kuru
Transmissible mink encephalopathy (mink)	Iatrogenic Creutzfeldt-Jakob disease
Bovine spongiform encephalopathy (BSE) (cattle)	Variant Creutzfeldt-Jakob disease
Exotic ungulate encephalopathy (e.g. kudu, nyala, gemsbok)	Familial Creutzfeldt-Jakob disease
Feline spongiform encephalopathy (exotic and domestic cats)	Gerstmann-Straussler-Scheinker disease (GSS)
	Fatal familial insomnia

further clinical cases (Ghani *et al.*, 2003). However, this projection is based on an assumption of a monophasic disease which may not be correct if differences in prion protein (PrP) codon 129 genotype lead to different incubation periods (*vide infra*) or if secondary transmissions are occurring through infected surgical instruments or blood, plasma or tissue products. Indeed, a recent retrospective study of 12 000 tonsillar samples in the UK revealed three positives, suggesting that as many as 3800 people aged 10–30 years (equivalent to around 11 000 in the total population) could be incubating variant CJD in the UK (Hilton *et al.*, 2004).

Finally, there are a number of familial forms of Prion disease including familial CJD, Gerstmann-Straussler-Scheinker disease (GSS) and fatal familial insomnia, which are related to single nucleotide polymorphisms in the prion protein gene (*PRNP*).

Prion diseases are therefore an unusual group of disorders which can arise spontaneously, can be transmitted via a variety of different routes and in which the propensity to, and clinical manifestations of, disease are strongly influenced by genetic polymorphism.

The molecular basis of prion diseases

Prion diseases are different from other forms of infectious agent in that no infection specific nucleic acids have yet been identified. Furthermore, treatment of infectious material with physical and chemical processes which would normally abrogate microbiological infectivity have little or no effect. Infectivity is, however, closely associated with a change in the conformation of the host PrP. This has led to the suggestion that conformationally altered PrP is an integral part of the infectious prion, either alone or in combination with other molecules (Prusiner, 1982). The normal prion protein human PrP^c is a 30–35 kD, 253 amino-acid glycoprotein with two N-linked glycosylation sites. It is synthesized through the endoplasmic reticulum and Golgi and is normally attached to the membrane through a glycosylphosphatidylinositol (GPI) anchor, though transmembrane anchorage has also recently been described. It is internalized via clathrin-coated pits, undergoing endocytosis and degradation with a half-life of 3–6 hours. The secondary structure consists of 3 α helices and a single β-pleated sheet, with the membrane distal region of the molecule being mainly unstructured. During the development of a prion disease, PrP undergoes a change in secondary structure with a substantial increase in the amount of β-pleated sheet (PrP^{Sc}). This changes the physicochemical and biological characteristics of the molecule, rendering it relatively resistant to degradation. In vitro treatment of PrP^{Sc} with proteinase-K, for example, removes only the unstructured membrane distal portion, leaving a 27–30 kD molecule rich in β-pleated sheet. PrP^{Sc} accumulates in the nervous system in prion diseases and is associated with neuronal death, reactive astrogliosis and a spongiform appearance. In addition to the more usual diffusely distributed PrP^{Sc} accumulation, a specific neuropathological feature of variant CJD is the presence of florid amyloid plaques consisting of fibrillar PrP aggregates. In patients with variant CJD, abnormal PrP also accumulates outside the nervous system on follicular dendritic cells (FDC) in the peripheral lymphoid tissue, including the tonsils, cervical, mediastinal and abdominal lymph nodes, gut-associated lymphoid tissue and spleen (Head *et al.*, 2004; Wadsworth *et al.*, 2001).

Polymorphism in the prion protein gene (*PRNP*), such as that which causes methionine or valine to be expressed at codon 129, can lead to differences in the propensity to develop disease, the incubation period and the clinical features. Thirty-seven per cent of the UK population are homozygous for the allele encoding methionine at this locus, 11% are homozygous for the allele encoding valine and 52% are heterozygous. In contrast, 80% of cases of sporadic CJD are methionine homozygotes at this locus (Palmer *et al.*, 1991) and all the clinical cases of variant CJD thus far examined are homozygous for methionine (Will, 2003). Polymorphisms in the *PRNP* gene also have a strong influence on disease characteristics in animal prion diseases. Studies in animal models have demonstrated the existence of multiple prion strains that interact with the PrP genotype of the host to determine susceptibility, incubation period and neuropathological features. It is clear from these studies that prion strains carry some form of information that can be transmitted unchanged between hosts with different PrP amino acid sequences, but the molecular basis of this information is not known. However, the conformation and glycosylation pattern of PrP^{Sc} differ according to the prion strain and there have been suggestions that these features carry strain determinants and pass them on to new PrP molecules. On the other hand, there may be other associated molecules that determine prion strain characteristics.

Although the molecular basis of prion strain variation is not understood, strain characterization in experimentally infected animals can be used to explore epidemiological links between prion diseases occurring naturally in different species. For example, when variant CJD and BSE are transmitted to standard inbred mouse lines, they produce closely similar incubation periods and neuropathological features in the mice. These differ from the

142

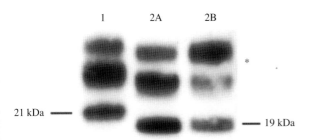

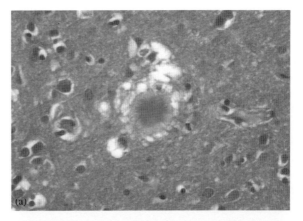

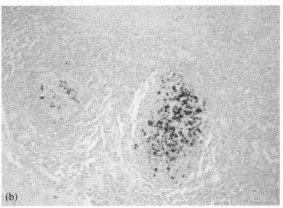

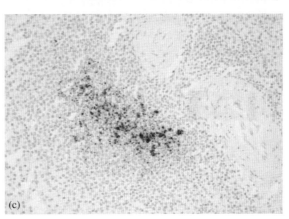

Figure 9.1 Characteristic Western blot profiles of protease-resistant prion protein (PrP^res) in samples of cerebral cortex from patients with either sporadic Creutzfeldt-Jakob disease (type 1 or type 2 A PrP^res) or variant Creutzfeldt-Jakob disease (type 2B PrP^res). PrP^res type 1 is defined as having a non-glycosylated (bottom band) with a molecular weight of ∼21kDa, and type 2 is defined as having a non-glycosylated (bottom band) of ∼19 kDa. The type 2 pattern is further sub-classified as 2A if the middle (monoglycosylated) or bottom (non-glycosylated) bands predominate or type 2B if the top (Marked *, diglycosylated) band predominates (with thanks to Dr Mark Head *et al.* (2004)).

incubation periods and neuropathology seen in mice infected with sporadic CJD or scrapie. These studies provide the strongest experimental evidence so far of a link between variant CJD and BSE (Bruce *et al.*, 1997). Prion strains also have different patterns of protease-resistant PrP fragment size on Western blot, the pattern being very similar in variant CJD and BSE and different from that seen in other types of CJD (Collinge *et al.*, 1996) (see Figure 9.1).

Pathophysiology of disease

In sporadic and familial forms of CJD the accumulation of infectious agent and PrP^Sc occurs predominantly in the nervous system, with minimal involvement of peripheral tissues. This is also the case for CJD associated with pituitary hormone treatment, even though infection has occurred by peripheral injection. In contrast, both infectivity (Bruce *et al.*, 2001) and PrP^Sc (Head *et al.*, 2004; Wadsworth *et al.*, 2001) are widely distributed in peripheral lymphoid tissues of variant CJD patients, suggesting that the potential for transmission via blood is higher for variant CJD than for sporadic CJD (see Figure 9.2).

Experimental peripheral transmission of scrapie or BSE in rodents and sheep results in the accumulation of infectivity and PrP^Sc in the spleen and lymph nodes from a very early stage, often long before either becomes detectable in the nervous system (Bruce *et al.*, 2000). In these experimental models, as in variant CJD, PrP^Sc accumulation is associated with follicular dendritic cells (FDCs) of the germinal centres of the secondary lymphoid tissues (McBride *et al.*, 1992). Further studies in mice have substantiated a critical role for FDCs in the pathogenesis of peripherally-transmitted prion diseases. Mice lacking FDCs as a result of genetic defects or transgenic manipulations fail to accumulate infectivity in their lymphoid systems and consequently have a low susceptibility to peripheral prion exposure (Mabbott and Bruce, 2001). B-cells are also critical but mainly because they provide essential maturation signals for FDCs, so that mice lacking B-cells also lack FDCs (Klein *et al.*, 1997). Even temporary inactivation of

Figure 9.2 (a) PrP accumulation in the brain as florid plaques (centre) in variant CJD. Haematoxylin and eosin stain, original magnification × 400. (b) PrP accumulation within a germinal centre in the tonsil in variant CJD. KG9 anti-PrP antibody, original magnification × 200. (c) PrP accumulation within a germinal centre in the spleen in variant CJD. 3F4 anti-PrP antibody, original magnification × 200. (See colour plate section).

FDCs using lymphotoxin β-receptor blockade (Mabbott *et al.*, 2000) or interference with the function of these cells by complement inactivation (Mabbott *et al.*, 2001) reduces the likelihood of peripheral transmission. It therefore appears likely that initial replication of peripherally transmitted prion diseases is dependent on complement mediated uptake by FDCs. Further studies have indicated that PrP expression by FDCs is also required for the accumulation of infectivity in lymphoid tissues (Brown *et al.*, 1999a). The mechanism by which prion infection spreads from

FDCs to the brain is not clear, although the pattern of spread would suggest transport along peripheral nerves rather than haematogenous spread (McBride *et al.*, 2001). However, as FDCs are intimately associated with circulating lymphocytes and other blood components it is likely that they release infectivity into the bloodstream, in either cell-associated or free forms.

As in experimentally infected animals, accumulation of abnormal PrP occurs in FDCs of peripheral lymphoid tissue in patients with variant CJD at a preclinical stage. A retrospective surveillance of tonsils and appendicectomy samples in the UK has shown a frequency of abnormal PrP accumulation of around 3/ 12 000 in 10–30 year old individuals (Hilton, 2004a). Two patients with variant CJD had demonstrable PrP^{Sc} in tonsil and appendicectomy samples removed at eight months and two years prior to the development of clinical disease (Hilton, *et al.* 2004b; 2002). It is therefore probable that high levels of infectivity are widespread in peripheral tissues of variant CJD patients, and that low levels may be present in blood, long before there are any clinical manifestations of disease.

Peripheral blood infectivity and the risk of transmission by blood and tissue products

Studies on PrP^c expression in normal samples show 100–300 ng/ ml in human peripheral blood with 68% in the plasma, 27% in the platelets, 3% in the mononuclear leucocytes and 2% in the erythrocyte compartments (Barclay *et al.*, 1999; MacGregor *et al.*, 1999). It was originally felt that the latter represented contamination with plasma, but more recent data suggests that different isoforms of PrP are expressed by different blood cells in man and animals, and that the human erythroid isoform of PrP is not detectable using some of the commonly used antibodies (Barclay *et al.*, 2002). The detection of PrP^{Sc} in peripheral blood is problematic for reasons that will be explored later in this chapter.

There have been numerous studies on the presence of peripheral blood infectivity in animals. Most of these have involved injecting small samples into indicator animals by the most efficient transmission route (intracerebral inoculation). As a generalization, no infectivity has been demonstrated using this approach in the peripheral blood in natural scrapie in sheep or goats, natural transmissible mink encephalopathy and natural or experimental BSE in cattle. Infectivity has, however, been demonstrated in the peripheral blood in experimental scrapie in sheep and rodents, experimental BSE and experimental GSS in rodents, during both the clinical and preclinical phases of disease (Brown, 2000; Brown *et al.*, 2001). The level of infectivity in the peripheral blood of prion infected rodents is many orders of magnitude less than that seen in the central nervous system and is estimated in experimental models to be around 100 infectious units/ml during the clinical phase of disease and 5–10 infectious units/ml during the incubation period. Studies on mice infected with the Fukuoka 1 strain of human GSS have shown a five-fold higher level of infectivity in the buffy coat (containing the leucocytes and platelets) compared with plasma (Brown *et al.*, 1998; 1999b). Similarly, plasma has more than a ten-fold higher concentration

of infectivity than any of the Cohn fractions derived from it in an experimental system. A similar distribution of infectivity, but at lower levels, has been described during the incubation period of the disease.

In a separate series of experiments, the 263 K scrapie infected hamster model demonstrated similar findings, but also showed that 5–7 times more buffy coat was required to transmit disease via an intravenous compared to an intracerebral route (Rohwer, 2000).

More recently, blood transfusion models in sheep have been developed. Although the efficiency of an intravenous prion inoculation is about ten-fold less than that of an intracerebral inoculation, this is more than offset by the much larger volumes of blood or blood fractions that can be tested by this route. Whole blood donations were withdrawn from sheep with natural scrapie or sheep experimentally infected with BSE by oral ingestion, during both the preclinical and clinical phases of disease. When the blood was transfused intravenously to further prion disease-free sheep, the rate of transmission of scrapie or BSE to the recipients was around 40%, demonstrating proof of the principle that blood transfusion can lead to transmission of prions (Houston *et al.*, 2000).

In man, there are five positive reports out of a total of 37 reported attempts to transmit sporadic CJD from the peripheral blood of individuals with clinical disease through intracerebral inoculation into rodents. However, there are criticisms surrounding the methodology in some of these reports and interestingly no transmission of sporadic CJD from human peripheral blood to primates by intracerebral inoculation has yet been described. Similarly, no transmission of variant CJD from peripheral blood of patients with clinical disease to either rodents or primates has yet been described, though limitations in the sensitivity of cross-species bioassays means that the presence of low levels of infectivity would go undetected in such assays.

Clinically there have been three anecdotal reports of patients who have developed sporadic CJD and have previously received blood components or plasma products. However, in none of these cases has the presence of sporadic CJD in the blood donors been demonstrated. In comparison, a series of epidemiological case control, look-back and surveillance studies over the last 20 years have shown no evidence of increased risk of sporadic CJD in blood or plasma product recipients (reviewed in Turner and Ironside, 1998).

The Transfusion Medicine Epidemiology Review (TMER) was set up in 1997 to investigate the possibility of a link between CJD and blood transfusion. The study involves the investigation of data in relation to blood donors and blood recipients who develop CJD (all types), and control donors and recipients. When the National CJD Surveillance Unit (NCJDSU) staff investigate cases of CJD, they ascertain whether the case was known to be a blood donor or had ever received a blood transfusion. Similar information is sought about the control cases. The information is provided by NCJDSU in a blinded fashion to the blood services, so that the blood services do not know whether the tracing exercise involves a CJD case or control.

The study is split into two arms: donors and recipients. For donors, NCJDSU supplies the details of the case to the relevant

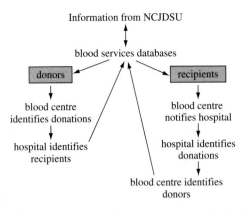

Information from NCJDSU

blood services databases

donors   recipients

blood centre identifies donations

hospital identifies recipients

blood centre notifies hospital

hospital identifies donations

blood centre identifies donors

Figure 9.3 Notification of donors or recipients who develop vCJD to the National CJD Surveillance Unit.

blood service, which then carries out a search of blood donor databases. Once records have been located, the blood donations given by the donor can be identified. The blood centre then carries out a look-back, requesting the recipient hospital(s) to trace the fate of the donation and to report back the details (name and date of birth) of any identified recipients. Those details are passed to NCJDSU for checking against the database of cases of CJD (see Figure 9.3).

In the case of recipients, it is necessary to know where (at which hospital) the blood transfusion took place. Provided that this information is available from the medical records or from relatives, NCJDSU notifies the details to the relevant blood service. The blood service then provides the information to the hospital blood transfusion laboratory and asks for details of the blood transfusion (date and unique identifier of the units transfused). Once that information has been obtained, the blood service can link the records back to the donors who provided the blood. The details of the donors are passed to NCJDSU and checked against the database of cases.

At NCJDSU, once details have been checked against the database of cases of CJD, a request is sent to the Office of National Statistics (ONS) for flagging of the individual's record. By this means, NCJDSU receives copies of death certificates for all cases in the study. Length of survival after blood transfusion (or blood donation) and cause of death are then available. It was through this mechanism that the association of cases of variant CJD in four recipients were linked to cases in donors (Llewelyn *et al.*, 2004; Peden *et al.*, 2004). The first donor case had been notified and investigated in 2000; the diagnosis of variant CJD was confirmed pathologically in 2001. One surviving recipient of non-leucodepleted red cells from a donation made by the donor in December 1996 was identified and details passed to NCJDSU. In December 2003, the death certificate for this individual was received from ONS; CJD was listed as a cause of death. The link between donor and recipient was made. The case was also notified clinically to the NCJDSU and neuropathological analysis established the diagnosis of variant CJD (Llewelyn *et al.*, 2004).

In 2004, another individual, identified as a recipient of non-leucodepleted red cells from a donor who subsequently died from variant CJD, died and underwent autopsy. This patient had not developed any clinical symptoms of variant CJD, there was no evidence of a spongiform encephalopathy in the brain or spinal cord and PrP^{Sc} was not detected in these tissues by Western blot. PrP^{Sc} was detected in the spleen by Western blot, and immunohistochemistry for PrP was positive in the spleen and in a cervical lymph node. The tonsil, appendix and gut-associated lymphoid tissues were all negative for PrP on immunohistochemistry. This case appears to represent a preclinical case of variant CJD infection following blood transfusion (Peden *et al.*, 2004). The patient was a heterozygote at codon 129 in the *PRNP* gene, indicating that this genotype is not resistant to variant CJD infection. The disease incubation period in this genotype may be more prolonged than for the methionine homozygotes, which might explain why no clinical cases of variant CJD in the codon 129 heterozygote population has yet been identified.

A third case was described in 2006; a patient developed variant CJD eight years after receiving a blood transfusion from a donor who developed variant CJD 20 months after the donation. The fourth and most recent case was described in 2007. A patient developed symptoms eight years after receiving blood from a donor who developed variant CJD 17 months after donation. This donor was also associated with one of the earlier transmissions.

Given the small number of cases of variant CJD who have been donors, and the poor long-term survival of some people who have required blood transfusion, there are only small numbers of surviving recipients of variant CJD donations. It is worth noting that only a small number of extant recipients have thus far reached the likely incubation period for secondary disease transmissions to manifest clinically. In contrast, there are larger numbers of long-term survivors in recipients of donations from individuals who later developed sporadic CJD. To date, no link has been demonstrated in the study between cases of sporadic CJD who have been blood donors or blood recipients.

Strategies to manage the risk of transmission

It is considered unlikely that sporadic CJD is transmissible by blood components or products, partly on account of the paucity of demonstrable PrP^{Sc} or infectivity in peripheral blood and partly because of the lack of evidence of clinical transmission over a period of more than 20 years. However, most countries do defer from donation volunteers thought to be at higher risk of iatrogenic or familial CJD as a precautionary measure. Variant CJD is known to be a different strain of TSE (transmissible spongiform encephalopathy) with evidence of peripheral lymphoid involvement and four cases of potential transmission by a blood component, and most blood transfusion services have chosen to adopt further strategies to manage this risk.

A number of issues need to be considered in evaluating the potential benefit and disadvantages of various risk management strategies. First, of course, is the likely efficacy of the strategy, both in reducing the risk of transmission of disease and in terms of the life years saved. Given the nature of the recipients of blood components, only 25% of whom survive longer than five years, and the long median incubation periods of peripherally-transmitted prion diseases, only a proportion of patients are likely to live sufficiently long to develop clinical disease should they become infected. The risks engendered by proposed risk management strategies also need to be considered, for example the potential risk of transmission of other infectious diseases from blood components sourced from other countries and the potential negative impact on the blood donor base, leading to critical blood component or plasma product shortages.

Donor selection

There are no epidemiological risk factors described thus far that would discriminate a high risk group for the development of variant CJD. For example, there is no evidence that cattle farmers, veterinary surgeons or abattoir workers are at higher risk of development of variant CJD than the general population. A number of countries have deferred donors who have spent more than a specified time in the UK or France. The time specified is dependent on the incidence of variant CJD in the indigenous population and the pattern with which the general population visit 'higher risk' countries, both of which impact upon the size of the marginal beneficial effect and the likely negative impact on the blood donor base. Many countries now permanently defer donors if they have spent more than a cumulative period of 3–6 months in the UK between 1980 and 1996.

There are a number of strategies which could reduce the risk potentially posed by individuals who are thought to be at risk of secondary transmission of variant CJD. For example, in the UK, individuals who think they may have received blood components since 1980 are deferred from blood donation, on the assumption that such individuals are at higher risk than the general population of incubating variant CJD. This has led to a loss of 5–10% of blood donations. Other possibilities include the deferral of plasma product recipients, those who have undergone any surgical procedures and those that have undergone other invasive medical procedures. The potential benefit for such deferral criteria needs to be weighed against the potential negative impact on the blood supply and the evidence that new blood donors recruited to replace those deferred are at higher risk of harbouring viral infections compared with established repeat donors.

Outsourcing blood and tissues from other countries

It is considered impractical to outsource the volume of red cell concentrates required from non-remunerated donors from a variant CJD/BSE free country, 2.5 million of which would be required for the UK per annum. In addition, it seems unlikely that platelets could be usefully sourced from other countries, in view of the difficulty in transporting them and their short shelf life. It might be practical to source clinical plasma and cryoprecipitate from outside the UK in view of the stability, long shelf life and the capacity to virus-inactivate the product. It may also be possible to source some components for selected groups of patients or on a temporary basis to offset the risk of shortages during implementation of other policies.

In the UK, a decision has been made to selectively source clinical plasma for a group of 'most vulnerable' recipients from outside the country, namely neonates and children up to 16 years old. The rationale for this age criterion is that neonates have a relatively high incidence of blood usage on account of prematurity and early surgical intervention to correct congenital abnormalities, that these patients have the longest potential lifespan in which to incubate variant CJD and a relatively low likelihood of contracting the disease via the food chain.

Development of a diagnostic/screening peripheral blood assay (see annexe at end of chapter for further details)

As previously described, no conventional immune response to the infectious agent is seen in prion diseases and no nucleic acid appears to be transmitted in association with these diseases. The usual approaches of serological and nucleic acid based screening techniques are therefore inapplicable in the context of CJD. There are a number of non-specific markers of CNS damage such as 14-3-3 and S100 which can be detected in the peripheral blood, but which are unlikely to be useful on account of the fact that they are associated with clinical neurological disease and such individuals would already be deferred from blood donation during donor selection.

Transcription of erythroid differentiation associated factor (EDAF) has recently been shown to be depressed in the peripheral blood and bone marrow of animals with experimentally transmitted prion diseases (Miele *et al.*, 2001), suggesting both involvement of the haematopoietic system in peripherally transmitted prion diseases and the possibility of developing a surrogate marker of disease, in much the same way that ALT was used in some countries before the development of specific tests for hepatitis C.

The gold standard, of course, is detection of PrP^{Sc} in the peripheral blood (MacGregor, 2001). However, there are a number of important concerns and issues. Thus far, only a handful of monoclonal antibodies have been described as being able to differentiate between PrP^{Sc} and PrP^c. Similarly, a number of other agents have been described as differentially binding to PrP^{Sc}. Many assays in development utilize physicochemical characteristics such as resistance to proteinase-K, resistance to heat degradation or changes in antibody binding affinity consequent upon conformational change with chaotropic agents. Preferentially, an assay should discriminate between PrP^{Sc} associated with variant CJD and that associated with other forms of the disease.

Analytical sensitivity is also highly problematic. If one assumes that the ratio of infectivity to PrP^{Sc} is similar in the peripheral blood of patients with variant CJD to that seen in experimental animal models, then 1–10 infectious units/ml of infectivity would reflect 0.1–0.01pg/ml of PrP^{Sc} in the context of 100–300ng/ml of PrP^c. The ratio of PrP^c to PrP^{Sc} in the peripheral blood would therefore be in the order of 1 million to one.

The route to validation of any such assay is also likely to prove problematic. One would normally validate a peripheral blood assay in patients with the relevant clinical disease. In variant CJD, however, at any one time there are only a handful of patients alive, they are severely neurologically compromised and it would be difficult to procure large volumes of peripheral blood for assay validation. It is likely that peripheral blood from experimental animal models and infected human brain and splenic homogenates spiked into normal human peripheral blood will take the place of peripheral blood samples from infected patients both for validation and to provide reagents for assay standardization. However, it should be borne in mind that infectivity in these model systems may be in a different physical form to that seen in human peripheral blood.

Specificity and sensitivity are dependent not only on the assay itself but also on the context in which it is being deployed. In the hypothetical scenario of an estimated prevalence of subclinical variant CJD of one/million, an assay with 99% sensitivity and specificity would detect one donor with variant CJD testing true positive on the assay per million donors per annum; 0.01 donors (one donor every 100 years) testing falsely negative on the assay, (i.e. who have variant CJD but test negative on the assay) per million donors per annum; the majority of donors testing negative in the absence of variant CJD (true negatives), but up to 10 000 blood donors per million tested per annum testing positive on the assay in the absence of disease (false-positive). This gives a negative predictive value of 99.9998% but a positive predictive value of 0.00089%. One would therefore face the prospect of informing and counselling a large number of donors, the vast majority of whom would not be incubating variant CJD. It is clear that as in screening strategies for other microbiological agents, good confirmatory assays, deploying detection techniques different from those used in the primary screening assay will be required before an assay can be introduced into routine practice.

Blood component processing

Universal leucodepletion was implemented in the UK in July 1998, predicated on the thesis that if infectivity is present in the peripheral blood of individuals during the incubation period of variant CJD then it is likely to be mainly associated with the buffy coat. As outlined earlier, there is some experimental evidence to support this view, including the involvement of the peripheral lymphoid system in the early stages of peripherally transmitted disease and a 4–5-fold higher level of infectivity in the buffy coat than in the plasma (Brown et al., 1998). However, leucodepletion does not remove non-cell associated infectivity from the plasma (Brown et al., 1999b) and it seems likely that, at best, the reduction in infectivity titre would be around ½ log infectivity (Gregori et al. 2004). Several commercial companies are currently developing prion filtration systems for blood. Other propositions that have been suggested include the use of apheresis rather than pooled recovered platelets, in order to reduce exposure of recipients to donors, the use of plasma-reduced platelets in optimal additive solution and further reduction in the amount of residual plasma in red cell concentrate.

Plasma products

The regulatory authorities in North America and Europe have taken the position that no batch recall will be initiated if a donor is found to develop sporadic CJD. However, in December 1997, in view of the uncertainty surrounding variant CJD, the UK Committee on the Safety of Medicines recommended batch recall if a donor develops variant CJD, and in May 1998 recommended discontinuation of the use of UK plasma for fractionation because of the risk of multiple batch recalls and consequent product shortages (please refer to Chapter 20).

In fact, studies using both endogenous infectivity models and spiking studies with prion infected brain homogenates show a reduction in PrP^{Sc} and infectivity at a number of different steps in the plasma fractionation process, including ethanol fractionation, chromatographic procedures, depth filtration and nanofiltration. It remains unclear as to whether these steps are cumulative in their effects or not (Foster, 2000).

Cell and tissue products

A wide variety of human-derived cell and tissue products are used as therapeutic products, including haematopoietic stem cells derived from bone marrow, mobilized peripheral blood and umbilical cord blood, bone products derived from both living and cadaveric donors, other musculo-skeletal tissue such as tendon and ligament, ocular tissue such as cornea and sclera, cardiac valves and amniotic membrane. The infectivity of most of these tissues has not been systematically studied and the risk of disease transmission is therefore difficult to assess. Again, certain processing steps such as morcellization and washing of bone to remove bone marrow could reduce the potential infectivity, though the pooling involved could have the opposite effect under some scenarios. Cadaveric donors could be subject to neurological or lymphoid tissue biopsy for evidence of prions prior to product release. The potential benefits of such measures have to be balanced against the potential negative impact on the therapeutic utility of the tissue itself.

Management of recipients of blood and tissue products from donors who develop CJD

It is not considered necessary to contact recipients of blood, plasma or tissue products if a donor goes on to develop sporadic CJD. However the possible transmission of variant CJD by blood transfusion has led to the recommendation that recipients of blood and plasma products should be identified and contacted in order that they themselves should not be a conduit for further transmission through blood, tissue or organ donation or contamination of surgical instruments. In the UK, the CJD Incidents Panel has proposed that any individual likely to have been exposed to more than 0.02 ID_{50} over a 12 month period (a 1% additional risk of exposure to an infectious dose), should be notified in order that public health precautions can be taken. Whilst blood component recipients will invariably fall into the notifiable group, the position with regard to recipients of plasma products is more variable. Some groups of patients, such as those with haemophilia, are likely to fall into the notifiable group; others, such as those who have received intravenous immunoglobulin, may be notifiable depending on how much of the affected product they received and some, such as those who have received a single dose of intramuscular immunoglobulin or albumin, are unlikely to be within the notifiable group.

Conclusion

Whilst the level of risk posed by variant CJD transmission by blood and tissue products remains unclear, further precautionary strategies are likely to be implemented. A balance needs to be struck against alternative risks, such as those of blood or plasma product shortages, the risk of transmission of other pathogens, deterioration in the therapeutic efficacy of the product itself, and financial and operational opportunity costs. Prudent use of blood, plasma and tissue products remains the most effective means both of reducing the risk of transmission of this disease and of offsetting the cost and negative impact of other measures on the blood supply.

Annexe

David J. Anstee and Gary Mallinson

Testing for prions

Development of a blood test for variant CJD

The first description of variant CJD in the UK population in 1996 (Will *et al.*, 1996) and the putative causal link with BSE highlighted the need for screening tests that could be used to prevent meat from infected cattle from entering the food chain. Since the abnormal form of prion protein (PrP^{Sc}), thought to be the causative agent of BSE and vCJD, is present in high concentrations in the brain of affected animals, the development of such tests was relatively straightforward. Monoclonal antibodies reactive with both normal prion protein (PrP^{C}) and PrP^{Sc} can be raised in mice genetically engineered to lack the normal prion protein gene and the greater resistance of PrP^{Sc} to protease digestion utilized to create a PrP^{Sc} specific immunoassay (see Figure 9.4). Assays of this type are widely used in Europe to test brain from slaughtered cattle before meat is released into the food chain (European Commission, 2006).

Evidence that infectivity is present in the blood of infected animals and that this could be transmitted by transfusion (Houston *et al.*, 2000) raised fears that vCJD can be transmitted by blood transfusion in man. Recent reports of probable transfusion-transmission (HPA, 2006; Llewelyn *et al.*, 2004; Peden *et al.*, 2004) suggest that blood is a relatively efficient medium for disease transmission and have intensified the need for a blood assay. However, the methods successfully developed for cattle brain cannot be directly applied to blood because PrP^{Sc} is present at

Immunoassay for PRP^{Sc} detection

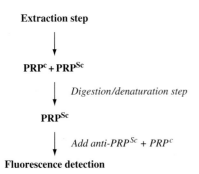

Figure 9.4 Immunoassay for PRP^{Sc} detection.

very low levels in blood, estimated at 1–10 infectious units/ml from animal studies (Brown *et al.*, 2001). A single infectious unit may be as few as 14–28 molecules of aggregated PrP (Silveira *et al.*, 2005), so any suitable assay has to be considerably more sensitive than those used for screening cattle. Furthermore, for such a test to be introduced into routine screening in transfusion services, it must be highly specific. High levels of false-positive reactions are not acceptable when blood donors testing positive will need to be counselled regarding the likelihood that they are at risk of developing an incurable neurodegenerative disease. Given the difficulty of the task, it seems probable that no one assay will give sufficient reassurance and the introduction of routine blood donor screening will depend on a combination of complementary assays being available. It will also be necessary to further analyse any potentially infected donations identified by the screening assays with confirmatory assays. Confirmatory assays need not be rapid and so in this circumstance it is possible to contemplate a more complex assay design in order to achieve greater precision.

A further significant hurdle impeding the development of blood tests arises because blood from vCJD-affected individuals is very limited in supply. Consequently, validating any putative test on human samples is very difficult. Assay developers, forced to use animal material because of the lack of human blood and tissue run the risk of developing a highly sensitive and specific test for animals that performs poorly with human blood samples. Despite these difficulties, a number of assays have been described recently that seem to be approaching the sensitivity required to detect prions in human blood and so, at the time of writing, there are reasons to be optimistic that suitable tests will be available in the near future.

All assays currently at an advanced stage of development are based on the detection of PrP^{Sc}. Surprisingly, in this era of widespread application of genomic and proteomic methods to disease, relatively few alternative surrogate markers to PrP^{Sc} have been reported. However, transcription of the erythroid-specific marker known variously as EDRF, ERAF and AHSP was identified as a surrogate marker of TSEs in animal models (Miele *et al.*, 2001).

PrP^{Sc} is an isoform of PrP^{C}. PrP^{C} is present in blood. Consequently, very sensitive nucleic acid techniques such as PCR cannot be used because PrP encoding mRNA is identical for both isoforms. Conventional immunoassays using monoclonal antibodies face similar difficulties. Very few monoclonal antibodies have been described that can discriminate between PrP^{C} and PrP^{Sc}. However, there are significant differences in the biochemical and biophysical properties of PrP^{Sc} and PrP^{C} and these differences can be exploited for assay development. PrP^{Sc} is relatively hydrophobic compared to PrP^{C} and PrP^{Sc} molecules have a tendency to form aggregates or fibrils. Aggregated PrP^{Sc} is partially resistant to proteases such as the serine protease proteinase K and controlled digestion of samples with proteinase K removes PrP^{C} whilst leaving PrP^{Sc} aggregates intact. However, there is a risk that some PrP^{Sc} may be digested by proteinase K and this might be a problem for blood samples where PrP^{Sc} levels are so low, particularly if the degree of PrP^{Sc} aggregation in blood is significantly less than that in other tissues like brain. For this reason, most of the assays currently under development do not use proteinase K digestion and rely on selective capture of PrP^{Sc} using a specific ligand or in vitro amplification of PrP^{Sc} by conversion of added PrP^C. Amplification of PrP^{Sc} by conversion of PrP^C in vitro seeks to replicate the autocatalytic conversion of PrP^C to PrP^{Sc} that most probably occurs in tissues during the disease process.

As blood samples from vCJD-affected individuals are not readily available, the first challenge for all putative tests is detection of human vCJD brain and spleen tissue diluted into human plasma. Fabricated samples such as these are far from ideal because the properties of PrP^{Sc} in brain or spleen, such as the size and amount of aggregated PrP^{Sc}, may be very different from that present in endogenous blood samples. An assay that is optimized to work well with diluted infected brain or spleen samples may perform poorly with blood samples from vCJD patients. Despite these limitations, exogenous samples provide a useful first step and a blinded panel of human brain and spleen samples in plasma is available from the National Institute of Biological Standards and Control, (NIBSC), UK (www.nibsc.ac.uk/cjd) for any company or academic institute wishing to assess the potential of a novel assay design. Assays that show promise can then be tested against blood samples from symptomatic and pre-symptomatic animals with BSE or scrapie and ultimately from human CJD-affected individuals.

The assays listed below, and summarized in Table 9.2, are blood-based diagnostic assays in development at the time of writing. All use plasma as the analyte.

Protein misfolding cyclic amplification (PMCA)

This assay utilizes the property of PrP^{Sc} to act as a template for conversion of PrP^C to PrP^{Sc}. In a process similar in concept to PCR, the analyte is subjected to repeated cycles of incubation in the presence of excess PrP^C then sonication. PrP^{Sc} in the sample recruits PrP^C to generate *de novo* PrP^{Sc} aggregates during the incubation phase. The aggregates are disrupted by sonication, producing new seed material for the next incubation phase. Amplification of PrP^{Sc} continues through each cycle until detectable levels of PrP^{Sc} are obtained (Saborio et al., 2001). In a recent report (Saa et al., 2006), PrP^{Sc} was detected in buffy coat from the blood of pre-symptomatic hamsters inoculated with scrapie (263K) well before onset of symptoms. Despite being a very powerful and sensitive technique, three significant hurdles have to be overcome before this assay could be considered as suitable for a routine screening assay. The assay is time consuming, some samples required up to seven rounds of 144 cycles for PrP^{Sc} detection and the incubation period for each cycle is 30 minutes (Saa et al., 2006). The assay requires a supply of host PrP^C and this is currently sourced from brain tissue from the same species as the initial analyte. Although it may be possible to substitute the source of PrP^C for human samples (Jones et al., 2007) it is becoming apparent that as yet unknown co-factors are required for efficient amplification. Finally, it is probable that the PrP^{Sc} generated by the assay will be infectious (Soto et al., 2005) and the assay could only be performed under strict biological containment. However, the existing PMCA assay could be suitable as a confirmatory assay for a more rapid but less specific test.

Misfolded protein diagnostic (MPD) assay

The MPD blood assay detects PrP^{Sc} by specific binding of a fluorescent conjugated, PrP derived, palandromic peptide. Binding of the peptide to PrP^{Sc} induces a conformational change in the peptide analogous to the transformation of PrP^C to PrP^{Sc}. The rearrangement of the peptide structure brings the fluorescent tags at either end of the peptide together and causes a detectable shift in the emission spectrum of the analyte. Each newly converted peptide is capable of inducing the same conformational change in other molecules of peptide in the reaction mixture, resulting in a rapid amplification of signal. The assay has been shown, in principle, to detect PrP^{Sc} in plasma from pre-symptomatic scrapie sheep, symptomatic cattle with BSE and human patients with sporadic and variant CJD (Grosset et al., 2005).

BioMérieux assay

This assay utilizes two chemical compounds to isolate and concentrate PrP^{Sc}. Samples are proteinase K treated to remove PrP^C then incubated with the antibiotic, streptomycin, which binds and precipitates PrP^{Sc}. Precipitated PrP^{Sc} is denatured and captured on a microplate coated with another PrP binding compound, Calix-6-Arene, and detected using a PrP-specific monoclonal antibody. This assay is able to detect PrP^{Sc} in blood samples from symptomatic cows with BSE and from humans with CJD.

15B3 assay

This assay uses a PrP^{Sc} specific monoclonal antibody (15B3) (Korth et al., 1997). Samples are incubated with 15B3 conjugated to a FACS compatible fluorescent label and analysed by flow cytometry. Positive results have been obtained from symptomatic sheep with scrapie.

Seprion ligand assay

Seprion is a PrP^{Sc} specific polyanionic polymer that is used to detect and concentrate PrP^{Sc}. The ligand is coated on magnetic beads, PrP^{Sc} is captured, eluted and denatured before detection in a routine EIA. The assay has detected PrP^{Sc} in symptomatic and asymptomatic sheep scrapie blood samples.

Peptoid assay

PrP^{Sc} capture and detection is achieved using PrP peptides from regions previously identified as important in the interaction between PrP^C and PrP^{Sc} (Peretz et al., 2001). PrP^{Sc} binding peptides, or similar modified peptides known as peptoids are conjugated to magnetic beads. PrP^{Sc} is captured from the sample using the beads, denatured and subsequently detected using a conventional EIA. The assay has been shown to detect PrP^{Sc} in human brain and spleen diluted into plasma.

Table 9.2 Blood Tests for vCJD.

Assay (company)	Detection of PrP^{Sc} in human brain/spleen diluted in plasma	Detection of PrP^{Sc} in the blood of animals or humans with TSE		
		Symptomatic animals	Asymptomatic animals	Blood from symptomatic humans
Protein misfolding cyclic amplification assay; PMCA (Amprion)	Yes	Yes (hamster)	Yes (hamster)	
Misfolded protein diagnostic assay (Adlyfe)	Yes	Yes (hamster, mouse, sheep, bovines)	Yes (hamster, sheep)	Yes (sCJD and vCJD)
BioMérieux assay (BioMérieux)	Yes	Yes (bovines)		Yes (iCJD, sCJD and vCJD)
15B3 assay (Prionics)	Yes	Yes (sheep)		
Seprion assay (Microsens)	Yes	Yes (sheep)	Yes (sheep)	
Peptoid assay (Chiron/ Novartis)	Yes			
Multimer detection system (PeopleBio)	Yes	Yes (hamster)		
Epitope protection assay (Amorfix)	Yes			
Immuno-PCR (Priontype)	Yes			

iCJD: iatrogenic CJD
sCJD: sporadic CJD
vCJD: variant CJD
Compiled from abstracts presented at scientific meetings and papers in peer reviewed journals between February 2005 and October 2006.

Multimer detection system

The multimer detection system assay will only detect aggregated PrP^{Sc}. PrP^{C} and PrP^{Sc} in the sample are captured onto a solid surface, such as a microplate, using a PrP specific monoclonal antibody. A second PrP specific antibody, recognizing an epitope on PrP overlapping that was recognized by the first antibody and conjugated to horseradish peroxidase, is then added. Bound PrP^{C} or PrP^{Sc} monomers cannot bind to the second antibody because its epitope is blocked by the first antibody and will not be detected. Aggregated PrP^{Sc} will have epitopes still available to bind the second antibody and will generate a signal. The assay has been shown to detect PrP^{Sc} in plasma from scrapie inoculated hamsters.

Epitope protection assay

In this assay, the sample is treated with peroxynitrite which chemically modifies a number of surface amino acids on PrP^{C} and PrP^{Sc}. The treatment destroys epitopes on the surface of PrP^{C} which are preserved in aggregated PrP^{Sc}. Once aggregated PrP^{Sc} is disrupted it can be detected by monoclonal antibodies that cannot bind to modified PrP^{C}. The assay has been shown to detect PrP^{Sc} in vCJD brain and spleen diluted in plasma.

Immuno-polymerase chain reaction

The assay cannot distinguish between PrP^{C} and PrP^{Sc} so a protease digestion stage is required to remove PrP^{C}. Residual PrP^{Sc} is bound to a solid matrix using a PrP specific monoclonal antibody. A second detection antibody is conjugated directly, or indirectly, to a length of DNA. The DNA segment can subsequently be used in a quantitative or qualitative PCR to amplify the detection signal. The assay has been shown to detect PrP^{Sc} from vCJD brain and spleen diluted into plasma.

Conclusion

At least three of the assays described above have been shown to detect PrP^{Sc} in blood from asymptomatic animals and two are reported to detect PrP^{Sc} in blood from patients with vCJD (see Table 9.2). However, it is not yet clear if any of these assays is robust enough in terms of reliability and ease of application to fulfil the requirements for rapid screening of large numbers of blood donors. The issue of confirmation of any reactive samples will also need to be addressed.

ANNEXE REFERENCES

Brown, P., Cervenakova, L. and Diringer H. (2001) Blood infectivity and the prospects for a diagnostic screening test in Creutzfeldt-Jakob disease. *J. Lab Clin. Med*, **137** (1), 5–13.

European Commission (EC) (2006) Regulation No 253/2006 amendment to Annexe X of EC Regulation 999/2001, Chapter C point 4.

Grosset, A., Moskowitz, K., Nelsen, C., *et al.* (2005) Rapid presymptomatic detection of PrP^{Sc} via conformationally responsive palindromic PrP peptides. *Peptides*, **26** (11), 2193–200.

Houston, F., Foster, J. D., Chong, A., *et al.* (2000) Transmission of BSE by blood transfusion in sheep. *Lancet*, **356** (9234), 999–1000.

HPA (2006) http://www.hpa.org.uk/hpa/news/articles/press_releases/2006/060209_cjd.htm

Jones, M., Peden, A. H., Prowse, C. V., *et al.* (2007) In vitro amplification and detection of variant Creutzfeldt-Jacob disease PrP^{Sc} *J. Pathol*, **213**, 21–6.

Korth, C., Stierli, B., Streit, P., *et al.* (1997) Prion (PrP^{Sc})-specific epitope defined by a monoclonal antibody. *Nature*, **390** (6655), 74–7.

Llewelyn, C. A., Hewitt, P. E., Knight, R. S., *et al.* (2004) Possible transmission of variant Creutzfeldt-Jakob disease by blood transfusion. *Lancet*, **363** (9407), 417–21.

Miele, G., Manson, J. and Clinton, M. (2001) A novel erythroid-specific marker of transmissible spongiform encephalopathies. *Nat. Med*, **7** (3), 361–4.

Peden, A. H., Head, M. W., Ritchie, D. L., *et al.* (2004) Preclinical vCJD after blood transfusion in a *PRNP* codon 129 heterozygous patient. *Lancet*, **364** (9433), 527–9.

Peretz, D., Williamson, R. A., Kaneko, K., *et al.* (2001) Antibodies inhibit prion propagation and clear cell cultures of prion infectivity. *Nature*, **412** (6848), 739–43.

Saa, P., Castilla, J. and Soto C. (2006) Presymptomatic detection of prions in blood. *Science*, **313** (5783), 92–4.

Saborio, G. P., Permanne, B. and Soto C. (2001) Sensitive detection of pathological prion protein by cyclic amplification of protein misfolding. *Nature*, **411** (6839), 810–3.

Silveira, J. R., Raymond, G. J., Hughson, A. G., *et al.* (2005) The most infectious prion protein particles. *Nature*, **437** (7056), 257–61.

Soto, C., Anderes, L., Suardi, S. *et al.* (2005) Pre-symptomatic detection of prions by cyclic amplification of protein misfolding. *FEBS Lett*, **579** (3), 638–42.

Will, R. G., Ironside, J. W., Zeidler, M., *et al.* (1996) A new variant of Creutzfeldt-Jakob disease in the UK. *Lancet*, **347** (2006), 921–5.

REFERENCES

Barclay, G. R., Hope, J., Barnard, G., *et al.* (1999) Distribution of cell associated prion protein in normal adult blood determined by flow cytometry. *Br J Hematol*, **107**, 804–14.

Barclay, G. R., Houston, F., Halliday, S., *et al.* (2002) Comparative analysis of normal prion protein expression on human, rodent and ruminant blood cells using a panel of anti-prion antibodies. *Transfusion*, **42**, 517–26.

Brown, K. L., Stewart, K., Ritchie, D. L., *et al.* (1999a) Scrapie replication in lymphoid tissues depends on prion protein-expressing follicular dendritic cells. *Nat Med*, **5**, 1308–12.

Brown, P. (2000) BSE and transmission through blood. *Lancet*, **356**, 955–6.

Brown, P., Cervenakova, L. and Diringer H. (2001) Blood infectivity and the prospects for a diagnostic screening test in Creutzfeldt-Jakob disease. *J Lab Clin Med*, **137**, 5–13.

Brown, P., Cervenakova, L., McShane, L. M., *et al.* (1999b) Further studies of blood infectivity in an experimental model of transmissible spongiform encephalopathy, with an explanation of why blood components do not transmit Creutzfeldt-Jakob disease in humans. *Transfusion*, **39**, 1169–78.

Brown, P., Preece, M. A., and Will, R. G. (1992) 'Friendly fire' in medicine: hormones, homografts and Creutzfeldt-Jakob disease. *Lancet*, **340**, 24–7.

Brown, P., Rohwer, R. G., Dunstan, B. C., *et al.* (1998) The distribution of infectivity in blood components and plasma derivatives in experimental models of transmissible spongiform encephalopathy, *Transfusion*, **38**, 810–6.

Bruce, M., Brown, K. L., Mabbott, N. A., *et al.* (2000) Follicular dendritic cells in TSE pathogenesis. *Immunol Today*, **21**, 442–6.

Bruce, M. E., McConnell, I., Will, R. G., *et al.* (2001) Detection of variant Creutzfeldt-Jakob disease infectivity in extraneural tissues. *Lancet*, **358**, 208–9.

Bruce, M. E., Will, R. G., Ironside, J. W., *et al.* (1997) Transmissions to mice indicate that 'new variant' CJD is caused by the BSE agent. *Nature*, **389**, 498–501.

Collinge, J., Sidle, K. C. L., Meads, J., *et al.* (1996) Molecular analysis of prion strain variation and the aetiology of 'new variant' CJD. *Nature*, **383**, 685–90.

Creutzfeldt, H. G. (1920) Uber eine eigenartige herdfomige Erkrankung des Zentralnervensystems. *Zeitschrift fur die gesamte Neurologie und Psychiatrie*, **57**, 1–18.

Donnelly, C. A., Ferguson, N. M., Ghani, A. C., *et al.* (2002) Implications of BSE infection screening data for the scale of the British BSE epidemic and current European infection levels. *Proc R Soc Lond B*, **269**, 2179–90.

Foster, P. R. (2000) Prions and blood products. *Ann Med*, **32**, 501–13.

Gajdusek, D. C. and Zigas, V. (1957) Degenerative disease of the central nervous system in New Guinea: epidemic of 'kuru' in the native population. *N Eng J Med*, **257**, 974–8.

Ghani, A. C., Donnelly, C. A., Ferguson, N. M., *et al.* (2003) Updated projections of future vCJD deaths in the UK. *BMC Infectious Diseases*, **3**, 8.

Gregori L, McCombie, N., Palmer, D., *et al.* (2004) Effectiveness of leucoreduction for removal of infectivity of transmissible spongiform encephalopathies from blood. *Lancet*, **364**, 529–31.

Head, M. W., Ritchie, D., Smith, N., *et al.* (2004) Peripheral tissue involvement in sporadic, iatrogenic and variant Creutzfeldt-Jakob disease: an immunohistochemical, quantitative and biochemical study. *Am J Pathol*, **164**, 143–53.

Hilton, D. A., Fathers, E., Edwards, P., *et al.* (2004b) Prion immunoreactivity in appendix before clinical onset of variant Creutzfeldt-Jakob disease. *Lancet*, **352**, 703–4.

Hilton, D. A., Ghani, A. C., Conyers, L., *et al.* (2002) Accumulation of prion protein in tonsil and appendix: review of tissue samples. *BMJ*, **325**, 633–4.

Hilton, D. A., Ghani, A. C., Conyers, L., *et al.* (2004a) Prevalence of lymphoreticular prion protein accumulation in UK tissue samples. *J Pathol*, **203**, 733–9.

Houston, F., Foster, J. D., Chong, A., *et al.* (2000) Transmission of BSE by blood transfusion in sheep. *Lancet*, **356**, 999–1000.

Jakob, A. (1921) Uber eine der multiplen Sklerose klinisch nahestehende Erkrankung des Zentralnervensystems (spastische Pseudosklerose) mit bemerkenswertem anatomischem Befunde. Mitteilung eines vierten Falles. *Med Klin*, **17**, 372–6.

Klein, M. A., Frigg, R., Flechsig, E., *et al.* (1997) A crucial role for B-cells in neuroinvasive scrapie. *Nature*, **390**, 687–90.

Llewelyn, C. A., Hewitt, P. E., Knight, R. S., *et al.* (2004) Possible transmission of variant Creutzfeldt-Jakob disease by blood transfusion. *Lancet*, **363**, 417–21.

Mabbott, N. A. and Bruce, M. E. (2001) The immunobiology of TSE diseases. *J Gen Virol*, **82**, 2307–18.

Mabbott, N. A., Bruce, M. E., Botto, M., *et al.* (2001) Temporary depletion of complement component C3 or genetic deficiency of C1q significantly delays onset of scrapie. *Nat Med*, **7**, 485–7.

Mabbott, N. A., Mackay, F., Minns, F., *et al.* (2000) Temporary inactivation of follicular dendritic cells delays neuroinvasion of scrapie. *Nat Med*, **6**, 719–20.

MacGregor, I. (2001) Prion protein and developments in its detection. *Transfusion*, **11**, 3–14.

MacGregor, I., Hope, J., Barnard, G., *et al.* (1999) The distribution of normal prion protein in human blood. *Vox Sang*, **77**, 88–96.

McBride, P. A., Eikelenboom, P., Kraal, G., *et al.* (1992) PrP protein is associated with follicular dendritic cells of spleens and lymph nodes in uninfected and scrapie-infected mice. *J Pathol*, **168**, 413–8.

McBride, P. A., Schultz-Schaeffer, W. J., Donaldson, M., *et al.* (2001) Early spread of scrapie from the gastrointestinal tract to the central nervous system involves autonomic fibres of the splanchnic and vagus nerves. *J Virol*, **75**, 9320–27.

Miele, G., Manson, J. and Clinton, M. (2001) A novel erythroid-specific marker of transmissible spongiform encephalopathies. *Nat Medicine*, **7**, 361–4.

National CJD Surveillance Unit, available at: www.cjd.ed.ac.uk/figures.htm, accessed 23 October 2007.

Palmer, M. S., Dryden, A. J., Hughes, J. T., *et al.* (1991) Homozygous prion protein genotype predisposes to sporadic Creutzfeldt-Jakob disease. *Nature*, **352**, 340–2.

Peden, A. H., Head, M. W., Ritchie, D. L., *et al.* (2004) Preclinical vCJD infection after blood transfusion in a *PRNP* codon 129 heterozygous patient. *Lancet*, **364** (9433), 527–9.

Prusiner, S. B. (1982) Novel proteinaceous infectious particles cause scrapie. *Science*, **216**, 136–44.

Rohwer, R. G. (2000) Titer, distribution and transmissibility of blood-borne TSE infectivity. Cambridge Healthtech Institute 6th Annual Meeting 'Blood Product Safety: TSE, Perception versus Reality'. Maclean, Virginia, USA.

Turner, M. L. and Ironside, J. W. (1998) New-variant Creutzfeldt-Jakob disease: the risk of transmission by blood transfusion. *Blood Rev*, **12**, 255–68.

Wadsworth, J. D. F., Joiner, S., Hill, A. F., *et al.* (2001) Tissue distribution of protease resistant prion protein in variant Creutzfeldt-Jakob disease using a highly sensitive immunoblotting assay. *Lancet*, **358**, 171–80.

Wells, G. A. H., Scott, A. C., Johnson, C. T., *et al.* (1987) A novel progressive spongiform encephalopathy in cattle. *Vet Rec*, **121**, 419–20.

Will, R. G. (2003) Acquired prion disease: iatrogenic CJD, variant CJD, kuru. *B Med Bull*, **66**, 255–65.

Will, R. G., Ironside, J. W., Zeidler, M., *et al.* (1996) A new variant of Creutzfeldt-Jakob disease in the UK. *Lancet*, **347**, 921–5.

10 BLOOD DONOR SELECTION AND QUALIFICATION

Virge James

Introduction: basic principles of blood donor selection

The basic principle of blood donor selection is simply stated: it should be safe for the donor to give blood and the donation should not harm the recipient.

The processes involved in achieving this deceptively simple aim are complex and so interwoven that no attempt can be made to separate out the criteria which might be considered specific for the microbiological safety of the donation.

Increasing public concern and litigation has led to many debates on the meaning of 'safe'. Calman (2001) draws attention to the importance of clarifying the language of risk; the relationship between safety and perception of safety is debated by many authors in the Millennium Festival of Medicine (2001) (please refer to Chapter 26). A new tool for communicating risk perception is introduced by Lee, et al. (1998). Sadly this excellent and clear method has not yet seen wider acceptance.

The term 'donor selection', with its implication that there is an abundance of potential donors from amongst whom the blood services have only to select those who meet their current pre-set criteria, is misleading and outdated. Today, it is the donor who selects the activities he/she participates in and therefore 'donor qualification', implying positive action by the donor might be a more appropriate term.

This chapter will examine the problems involved in setting and implementing the selection/qualification criteria, highlight inconsistencies and seek solutions. Not only the safety of the donor and recipient but also the availability of sufficient quantities of blood and blood components must be ensured. Achieving a balance between safety and sufficiency remains the demanding task of all blood services. Goodenough et al. (2003) look to future solutions. Simon (2003) gives a personal view of the factors contributing to avoidable loss of blood donors and urges the services to 'reopen the gates of donation'.

There are numerous stages between recruiting donors from the general population to obtaining a usable donation: education of the general public; marketing and recruitment of potential donors; provision of understandable information to potential donors about blood donation and transfusion; registration of donors; provision of more detailed information about the processes of donation to actual donors; obtaining consent to donation; donor health screening by physical examinations, tests, questionnaires and interviews; the application of selection/qualification guidelines based on all the information gathered; and only finally does the collection of the donation take place.

At each stage there is a loss of potential donors which must be minimized by ensuring sensible criteria are well implemented. Educated and continuously well trained staff are essential to the process.

Recruitment to registration

The fundamental requirement, that the donors understand what is involved in the donation process and accept their own responsibility to reduce risk to themselves and others, involves legal, ethical, political and psychological considerations.

The voluntary non-remunerated donor

Domen (1995) and Davey (2004) argue that the most important advance in blood safety in the past 50 years is the conversion to a voluntary donor blood supply. The Council of Europe has promoted voluntary blood donation since the 1950s and its definition: 'donation is considered voluntary and non-remunerated if the person gives blood, plasma or cellular components of his/her own free will and receives no payment for it, either in the form of cash, or in kind which could be considered a substitute for money' (Council of Europe, 2003) has been adopted throughout the world. Such donors have no reason to be anything but truthful about their identity, age or medical history and, even though their motivation may be complex, they are more likely to donate for altruistic reasons than any personal gain and thus are less likely to conceal issues which might affect their eligibility to donate.

The term 'non-remunerated' is used to distinguish between financial and other types of reward. Unpaid donors could still receive highly motivating remuneration. Small tokens of recognition such as keyrings, caps, logo bearing T-shirts, the reimbursement of travel expenses and parking fees are not considered as such, but food, food coupons, tickets for entertainments, sponsorship, free health checks for donors and family, free medical treatment, and days off work are forms of motivating remuneration. The donors may not be paid but they receive goods or services for which they would otherwise have to pay. In the USA the distinction is simplified to paid and volunteer donors; paid donors are those who receive cash or any item that could be converted to cash and guidance on evaluation of this is provided (FDA compliance policy guide, 2002).

Many different systems operate in the blood industry and different types of donors offer different challenges for ensuring blood safety.

The plasma industry and many platelet providers rely on paid donors. The plasma industry has many safeguards in testing and

Transfusion Microbiology, eds John A. J. Barbara, Fiona A. M. Regan and Marcela C. Contreras. Published by Cambridge University Press. © Cambridge University Press 2008.

processing (e.g. viral inactivation to ensure safety of plasma fractions) but these cannot all be applied for blood components which undergo no further processing.

Replacement donors are donors who donate to replace blood transfused to a patient. They are generally recruited by the patient, their doctor, or family. Such donors are usually family or friends of the patient but may also be 'professional' donors who receive payment either from the patient or the institution requiring the blood.

Directed donations are donations given for specific named patients. Many countries discourage this practice for safety and legal reasons. The UK viewpoint is that: donated blood has reached a high safety standard which directed donations may not meet; there are concerns about infection, transfusion-associated grafts vs. host disease and other immunological complications; and 'it is important not to create another avoidable risk for the patient'. These risks are set out by McClelland (2001).

Directed donations are usually between family or friends and tend to involve 'once only' first-time donors. Some countries are heavily dependent on this system, despite there being a higher incidence of infectious markers in such donors. Clear data is difficult to obtain due to a lack of uniformity of definitions and correct information.

Whilst there is widespread agreement that all blood services should work towards achieving a non-remunerated volunteer donor base, this may be an unrealistic target. The European Union Directive (2002) states: 'voluntary and unpaid donations are a factor which can contribute to a high safety standard for blood components and therefore to the protection of human health'. The 25 member states of the EU are tasked with promoting and encouraging voluntary unpaid donations. Even this directive cannot insist on a voluntary system for fear of lack of availability of blood.

Blood donor registers

Donor registers, whether paper based or electronic, local or national are a basic and essential requirement taken for granted by the developed transfusion services. These registers enable identification of donors, provide contact information and donation history, all vital to a safe blood supply. It is a fact that repeat, known donors are safer than first-time donors.

In many parts of the world, registers either do not exist or are very rudimentary. There may be many reasons for this: lack of good communication systems, a very mobile population, donors with no fixed abodes and lack of organized blood services. In these circumstances it is not surprising that it is not possible to make the most efficient use of donors who appear from time to time, often at different locations. Hence, attempts to apply and maintain records of donor particulars, qualification criteria and results of any previous tests are haphazard. Resources devoted to creating and maintaining such registers in developing countries may contribute more to blood safety than the provision of ever more complex tests.

Informed consent

Donors must consent to donation and, by definition, consent has to be 'informed'.

Donors must therefore understand what is involved both for themselves and the blood recipient, before they can consent to donation. This self-evident consideration has been incorporated into the law of the 25 European Union countries. The EU Commission Directive (2004) states that donors must be given: 'specific information on the nature of the procedures involved in ... donation and their associated risks'. The legal minimum age of donation depends on the considered capacity of the donor to give consent.

Realistically, however, can all the different possible consequences of donation be fully understood by anyone? Are they all known and documented?

Trouern Trend *et al.* (1999) published a multicentre study of vaso-vagal reactions in blood donors, but there has been no continuous systematic collection of such data except at local levels. Initiatives are now in progress through haemovigilance networks. The results of this collection of data according to standard definitions will inform the future formulation of consent to donation.

Consent for use of the donation for purposes other than clinical transfusion, for example reagents or research, has also to be carefully explained and sometimes results in refusal.

Consent to tests

Blood donors must consent to all the tests that may be performed on their donation and agree to being informed of the results of tests which may have consequences for them. In the interest of increasing blood safety, numerous screening tests have been introduced over the years. The introduction of these tests has seldom considered the consequences for the donors, yet every test has the potential of turning a well person into a patient. Often this is to the benefit of the donor, like finding an unsuspected iron deficiency. On the other hand, it may often result in many years of anxiety, such as finding repeat reactive or indeterminate microbiology test results. Sadly, the final psychological and social outcome for such donors remains uninvestigated and therefore unknown.

It is not just microbiology tests which pose problems for obtaining informed consent; even determining the blood group or finding unexpected antibodies to red cells can lead to problems within families.

Taking all these features into consideration, obtaining real 'informed consent' becomes an impossibility. The inevitable introduction of a screening test for vCJD will challenge such understanding to the full. Currently, few donors refuse the consent requested from them; this may change with the advent of a screening test for a condition which we know so little about (please refer to Chapter 9).

Confidentiality

Confidentiality is another goal difficult to achieve. Whilst all services inform donors that confidentiality will be maintained and indeed it is now enshrined in laws governing most blood services, in practice this is very difficult due to the public nature of donor sessions, the multiplicity of staff involved and the necessity of keeping attributable records in any health care establishment.

Registration to donation

Once registered on a data base, the donor proceeds through various assessments to donation. The exact sequence of events and types of assessments vary, but can be divided into physical examinations and tests, followed by medical history and lifestyle details elicited by questions and interviews. The latter developed originally for conditions where suitable laboratory tests either did not exist or were found wanting. Prior to the 1980s, when it was shown that HIV was blood-borne, such interviews, if they existed at all, were rudimentary. Now they provide a major means of assessing lifestyles and risk of donors transmitting infectious agents.

Physical examination

An essential requisite for donation is that the subject is fit and healthy. Full medical examination is impossible in most donation settings and generally unnecessary for volunteer non-remunerated donors. The body temperature, pulse and blood pressure may be taken; heart and lung auscultation and chest X-ray may be performed in some countries. The value of such examinations is debatable. The body temperature, pulse and heart rates measured in a donation environment by primitive means may not be accurate nor reveal underlying disease. The levels set for acceptable blood pressure in donors (180 mm Hg systolic and 100 mm Hg diastolic, according to the Council of Europe Guide) are not based on any evidence of harm to donors; further it is acknowledged that accurate blood pressure estimations cannot be achieved at blood donor sessions.

The performance of chest X-rays to detect tuberculosis in countries with a high incidence of tuberculosis may bear little relationship to ensuring the safety of the donation.

Laboratory tests

The tests carried out vary from a haemoglobin (Hb) level, which is universal, either immediately before or following donation, to numerous laboratory tests.

The current Council of Europe (CoE) recommendation and EU law set minimum haemoglobin levels of 12.5 g/dl for females and 13.5 g/dl for males. The evidence base for these minimum high levels is lacking. It is currently undergoing re-evaluation, as deferring otherwise suitable donors is no longer an option for most services. Newman (2004) suggests changed management of female donors and James et al. (2003) reported a dual Hb screening system which reduced donor loss in the UK.

Donor questionnaires and interview

The medical history is generally taken by asking donors questions in written, verbal or electronic format. The questions are intended to elicit information relevant to donation, about the donor's health and lifestyle. Long lists of various illnesses and behaviours to be denied are decreasing and more carefully worded questionnaires, aimed at eliciting information which can be further explored in a one-to-one private interview have been developed, as discussed by James et al. (1999). Much effort, mostly unpublished, has been invested in finding appropriate formulations for questionnaires and different means of applying them.

Once answers to questions are obtained, the decision to accept or defer the donor is made by the interviewing health care professional on the basis of guidelines or donor selection criteria; these may be very elaborate or rudimentary and inevitably vary from country to country according to the prevailing epidemiology and socio-economic systems. No set of guidelines, however lengthy, can address all the issues which a donor might present; therefore, often individual 'ad hoc' decisions based on generalities are made. The current guidelines used in the UK can be found at www.transfusionguidelines.org.uk.

Development of donor selection guidelines and criteria

The guidelines and criteria have developed through time-honoured custom and practice and are generally based on pragmatic medical common sense, the precautionary principle, knowledge of other countries' guidelines and individual 'expert' opinion. According to the Field and Lohr classification (1990), most are evidence level III and IV, that is non-experimental descriptive studies and expert reports and opinions. In view of the shrinking volunteer donor base, deferral of donors for weak criteria is no longer acceptable and efforts should be made to strengthen the evidence base used. The findings of audits of deferred donors, of post-donation information received from donors and of investigation of post-transfusion problems at all stages of the processes involved, should be used as a basis to adapt the wording of questionnaires as well as to change the selection criteria themselves.

Donor selection/qualification criteria

These criteria may be grouped into six distinct categories:
(1) Donors whose own health might be damaged by donating
(2) Donors with a transfusion-transmissible infection
(3) Donors at risk of a transfusion-transmissible infection
(4) Donors with a condition where transmissibility by blood is unknown
(5) Donors at risk of such a condition
(6) Sensitive physical/social considerations: non-suitable donors.

Donors whose own health might be damaged by donating

Taken to the extreme, every donor's health may be damaged by donating. An unexpected delayed faint could result in a fatal accident.

Donor selection criteria aim to reduce risk by using arbitrary deferral times for donors with hazardous occupations or hobbies, where a delayed faint might have serious consequences. The lists of such occupations and hobbies are never comprehensive and seldom comprehensible to either donors or staff.

Since weight is related to blood volume, no donor should give more blood than 13% of the estimated blood volume. In the UK, where the volume of blood collected is 450 ml, the minimum acceptable weight is 50 kg.

Most deferral criteria under this heading come from custom and practice. Examples are deferrals for recent pregnancy, history of convulsions, diabetes and asthma. The worry is that donation could precipitate adverse reactions. Knowledge of the medication donors are taking becomes important mainly to ascertain an underlying illness but also to prevent harm to recipients from ill understood effects of some metabolites (e.g. teratogenic drugs).

As more and more medications come onto the market, particularly for prophylactic use, more and more ad hoc decisions are made, although most services try to maintain updated lists and somewhat arbitrary deferral times, even if attempts are made to take account of the pharmacodynamics of the drugs involved.

Basing these particular criteria on better evidence would result in the saving of numerous donations and, by reducing the numbers of new donors required, make a substantial contribution to blood safety. Better evidence could be obtained by comparing outcomes in systems where differing criteria are in use, (e.g. deferral for a recent pregnancy varies from six weeks to one year). Energy expended in this non-glamorous field of research would bring sound dividends.

Donors with a transfusion-transmissible infection

Elimination of blood-borne infections is still perceived to dominate donor selection criteria. They are the easiest to apply since they are clear cut. Donors found positive for any of the mandatory microbiology tests (e.g. HIV, HBV, HCV) are permanently deferred.

Difficulties arise when test results are not clear cut (repeat reactive results) or are difficult to interpret (e.g. tests for syphilis). (Please refer to Chapter 12.)

AuBuchon (2004) points out that by concentrating on these infections, risks of much greater magnitude (e.g. transfusion-related acute lung injury, bacterial contamination and administration of the wrong transfusion) are ignored. Donor selection may have a role to play in reducing bacterial contamination, for example the deferral of donors with eczema who are considered to have a higher bacterial contamination rate with skin flora. The relevance of transmissible infections which do not appear to cause illness, such as SEN-V, GB virus and HHV8 is debated by Dodd and Leiby (2004). (Please refer to Chapter 6)

Donors at risk of a transfusion-transmissible infection

The challenges here are two-fold: first eliciting relevant information and second, assessing the actual risk; both are difficult.

Eliciting relevant information involves questions about lifestyle: travel, occupation, living conditions, sexual behaviour, drug abuse and body piercings. It also involves a careful history of medical treatments, such as acupuncture, blood transfusion, transplantation, biopsies and immunizations.

Assessing the actual risk is a developing science and, on the whole, the precautionary principle is applied. Emerging diseases, unusual infections associated with foreign travel and worries about biological weapons add daily to the changing criteria.

The incidence of TRALI could be greatly reduced if plasma from multiparous women was not used for transfusion.

- Travel: an accurate travel history is required for many of these transmissible infectious. However, the practicalities of obtaining such a history in much travelled donors, taking account not only of places visited but places been through, the understanding of donors and staff, and the speed at which this information has to be acquired at a donor session makes the problems apparent. Deferrals are based either on the results of tests where they exist, or sometimes involve time scales, or are worked out on complex risk assessments (time and length of residence in UK for vCJD risk). Even where appropriate tests exist, such as for malaria, *Trypanosoma cruzi*, or West Nile virus, there is disagreement about the value of a particular test as an indication of definite infection risk. Simple deferral on the basis of travel history does risk estranging a far greater number of donors than those who actually pose a real risk.
- Occupation: the increased risk of sustaining injury after donation and risk of exposure to infections before donation has to be assessed. Serving with the armed forces and being a member of aircrew carry higher risks of acquisition of tropical disease. On the whole it is not the occupation itself but the level of associated risk that matters.
- Living conditions: living conditions are thought to be relevant in the context of *T. cruzi*, household contacts of HBV and in relation to the increased risk of HIV, HBV and HCV in institutions or prisons.
- Drug injecting behaviour: the widespread native of intravenous drug misuse was revealed when HCV screening of all blood donations was instituted. Eliciting the information from prospective donors is crucial.
- Sexual behaviour: the relevance of sexual behaviour to the acquisition of TTI came into focus in the early 1980s with the advent of AIDS.

The assessment of these risks for any one individual remains a very difficult and divisive issue. Throughout Europe there is currently a permanent ban on men who have sex with men. Soldan and Sinka, 2003 evaluated the risks posed in the UK and reached the conclusion that permanent deferral was warranted. The risk assessments are under constant review. The European Commission Directive (2004) has left the issue open to national interpretation by requiring 'permanent deferral for persons whose sexual behaviour puts them at high risk of acquiring severe infectious diseases that can be transmitted by blood'.

- Medical interventions: permanent deferrals apply to people who have been exposed to iatrogenic risk of CJD by growth hormone injections or dura mater grafts in a certain time period; most countries exclude previously transfused donors (in particular if the transfusion was in the UK); more controversial criteria apply to donors who have had acupuncture treatment or gastrointestinal biopsy, as the risk from these procedures depends on the prevailing sterilization procedures. Donors who have had any variety of xenotransplant are also excluded, although a clear definition of xenotransplant has not been reached, let alone one suitable for eliciting at a donor session. There is a dearth of data on the effects of recent immunizations. A deferral period of four weeks following vaccination with attenuated viruses or bacteria and no deferral for vaccination with inactivated/killed viruses are common practice, albeit lacking in any evidence base. A seven-day deferral for HBsAg immunization is used for operational reasons to avoid temporary reactive results with current highly sensitive assays.

Donors with a condition where transmissibility by blood is unknown

These medical conditions and infectious diseases tax all guideline developers. How far can one carry the 'precautionary' principle without jeopardizing the blood supply?

One example is the generally permanent deferral of donors with a history of a malignancy, other than carcinoma in situ, even when successfully treated, for fear of transmissibility. Many donors may have malignancies unbeknown to them at the time of donation, but look-back studies, which would indeed be very difficult to conduct, are not reported. Currently, there is no evidence for the blood-borne transmission of any solid malignancy. However, the application of the precautionary principle in the UK in the face of vCJD, prior to evidence of its transmissibility by blood reinforces the value of this principle in the face of the unknown but possible.

Donors at risk of acquiring a condition where transmissibility is unknown

Here one can only pose questions. The worldwide blood services' reaction to SARS demonstrated the problems that can develop at speeds similar to travel. Not only emerging diseases fall in this category but also well-known illnesses. Should female donors with a family history of breast cancer be deferred? Should those with the genetic tendency to developing such malignancies be deferred? Should all smokers be deferred?

These questions pose ethical problems, which remain unresolved.

Social considerations

Every transfusion service has experience of donors who are deemed 'not suitable' for what might be considered social reasons. These are people who disrupt donor sessions due to behavioural problems or mental ill health; donors who cause anxiety to other donors and staff because of poor personal hygiene; donors whose obesity makes veins difficult to reach; donors whose physical disability would cause problems should they faint or the venue need evacuation.

Every effort must be made to make donation accessible to people with communication problems. However, donors with learning disabilities or donors who lack an understanding of the prevailing language cannot give informed consent to donation.

Guidelines in this sensitive area are often deemed discriminatory and may remain unwritten and left to individual judgement at the time.

Applying the guidelines

Assuming that carefully worded questionnaires and well written guidelines are in place, the final step of applying the guidelines correctly rests with the staff involved and their decision-making processes at the time.

The education of staff is of prime importance. Training which emphasizes the task should not be confused with education, which leads to an understanding of the relevance of the task.

Conclusion

Although the emphasis in blood safety has been on donation testing procedures and is now moving towards pathogen reduction technology and correct administration of transfusions, the role of appropriate donor selection/qualification criteria should not be underestimated as a means of building quality into the process. The evidence base for these selection or qualification criteria needs to be developed and this could be done by more collaboration between countries where differing criteria are in use. Correct application of well considered criteria would lead to a safer blood supply and help ensure availability by reducing the risk of blood-borne diseases and minimizing the loss of suitable donors.

REFERENCES

AuBuchon, J.P. (2004) Managing change to improve transfusion safety. *Transfusion*, 11 (44), 1377–83.

Calman, K.C. (2001) The language of risk: a question of trust. *Transfusion*, 41(11), 1326–8.

Food and Drugs Agency (2002) Compliance Policy guide for FDA staff and industry blood donor classification statement (available at: www.fda.gov).

Davey, R.J. (2004) Recruiting blood donors: challenges and opportunities. *Transfusion*, 44, 597–600.

Dodd, R.Y. and Leiby, D.A. (2004) Emerging infectious threats to the blood supply. *Ann Rev Med*, 55, 191–207.

Domen, R.E. (1995) Paid-versus-volunteer blood donation in the United States: a historical review. *Transfusion Medicine Reviews*, 9, 53–9.

EU Directive 2002/98/EC *Official Journal of the European Union* L33/30 8.2.2003.

EU Commission Directive 2004/33/EC *Official Journal of the European Union* L91/25 30.3.2004.

Field, M.J. and Lohr, K.N. (eds) (1990) *Institute of Medicine Committee to Advise the Public Health Service in Clinical Practice Guidelines: Directions for a New Program*. Washington, DC, National Academy Press.

Goodnough, L.T., Shander, A. and Brecher, M.E. (2003) Transfusion medicine: looking to the future. *Lancet*, 361, 161–9.

Council of Europe (2003) Guide to the preparation, use and quality assurance of blood components, 10th edn. Strasburg, Council of Europe.

James, V., Hewitt, P.E. and Barbara, J.A.J., *et al.* (1999) How understanding donor behaviour should shape donor selection. *Transfus Med Rev*, 13, 49–64.

James, V., Jones, K.F., Turner, E.H., *et al.* (2003) Statistical analysis of inappropriate results from current Hb screening methods for blood donors. *Transfusion*, 43, 400–404.

Lee, D.H., Paling, J.E. and Blajchman, M.A. (1998) A new tool for communicating transfusion risk information. *Transfusion*, 38(2), 184–8.

McClelland, B. (ed.) (2001) *Handbook of Transfusion Medicine*, TSO 3rd edn. London, The Stationery Office.

Millennium Festival of Medicine (2001) *Transfusion Med*, 11, 119–45.

Newman, B.H. (2004) Adjusting our management of female blood donors: the key to an adequate blood supply. *Transfusion*, 44, 591–6.

Simon, T.L. (2003) Where have all the donors gone? A personal reflection on the crisis in America's volunteer blood program. *Transfusion*, 43(2), 273–9.

Soldan, K. and Sinka, K. (2003) Evaluation of the de-selection of men, who have had sex with men, from blood donation in England. *Vox Sang*, 84, 265–73.

Trouern Trend, J.J., Cable, R.G., Badon, S.J., *et al.* (1999) A case controlled multi-centre study of vasovagal reactions in blood donors: influence of sex, age, donation status, weight, blood pressure and pulse. *Transfusion*, 39, 316–20.

www.transfusionguidelines.org.uk

11 CURRENT SEROLOGICAL METHODS OF TESTING AND AUTOMATION

Peter D. Rogan

Introduction and history

Despite the increasing importance of nucleic acid testing (NAT) for the direct detection of viraemia, the main methods of testing blood donors for evidence of infection continue to rely on detection of antigens produced by pathogens or antibodies raised against them. From the earliest cardiolipin tests for syphilis, introduced before the Second World War, to the most modern and sophisticated automated systems, this principle has not changed. The first viral marker to be conclusively associated with transfusion-transmitted infection was the so-called Australia antigen, now called HBsAg (Blumberg *et al.*, 1965). Within five years of publication of his findings, most major blood centres, at least in the developed world, were routinely screening donations for this marker. The earliest tests were immuno-diffusion and counter immuno-electro-osmopheresis (CIEOP). Poor specificity and sensitivity, along with the continued inability to culture hepatitis-causing viruses in the laboratory, led to the development of increasingly sophisticated and sensitive tests, ranging from haemagglutination assays to solid phase radiometric assays. The development of EIA (enzyme linked immuno-sorbent assay) by Engvall and Perlmann (1971) and Van Weemen and Schuurs (1971) laid the foundation for modern test methods, allowing for development of assays that could be automated, and facilitating compliance with GMP (good manufacturing practice), the foundation of the quality and regulatory systems used by many countries to ensure the highest quality of test performance. It is worth noting that diagnostic tests (e.g. as used in hospital laboratories) are not necessarily directly transferrable to the routine mass screening context of a blood centre. Nevertheless, there is considerable overlap. Some of the special demands made by blood centre screening include:

- High sensitivity
- Equally high specificity
- Amenability to automation
- Full process control
- Simplicity (for high throughput)
- Rapid turnaround time
- Full information tracking
- Low cost if possible.

The range of tests performed on blood donors varies greatly from country to country. Most countries, as a minimum, perform tests for HBsAg, antibodies to HIV1 and 2 and antibodies to HCV. In addition, many countries are still required to perform testing for antibodies to *Treponema pallidum*, the causative agent of syphilis. Increasing numbers of countries, at least in the developed world, are introducing tests for antibodies to HTLV I/II and at least some, including the USA, perform (or have performed up to the introduction of NAT for HIV) HIV p24 antigen testing. Cytomegalovirus antibody testing is performed on selected donors in several countries to protect at risk immunocompromised patient groups, such as low birth weight neonates and stem cell transplant recipients, from transfusion-transmitted CMV infection. Although some countries rely on leucoreduction methods to protect against CMV, it is still a matter of controversy as to which of the two methods is best (Vamvakas, 2005). Screening for parvovirus B19 is now under consideration in some countries and West Nile virus (WNV) is being tested for in countries where the virus has posed an infectious risk. Since this is an acute infection with no carrier state, testing for this agent is by NAT. (Please refer to Chapters 6 and 15.)

Testing for parasites is also relevant to specific areas of the world. In Central and Southern America, antibodies to *Trypanosoma cruzi* are routinely tested for in all (or most) blood donors, whereas in the UK and some other countries, such testing will be selective, based on a history of travel or residence in an endemic area, to allow seronegative donors, who would otherwise be debarred from donating, to do so. A similar strategy is in place in the UK and France for donors who have visited or been resident in a malaria endemic area, or suffered from a febrile illness which has been diagnosed as, or is strongly indicative of, malarial infection. Again, the option is to test for antibodies to malaria in order to allow the early reinstatement of donors as a way of increasing the eligible donor population. The UK approach is to carefully question donors about their travel, illness and residence history, and in the case of *T. cruzi* their mother's residence history. Where a donor reports a potential exposure to malaria, he/she cannot donate for at least six months after the last known exposure. Red cells may only be used if a negative test for malaria antibodies is obtained by an approved test method, currently EIA. Without a valid test, visitors to malarious areas are deferred for 12 months from return to the UK. Long-term residents of a malarial endemic area (who have lived more than six months in the area) are deferred for at least five years after the last exposure. Donors who have had malaria are permanently excluded unless malaria antibody negative at least six months after cessation of symptoms or treatment, and the last visit to a malarious area. Donors with an undiagnosed febrile illness and who have recently been in a malarious area are deferred for 12 months unless malarial antibody negative at six months. Donors who have returned from a *T. cruzi* risk area are deferred for at least six months before testing for antibody to *T. cruzi* using a validated test. Several EIA and other tests are available. Even if blood donations are not taken, a negative result on a sample would qualify the donor to attend for

Transfusion Microbiology, eds John A. J. Barbara, Fiona A. M. Regan and Marcela C. Contreras. Published by Cambridge University Press. © Cambridge University Press 2008.

future donations. Where testing is not available, or if the result is positive, donors are permanently excluded.

Principles of current tests

The term 'generation' when applied to assays (e.g. 'first generation') does not strictly apply either to chronological development or to increasing sensitivity, but to technological development (which tends to associate with enhancing sensitivity and detection range).

Solid phase immunoassays

Solid phase immunoassays rely on the manipulation of a solid phase, usually in the form of a plastic bead or the interior of a plastic micro-titration plate well, to which the coating antigen or antibody has been attached. Target antibody or antigen in donor sample (either serum or plasma) will attach to the coating molecule on the solid phase, after appropriate incubation. The solid phase is then washed to remove sample and unbound proteins before adding a specific conjugate reagent to the solid phase. This will be a hybrid molecule consisting of specific antigen or antibody (to attach to the target molecule bound to the solid phase) and a marker to allow detection of the reaction. Again, after suitable incubation, the solid phase is washed to remove unbound conjugate, before the final detection of the marker, and thus the reaction. Radio-immune assay (RIA) uses a radio-labelled conjugate, most commonly ^{125}I. When present, this emits γ radiation which can be detected in an appropriate γ counter. Because the half-life of ^{125}I is only short (about 58 days) the environmental impact is quite small, but there are health and safety issues when handling, storing and disposing of radioactive material. Also, a short half-life means a short shelf life, so a good, short supply chain is essential, and often impossible in remote sites. This type of test is much harder to automate in larger testing sites because of the limitations of counting multiple samples. Special equipment is required to eliminate cross-talk (activity in one well being detected in another) and an average counting time of one minute relegate this technically excellent methodology to specialist confirmatory and research laboratories.

Enzyme-immunoassay uses an enzyme labelled conjugate. The enzyme is detected by use of a chromogenic substrate, which gives a colour reaction which can be read by eye, and photometrically in a plate reader or similar device. By far the most common enzyme used is horseradish peroxidase (HRP). This is readily available and robust. Safe substrates are available. O phenyl diamine (OPD) which gives an orange/brown colour, and 3,3′,5,5′ tetra-methyl benzidine (TMB), which gives a blue colour, turning yellow on addition of acid stop solution, are the most widely used substrates. Alkaline phosphatase may be used where HRP is not suitable. In addition, some assays use amplification techniques to speed up the reaction or to improve signal to background ratios for weak reacting samples, and therefore increase sensitivity. A number of methods have been used but the commonest in routine use uses a two step conjugate system. The primary conjugate antibody or antigen is tagged with biotin

rather than enzyme. This may be called a probe in some systems. A second component, consisting of enzyme labelled anti-biotin or enzyme labelled streptavidin is then added, and binds to the biotin, if present. This two-step method allows several molecules of enzyme to be attached to one antibody or antigen molecule, giving enhanced colour production in weak reactors. Enzyme linked immunosorbent assay is the form of enzyme immunoassay (EIA) which has formed the basis of mass screening for the past 25 years and fully automated EIA systems are becoming more common. Most notably, test kits consist of coated micro-well strips which can be loaded with sample and reagents using automated samplers and incubated and manipulated by automated processors before reading final results on spectro-photometric equipment, under computer control, with on-board data reduction software. This gives the total process control and positive sample identification required by modern blood testing laboratories operating under GMP or similar regulations. The kits are such that tests can be manually performed and results read by eye, so the technology is still available to remote sites which may not have access to automated and semi-automated equipment.

Fluorescence immunoassay (FIA) uses a conjugate labelled with a fluorochrome, such as fluorescein isothiocyanate (FITC), which is detected by its ability to fluoresce when exposed to ultraviolet light. Slide-based antibody tests may be used for detection of antibodies to syphilis or malaria but are very labour intensive and not suitable for large-scale screening. Their use tends to be restricted to confirmatory work in specialist laboratories. Although special micro-titre plates and plate readers are available for FIA based tests, their high cost means they have not been widely used for routine assays required in blood donation screening. Some fully automated immunoassay systems use an enzyme linked fluorescence detection system (see below).

Solid phase antigen tests

Enzyme linked immuno-sorbent assay (ELISA) has been the test of choice for detecting hepatitis B surface antigen (HBsAg) for many years. Modern tests are highly specific and are capable of detecting HBsAg levels of less than 0.2 IU/ml sample (0.1ng/ml). More recently, HIV1 p24 antigen testing has been introduced in a number of countries, notably the USA, in an effort to improve early window-period detection of HIV infected donors. Ortho Clinical Diagnostics have recently introduced an HCV antigen test, as a possible alternative to nucleic acid testing. It is supplied in two assay formats: a free antigen test for early window-period detection of HCV infected individuals, as required in blood screening, and a total antigen test for estimating viral load in HCV infected patients. The specific antigen detection principle is similar for all three antigens (see Figure 11.1). For detection of antigen, the solid phase is coated with specific antibody. When incubated with sample, antigen in the sample will bind to the antibody on the solid phase. The solid phase is then washed to remove excess sample and unbound protein. After addition of enzyme labelled conjugate antibody, the test is re-incubated. Conjugate will bind to any antigen present on the solid phase, unbound conjugate

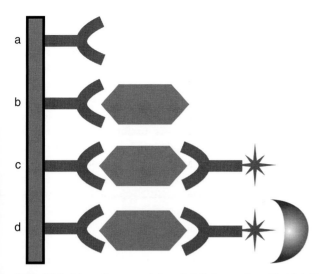

Figure 11.1. Schematic representation of solid phase antigen EIA. (a) Antibody coated solid phase, to which sample is added. (b) Antigen from sample bound to antibody on solid phase after incubation, unbound sample washed away, then conjugate added. (c) Enzyme labelled conjugate antibody bound to antigen after incubation, unbound conjugate washed away. (d) Substrate gives colour reaction in presence of enzyme, indicating a positive reaction.

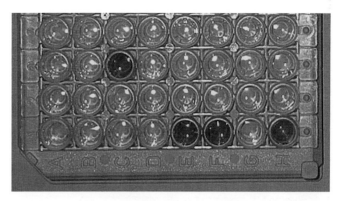

Figure 11.2 EIA HBsAg test. Row 1 contains controls; wells A–D, negative; wells E and F positive; well G, reference negative; well H, reference positive 0.2 IU/ml HBsAg sub-type ad. All wells in rows 2–4 are test samples; well C3 is positive.

being washed away. The reaction is visualized by addition of a chromogenic substrate containing hydrogen peroxide and either OPD or TMB. If enzyme is present, indicating a positive reaction, then a colour will form, which, after stopping the reaction with dilute sulphuric acid, can be read by visual inspection or by use of a colourimetric plate reader. (See Figure 11.2). The use of monoclonal antibodies for solid phase and conjugate in HBsAg testing means that steps one and two can be combined. Adding sample and conjugate at the same time is not possible when polyclonal antibodies are used for both solid phase and conjugate, as antigen binds preferentially to the liquid phase, conjugate antibody, effectively neutralizing the test. By selecting antibodies against different epitopes of the major *a* determinant of the HBsAg molecule, conjugate can be added to the reaction well at the same time as the sample, simplifying the procedure by reducing the number of incubation and washing stages. Use of monoclonal antibodies also improves specificity as false reactions due to heterophile antibodies are reduced. When animal polyclonal antibodies are used, the solid phase and conjugate antibodies must be from different animals to avoid the possibility of heterophile antibodies in donor sera cross-linking the two antibodies and giving a spurious reaction.

Concern has been expressed that monoclonal antibodies may be too specific, and may fail to detect *a* determinant (antibody escape) mutant strains of hepatitis B (Jongerius *et al.*, 1998). These are invariably point mutations at position 145 of the *a* determinant sequence of the viral DNA, with or without mutations at other points, which may lead to conformational changes in the shape of the immuno-dominant proteins (Carman and Thomas, 1991; Carman *et al.*, 1993). To reduce the possibility of this, many kit manufacturers use several monoclonal antibodies against the most conserved regions of the *a* determinant. Test kit

evaluations have demonstrated variability in ability to detect mutant strains (Zaaijer *et al.*, 2001). Currently test kits generally accepted as suitable have been modified in order that they can detect mutants identified to date.

The specificity of samples giving reactive results in antigen tests may be confirmed using specific neutralization studies. Aliquots of sample (which may need pre-dilution if the initial reaction is very strong) are pre-incubated with potent specific antibody or inert serum; then both treated aliquots are re-tested by the original antigen test. A genuine reaction is confirmed if the aliquot exposed to specific antibody gives a negative result, or a considerably weaker one (usually considered as at least 50% reduction) than the original untreated sample, while the aliquot treated with inert serum shows no significant reduction in reaction strength. (See Chapter 12.) If the inert serum also causes significant reduction, then the possibility that the result is not genuine must be considered and further investigations performed.

Solid phase antibody tests

Antibody tests may be used for several different reasons in the differential diagnosis of microbial infections. Antibody response also varies between micro-organisms, some eliciting mono-specific antibodies to simple antigens, others eliciting multi-specific antibodies to complex antigenic structures representing different components of the microbial structure, or even different parts of its life cycle. Determination of immunity requires detection of IgG antibodies to those antigens which stimulate production of protective antibody. For example, in hepatitis B infection, production of antibodies to HBsAg (anti-HBs) confers protection against future infection, whereas production of antibody against viral core protein (anti-HBc) does not. Detection of IgM antibody is required when determining whether an infection is recent, as IgM is the first immunoglobulin class produced after a specific immunizing incident. Antibody tests for determining whether blood donors have previously been exposed to infectious agent must detect IgG antibodies against all known strains of the agent, including mutants, to confer the greatest protection. For

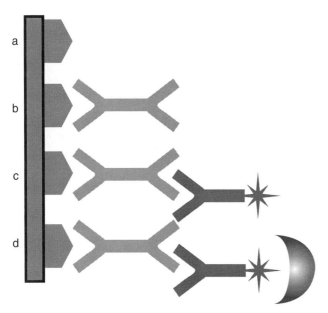

Figure 11.3 Schematic representation of solid phase antiglobulin EIA (a) Antigen coated solid phase, to which diluted sample is added. (b) Antibody from sample bound to antigen on solid phase after incubation, unbound sample washed away, then conjugate added. (c) Enzyme labelled antiglobulin conjugate bound to antigen after incubation, unbound conjugate washed away. (d) Substrate gives colour reaction in presence of enzyme, indicating a positive reaction.

example, modern anti-HIV tests will detect antibodies to several components of HIV1, including sub-type O, and also components of HIV2. Failure to include a specific HIV O peptide may cause false-negative reactions in donors or patients infected with HIV1 subtype O (Gürtler *et al.*, 1995; Loussert-Ajaka *et al.*, 1994). Ideally, screening tests for blood donors should also detect IgM, to reduce the window period, early in infection, when the donor may be capable of transmitting disease, but giving a negative IgG antibody test.

A number of different methods of solid phase antibody tests, each with its own strengths and weaknesses, have been developed. All are, or have been, used successfully for screening blood donors. There are four classes of immunoassay, although some recently emerging assays combine elements of more than one, in order to improve performance.

Antiglobulin test The solid phase is coated with specific antigen(s). Sample, which has been pre-diluted in a special sample diluent, is added to the solid phase and incubated. Specific antibody in the sample will bind to the antigen on the solid phase. Unbound protein and excess sample are then washed away before adding conjugate. Conjugate consists of enzyme labelled anti-human globulin reagent. It may be specific anti-human IgG, specific anti-human IgM, or a combination of both. On incubation, the anti-globulin attaches to any antibody bound to the solid phase. After unbound conjugate is washed away, the reaction is visualized by adding chromogenic substrate. (See Figure 11.3.)

Advantages Antiglobulin reagents are generic reagents which will react with any human antibody. Therefore, the same reagent, with associated wash buffers and substrates, can be used in a variety of different antibody tests. This allows manufacturers to reduce their overheads, and testers to have simplified procedures, with common reagents. Use of specific anti-IgG and anti-IgM tests allows for differential diagnosis of viral infection. Combined anti-IgG/-IgM tests are useful screening tests for blood donor screening. Only small sample volumes are required. Antiglobulin tests may be used for simultaneously testing for several antibody specificities, for example HIV1 gag and core proteins, plus HIV1 subtype O, + HIV2 gag and core; HCV c-22, c-33, NS5.

Disadvantages Binding of non-specific antibodies can give false-positive results. Coating antigens derived from viral lysates, where human cell lines have been used in the culture, may contain human leucocyte (HLA) antigens which will bind HLA antibodies in the sample. Antiglobulin conjugate will bind to these antibodies as readily as to virus specific ones, giving false-positive reactions. The majority of kits in use now rely on recombinant or synthetic peptide antigens so this problem is much diminished. Anti-IgM kits have been historically very prone to interference from rheumatoid factor, an IgM auto-antibody directed against IgG. This has required pre-treatment of the sample before performing anti-IgM tests. Use of monoclonal antiglobulin reagents and addition of adsorbing components such as aggregated IgG to the specimen diluent has greatly improved specificity. Use of small volume of sample with sample pre-dilution may tax some automated diluters.

Examples of uses in donor screening include: all available solid phase anti-HCV tests that are of the antiglobulin type, invariably detecting IgG antibodies only. In HCV infection, IgG and IgM appear almost at the same time so it is thought that there is little benefit in detecting IgM antibody, especially if nucleic acid detection of HCV is also performed (Kitchen and Barbara, 1997). Antiglobulin tests may also be used to detect IgG/IgM (so-called total antibody), antibodies to hepatitis B core (anti-HBc) and also CMV.

Antigen sandwich assay As with the antiglobulin assay format, the solid phase is coated with specific antigen(s) to which antibody in the sample will bind on incubation. Unbound proteins and excess sample are then washed away. Conjugate is made from the same antigen(s) used in coating the solid phase, but in solution and labelled with enzyme. On incubation this binds to any specific antibody already attached to the solid phase to give the antigen/antibody/antigen sandwich which gives the assay its name. After washing to remove unbound conjugate, chromogenic substrate is added and if enzyme is added, a colour develops indicating a positive reaction. (See Figure 11.4.)

Advantages Antigen sandwich assays are highly specific assays and are capable of detecting both IgG and IgM immunoglobulins, making them ideal for donor screening. Antigen sandwich assays may be used for simultaneously testing for several antibody

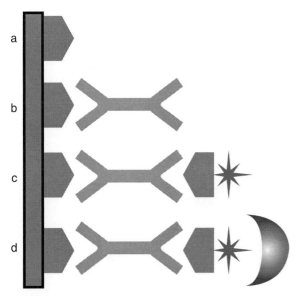

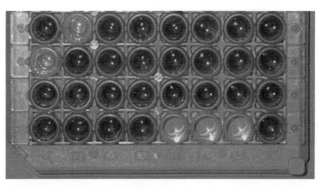

Figure 11.5 Competitive antibody EIA. Row 1 contains controls; wells A–D, negative; wells E–G, positive. All wells in rows 2–4 are test samples. Wells A3 and B4 are positive.

Figure 11.4 Schematic representation of solid phase antigen sandwich EIA. (a) Antigen coated solid phase, to which sample is added. (b) Antibody from sample bound to antigen on solid phase after incubation, unbound sample washed away, then conjugate added. (c) Enzyme labelled antigen conjugate bound to antigen after incubation, unbound conjugate washed away. (d) Substrate gives colour reaction in presence of enzyme, indicating a positive reaction.

specificities, for example HIV1 *gag* and core proteins, plus HIV1 subtype O, + HIV2 *gag* and core; HCV c-22, c-33, NS5.

Disadvantages Antigen conjugates are specific to one test type so are only economical to produce for assays where large-scale production is possible. Some viral antigens are fairly labile and may not withstand the conjugation process. Examples of uses in donor screening include most modern anti-HIV1 +2 solid phase immunoassays that are of the antigen sandwich type, as are many anti-HTLV1 +2 kits. They may also be used for syphilis (*T. pallidum*) antibody and anti-HBc detection.

Particle agglutination assays (see page 166) are also (simplified) examples of 'sandwich assays'.

Competitive immunoassays The solid phase is coated with specific antigen. The conjugate is an antibody-enzyme complex, but the specificity of the antibody is the same as that of the antibody under test. For example, if the assay is for detecting CMV antibodies, then the conjugate is enzyme labelled anti-CMV. Both sample and conjugate are added at the same time. Upon incubation, if no antibody is present in the sample, the conjugate antibody will bind directly to the coating antigens. After washing and addition of chromogenic substrate, a colour will develop. If antibody is present in the sample, then it, too, will attempt to bind to the coating antigen, in competition with the conjugate antibody. The dynamics of the assay are adjusted so that even a small amount of antibody in the sample will win the competition, thus blocking uptake of enzyme labelled

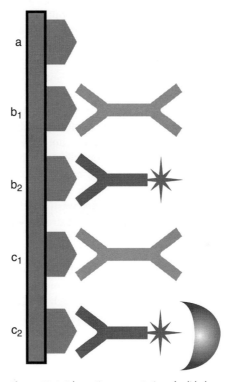

Figure 11.6 Schematic representation of solid phase competitive antibody EIA. (a) Antigen coated solid phase, to which sample and antibody conjugate are added. (b) Antibody from sample (b1) or conjugate (b2) bound to antigen on solid phase after incubation. Sample antibody blocks attachment of conjugate antibody. (c) Substrate gives colour reaction in presence of enzyme, indicating a negative reaction (c2). No colour is developed if enzyme is absent, indicating a positive reaction (c1).

conjugate. After washing and addition of chromogenic substrate, little or no colour develops. (See Figure 11.5.) Competitive assays differ from other assay formats because negative reactions lead to colour formation, while positive reactions lead to the partial or total abolition of colour development. (See Figure 11.6.)

Advantages Conjugate and sample are added at the same time, reducing incubation and washing steps. Test performance can be very rapid, with some manufacturers producing kits which can give results in 60 minutes or less. The method detects both IgG and IgM immunoglobulins though sensitivity to IgM antibodies is not as good as with IgM specific assay methods.

Disadvantages Competitive immunoassays are not suitable for detecting antibodies to several antigens at once, such as HIV1 +2. The competitive nature of the test means that if multiple antigens were present on the solid phase, all would need to be blocked to allow for a positive result. If any weren't blocked, sufficient conjugate would bind to produce a colour signal which would be interpreted as a negative result. Examples of uses in donor screening include competitive assays that are frequently used for detecting antibodies to *T. pallidum*, CMV and hepatitis B core antigen (anti-HBc). Specific anti-HIV1 and anti-HIV2 tests are also available which are useful in the differential diagnosis of a test sample found positive in a combined anti-HIV1/HIV2 screening assay.

Antibody capture assays These are a variation on the antiglobulin test. The solid phase is coated with anti-human globulin. This may be anti-IgG, anti-IgM or a mixture. When incubated with sample, antibodies of the appropriate immunoglobulin class, of any specificity, will bind. Unbound protein and excess sample will be washed away. The conjugate consists of specific antigens labelled with enzyme. On incubation, conjugate will bind only if the specific antibody is present in the mixture of antibodies attached to the solid phase. After washing, the reaction is visualized by addition of chromogenic substrate. (See Figure 11.7.)

Advantages The plate is generic, so can be used as the base for a range of assays, with common wash buffers and chromogenic substrates, but with specific antigen conjugates for each specificity. It can detect specific IgG and IgM classes for differential diagnosis.

Disadvantages Antibody capture assays combine some of the disadvantages of both antiglobulin assays (as they may be prone to false-positive IgM tests in the presence of rheumatoid factor) and antigen capture assays (antigen conjugates may be difficult or expensive to produce). Sensitivity is poor in samples from early seroconverters as the small amount of specific antibody present may be swamped by large amounts of other antibody molecules binding to the solid phase. Examples of uses in donor screening include syphilis antibodies and anti-HBc IgM.

Combination assays A number of manufacturers are now producing assay kits which make use of more than one method to improve performance, especially in the early detection of newly infected individuals. Some syphilis tests, for example Murex ICE (Abbott) use antibody capture combined with antigen sandwich. Several manufacturers, such as Abbott, Bio-Rad and Organon, are now producing anti-HIV1 +2 kits which

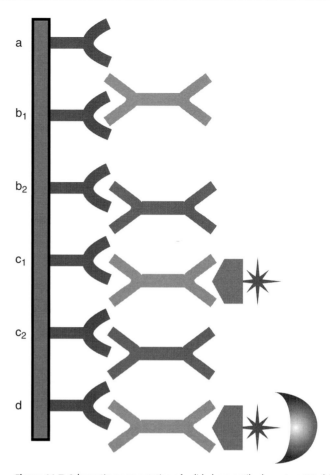

Figure 11.7 Schematic representation of solid phase antibody capture EIA. (a) Antiglobulin (anti-IgG and/or anti-IgM) coated solid phase, to which diluted sample is added. (b) Specific antibody (b1) and other antibody specificities (b2) from sample bound to antigen on solid phase after incubation, unbound sample washed away, then conjugate added. (c) Enzyme labelled antigen conjugate bound to specific antibody (c1) but not other antibody specificities (c2) after incubation, unbound conjugate washed away. (d) Substrate gives colour reaction in presence of enzyme, indicating a positive reaction.

simultaneously detect HIV1 p24 antigen. The antibody part is antigen sandwich, and the antigen detection uses monoclonal antibodies to HIV1 p24 on the solid phase. This improves early detection of infection and allows countries which require HIV1 p24 testing to do so, without use of a separate kit, with the extra cost and staffing resources that such additional testing requires (Hashida *et al.* 1996). Combined assays literally use the same principles as the individual component assays, built into one test.

Performance of enzyme linked immunosorbent assay tests: some practical considerations

Selection of test kits
For each assay required there are literally dozens of manufacturers. Not all kits available are suitable for donor screening. Some may not meet the required sensitivity standards. Others may be sensitive but have poor specificity, which leads to loss of

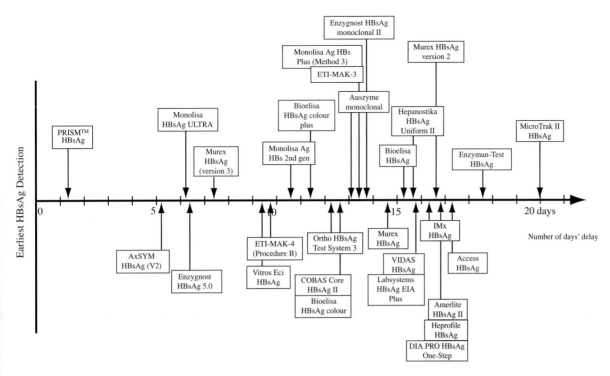

Based on the analysis of 16 seroconversion panels. The origin of the horizontal axis represents the earliest recorded detection of HBsAg.

Figure 11.8 Comparative sensitivity of HBsAg test kits against commercial conversion panels.

product and difficulty in counselling donors. Ease of use, user friendly components and speed of test performance are also factors which may be considered in selecting a kit. In the UK, only approved test kits may be used for donor screening. The Kit Evaluation Group (KEG) has representatives from the UK blood services and the Health Protection Agency. It is responsible for arranging detailed testing of new and reformulated kits to ensure they meet the standards of sensitivity and specificity required by the UK blood services (Barbara *et al.*, 2006). Figures 11.8 and 11.9 show comparative sensitivity of HBsAg and anti-HIV1 + 2 test kits when tested against a series of commercially available seroconversion panels. There are only three anti-HCV kits available in the UK (apart from variants used on automated equipment, see below for section on 'Newer technologies'). Sensitivity is less important due to the requirement to perform HCV RNA testing. Approval by KEG of a given kit is not meant as an endorsement for the kit, merely confirmation that it meets the standards required by the UK blood services.

Performance of assays

Although it is possible to perform and read EIA tests manually, especially for micro-plate based assays, it is only possible to achieve optimum performance and sensitivity using some kind of automated or semi-automated apparatus. Washing is critical, as any residual components may lead to false-positive reactions. The majority of initial reactive samples are not confirmably positive. The initial spurious result is invariably due to technical error, either unsatisfactory washing or careless adding of reagents, causing splashing. Nevertheless, most manufacturers (and blood services) recommend that repeat testing is performed in

duplicate and only if both replicates are clearly negative is the final interpretation deemed to be negative for that marker and the product released. Otherwise the result is presumed to be positive, all products are discarded and confirmatory testing arranged. While strongly reactive wells are clearly visible to the unaided eye, weakly reactive ones may not be, especially if using a competitive type assay where negatives are coloured and positive results lead to a reduction or abolition of colour development. Use of independent standards of known activity may be useful in setting sensitivity limits. Supplies of standards for single activities and multi-specificity markers are available from several sources, such as the UK National Institute for Biological Standards and Control (NIBSC) and Boston Biomedica Inc (BBI). Again, these are designed, not just to confirm sensitivity in a single run, but to monitor system performance over time, so a numerical value is required to achieve this. Manufacturers always provide a cut-off calculation and quality checking algorithms for their assay. Although any cut-off is a compromise between sensitivity and specificity, it is based on extensive pre-production testing when the parameters of the assay performance are optimized. Manual reading, without a numerical result, will not allow either correct use of manufacturers' instructions or statistical process monitoring of performance. For a more extensive discussion of automation and quality systems, please see Chapter 17 on quality/error free pathways.

Automation

The best way to achieve consistent test performance and proof of performance to manufacturers' instructions, is to use some kind of automation. Equipment is available from several suppliers

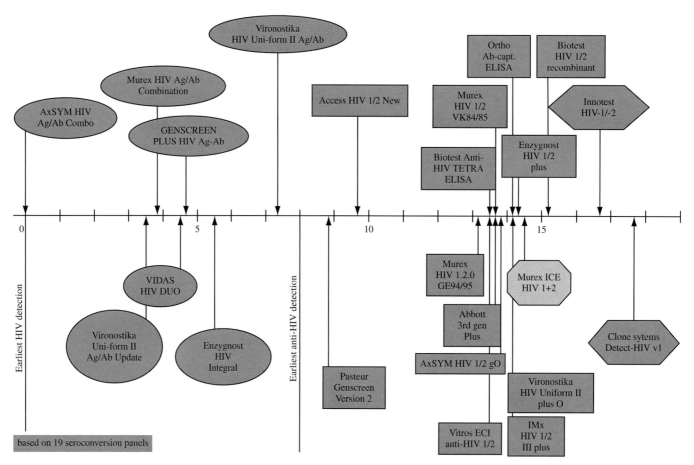

Figure 11.9 Comparative sensitivity of anti-HIV1 +2 and anti-HIV/p24 antigen combi-test kits against commercial seroconversion panels.

designed to automate all or part of the testing process. These include robotic samplers (see Figure 11.10) which dispense samples, controls and diluents into plates under computer control with barcode identification of samples, control and test plates to allow positive sample identification. These may link to readers or to other automation. Plate processors (see Figure 11.11) look after the incubation, washing and reagent dispensing functions and include a reader for final OD determination. Data reduction software may be included, but more commonly the raw data is exported to third-party software. Fully automated systems (see Figure 11.12) include both sampling, plate processing and data reduction. These have been slow, low capacity instruments designed for reference laboratories or laboratories with small workloads. Systems are now becoming available which have the throughput required of larger testing laboratories and incorporate all of the checks required for GMP compliance.

Particle agglutination assays

Simply put, inert particles are coupled to purified antigen (when screening for antibody) or specific antibody (when screening for antigen). Coated particle suspensions are mixed with donor serum or plasma and allowed to react for a predetermined

time. In some cases, constant rotation of the test is required. After a predetermined time the test is examined. For non-reactive samples the particles may remain in suspension. For reactive samples the particles will clump due to the cross-linking with reactant (antigen or antibody) in the sample. (See Figure 11.13.) A number of different particles may be used for different assays.

Carbon particles

These are used extensively for testing for syphilis antibodies using non-treponemal antigens. Tests are quick, cheap and easy to perform, requiring minimal equipment. Commonest forms are VDRL (Venereal Disease Reference Laboratory) and RPR (Rapid plasma reagin) tests (see Figure 11.14). Some versions can be automated, though the reliability of these tests has been questioned. Although the method of choice for many countries, the relatively high numbers of false-positive and -negative reactions has led to their efficacy as donor testing methods being called into doubt (Muller, 1981). Further, the extreme rarity of post-transfusion syphilis has led to the questioning of the need for syphilis testing altogether. Generally, in Europe, for those countries where testing is required, alternative, specific treponemal testing methods have been employed.

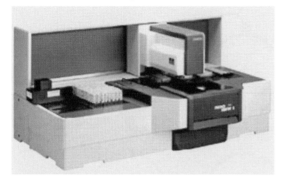

Hamilton Microlab AT Plus

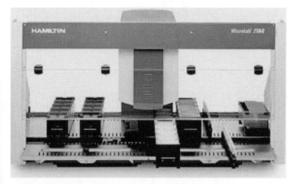

Hamilton Star

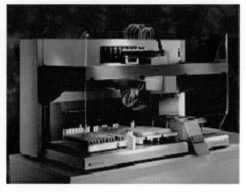

Tecan Genesis

Figure 11.10 Examples of robotic samplers.

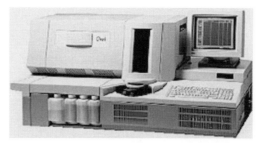

Bio-Tek Omni

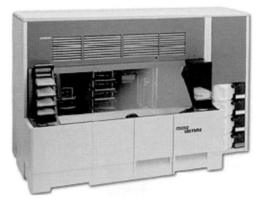

Hamilton FAME

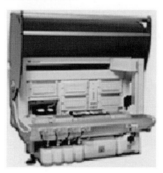

Bio-Kit BEST 2000

Figure 11.11 Examples of automated plate processors.

Latex particles

These use exactly the same principles as the carbon based tests, but use white, rather than black particles. The uniformity of size and density of latex particles is easier to control, so variation between different production lots is said to be better than for carbon particles. Although it is possible to test for HBsAg by this method, it would not meet the sensitivity requirements of most developed countries. However, its price, ease of training and use, and requirement for only basic instrumentation has led to its use in some developing countries.

Haemagglutination tests

Animal red cells have proven to be a very useful carrier for antigen or antibody tests. The permeability of the membrane makes it relatively easy to incorporate antibodies or antigens by use of tannic acid. Cells can also be pre-fixed with glutyraldehyde or formaldehyde to allow long-term storage in the liquid or freeze dried state. Allowing cell and donor serum mixture to react in plastic micro-titration trays leads to a very specific settling pattern (see Figure 11.15). Negative samples or controls produce a very tight button of cells at the bottom of the well, while positive reactors cause the cells to agglutinate, producing a carpet of cells across the bottom of the well. These results are both easy to interpret by eye and can be read by scanning plate readers, which, when coupled to a robotic sample dispenser, gives a GMP compliant automated process. Some tests can be fully automated by incorporation into a blood grouping analyser such as the Olympus PK7200 (Olympus), the primary instrument used in large testing centres worldwide. This allows for a testing process with full process control. Haemagglutination antibody assays of this type may be referred to as passive or indirect haemagglutination assays (PHA, IHA) because the specific antigen is not a

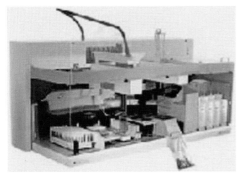

Tecan Genesis RMP

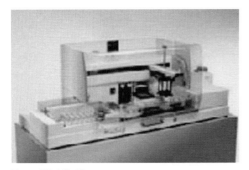

Tecan Mini-Swift

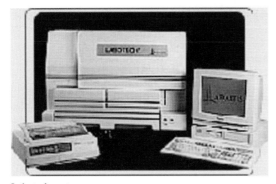

Labotech system

Figure 11.12 Examples of fully automated systems, including both sample handling and plate processing in one unit.

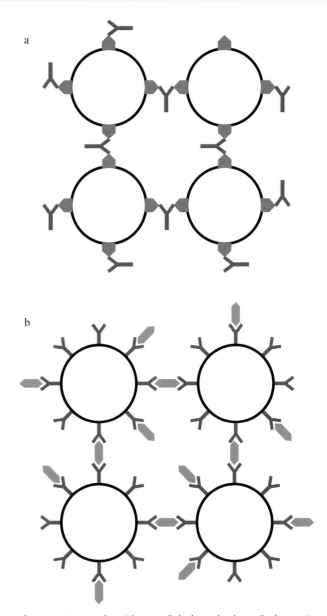

a

b

Figure 11.13 Coated particles cross-linked together by antibody or antigen in donor sample to form an aggregate or agglutinate which is visible to the naked eye.

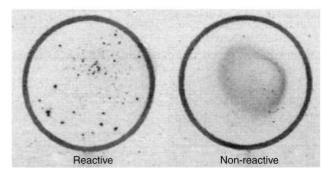

Reactive   Non-reactive

Figure 11.14 Rapid Plasma Reagin (RPR) test for syphilis antibodies in serum or plasma. Carbon coated particles are mixed with sample. If antibodies are present the particles clump together, in non-reactive samples they remain dispersed.

natural part of the red cell membrane's antigenic structure. Assays where antibody has been incorporated into the red cell membrane, in order to detect antigen, may be referred to as reverse passive haemagglutination assays (RPHA).

Although human red cells have been used in such tests their sensitivity to cold agglutinins, found in many normal donor sera, makes them unpopular due to specificity concerns. Animal red cells are used for preference. Sheep red cells are commonly used for detecting antibodies to syphilis, but due to relatively high rates of heterophile antibodies to sheep proteins, may give specificity problems unless samples are pre-treated with an absorbing diluent. Avian red blood cells, especially chick cells, are the most commonly used cells in PHA tests. They are nucleated, so settle faster than mammalian cells, and incidences of heterophile antibodies are lower, increasing specificity.

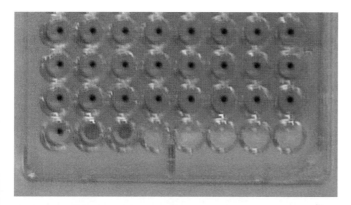

Figure 11.15 Part of a micro-titration plate showing TPHA tests. Row 1, controls: (left to right) negative, positive, independent weak positive. Rows 2–4, negative donor samples.

Syphilis antibodies *T. pallidum* haemagglutination assay (TPHA) is widely used in Europe for testing blood donors for the presence of antibodies to syphilis. Unlike cardiolipin based tests, red cells are coated with specific treponemal antigens (Nichols strain) leading both to greater specificity and much improved sensitivity, especially in the early stages of primary syphilis, with claims of 98% of patient sera reacting within two weeks of infection (Müller, 1981). The test is both rapid and easy to perform, with chick cell based assays giving results in one hour (see Figure 11.15). It may be automated in micro-titration trays and several companies provide assays optimized for use on Olympus grouping machines. Other treponemal infections, such as Pinta (*T. arateum)* and Yaws (*T. pertenue*), may cross-react with TPHA so must be borne in mind when investigating TPHA positive patients in donors in parts of the world2 where such diseases are or have been common.

Hepatitis Reverse passive haemagglutination assay tests for hepatitis B surface antigen (HBsAg) have been widely used for screening blood donors. Although largely superseded by solid phase assays due to sensitivity issues, they are still useful in areas where HBV is endemic and the method has been modified to provide semi-automated testing, including use on Olympus grouping machines. Antibody tests for antibody to HBsAg (anti-HBs) and antibody to hepatitis B core antigen (anti-HBc) tests have also been produced. Anti-HBc was used as a surrogate test for non-A non-B (NANB) hepatitis in several countries (Barbara, 1983) and currently may be used to enhance hepatitis B detection in the core window period. Like other viruses, HBV has a window period after infection but before detectable markers are present when the donor may be infectious. In addition, as antigen is screened for, in acute HBV infection there is a second window period (the core window) when HBsAg becomes undetectable but the donor may still be infectious until sufficient anti-HBs has developed to confer immunity. Such donors may be detected by screening for anti-HBc. If positive, immune and potentially infectious donors may be distinguished by quantitative anti-HBs determination. Anti-HBs may be used both to confirm the immune status of HBsAg negative, anti-HBc positive blood

donors and to screen and monitor antibody levels in donors selected for the provision of source plasma for hepatitis B immune globulin (HBIG). The now defunct Japanese Green Cross produced a PHA test for anti-HCV strictly for use in Japan, though this is no longer available. Many other kits are available, although these are generally not of use in the screening of blood donors.

Particle agglutination tests
Fujirebio Inc. have produced the Serodia® range of particle agglutination assays. These use coloured latex particles as the solid phase. The particles are approximately the same size and density as red blood cells, so performance and reading of tests, including automation, is very similar to that for haemagglutination assays. It is claimed that specificity is much better than haemagglutination assays and lot to lot variation is much lower. Included in the range of tests are anti-HIV1, anti-HIV1 +2, anti-HTLV1, anti-HCV, antibodies to syphilis (TPPA, *T. pallidum* particle agglutination test), an Olympus PK7200 version of the TPPA, antibodies to CMV and antibodies to *Trypanosoma cruzi*, the causative agent of Chagas' disease. These tests are easy to perform with minimal equipment, so fit in with the needs of developing countries, especially in remote areas, yet can be automated to provide the GMP compliance required by developed counties. Because of cross-licensing agreements, not all kits may be available in all countries.

Newer technologies

Modern requirements for donor testing place increasing demands on limited resources. Ever more stringent standards for GMP and error free systems require increasingly sophisticated technology with high throughput and full audit trail. The high cost of such systems makes them practicable only for large-scale testing. In England, for example, donor testing only occurs in ten testing sites, with annual workloads of between 150 000 and 300 000 donations, with staff and extended working days to manage the workload in a timely manner. This model is true of many other countries, including the rest of the UK, much of Europe, American Red Cross and other US commercial testing laboratories, and Australia. Smaller hospital based and community blood banks are still common, however, in Europe, USA and many developing nations. These may handle only small numbers of donation samples daily, so cannot reasonably justify the cost of large testing instruments. Hospital based units may be able to take advantage of existing instrumentation in other sections of the hospital pathology department. Several clinical immunology and chemistry analysers offer infectious disease testing profiles giving rapid result turnaround and full automation. The principles of the tests are still based on solid phase immunoassay, but the solid phases are tailored to match the instrument. Novel methods of visualizing the reaction are also utilized, including enzymatic and non-enzymatic chemiluminescence and fluorescence. Not all instruments offer a full range of markers and there may be restrictions on what tests are available by country. For

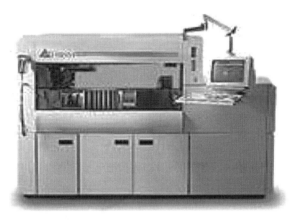

Figure 11.16 Abbott PRISM system.

example, US Food and Drug Agency (FDA) licensing restrictions may mean assays available in Europe may not be available in North America. All of these instruments use a solid phase based test system.

Abbott PRISM (Abbott Diagnostics Division)

This is a sophisticated fully automated high throughput instrument, designed specifically for the blood donation screening market (see Figure 11.16). It offers full GMP compliance and is capable of processing 180 samples an hour. The end to end process, from sampling to result calculation, is just under an hour, so it is very fast when handling urgent (stat) samples. It is a six-channel instrument. The usual configuration is to have five assay channels and a back-up channel, which can be configured for any assay, in the event of a channel failure. This gives great flexibility and allows the instrument to be quickly brought back into use by the operator after channel failure, greatly reducing reliance on service engineers. The primary assay panel is HBsAg, anti-HBc, anti-HIV1/HIV2 (with extra peptide to improve detection of antibodies to HIV1 sub-type O), anti-HCV and anti-HTLV1/HTLV2. In addition, there is an HBsAg confirmatory neutralization test, and anti-HBs and HIV1 p24 antigen tests are available in some countries. An anti-HIV1/HIV2, HIV1 p24 antigen combi-test is also available and will allow the simultaneous detection of both antibodies and antigen to HIV in a single test. The principle of the Abbott PRISM is based on the use of microscopic latex micro-particles for the solid phase. These are coated with antigens or antibodies as appropriate. When mixed with sample they have an extremely large surface area in contact with the sample and therefore taking part in the reaction, compared with other solid phases such as micro-wells. This makes the initial reaction very fast. The micro-particles are then immobilized on a glass fibre matrix where they can be washed and other reagents added as required. The second innovation is in the use of a non-enzymatic conjugate. Instead, an ester of acridinium is used. This is chemiluminescent in the presence of hydrogen peroxide in alkaline conditions. This activator solution is added in lieu of chromagenic substrate. If a

reaction has occurred, and acridinium is present, a pulse of light is emitted and detected by a photo-multiplier tube (PMT). Unlike EIA, which requires 10–30 minutes for colour to develop, the chemiluminescent event is virtually instantaneous (flash chemiluminescence), again contributing to the overall speed of the process. Further, by using a PMT, which gives measurement in counts per minute (CPM), rather than a photometer, which gives results in optical density (OD) units, the assay is linear against a considerable range of concentrations, so semi-quantitative data can be obtained without diluting the sample. Apart from the unusual solid phase and detection systems, the principles of the assays are no different from other solid phase assays. The HBsAg test is a sandwich assay; the anti-HCV is an IgG antiglobulin assay; the anti-HIV1/HIV2 and anti-HTLV1/HTLV2 tests are antigen sandwich assays; and the anti-HBc test is a competitive assay. The HIV antibody/antigen combi-test uses antibody and antigen sandwich assays in a single system. Particularly useful in the highly regulated area of donor testing are the built-in GMP functions. All reagents are barcoded and master lot details are stored on board which blocks use of expired reagents, reagents from different lots, and does not allow reagents to be loaded in the wrong position. Sample and reagent addition and volumes are dynamically monitored, and failures are stored in an event log and an alarm sounded, without stopping the instrument, making it truly "walk-away". Reaction temperature is also monitored dynamically. Finally, the manufacturer defines which calibration checks are required, and how often, and provides the tools with which to perform them.

Axsym (Abbott Laboratories)

This is a fully automated immunoassay system widely used throughout the world. It is a medium capacity unit (120 tests per hour) which offers a range of assays for infectious disease markers based on micro-particle enzyme immuno-fluorescence using alkaline phosphatase as the conjugate enzyme and four methyl umbelliferyl phosphate (MUP) as the substrate. If the enzyme is present a phosphate group is cleaved from the substrate to produce methylumelliferone (MU) which is fluorescent. Assays of interest to blood screening laboratories include HBsAg, Anti-HBc, anti-HCV, anti-HIV1+2, HIV antibody/antigen combi-test and CMV. The machine is single channel, so only one assay can be performed at a time, but would be perfectly capable of handling a small laboratory's needs.

Architect (Abbott Laboratories)

This is the 'big brother' of Axsym, consisting of modular units which can be combined to make a very large throughput instrument capable of performing both chemistry and immunoassay functions. The principles of the assay are similar to Axsym but use acridinium based chemiluminescence. The assay range is also similar to that of Axsym but anti-HTLV1/2 is also available.

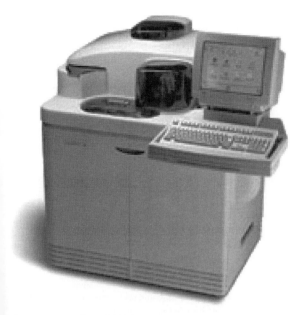

Figure 11.17 Ortho VITROS Eci system.

VITROS Eci (Ortho Clinical Diagnostics)

This is a low throughput (90 tests per hour) immunoassay unit (see Figure 11.17). It uses enhanced chemiluminescence assays for its infectious disease marker range, which includes HBsAg, anti-HBc, anti-HIV1 +2 and anti-HCV.

Vidas (BioMérieux)

This system is widely used in both routine and reference laboratories. It can be used to test multiple markers on a sample or to test multiple samples for a marker, or a combination of the two. The assays are based on a unique cassette system including a sample tip and all reagents for one assay. The tip is used not just to aspirate sample but also acts as the solid phase, the inside surface being coated with antibody or antigen as appropriate. The cassette contains wash and conjugate solutions which are aspirated into the tip as required. Used material is dispensed back into the cassette chambers so no waste goes down into the sewage system. Not only is this environmentally friendly but the lack of fluidics to pump reagents simplifies the instrument layout, improving reliability. The final signal detection is based on MUP, the reacted substrate being placed in the last chamber of the cassette which has an optical surface to allow detection of any fluorescence. Assays in the range include HBsAg, anti-HBc, anti-HIV1 +2/HIV antigen combi-test and HIV1 p24 antigen.

Roche Cobas Core II (Hoffman-La Roche)

This is a medium capacity analyser with both routine and stat functions. It is a compact desk top analyser with a fast result turnaround time and an average throughput of about 150 tests per hour. One useful feature of its software is its ability to automatically re-schedule screen reactives and re-test them in duplicate. Reactions are based on a polystyrene bead as the solid phase. Available assays include HBsAg, anti-HBc, anti-HIV1 +2/HIV antigen combi-test, HIV antigen, anti-HTLV1/2 and anti-CMV IgG. HCV is not included because of associated patent issues.

Access (Beckman)

This medium capacity analyser uses magnetic particles as the solid phase. It allows rapid separation from reagents and wash solutions, which coupled with a chemiluminescent signal give a fast reaction. The range of assays includes HBsAg, anti-HBc and anti-HIV1 +2.

Advia Centaur (Bayer)

This high throughput (up to 200 tests per hour) immunoassay instrument, with a rapid (18-minute) reaction time and virtually no start-up time is very flexible in routine use. Like the Cobas Core, repeat testing can be programmed as an automatic function. The assay range includes HBsAg, anti-HBc, anti-HCV and anti-HIV1 +2.

The list of instruments described represents the most popular instruments available at the time of writing, though many others are available and may offer a useful testing facility. Each have their own strengths and weaknesses when applied to blood donation screening. None offers the full range of assays required but nevertheless, if available to the smaller laboratory, will play a role in offering high quality testing capacity while relieving pressure on the donation testing laboratory, releasing staff to concentrate on those tests not covered by available instrumentation. In a busy hospital laboratory there may be conflict between donation screening and clinical testing which may increase pressure on a busy immunoassay department. This, too, needs to be accounted for when determining the optimum testing strategy in smaller community or hospital blood banks.

From immuno-diffusion to Abbott PRISM, the development of donation strategies has had the goal of improving performance, by increasing sensitivity, improving specificity and building GMP into the instrument. Nevertheless, the basic premise of detecting antibody or antigen has not changed since Blumberg first discovered Australia antigen (Blumberg, *et al.*, 1965). No matter how much technology improves, serological testing can never give 100% guarantee of donor safety because the human body requires time to produce these markers in measurable amounts, and a new pathogen may always be just around the corner. The increasing use of direct nucleic acid detection of viral DNA and RNA, coupled with improving methods of pathogen reduction will inevitably lead to more scientists asking the question, 'Do we actually need serological testing methods any more?' However, until pathogen reduction becomes available for all components and manufacturers can allay concerns about potential side effects and cost-effectiveness, serological methods will remain the 'primary tools' (Alter *et al.*, 2003; Stramer *et al.*, 2004) for testing.

REFERENCES

Abbott Laboratories, Diagnostic Division, 100 Abbott Park Road, Abbott Park, IL60064-3500, USA (available at: www.abbott.com).

Alter, M. J., Kuhnert, W. L. and Finelli, L. (2003) Guidelines for laboratory testing and result reporting of antibody to hepatitis C virus. *MMWR Recomm Rep*, **52** (RR-3), 1–13.

Barbara, J. A. J. (1983) *Microbiology in blood transfusion*, p. 72. Bristol, John Wright & Sons Ltd.

Barbara, J., Ramskill, S., Perry, K., *et al.* (2006) The National Blood Service (England) approach to evaluation of kits for detecting infectious agents. *Transfus Med Rev*, **21** (2), 147–58.

Bayer Healthcare, LCC Diagnostic Division, 511 Benedict Avenue, Tarrytown, NY 10591, USA (available at: www.labnews.com).

BioMérieux sa, F-69280 Marcy l'Etoile, France (available at: www.biomerieux.com).

Blumberg, B. S., Alter, H. J. and Visnich, S. (1965) A 'new' antigen in leukaemia sera. *J Am Med Assoc*, **191**, 541.

Carman, W. F. and Thomas, H. C. (1991) Genetically defined variants of hepatitis B virus. *Rev Med Virol*, **1**, 29–39.

Carman, W., Thomas, H. and Domingo, E. (1993) Viral genetic variation: hepatitis B virus as a clinical example. *Lancet*, **341**, 349–53.

Engvall, E. and Perlmann, P. (1971) Enzyme-linked Immunosorbent Assay (ELISA) – quantitative assay of immunoglobulin G. *Immunochemistry*, **8** 870–4.

F. Hoffmann-La Roche Ltd, Group Headquarters, Grenzacherstrasse 124, CH-4070 Basel, Switzerland (available at: www.roche.com).

Fujirebio Inc, 2–62–5, Nihombashi-hamacho, Chuo-ku, Tokyo 103–0007, Japan (available at: www.fujirebio.co.jp).

Gürtler, L. G., Zekeng, L., Simon, F., *et al.* (1995) Reactivity of five anti-HIV1 subtype O specimens with six different anti-HIV screening ELISAs and three immunoblots. *J Virol Methods*, **51**, 177–84.

Hashida, S., Hashinaka, K., Nishikata, I., *et al.* (1996) Earlier diagnosis of HIV-1 infection by simultaneous detection of p24 antigen and antibody IgGs to p17 and reverse transcriptase in serum with enzyme immunoassay. *J Clin Lab Anal*, **10**, 213–9.

Jongerius, J. M., Wester M., Cuypers, H. T., *et al.* (1998) New hepatitis B virus mutant form in a blood donor that is undetectable in several hepatitis B surface antigen screening assays. *Transfusion*, **38**, 56–9.

Kitchen, A. D. and Barbara, J. A. J. (1997) The development of tests for antibody to hepatitis C virus. In *The Molecular Medicine of Viral Hepatitis*, eds T. J. Harrison and A. J. Zuckerman. Chichester, John Wiley and Sons Ltd.

Loussert-Ajaka, I., Ly, T. D., Chaix, M.L., *et al.* (1994) HIV-1/HIV-2 seronegativity in HIV-1 subtype O infected patients. *Lancet*, **343**, 1393–4.

Müller, F. in International Forum (1981) Does it make sense for blood transfusion services to continue the time-honoured syphilis screening with cardiolipin antigen? *Vox Sang*, **41**, 188.

Ortho Clinical Diagnostics, Mandeville House, 62 The Broadway, Amersham, Bucks, HP7 0HJ, United Kingdom (available at: www.jnjgateway.com).

Stramer, S. L., Glynn, S. A., Kleinman, S. H., *et al.* (2004) Detection of HIV-1 and HCV infections among antibody-negative blood donors by nucleic acid-amplification testing. *N Eng J Med*, **351**, 760–8.

Vamvakas, E. C. (2005) Is white blood cell reduction equivalent to antibody screening in preventing transmission of cytomegalovirus by transfusion? A review of the literature and meta-analysis. *Trans Med Rev*, **19** (3), 181–99.

Van Weemen, B. K. and Schuurs, A. H. W. M. (1971) Immunoassay using antigen-enzyme conjugates. *FEBS Letters*, **15**, 232–6.

Zaaijer, H. L., Vrielink, H. and Koot, M. (2001) Early detection of hepatitis B surface antigen and detection of HBsAg mutants: a comparison of five assays. *Vox Sang*, **81**, 219–21.

CONFIRMATORY TESTING AND DONOR RE-ADMISSION

Alan D. Kitchen and Brian C. Dow

Introduction

The major focus in ensuring the microbiological safety of the blood supply relies heavily on the primary screening of donated blood. Although routine donor screening assays are highly sensitive, this sensitivity is often achieved at the expense of specificity (0.05–0.5%) (Dow, 2000).

Blood donations found to be initially reactive at donor testing sites should be repeat tested in duplicate. Should any of the repeat tests result in reactivity, the donation is classified as 'repeatedly reactive', the donor is flagged on the donor database and samples are submitted to the designated national reference laboratory or other designated facility. Regardless of confirmatory test results, the donation and all its associated components will be excluded from transfusion.

Throughout the world, blood services have differing policies with regard to confirmation of microbiology reactive donations. Most developed countries' services are capable of performing adequate confirmation of reactive donations. However, some services use an alternative strategy of reporting reactivity directly to the donors, often resulting in considerable donor anxiety and potential personal expense to reach a confirmatory conclusion. Obviously, in areas of high endemicity, there is a higher predictive value associated with a repeat reactive result and in this situation, simpler confirmatory algorithms can be utilized. Generally though, in developed countries, donors have relatively low prevalences of infection and therefore more complex confirmatory algorithms, like those described in this chapter, are often necessary before notification to the apparently healthy volunteer donor.

The vast majority (90–99%) of repeatedly reactive donations are probably reacting non-specifically in the test system. The principal role of the confirmatory laboratory is to ascertain which of these reactives represent true positivity. Confirmatory laboratory personnel are/must be highly skilled in the performance of numerous assays and in their interpretations.

Principles of confirmatory testing

Key factors to consider are:

(1) The nature of the samples being referred – blood donors consider themselves to be normal healthy individuals, therefore confirmatory algorithms for samples from high-risk patients are not usually appropriate.

(2) The screening strategy being used – generally repeat reactivity is required.

(3) The screening test being used – confirmatory tests should have an advantage on sensitivity.

(4) The prevalence (level of disease) and incidence (rate of new infection) of the particular infection in the screening population.

(5) The use that will be made of confirmatory results, for example confirmed positive donors might, in some organizations, be referred directly to appropriate physicians.

(6) The need to obtain a second sample from confirmed positive donors to confirm donor identity and also confirm infection status.

Donors with no demonstrable reactivity in the initial confirmatory tests are relatively straightforward to deal with, but there are many donors (up to 90–99%) who are ultimately confirmed as having no evidence of infection, but who do demonstrate some spurious reactivity on some assays, reactivity that may be identical to the reactivity seen in early or recently acquired infection or following an atypical immune response to infection. It is clearly essential that the confirmatory testing performed can distinguish between such spurious, and often intermittent, false reactivity and any presentation of reactivity marking true infection.

Effective confirmation requires effective and reliable confirmatory algorithms (Dow, 1999). To be effective, the algorithms must reflect the types of samples referred, the incidence and prevalence of infection in the screening population, the screening strategies adopted and the overall performance of the assays used both for screening and confirmation. To be reliable, the algorithms must be scientifically valid and must not be unduly complex. Confirming true infection in donors entails undertaking sufficient and appropriate tests to demonstrate infection unequivocally. Confirmatory algorithms must therefore be designed to ensure that all confirmed positive donors are identified but that no non-specifically reacting positive donor is classified as 'confirmed positive'. Algorithm design is therefore something that is very specific to the situation, but at the same time has some broad generic components. Some algorithms may be suitable for certain populations but may be totally inappropriate in others.

Ideally, algorithms allow correct conclusions to be reached at an early stage of the confirmatory process. A sequential stepwise approach is needed that provides a useful and appropriate answer at each step, using the minimum level of complexity to give the maximum accuracy and reliability of results.

Whilst in general serological methods should confirm serological screening and nucleic acid testing (NAT) should confirm NAT screening, there are many instances where serology can confirm infection in NAT reactive samples and vice versa.

It is also important for reference laboratory staff to identify unusual test reactivities that may best be resolved by immediately

Transfusion Microbiology, eds John A. J. Barbara, Fiona A. M. Regan and Marcela C. Contreras. Published by Cambridge University Press. © Cambridge University Press 2008.

obtaining a fresh sample from the donor, who, if in the process of seroconversion in a true infection, will have then developed unambiguous levels of reactivity.

Primary level confirmatory tests

Most confirmatory algorithms will have an initial level using alternative highly specific EIAs of comparable or greater sensitivity than the primary screening assay. Negative results would be reported (and eventually allow actual re-entry of the donor), whilst reactivity in one or both assays will undoubtedly lead to second level tests.

Ideally, the choice of alternative EIAs will utilize kits that include different source materials (to minimize the possibility of cross reactivity) and use different EIA principles (indirect, competitive, capture or sandwich) (Dow, 2000). (Please refer to Chapter 11.) Tests are regularly reviewed by the confirmatory laboratories. These laboratories are expected to continually assess new alternate assays and have a controlled process for altering algorithms by substitution or addition of new assays.

Secondary level confirmatory tests

The costs of secondary level confirmatory tests are considerable, but good algorithms should filter the number of referrals to those donations that are expected to confirm positive. Such tests will include neutralization tests to confirm antigen reactivity (e.g. HBsAg) and immunoblots to reveal the spectrum of antibody reactivity. A positive result at this stage should lead to counselling of the particular donor, collection of a second confirmatory sample (to confirm donor identity and also infection status) and making arrangements for referral to an appropriate specialist for further management, with the donor's agreement. (Please refer to Chapter 23.)

However, it has to be accepted that no matter how good the algorithm is there will always be a population of donors, albeit small, who cannot be confirmed as either clearly positive or negative. In a donor population where there is a specific selection process, and with ambiguous reactivity, no clinical history and therefore the presumption of health in the donor, a follow-up sample in three to six months becomes even more important.

In cases where the donor is highly likely not to be infected, but where there is a significant pattern of reactivity that does not change over an extended period of time it may be that the donor simply can no longer be considered suitable to donate. In cases where there is a less significant pattern which again does not change or gradually disappears over time, then it could be considered quite reasonable to reinstate the donor, assuming that the donor was not reactive in the screening test used.

Tertiary level confirmatory tests

Tertiary level tests will seldom be absolutely necessary but can be supplemental to the confirmatory investigation.

An example is the use of HCV NAT in testing confirmed anti-HCV positive donors. Such a result can be helpful in determining whether priority should be given to donor referral to a gastroenterologist.

Confirmatory algorithms

Each microbiological marker is treated separately, as it is unusual for a donation to be reactive in more than one screening assay. Example generic algorithms are shown to help illustrate the principles. Confirmatory laboratories are constantly striving to improve the reliability and predictability of their algorithms in order to ensure accurate results. Thus, these laboratories will replace less sensitive and specific assays with newer, better assays.

Hepatitis B

Please refer back to Chapter 1.

An example of a HBsAg confirmatory algorithm is shown in Figure 12.1. This shows an algorithm for specimens originally screened using a dedicated blood screening analyzer. Reference testing would be based upon alternative microplate EIAs with specific neutralization. Anti-HBc tests may be performed on all referrals. An HBsAg negative, anti-HBc positive, result may be seen in some populations and therefore including anti-HBc in the primary level of the algorithm may generate problems (Grob et al., 2000).

Once a confirmed HBsAg neutralization test has been obtained, testing for HBeAg/anti-HBe and anti-HBc IgM can be of considerable help in advising the donor of his/her infectivity state. A low level HBsAg confirmed positive, anti-HBc negative, result (in the absence of HBe markers) would indicate possible recent hepatitis B vaccination (Dow et al., 2002; Salker et al., 2001) or early acute hepatitis B infection. In this situation use of HBV PCR may be useful – HBV DNA negative indicating probable recent vaccination and HBV DNA positive indicating early acute HBV infection. A history should be sought from the donor.

Hepatitis C

Antibody (anti-hepatitis C virus)

Please refer back to Chapter 1.

An example of an algorithm for anti-HCV confirmation is shown in Figure 12.2. The choice of alternate EIAs can best be illustrated by determining the percentage of referred reactive samples (e.g. by PRISM) that are reactive by an alternate EIA and are eventually confirmed positive (see Table 12.1). The use of alternative assays may be restricted by the assays available in different countries, depending upon licensing and intellectual property agreements. Additionally, this is further complicated when HCV Ag/Ab assays are used. In this situation the confirmation must include an antigen component in at least one assay. Whether one, two or even three alternative assays are used depends upon the performance of the screening assay, the prevalence of HCV and the predictivness of the alternate assays.

Recombinant immunoblot assay-3 (see Figure 12.3) has been referred to as the 'gold standard' confirmatory assay for anti-HCV

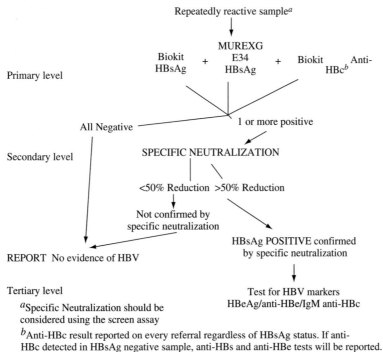

Figure 12.1 Algorithm for HBV confirmatory testing.

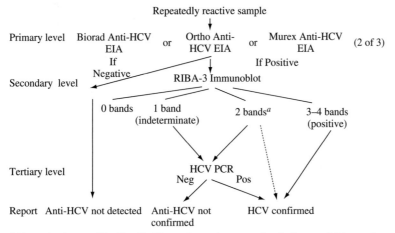

Figure 12.2 Algorithm for HCV confirmatory testing.

(Dow *et al.*, 1996). Unfortunately, this immunoblot is not entirely specific. Around 0.5 to 5% of screen negative samples will exhibit a line on this assay (Kitchen and Tucker, 1995). The experience with this assay has demonstrated that samples with two bands should not be considered diagnostic unless there is clear reactivity in alternate EIAs or HCV RNA is detected. Most immunoblots have some interpretation problems if the results are not looked at in the context of the other confirmatory results. Using the manufacturer's protocols without due consideration may lead to over-interpretation, for example, samples exhibiting a 2+ intensity band or reactive in two bands (even from the same region) are often deemed to be positive. In general experience has shown that

in the case of HCV confirmation, to avoid incorrect conclusions a more conservative minimum interpretation criterion would be evidence of reactivity to at least two bands *from different regions* of the HCV genome in addition to reactivity in alternative EIAs.

Hepatitis C virus NAT will not confirm antibody, but will confirm HCV infectivity and therefore may add to the final report in some cases. It should be remembered that 20–30% of confirmed anti-HCV positive donors will be HCV NAT negative. Hepatitis C virus serotype or genotype testing can be useful to determine whether an HCV positive donor is likely to benefit from antiviral therapy, but is costly and generally not available with transfusion services.

Table 12.1 Anti-HCV preliminary level strategies to filter 296 prism HCV reactive samples of which 32 confirmed positives were detected by all 3 assays.

Strategy	Assay		
One Alternate EIA	Murex	Ortho	Biorad
296	80	93	108
	(40%)	(34%)	(29%)
Two Alternate EIA	Murex/Ortho	Murex/Biorad	Biorad/Ortho
296	52	56	74
	(61%)	(575%)	(32%)
Three Alternate EIA	Murex/Ortho/Biorad		
296	43		
	(74%)		

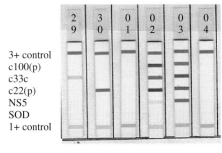

Figure 12.3 RIBA-3 HCV immunoblot

29 indeterminate

30 indeterminate

01 negative

02 positive

03 positive control

04 negative control.

(See colour plate section).

Hepatitis C virus ribonucleic acid

The confirmation of seronegative HCV NAT reactivity can be quite involved. Ideally, the reference laboratory should have an alternative HCV NAT test at its disposal. If screening laboratories utilize different technologies the exchange of sample may also provide independent confirmation.

Hepatitis C virus antigen serological assays have been reported to be almost as sensitive as HCV NAT (Courouce *et al.*, 2000; Lee *et al.*, 2001) but have limited use in confirmation (Dow *et al.*, 2004). In the latter circumstance, obtaining a follow-up sample from the donor can demonstrate development of HCV antibodies, thus confirming HCV infection.

Human immunodeficiency virus

Please refer back to Chapter 4.

Figure 12.4 shows an example of an HIV confirmatory algorithm. At the primary level, two alternative HIV combi (HIV Ag/Ab) assays provide the first filter. If either test is reactive, a second line of confirmation would ideally determine the activity present (anti HIV-1, anti HIV-2 or p24 antigen) based upon more discrete and specific tests. Anti-HIV-1 activity would be confirmed using HIV Western blot (see Figure 12.5), anti-HIV-2 using an HIV-2 Western blot and p24 antigen activity using a neutralization test.

In the scenario where HIV antigen tests are reactive, neutralization tests should be performed, but are not always reliable. In this particular situation, if Western blot fails to confirm, then HIV-NAT could provide additional data. Human immunodeficiency virus genotyping can provide important epidemiological information that may help in assessing the potential need for modification to donor deferral criteria, and in determining the possible mode of HIV acquisition.

Syphilis

Please refer back to Chapter 7.

Figure 12.6 shows a typical syphilis confirmatory algorithm. Many blood services use *Treponema pallidum* haemagglutination assays (TPHA) to screen blood donors. Therefore, the use of two EIA assays (sandwich, indirect or individual capture) at confirmatory laboratories ensures an independent means of confirmation, ruling out cross-reacting erythrocyte antibodies. If either EIA is reactive, TPHA titre, VDRL, specific IgM and blots (Figure 12.7) should be performed to determine the infection status of the individual. VDRL titre and an IgM EIA are important to identify recent (probably untreated) infection which requires prompt management.

Human T-cell lymphotropic virus

Please refer back to Chapter 4.

In general, anti-HTLV assays demonstrate good specifity and therefore the reactive rates are relatively low. Primary level confirmatory testing may be performed using alternate EIAs, followed by secondary level immunoblotting (Figure 12.8). This is generally sufficient. Most HTLV screening assays now incorporate HTLV-II components in addition to the usual HTLV-I antigens. Additionally the immunoblot assays commercially available can differentiate between HTLV-I and HTLV-II infections by utilizing specific protein bands derived from the envelope region (gp46) of the genome.

Importantly, HTLV immunoblots, unlike HIV and HCV immunoblots, do not suffer from significant numbers of indeterminate spurious results. Donors exhibiting persistent indeterminate results can be tested by HTLV NAT to determine if they are truly infected but few are expected to be positive.

Inconclusive and indeterminate results

Although only a small proportion of referred samples will require a more detailed secondary examination and possibly some additional testing, these samples are the ones that require a significant amount of resources to try to clarify their status. These samples have already demonstrated reactivity in a range of assays

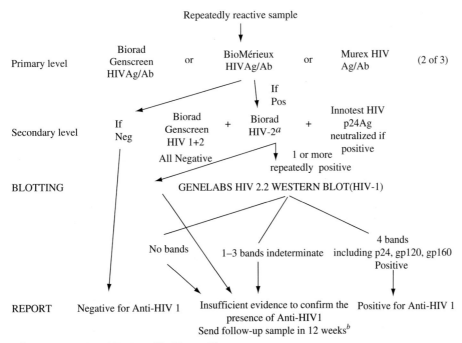

Figure 12.4 Algorithm for HIV confirmatory testing.

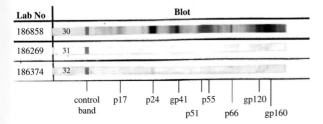

Figure 12.5 HIV Western blot (Genelabs HIV 2.2)
strip 30 confirmed positive
strip 31 negative
strip 32 indeterminate (p24).
(See colour plate section).

assay, reactivity in just a single assay may indeed indicate the presence of low level analyte, indicating an early, or even possibly a late resolving, infection. A follow-up sample taken after a few weeks will elucidate and confirm the situation. However, where a similar situation occurs with an assay that is not particularly sensitive or indeed is known to have limited specificity, or where the results are variable with little if any consistency, then such a result should be considered in a different way, more likely to be due to non-specific reactivity rather than reflecting true, but low level, infection. In either situation, only a certain level of information can be obtained from testing the index sample. Additional useful information can only come from a further sample taken a few weeks later.

and they may now demonstrate additional false reactivity that can significantly complicate investigations and be harder to resolve.

The range of such problem results is considerable but can be broken down into three broad groups of problems:

- Disparate EIA results
- Spurious blot/line assay bands
- Atypical overall patterns.

Disparate EIA results

All EIAs have defined levels of sensitivity and specificity. It is therefore expected that some assays will be slightly more sensitive and some more specific. Where it is known that an assay has a higher sensitivity and consistent results are obtained with the

Spurious blot/line assay bands

This is probably the most common situation when performing blots and line assays on low-risk donor samples. The advantage of the blot/line assay can be negated if its limitations are not fully understood. Blot/line patterns are generally clearly positive when testing samples from truly infected individuals, but when testing samples from uninfected individuals, either those that are reactive or those that are non-reactive on certain screening assays, sometimes one, two or even three bands/lines may appear because of cross-reactivity or other factors that result in specific or non-specific binding of antibodies to the immobilized proteins. Interpretation of blot/line assays is difficult in such situations, with a tendency to over interpret. For such samples, where the primary EIA results are consistent and in good agreement,

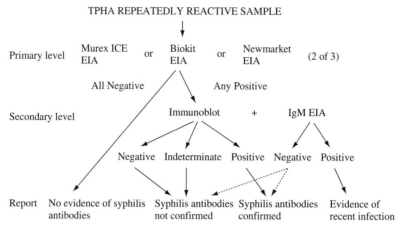

Figure 12.6 Algorithm for syphilis confirmation.

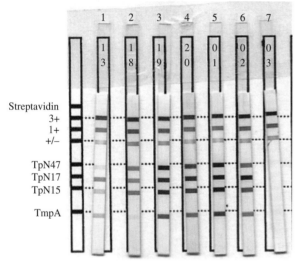

Figure 12.7 Syphilis immunoblot (INNOLIA)
strips 13 to 02 confirmed positive
strip 03 negative. (See colour plate section).

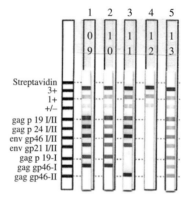

Figure 12.8 HTLV immunoblot (INNOLIA)
strips 09 and 10 confirmed HTLV-I
strip 11 confirmed HTLV-II.
strip 12 negative
strip 13 positive control.

there is a greater probability that the blot results are significant. Where the EIA results are clearly inconsistent the blot results need extreme caution in their interpretation.

In general, blot/line assays are not techniques that should be used early on in any investigation; their use is more effective and less prone to confounding conclusions if used in a more restricted way as the final investigations in any algorithm. This may not always be possible if suitable alternative techniques/assays are not available, for example in the case of HCV where the number and variety of serological tests available is very limited.

Atypical overall patterns

Atypical overall patterns are common. Although most are non-specific, within this group there are going to be some samples from donors who are truly infected. This group of samples are those that demonstrate reactivity, but the overall pattern is not

clear and does not fit any expected pattern for the particular marker under investigation. These samples are problematical. It can be very hard to determine the true status of donors who give such results, as there is often no clear dividing line between specific, but atypical reactivity reflecting true infection, and non-specific reactivity in a number of assays, which does not reflect infection. Indeed when testing seroconversion panels it is very easy to demonstrate that particular patterns of non-specific reactivity seen in some samples from non-infected individuals can resemble those seen early in infection. In addition, seroreversion can also result in atypical patterns. For example, it is very likely that many cases of long past acute HCV infection where seroreversion has occurred would not be detected on testing of a single donor sample. The results would resemble the non-specific reactivity seen in many non-infected donors. Only detailed history taking and the testing of previous (archived) samples would identify that those donors had been infected previously with HCV, but even then, may not if infection had occurred and resolved prior to the individual becoming an active donor. In blood screening and confirmatory testing, HCV is still the most problematical infectious agent, followed by HIV, syphilis, HBV and HTLV.

A further confounding issue when interpreting confirmatory results is that of non-specific reactivity concurrent with specific reactivity. Although cases of non-specific reactivity in acute or chronically infected donors are rare, examples of non-specific reactivity in donors who may have previously been infected but who have now cleared their infection are more common. For example, donors with resolving or resolved HBV infection have been identified with concurrent non-specific reactivity in HBsAg assays, giving a picture of HBsAg in the presence of high titre anti-HBs.

Causes of non-specific reactivity

Understanding the types and causes of non-specific reactivity is essential when performing confirmatory testing. Non-specific reactivity can be divided into three broad groups:

- Reactivity that is associated with a particular sample or one or two sequential samples only
- Reactivity that persists from sample to sample
- Reactivity associated with fresh samples only.

Unfortunately, these groupings are not clean divisions and there is significant overlap between them. They do, however, enable the basic differences and causes to be considered and enable the confirmatory algorithms to be developed accordingly.

Reactivity that is associated with a particular sample, or one or two sequential samples only

Transient reactivity is the most common presentation of the non-specific reactivity seen in screen reactive donor samples. This reactivity presents as clear reactivity, most commonly in some, but not all assays, may be seen in one sample or possibly persists for a few months, but which then disappears completely. The reasons for this are numerous, but centre on the appearance of a specific, potentially identifiable, antibody, which, however, is not specific for the particular infectious agent under investigation. People are constantly exposed to a wide range of stimuli to the immune system and there is a constant production of antibodies to a wide range of antigens, most of which rise in titre for a short while and then fall away. Some of these antibodies may closely resemble the specific antibodies that an assay detects, sufficiently closely to cross-react in the assay. As the levels of these antibodies then fall, the cross-reaction disappears. A frequently cited cause of transient increases in non-specific reactivity in low-risk populations is that of mass vaccination programmes, for example 'flu' vaccinations in adults. This transient reactivity is relatively simple to deal with as it disappears and generally does not return. Donor status can easily be confirmed and donors reinstated.

Reactivity that persists from sample to sample

Reactivity persisting from sample to sample can usually be considered to be inherent to the donor. This reactivity is most often due to the presence of specific antibodies in the donor, not specific to the infectious agent under investigation, but specific to a component or components of the assay(s). These specific antibodies are generally either anti-species, common examples are anti-mouse and anti-horse, or antibodies against components of the cloning and expression systems used in the production of the recombinant antigen used, common examples being antibodies to *Escherichia coli* or *Saccharomyces cervisae*. Anti-species antibodies are not uncommon in healthy individuals and, if present, they can react with core components of assays. Many antibodies used are of animal origin; diluents and coating buffers use animal albumin or serum products. Microbial antibodies are also common, often with more variable titres than species antibodies, and where present may cross-react with residual recombinant vector protein. Many recombinant antigens are produced with some vector sequences still attached. There are many good reasons for this (stability, tertiary and quaternary structure, etc.), but this can then lead to cross-reactions with microbial antibodies present in some samples. Such reactivity is generally at high level and is persistent, and is thus problematical with several assays. The problems can be resolved by careful choice of screening assay, avoiding those containing the specific species-derived materials.

Reactivity associated with fresh samples only

Some samples demonstrate non-specific reactivity that only appears when fresh samples are tested. In rare cases, reactivity which disappears following simple refrigeration occurs in samples. However, most samples tested by transfusion services have been stored at 4°C for at least a short period. More commonly, non-specific reactivity is seen which disappears after freeze/thawing the sample. There are many potential substances/factors which can cause this, but in these cases one freeze/thaw cycle is sufficient to remove the reactivity. Additionally, similar situations may be seen with plasma and serum samples, in general plasma samples being more problematical than serum.

The use of additional samples

There are occasions when the index donor sample no longer yields useful information. At this point no more testing of the index sample should be performed; the only option is to test a further sample from the donor. This may either be a fresh 'follow-up' sample or an archive sample if available. Depending upon the results obtained and donor history, archive samples (if available), can be more useful than follow-up samples. One common situation is the finding of strong non-specific screen reactivity in an existing donor, generally following a change of screening assay. Testing of archive samples can show that the reactivity has been present for some while, very often present in all the previous donations, and helps to validate the confirmatory findings. On the other hand, in cases of suspected early infection, a subsequent sample taken 4–6 weeks later usually resolves whether the donor is truly infected or not.

Donor re-admission

It must be remembered that the expectation in any properly organized blood transfusion service functioning in a country with a developed health care system, is that the donations collected are from appropriately selected healthy, uninfected donors. The donor selection procedures followed are designed to act as a primary filter to identify and defer donors who may carry a risk of infection. Thus, the majority of reactive donations would not normally be expected to indicate true infection, they would be non-specifically reactive. The positive predictive value of screening tests is of greater importance when the rate of true infection is very close to that found on screening blood donors. For instance, where the repeat reactive rate for a test (e.g. HBsAg or anti-HCV) is 1 in 1000 , and the rate of true infection in new donors is around 1 in 1000, then the positive predictive value is around 100%. However, if the rate of true infection in established donors is 1 in 50 000, then the positive predictive value will be around 2% (i.e. 98% of repeat reactivity is false). There are many reasons for non-specific reactivity in sample populations, and indeed the test itself may show consistent reactivity with certain samples, but whatever the reactivity is due to, it does not reflect true infection. Once it has been established that the majority of screen reactive donations are not from truly infected donors, it becomes easier to understand how the confirmatory testing becomes a donor management exercise. Most transfusion services in developed countries have finally realized that it is far more efficient and effective to develop pools of regular donors rather than continually trying to recruit new donors. Obviously, there is always a turnover of donors, but recruitment is expensive, whereas building and maintaining a solid base of regular donors is cheaper and a far better basis for a sustainable service; established donors are also inherently less of a microbial risk (please refer to Chapter 25). Thus, the loss of donors due to false reactivity on the primary screening tests is something that blood services wish to minimize. However, even using highly specific assays there will always be a small percentage of donors who are falsely reactive. On their own the numbers are small, but they accumulate on a day-by-day basis, and, if no action is taken, the donor base can slowly, but inexorably, be eroded. In addition, the loss of a single donor can result in the annual loss of up to three or four donations, depending upon donation interval. Confirmatory testing of reactive donors is therefore a means by which falsely reactive donors can be identified and, using an appropriate strategy, be reinstated.

In the UK, confirmed infection occurs in less than 5% of the donor samples referred to the transfusion microbiology reference laboratories. Although a number of donors demonstrate repeatable non-specific reactivity across a number of different assays and have to be deferred, more than 90% of referrals are from donors who are not infected, have clearly demonstrable non-specific reactivity with the screening assays and who could, and in most cases can, be reinstated.

Unconfirmed donors have several means of re-entry onto the donor panel. The underlying logic of a minimum deferral period of 12 weeks before re-entry can be considered, should allow a normal individual (below the threshold of confirmatory testing at the time of the index donation) to develop detectable markers of infection if truly infected. Samples from previously repeatedly reactive but unconfirmed donors are often subject to fewer confirmatory tests than for their original index donations. The current UK Blood Transfusion Guidelines (2002) give instructions on algorithms to be used for donor re-entry. After 12 weeks, a 'flagged' unconfirmed donor could be resampled and, if found negative by mandatory markers at the testing centre and also negative for the original specificity by the reference laboratory, then they could be reinstated. If the testing centre still records a reactive result and if the reference laboratory records a negative conclusion, an alternative assay of equivalent sensitivity (please refer to Chapter 17, Quality in Screening) may be used on subsequent donations to allow donor re-entry. In practice this means donations known to be reactive against screening assay (A) will be transported to a site using an alternative screening assay (B) for donation testing. For this system to operate efficiently it is essential that secure mechanisms are in place to ensure alternative assays are suitably sensitive, and that index donations are barred from such testing. A national (or nationally coordinated) blood service makes such a policy possible.

Confirmatory laboratories should consider a minimal approach to allow maximal donor re-entry if the donor has now been found negative at the testing centre. Choice of assay can be crucial. Assays should be selected based on the minimum amount of cross-reactivity.

The UK Blood Services Microbiology Kit Evaluation Groups oversee the evaluations of new candidate microbiological donor screening assays. The groups are responsible for assessing the suitability of candidate assays (as well as currently used assays) for donor screening. Sensitivity evaluations are performed using at least 200 (often as many as 500) examples of samples positive for the marker (covering appropriate genotypes prevalent in the general population). This will include 'tricky' or weak positive samples that poorer 'unapproved' assays are known to fail to detect. Specificity is assessed by testing at least 2000 routine donor samples (serum and plasma). Only those assays that clearly demonstrate equal or better sensitivity than the existing screening assays are considered worthy of approval. Acceptable specificity is also determined by comparison with existing screening assays. It is important that both sensitivity and at least part of the specificity evaluations are conducted with the same batch of tests. An additional batch of tests should also be included in the evaluation to ascertain whether there is any significant batch to batch variation. (Please refer to Chapter 17.)

Hepatitis B virus

This involves a primary level screen of two sensitive HBsAg assays plus anti-HBc test-if all are negative, consider reinstatement.

Hepatitis C virus

Test using a primary level screen of two alternative HCV Ab or Ag/Ab combi-assays.

Human immunodeficiency virus

A primary level screen of two alternative HIV Ag/Ab combi-assays.

Syphilis

A primary level screen of two alternative syphilis assays (ideally EIAs).

Unfortunately, some (probably) uninfected donors persistently react in more than one screening assay and are unable to follow the option of an alternative screening assay. Blood services are best to advise such donors of their false reactivity in current screening tests and defer them until such time as the particular donor screening assay is replaced.

Importance of confirmatory testing of blood donors, beyond the safety of individual donations

There are a number of reasons why confirmatory testing is important to any blood transfusion service (BTS), some very clear and others less so. Primarily, confirmatory testing is concerned with donor management, but in addition, the health of the donor, always a concern to any BTS, must be considered. In low incidence/prevalence countries most screen reactive blood donors are not truly infected, and the potential wastage of donors due to non-specific reactivity is high. Although most screening assays currently available from the major global diagnostic companies are of high quality, with good sensitivity and specificity, to ensure high sensitivity there may still be some compromise with specificity. Thus, non-specific reactions need to be identified and the donors handled (managed) appropriately, and donors confirmed to be truly infected also need to be identified and treated appropriately. These donors need to be counselled and referred for the appropriate clinical care. Partners and close contacts also need to be protected, and this can be extended to the protection of the general population. There is therefore a public health aspect to the confirmatory process. Also, there is further benefit to the blood transfusion service itself in the monitoring of infection rates in blood donors, as well as the better understanding of donor behaviour and risk activities. Knowing and understanding infection rates in blood donors enables a service to ensure that its screening strategies are up-to-date and effective. For example, a rising incidence of infection theoretically increases the probability of donation from recently infected donors and this may require additional testing or other change in strategy to ensure that such early infections are picked up on screening. Conversely, a falling or low incidence and a low prevalence of infection may also require a change in strategy, for example the use of pooled testing rather than individual donations.

Interview of such donors can provide information on the possible routes of infection and the effectiveness of the donor selection procedures; why did the donor donate, did they already know that they were infected, should they have been excluded by the donor exclusion criteria in use? Such information helps to understand disease patterns in 'healthy individuals', can be used to improve the selection criteria themselves and help to ensure that the way in which the criteria are presented to both staff and donors is clear and that the exclusion process works effectively.

Effective confirmation of screening reactivity is thus an essential activity for any high quality transfusion service, serving to help in the management of donors and in the understanding of blood-borne diseases in the donor population.

Further functions of the transfusion microbiology reference laboratory

In addition to the core activities of confirmation and donor re-admission, transfusion microbiology laboratories are involved in other functions.

The transfusion microbiology reference laboratories are expected to conduct the investigation of any suspected case of transfusion-transmitted infection (TTI). In addition to utilizing 'state of the art' serological tests, NAT may be necessary on archive samples from implicated donations and/or follow up samples from implicated donors. The outcomes of these investigations are reported to the appropriate medical personnel and to the relevant haemovigilance scheme, for example SHOT. It is noteworthy that reference laboratories often perform tests for extra products/services provided by blood services, for example for tissue services (bones, heart valves), for stem cells, cord blood, etc which do not fit comfortably into the primary screening procedures. Trials of new products or services invariably utilize the reference laboratories to ensure patients show no development of blood-borne virus markers.

Transfusion microbiology reference laboratories have to ensure they keep abreast of all test developments. Therefore, these laboratories often assist in the development of commercial kits and undertake evaluations of both developmental and launched commercial kits.

Over the past decade the UK reference laboratories have also become heavily involved in either the provision of batch pre-acceptance panels to donor testing sites, or alternatively the actual batch pre-acceptance testing performed on a centralized basis (Newham and Kitchen, 2003).

The provision of accurate microbiological testing statistics and donor epidemiology is often facilitated through the laboratories. Lastly, the laboratories provide advice to many within and outwith their organizations.

Conclusion

Confirmatory testing in transfusion microbiology is a very specific and specialized activity which has significant value to any transfusion service. The recovery of screen reactive, but confirmed negative donors is now critical to transfusion services who find it increasingly more difficult to recruit and retain new donors. There is, however, a fine balance between retaining an active donor panel and ensuring the ultimate safety of the blood supply. The use of well selected confirmatory tests together with skilled interpretation ensures that this safety is not compromised, yet maximizes the volunteer donor base.

Finally, one cannot underestimate the importance of ensuring that counselled donors are indeed truly infected. To get this wrong would cause stress to the donor and could lead to adverse publicity with adverse repercussions to the blood service.

REFERENCES

Allain, J. P., Kitchen, A., Aloysius, S., *et al.* (1996) Safety and efficacy of hepatitis C virus antibody screening of blood donors with two sequential screening assays. *Transfusion*, **36**, 401–5.

Courouce, A. M., Le Marrec, N. and Boucherdeau, F. (2000) Efficacy of HCV core antigen detection during the preseroconversion period. *Transfusion*, **40**, 1198–1202.

Dow, B. C. (1999) Microbiology confirmatory tests for blood donors. *Blood Rev*, **13**, 91–104.

Dow, B. C. (2000) 'Noise' in microbiological screening assays. *Transfus Med*, **10**, 97–106.

Dow, B. C., Buchanan, I., Munro, H., *et al.* (1996) Relevance of RIBA-3 supplementary test to HCV PCR positivity and genotypes for HCV confirmation of blood donors. *J Med Virol*, **49**, 132–6.

Dow, B. C., Munro, H., Buchanan, I., *et al.* (2004) Acute hepatitis C virus seroconversion in a Scottish blood donor: HCV antigen is not comparable with HCV nucleic acid amplification technology screening. *Vox Sang*, **86**, 15–20.

Dow, B. C., Munro, H., Ferguson, K., *et al.* (2001) HTLV antibody screening using mini-pools. *Transfus Med*, **11**, 419–22.

Dow, B. C., Yates, P., Galea, G., *et al.* (2002) Hepatitis B vaccinees may be mistaken for confirmed hepatitis B surface antigen-positive blood donors. *Vox Sang*, **82**, 15–17.

Grob, P., Jilg, W., Bornhak, H., *et al.* (2000) Serological pattern 'anti-HBc alone': report on a workshop. *J Med Virol*, **62**, 450–5.

Kitchen, A. D. and Tucker, N. V. (1995) The specificity of anti-HCV supplementary assays. *Vox Sang*, **69**, 100–103.

Lee, S. R., Peterson, J., Niven, P., *et al.* (2001) Efficacy of a hepatitis C virus core antigen enzyme-linked immunosorbent assay for the identification of 'window-phase' blood donations. *Vox Sang*, **80**, 19–23.

Newham, J. A. and Kitchen, A. D. (2003) Lot release of microbiology blood screening kits in the English National Blood Service. *Transfus Med*, **13** (1), 55.

Salker, R., Howell, D. R., Moore, M. C., *et al.* (2001) Early acute hepatitis B infection and hepatitis B vaccination in blood donors. *Transfus Med*, **11**, 463.

UK BTS/NIBSC Joint Professional Advisory Committee (2002) Guidelines for the Blood Transfusion Service. 6th edn. Norwich, The Stationery Office.

13 THE STRATEGY FOR APPLICATIONS OF NUCLEIC ACID TESTING

Paul R. Grant and Richard S. Tedder

Although blood transfusion is appropriately considered a lifesaving procedure it remains, as has been recognized for more than six decades, a procedure which carries risks of transmission of infection from donor to the recipient. These risks are best considered in terms of first, the administration of a (usually) small number of discreet whole blood units, and second, blood components, that is, the practice of blood transfusion, as compared with the replacement of a deficient plasma constituent by a blood product containing material from many, often thousands of donors, which has been purified from a starting plasma pool, that is, the use of a blood product. The essential mantra for transfusion safety remains first, 'know your donor' and second, 'test your donor'. Both are essential for the safety of blood and blood components which remain difficult to subject to terminal product sterilization. For blood products, on the other hand, the operational side of manufacture has led to derogation of 'know your donor' in favour of 'test your donor' and paradoxically it is in this area that the application of nucleic acid testing (NAT) has had most impact. This is perhaps understandable given the non-biological 'amplification' of microbial transmission in blood product usage, whereby a single donor may effectively contaminate and render infectious all products from a pool containing plasma from thousands of otherwise acceptable donors. This is best exemplified by post-transfusion hepatitis in first-time recipients of native blood products.

The first step along the NAT pathway was the acceptance in 1998 by the European Agency for the Evaluation of Medicine (EMEA) of the recommendation by the Committee for Proprietary Medicinal Products (CPMP) to introduce NAT for the hepatitis C virus (HCV) RNA in plasma pools (CPMP/BWP/390/97), which in turn arose through an entirely predictable transmission of HCV by an intravenous immunoglobulin preparation earlier in the decade. This legislature required pre-acceptance testing of pools for HCV RNA and remains the first step in a pathway which has led to the testing of pools for a number of blood-borne viruses, the choice of which varies from country to country. The cost of these endeavours is enormous and, given the ability to apply stringent pathogen reduction and viral inactivation procedures to the final product, has to be of questionable cost-effectiveness. Political pressures and market forces combine to disincline national authorities from examining the essential issue of value for money. The anomaly of this situation would have become less grotesque if the data on NAT could have been used to impact upon the safety of blood and blood component usage. This has only been a relatively recent development with the advent of donor nucleic acid screening in real time. Nevertheless, even where NAT can be applied to routine

transfusion practice, low prevalence countries may elect not to use NAT in view of both recent advances in serological testing, principally combined antigen/antibody assays, and national studies examining the cost of prevention of each single case of a given post-transfusion infection. In practical terms, the identification of an infected donor by NAT implies that the donor will have escaped detection by conventional donor screening using immunologically-based assays. Such donations are widely referred to as being 'window donations'.

For those working in donor screening laboratories, the obliging transmissible agent will have a number of key parameters including a discernable, early and overt clinical illness; overt and invariant epidemiology; a carrier state which is routinely expressed; and finally secure and invariant markers for detection. Casting back over years of experience with that most obliging of agents, hepatitis B (HBV), even this infection fails to fulfil all of these criteria. Furthermore, in the current new philosophy/legislation framework of 'zero risk', new and emerging infections that plague transfusion microbiology include acute viral infections (especially if the frequency of infection is high), which are an altogether more difficult set of transmissible candidates, where the need to control them can be used to justify continuing with the development of NAT procedures. Indeed, in the absence of NAT, testing for such agents would not have been possible as the presence of antibody indicates clearance of the agent. Nevertheless, the questions relevant to NAT must remain 'Can it be achieved?' 'Can it be afforded?' And finally, 'Is it relevant?'

Window-period donations arise when the donation is taken from an infected donor who has not developed serologically detectable markers. The implication is that this will occur early in the incubation period, if the serological test uses antigen detection at a time between the eclipse period, when transmission is not yet possible, and the development of antigenaemia. Not all window-period infections may fall into this category and in theory for any infection, and for HBV in particular, an infected host may remain viraemic after clearance of detectable antigenaemia. Of course, if antibody to hepatitis B core antigen (anti-HBc) were used routinely such infections would be detectable. However, for HIV and HCV the loss of serum antigen coincides with the development of detectable antibody. Clearly, as described elsewhere in this book, the rate of rise or 'burst' of viraemia, also referred to as viral dynamics, will affect how long it will take and how easy it will be to implement NAT and also define the temporal difference between detection by NAT and by antigen testing. Similarly, the rate of decline of both viraemia and antigenaemia in relation to the developing antibody response will define the possible second window of the recovery from acute infection.

These factors are of relevance both to the evolution of markers in those blood-borne viruses which cause carrier states and in the acute infections which resolve spontaneously (in part at least) where the continued existence of circulating virus in the face of antibody becomes a diagnostic problem for transfusion practice.

Putting these considerations aside, the various NAT methods have three component steps in common:

(1) Sample preparation, including viral concentration and nucleic acid extraction
(2) Amplification of the target DNA or RNA
(3) Detection of the amplified product.

Each component requires controlling for sensitivity, specificity and robustness. Sensitivity should be defined against international standards and refer not simply to the 'detection' sensitivity but to the level of genomic input which will be detected at various thresholds, for example thresholds for giving a reaction 50% of the time and thresholds for 95% of the time by probit analysis. In these standardizations it is important to use a relevant matrix for the dispersal of the targets; this is best defined by the analyte which is to be used for testing. Pooled citrate or EDTA plasma are good examples. Similarly, the best target for these studies will match the physicochemical properties of the natural target, usually afforded by high titre plasma of human origin. Though molecularly defined synthetic targets have a powerful attraction they do little to prove the fidelity of a system as they differ widely from the native target and will behave anomalously in different extraction procedures, causing confusion when comparisons are undertaken. Sensitivity studies should also address the stochiometry of the whole assay, in other words plasma input volumes, extract volumes and proportions used for the NAT.

Since in practice the majority of viral NAT undertaken in blood services in high Human Development Index (HDI) countries will generate negative results, it is vitally important that these negative results are shown to be valid. This implies a somewhat different view from that adopted by current manufacturers. Whilst in many manufacturers' kits an internal control (IC) target is used to show that the amplification is functional, the acceptability threshold is set so low as frequently to allow a significant loss of sensitivity and certainly does not control for the sensitivity of the extraction process unless the IC goes into the extraction procedure itself. With the advent of the TaqMan style of homogenous amplification assays, there is more than sufficient precision to allow very careful analysis of the behaviour of the IC as well as the assay as a whole. The requirement for specific (or 'positive') sample identification and accurate software analysis of the assay are also essential components of any NAT protocol. This is addressed by the move to the 'black box' closed system so desired by the diagnostic industry manufacturers, but at the cost of resigning any and all control of such systems to the manufacturer, which is something we should do reluctantly.

Nucleic acid extraction

Turning now to each component, the various extraction methods generally have a viral lysis step in which the protein coat of the virus is disrupted and the nucleic acid is released and rendered available for purification. The viral nucleic acid is then purified by biochemical methods, captured by either sequence specific probe capture methods or non-specific binding of nucleic acids to silica particles or other solid phases. Once the nucleic acid is captured in this way the lysis buffer and other impurities are washed away and the nucleic acid is re-suspended. These steps are routinely performed by robotic sample handling platforms. Amplification is then achieved by one of the several methods that will be discussed later. Typically, these will generate up to a billion-fold amplification of the target nucleic acid sequence, enabling detection of ten or fewer copies of viral nucleic acid in the starting sample. The amplified sequences can then be detected by a variety of methods including colourimetric, chemiluminescent or fluorescent technologies.

Polymerase chain reaction (PCR) amplification

Polymerase chain reaction was the first DNA amplification method devised and is still the most versatile and widely used NAT technique. It was devised by Kary Mullis of Cetus Corporation (Emeryville, CA, USA) (Mullis and Faloona, 1987; Mullis et al., 1986) who received the 1993 Nobel Prize in chemistry in recognition. Polymerase chain reaction was first described for the amplification of the beta globin gene in the diagnosis of sickle cell anaemia (Saiki et al., 1985). The polymerase enzyme was destroyed by the temperature required for denaturation and therefore had to be replaced after each PCR cycle. However, the discovery of a thermostable polymerase enzyme from a bacteria that lives in hot pools, Thermus aquaticus (Taq) allowed the PCR process to be repeated for many cycles without the need to replace the enzyme (Saiki et al., 1988).

Polymerase chain reaction may be used to detect the DNA sequences of viruses directly (Kaneko et al., 1989; Larzul et al., 1988; Ou et al., 1988). However, for detection of RNA viruses such as HCV, a reverse transcription (RT) step must be used (Garson et al., 1990; Murakawa et al., 1988). Reverse transcription of an RNA target is carried out to generate complementary DNA (cDNA) which can then be used as a template for PCR (Kawasaki et al., 1988). For such assays the IC will be RNA rather than DNA in order to control for the RT step.

The main steps of PCR are shown in Figure 13.1. Target DNA or cDNA molecules are denatured into single strands by heating the reaction mixture to around 94 °C; the temperature is then reduced to allow synthetic oligonucleotide primers, complementary to the area of interest, to bind to each of the single-stranded DNA molecules. The temperature is then raised to the optimum for strand extension by Taq polymerase (Mullis and Faloona, 1987). Two such primers, binding to the sense and antisense strands are used to copy the complementary sequence of the target DNA. By cycling the temperature between denaturation, primer annealing and extension steps for 30 or more cycles, a greater than 10^9 fold amplification of the target sequence can be achieved. The amplified sequences (amplicons) can be detected by a number of methods such as visualization with ethidium bromide on an agarose gel, or by using sequence specific probes labelled with radioactive or chemiluminescent

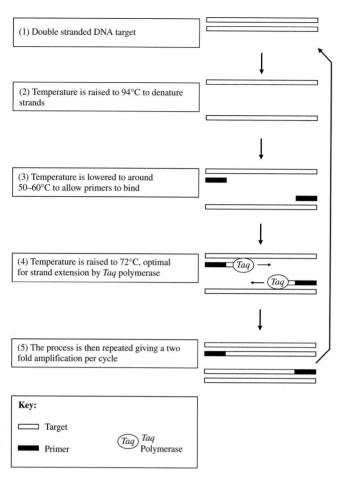

(1) Double stranded DNA target

(2) Temperature is raised to 94°C to denature strands

(3) Temperature is lowered to around 50–60°C to allow primers to bind

(4) Temperature is raised to 72°C, optimal for strand extension by *Taq* polymerase

(5) The process is then repeated giving a two fold amplification per cycle

Key:

☐ Target
■ Primer
(*Taq*) *Taq* Polymerase

Figure 13.1 Polymerase chain reaction (PCR).

tags with enzymes which can catalyse colour change or light production reactions.

Roche Molecular Systems Inc. (Pleasanton, CA, USA) purchased the patent rights to PCR from Cetus in 1991 and has developed commercial assays for the detection or quantification of several viruses in peripheral blood mononuclear cells, plasma or other fluids (Gerken *et al.*, 1998; Long *et al.*, 1998; Sun *et al.*, 1998; Vrielink *et al.*, 1997; Young *et al.*, 1993). Each assay is capable of detecting as few as one to 100 molecules of target DNA or RNA in the processed sample volume, and each uses primers and probes recognizing the conserved sequences of one or more viral genes to ensure the detection of most known variants. In these assays the probes are used to detect solid phase captured amplicons by enzymatic colourimetric or chemiluminescent reactions.

Real-time PCR

Real-time PCR is based on the conventional PCR reaction for the amplification of target molecules; the difference is that the amount of PCR amplicon is measured during the reaction, that is, in real time, rather than at the end of the reaction, achieving a homogenous assay able to amplify and detect in the same tube. There are several methods by which this can be achieved but the best known is TaqMan PCR (Lee *et al.*, 1993).

In a TaqMan PCR the amount of amplicon is measured using a dual fluorescent-labelled oligonucleotide probe. The probe has a fluorescent dye with a different excitation and emission wavelength attached to each end; these dyes are designated reporter and quencher. The excitation wavelength of the quencher is similar to the emission wavelength of the reporter and so when the reporter and quencher are held in close proximity the energy emitted by the reporter is absorbed by the quencher in a process known as fluorescence resonance energy transfer (FRET) (Forster, 1948).

The dual labelled probe is designed so that its melting temperature is higher than that of the two primers. This ensures that when the temperature is reduced between the denaturation and annealing steps of the PCR the probe will bind to the target sequence before the primers. During primer extension the bound dual labelled probe is hydrolysed by the 5′ exonuclease activity of the *Taq* polymerase (Holland *et al.*, 1991). As the dual labelled probe is hydrolysed the reporter and quencher dyes are released and so FRET no longer occurs and the light is emitted by the reporter fluorophore. The dual labelled probe is hydrolysed during each round of PCR and so the fluorescence emitted by the un-quenched reporter increases. The increase in fluorescence at the emission wavelength of the reporter dye is measured after each cycle of PCR and is proportional to the amount of amplicon generated in the reaction. The TaqMan process is shown in Figure 13.2.

A variation called kinetic PCR (kPCR) has also been developed which is based on the intercalation of ethidium bromide or SYBR Green dyes (included in each PCR reaction tube) into the double-stranded DNA that accumulates during each PCR cycle (Higuchi *et al.*, 1993). This results in exponentially increasing fluorescence in the tube that parallels PCR product formation and can be monitored in real time.

The advantage of these systems is that amplification and detection of nucleic acid is fully automated, occurring in a closed tube. There is no need for post-PCR amplicon manipulation, which reduces the time taken for results and minimizes the possibility of contamination of other samples by amplicons.

Transcription mediated amplification (TMA)

Transcription mediated amplification is an isothermal amplification method that is patented by Gen Probe Inc. (San Diego, CA, USA). Viral sequences are captured from plasma by oligonucleotide capture. It uses two enzymes, reverse transcriptase and RNA polymerase to achieve greater than one billion-fold amplification without thermal cycling (McDonough *et al.*, 1998). A primer with an RNA polymerase promoter sequence attached is used to anneal to the RNA template and prime cDNA synthesis with reverse transcriptase. The RNA is then degraded with RNAse H activity to leave a single strand of DNA which includes the promoter sequence. Another primer is then used to generate the complementary strand. The RNA polymerase enzyme generates 100 to 1000 RNA copies from the DNA template which go through the process again (see Figure 13.3).

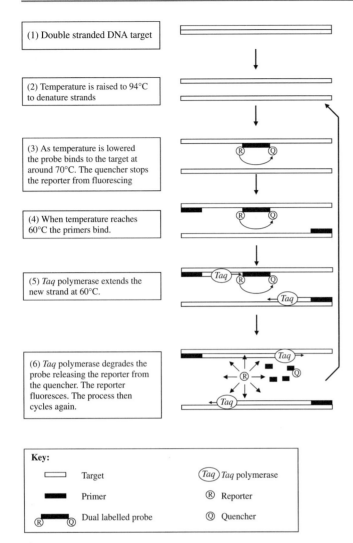

(1) Double stranded DNA target

(2) Temperature is raised to 94°C to denature strands

(3) As temperature is lowered the probe binds to the target at around 70°C. The quencher stops the reporter from fluorescing

(4) When temperature reaches 60°C the primers bind.

(5) *Taq* polymerase extends the new strand at 60°C.

(6) *Taq* polymerase degrades the probe releasing the reporter from the quencher. The reporter fluoresces. The process then cycles again.

Key:

▭	Target	Ⓣaq	*Taq* polymerase
▬	Primer	Ⓡ	Reporter
Ⓡ▬Ⓠ	Dual labelled probe	Ⓠ	Quencher

Figure 13.2 TaqMan assay.

As both enzymes require the same temperature to function, the reaction occurs auto-catalytically under isothermal conditions, with the majority of the amplicon being RNA transcripts.

Nucleic acid sequence based amplification (NASBA)

Another isothermal amplification system, nucleic acid sequence-based amplification (NASBA) is patented by Organon Teknika (Boxtel, the Netherlands) (Compton, 1991; Kievits *et al.*, 1991). NASBA kits are available for HIV-1 and CMV as well as a basic kit that can be adapted to other viruses by the user (Deiman *et al.*, 2002). Nucleic acid sequence-based amplification is not used for blood screening, but the extraction technology which uses the chaotropic salt guanidinium isothiocyanate and silica particles (Boom *et al.*, 1990), may be automated with the NucliSens Extractor (Buul *et al.*, 1998). This extraction method has been used by the blood services of several countries for in-house developed NAT methods as the NucliSens Extractor will extract any DNA or RNA from up to 2 ml sample volume, which can then be used in a variety of amplification and detection methods.

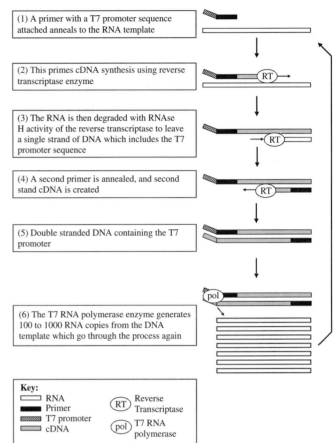

(1) A primer with a T7 promoter sequence attached anneals to the RNA template

(2) This primes cDNA synthesis using reverse transcriptase enzyme

(3) The RNA is then degraded with RNAse H activity of the reverse transcriptase to leave a single strand of DNA which includes the T7 promoter sequence

(4) A second primer is annealed, and second stand cDNA is created

(5) Double stranded DNA containing the T7 promoter

(6) The T7 RNA polymerase enzyme generates 100 to 1000 RNA copies from the DNA template which go through the process again

Key:

▭	RNA	RT	Reverse Transcriptase
▬	Primer		
▨	T7 promoter	pol	T7 RNA polymerase
▭	cDNA		

Figure 13.3 Transcription mediated amplification (TMA).

Ligase chain reaction (LCR)

Ligase chain reaction uses two pairs of probes complementary to each other that hybridize adjacent to each other on each strand of the target nucleic acid sequence. Each pair is then joined together by the nick repair mechanism of DNA ligase (Wu and Wallace, 1989). After denaturation both the single stranded target sequence and the ligated probes can act as a template for annealing of further probe sets. Using a thermostable DNA ligase, the reaction can be cycled as in PCR to denature the strands and re-anneal the probes (see Figure 13.4), achieving exponential amplification (Barany, 1991).

Abbott Laboratories (Abbott Park, IL, USA) currently markets LCR assays for *HIV1 RNA, Chlamydia trachomatis* and *Neisseria gonorrhoeae* using an automated instrument, the LCx analyser, but at present LCR is not used for screening for blood-borne pathogens.

Branched DNA signal amplification assay (bDNA)

The branched DNA (bDNA) technique was developed by Chiron Corporation (Emeryville, CA, USA), but this technology is now owned and marketed by Bayer Corporation (Emeryville, CA, USA). The bDNA assays are based on the principle of amplifying the signal from annealed DNA probes through the formation

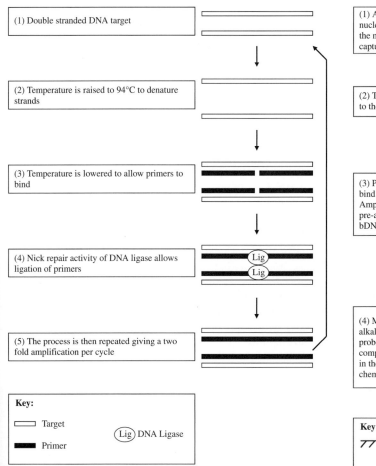

(1) Double stranded DNA target

(2) Temperature is raised to 94°C to denature strands

(3) Temperature is lowered to allow primers to bind

(4) Nick repair activity of DNA ligase allows ligation of primers

(5) The process is then repeated giving a two fold amplification per cycle

Key:

☐ Target

(Lig) DNA Ligase

■ Primer

Figure 13.4 Ligase chain reaction (LCR).

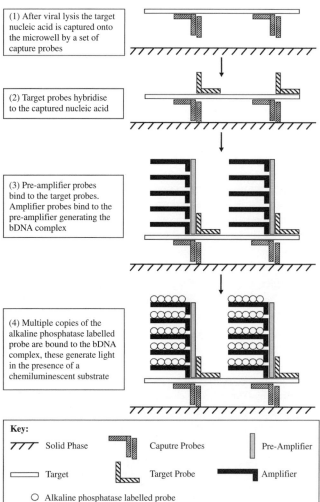

(1) After viral lysis the target nucleic acid is captured onto the microwell by a set of capture probes

(2) Target probes hybridise to the captured nucleic acid

(3) Pre-amplifier probes bind to the target probes. Amplifier probes bind to the pre-amplifier generating the bDNA complex

(4) Multiple copies of the alkaline phosphatase labelled probe are bound to the bDNA complex, these generate light in the presence of a chemiluminescent substrate

Key:

⁄⁄⁄ Solid Phase

☐ Target

○ Alkaline phosphatase labelled probe

Caputre Probes

Target Probe

Pre-Amplifier

Amplifier

Figure 13.5 Branched DNA signal amplification.

of a controlled network of synthetic oligonucleotide probes, rather than amplification of the target nucleic acid (Urdea, 1997). The method involves a series of hybridizations of target probes specific to the sequence of interest (e.g. the HIV assay uses 39 binding sites to *gag* or *pol* sequences) (see Figure 13.5). A subset of the probes mediate capture of the target molecules to a capture oligo modified microplate, while the second set bind to target as well as to a bDNA amplifier molecule. The bDNA amplifier is a chemically synthesized structure containing 45 copies of a sequence that can bind a labelled probe, but just one copy of a sequence that binds to target probes. Multiple copies of bDNA amplifiers are bound to the probe-target complex on the microplate to incorporate up to 1800 labelled (alkaline phosphatase) probes on each target sequence. A chemiluminescent substrate, dioxetane, is used to generate a visible light signal that is quantified with the use of a luminometer.

Control of contamination

Because NAT methods are so sensitive, they are susceptible to contamination, causing false-positive results. There are two forms of contamination, sample to sample and amplicon contamination. Sample to sample contamination occurs when a positive sample containing very high target copy numbers is processed next to negative samples and their contamination is caused by splashes or aerosols. The contaminated sample will contain native target indistinguishable from street virus and can be difficult to identify. Samples with very low viral titres tested at the same time as samples with very high titres can lead to suspicion of contamination, but this can only be proven by sequencing linkage studies.

Amplicon contamination is caused by PCR products (amplicons) getting into the samples or reagents of subsequent assay runs. Strict procedures are employed by laboratories to avoid contamination (Kwok and Higuchi, 1989), the most important of which is physical separation of the pre- and post-amplification areas. Ideally these take place in different rooms and with a strict one way flow from pre- to post-amplification. The post-amplification area should have dedicated equipment, so that racks, pipettes, notebooks, etc. contaminated with amplicons are not used in the pre-amplification area. Separate laboratory coats and gloves should be used, dedicated to each area, and never worn in or carried from post- to pre-amplification areas. Contaminating DNA may be removed by 10% bleach (Prince and Andrus, 1992) or UV irradiation (Sarkar and Sommer, 1990).

An enzymatic method to avoid amplicon contamination may also be employed (Longo *et al.*, 1990). If the dNTP uracil is used in the PCR reaction in place of thymidine, then the amplicons generated will be susceptible to enzymatic degradation by Uracil N-Glycosilase (UNG). The UNG enzyme is added to the PCR reaction and degrades any amplicons from previous reactions without degrading the target DNA which will contain thymidine.

Use of controls

There are many types of controls used in NAT assays. As described above, positive controls are known positive native material dispersed in an appropriate matrix which is extracted, amplified and detected with the clinical samples. This control ensures that the overall process has worked correctly and controls for a major failure at any step. This is particularly important when the samples are expected to be negative. Positive controls are generally at a medium to high level which would be expected to be easily detected. However, they may also be at a low level to check that the sensitivity of the assay was adequate. It is also conventional to have a GO/NO GO run control which should be stronger than the PROBIT 95% level and which has to be detected for the assay run to be valid.

Monitoring controls may also be used which are set at or below the limit of detection of the assay so that they will have around a 50% chance of being detected. These monitoring controls have no use in the validation of an individual assay run, but over time their percentage detection rate may reveal changes in the sensitivity of the assay caused by different batches of reagents or different equipment.

In a quantitative assay a dilution series of a positive control can be used to generate a calibration curve against which any positive clinical samples may be checked to determine titre.

Several international NAT standards have been introduced which can be used to calibrate secondary standards (Holmes *et al.*, 2001; Saldanha *et al.*, 1999; 2001; 2002; 2005). These international standards are positive materials that have been quantified by laboratories around the world and assigned an arbitrary unit. This contrasts with the early stages of NAT usage when each individual laboratory or assay manufacturer had quantified their own assay standards in different ways, so that the same sample tested by different methods could give different results in target copies per ml. Assay sensitivities were also quoted in copies per ml and varied depending on how the standards used had been quantified. With the availability of international NAT standards, individual secondary standards can be calibrated in international units per ml and will be the same throughout the world (Davis *et al.*, 2003; Saldanha *et al.*, 2000).

Run controls are used in quantitative assays to ensure that the calibration curve is accurate and that clinical samples are assigned the correct viral load. Run controls are pre-aliquotted in large numbers so that the same material is run in every assay, and should give the same result each time; any variation in the viral load calculated for the run controls indicates a problem with that particular assay run.

Negative controls are known negative material which is extracted, amplified and detected with the clinical samples. These controls are a contamination check; they should be negative and so if they are found to be positive they indicate contamination of the assay, and any other positive samples on the run must be regarded with suspicion.

ICs consist of a different target or artificial construct which is introduced with the samples or into one of the reagents during the extraction process. They are extracted and amplified with the clinical samples but have a different detector so that they may be distinguished from the target-positive samples. These controls act to detect any inhibition in individual samples, or the failure of the NAT process for any particular sample. Some clinical samples contain substances that will inhibit the NAT process (Abu al-Soud and Radstrom, 2001), giving a falsely negative result. However, if an internal control is used this will also be negative, showing that the sample was inhibitory. The internal control will also show up an individual extraction or amplification failure, which affects only a single sample and not the whole assay. In qualitative assays the internal control is usually at a very low level so that it does not compete for reagents with the target. A very strongly positive target sample may make the internal control negative, but this does not invalidate the result as the internal control is only intended to validate that negative results really are target negative.

Sample pooling

Please refer to Chapter 14.

For NAT of blood donations destined for transfusion, samples can be pooled together prior to testing. This allows blood centres to screen a large number of blood donations with relatively few tests and in a timely fashion, despite minimizing the numbers of costly testing laboratories. This is practical because the number of positive samples is expected to be low, therefore the number of positive sample pools is few. The two widely used commercial NAT systems, Roche AmpliScreen (Sun *et al.*, 1999) and Gen-Probe/Chiron Procleix (McDonough *et al.*, 1998), use pools of 24 and 16 blood samples per test respectively. Larger pool sizes of 48 or 96 samples per pool can also be used with in-house assays or modified Roche AMPLICOR/AmpliScreen assays (Beld *et al.*, 2000; Grant *et al.*, 2002; Jarvis *et al.*, 2000; Meng *et al.*, 2001; Roth *et al.*, 1999).

When a pool is found to be positive, sub-pools or the individual donations within the pool must be tested to determine which one was positive and to release the rest. For the smaller pools this can be done by testing sub-pools, for example a reactive minipool of 24 donations would be split into four sub-pools of six donations each; these would be tested and finally the six donations in the reactive sub-pool would be tested. For larger pools such as those of 48 or 96 donations, 'cross pools' are used. If the donations are arranged in a 96 sample 8 by 12 format matrix, then each row and each column can be pooled, giving 12 cross-pools of 8 donations each, and 8 cross-pools of 12 donations each. These row and column pools are tested and where the positive row and positive column pools intersect, the positive donation is found (Mortimer, 1997). The same principle can be used for 48 sample minipools with an eight by six matrix.

The problem with pooling is that the greater the number of samples pooled for each test, the smaller the volume of each individual sample that is tested, resulting in a reduction in the sensitivity of detection. This reduction in sensitivity has led to samples with very low level of virus being undetected by pooled NAT (Delwart *et al.*, 2004; Najioullah *et al.*, 2004; Schuttler *et al.*, 2000), which may have been detected if they had been tested by single NAT. The cost of testing would obviously be increased with a move from mini-pool testing (MP NAT) to individual donation (ID NAT) testing, not only due to the increased number of tests required but also the increased infrastructure to enable this testing in a timely manner. With the cost to benefit ratio of NAT being questionable for MP NAT, it would be even more so for ID NAT, as the residual risk after mini-pool NAT is so low. The risk also depends on how likely any given sample is to have a very low level of virus which would not be detected by mini-pool testing but which would be detected by individual testing. This likelihood depends on the virus in question. For example, HIV-1 and especially HCV both rise quickly to high levels of virus during replication and therefore the 'window' between MP NAT and ID NAT may only be a few hours. For HBV it may be longer as this virus is often present in low levels and has a slower 'burst'. One virus for which ID NAT has been feasible is West Nile virus. Since this is often present at low titres it has been shown to have been undetected in some instances by MP NAT (Macedo *et al.*, 2004). Because of the epidemic nature of WNV it has been possible to generate a strict set of criteria for switching from MP NAT to ID NAT in particular blood centres for a few weeks when the virus has a very high incidence (Custer *et al.*, 2004).

Multiplexing

In order to reduce the work burden on the testing laboratory there are increasing moves to provide assays which are able to test for and signal the presence of more than one molecular species in a single tube. Not surprisingly, in transfusion practice this often includes the three major blood-borne viruses of HBV, HCV and HIV. With the possibility of up to five fluorophores with discrete wavelengths, it is possible to assay for three targets in one tube with each being individually identified. However, for transfusion practice it is sufficient to have a common fluorophore since any positive reaction will lead to rejection of the donation and identification of the particular blood-borne virus can be subsequently undertaken. In the diagnostic laboratory the problem of cross competition and resulting loss of sensitivity for one species in the face of a strong signal of another species remains a potential problem.

The most widely used commercial blood screening multiplex NAT assay in use is the Procleix TMA assay for HIV-1 and HCV (Giachetti *et al.*, 2002). This assay was developed by Gen-Probe Inc., the inventors of TMA, and is distributed by Chiron Corporation. Either HIV-1 or HCV RNA is extracted from the plasma of individual or pooled donations by a magnetic particle assisted oligo capture method. Amplification of either target is then achieved by TMA. As the assay does not distinguish between HIV and HCV, a reactive sample has to be re-tested by individual assays for HIV and HCV to determine which virus(es) the reactive sample contained.

Another multiplex system developed by Roche Diagnostics in Japan for use by the Japanese Red Cross (AMPLINAT MPX assay) can test for HCV, HBV and HIV simultaneously in pools of 50 blood donations (Meng *et al.*, 2001; Mine *et al.*, 2003). As with the TMA multiplex test, discriminatory assays must be used to find which virus is present in any reactive sample.

Conclusion

Nucleic acid testing blood screening systems, which initially targeted HCV, but now more generally detect blood-borne viruses, have been successfully implemented in blood banks and blood services around the world. Current NAT systems generally screen pooled donations, with pool sizes ranging from 16 to 96 donations. At present, yields for HCV NAT positive, antibody negative donations range from approximately one per million donations in Europe to four per million in the USA (Busch *et al.*, 2005). For HIV-1 the yield is lower, at approximately 0.3 positive donations per million worldwide. However, even with NAT there is still a risk of infected blood being transfused at the end of the eclipse period, early in the burst phase, when the viral levels are below that which can be detected by NAT although the blood may still be infectious. This possibility is heightened by the large inoculum which a transfusion presents. It is questionable whether striving for even more sensitivity in the tests used in order to detect infections even earlier can be justified. By switching from MP-NAT to ID-NAT the effective sensitivity will be increased (at dimishing yield), but the costs would also rise not only with the number of tests required but also for the increased infrastructure, raising yet further the already enormous costs for each quality adjusted life year gained by screening activity. With the current technology, many testing sites would simply be unable to NAT screen every blood donation on an individual basis. More cost-effective benefit may be gained by introducing tests for other target modalities such as combined antibody/antigen assays and by considering judicious use of multivariate single tube testing afforded by multiplex NAT assays. Either way, NAT must not be allowed to further distort health economics.

REFERENCES

Abu al-Soud, W. and Radstrom, P. (2001) Purification and characterization of PCR-inhibitory components in blood cells. *J Clin Microbiol*, **39**, 85–93.

Barany, F. (1991) Genetic disease detection and DNA amplification using cloned thermostable ligase. *Proc Natl Acad Sci USA*, **88**, 189–93.

Beld, M., Habibuw, M. R., Rebers, S. P., *et al.* (2000) Evaluation of automated RNA-extraction technology and a qualitative HCV assay for sensitivity and detection of HCV RNA in pool-screening systems. *Transfusion*, **40**, 575–9.

Boom, R., Sol, C. J., Salimans, M. M., *et al.* (1990) Rapid and simple method for purification of nucleic acids. *J Clin Microbiol*, **28**, 495–503.

Busch, M. P., Stramer, S. L., Strong, D. M., *et al.* (2005) International Forum: 2. *Vox Sang*, **88**, 298–301.

Buul, C. van, Cuypers, H., Lelie, P., *et al.* (1998) The NucliSens (TM) Extractor for automated nucleic acid isolation. *Infusionstherapie und Transfusionsmedizin*, **25**, 147–51.

Compton, J. (1991) Nucleic acid sequence-based amplification. *Nature*, **350**, 91–2.

Custer, B., Tomasulo, P. A., Murphy, E. L., *et al.* (2004) Triggers for switching from minipool testing by nucleic acid technology to individual-donation nucleic acid testing for West Nile virus: analysis of 2003 data to inform 2004 decision making. *Transfusion*, 44, 1547–54.

Davis, C., Heath, A., Best, S., *et al.* (2003) Calibration of HIV-1 working reagents for nucleic acid amplification techniques against the 1st international standard for HIV-1 RNA. *J Virol Methods*, 107, 37–44.

Deiman, B., van Aarle, P. and Sillekens, P. (2002) Characteristics and applications of nucleic acid sequence-based amplification (NASBA). *Mol Biotechnol*, 20, 163–79.

Delwart, E.L., Kalmin, N.D., Jones, T.S., *et al.* (2004) First report of human immunodeficiency virus transmission via an RNA-screened blood donation. *Vox Sang*, 86, 171–7.

Forster, T. (1948) Zwischenmolekulare Energiewanderung und Fluoreszenz. *Annals of Physics*, 2, 55–75.

Garson, J.A., Tedder, R.S., Briggs, M., *et al.* (1990) Detection of hepatitis C viral sequences in blood donations by 'nested' polymerase chain reaction and prediction of infectivity. *Lancet*, 335, 1419–22.

Gerken, G., Gomes, J., Lampertico, P., *et al.* (1998) Clinical evaluation and applications of the Amplicor HBV Monitor test, a quantitative HBV DNA PCR assay. *J Virol Methods*, 74, 155–65.

Giachetti, C., Linnen, J.M., Kolk, D.P., *et al.* (2002) Highly sensitive multiplex assay for detection of human immunodeficiency virus type 1 and hepatitis C virus RNA. *Journal of Clinical Microbiology*, 40, 2408–19.

Grant, P.R., Sims, C.M., Krieg-Schneider, F., *et al.* (2002) Automated screening of blood donations for hepatitis C virus RNA using the Qiagen BioRobot 9604 and the Roche COBAS HCV Amplicor assay. *Vox Sang*, 82, 169–76.

Higuchi, R., Fockler, C., Dollinger, G., *et al.* (1993) Kinetic PCR analysis: real-time monitoring of DNA amplification reactions. *Biotechnology (NY)*, 11, 1026–30.

Holland, P.M., Abramson, R.D., Watson, R., *et al.* (1991) Detection of specific polymerase chain reaction product by utilizing the 5′–3′ exonuclease activity of thermus aquaticus DNA polymerase. *Proc Natl Acad Sci USA*, 88, 7276–80.

Holmes, H., Davis, C., Heath, A., *et al.* (2001) An international collaborative study to establish the first international standard for HIV-1 RNA for use in nucleic acid-based techniques. *J Virol Methods*, 92, 141–50.

Jarvis, L., Cleland, A., Simmonds, P., *et al.* (2000) Screening blood donations for hepatitis C virus by polymerase chain reaction (letter). *Vox Sang*, 78, 57–8.

Kaneko, S., Miller, R.H., Feinstone, S.M., *et al.* (1989) Detection of serum hepatitis B virus DNA in patients with chronic hepatitis using the polymerase chain reaction assay. *Proc Natl Acad Sci USA*, 86, 312–6.

Kawasaki, E.S., Clark, S.S., Coyne, M.Y., *et al.* (1988) Diagnosis of chronic myeloid and acute lymphocytic leukemias by detection of leukemia-specific mRNA sequences amplified in vitro. *Proc Natl Acad Sci USA*, 85, 5698–702.

Kievits, T., van Gemen, B., van Strijp, D., *et al.* (1991) NASBA isothermal enzymatic in vitro nucleic acid amplification optimized for the diagnosis of HIV-1 infection. *J Virol Methods*, 35, 273–86.

Kwok, S. and Higuchi, R. (1989) Avoiding false positives with PCR. *Nature*, 339, 237–8.

Larzul, D., Guigue, F., Sninsky, J.J., *et al.* (1988) Detection of hepatitis B virus sequences in serum by using in vitro enzymatic amplification. *J Virol Methods*, 20, 227–37.

Lee, L.G., Connell, C.R. and Bloch, W. (1993) Allelic discrimination by nick-translation PCR with fluorogenic probes. *Nucleic Acids Res*, 21, 3761–6.

Long, C.M., Drew, L., Miner, R., *et al.* (1998) Detection of cytomegalovirus in plasma and cerebrospinal fluid specimens from human immunodeficiency virus-infected patients by the AMPLICOR CMV test. *J Clin Microbiol*, 36, 2434–8.

Longo, M.C., Berninger, M.S. and Hartley, J.L. (1990) Use of uracil DNA glycosylase to control carry-over contamination in polymerase chain reactions. *Gene*, 93, 125–8.

Macedo, D.O., Beecham, B.D., Montgomery, S.P., *et al.* (2004) West Nile virus blood transfusion-related infection despite nucleic acid testing. *Transfusion*, 44, 1695–9.

McDonough, S.H., Giachetti, C., Yang, Y., *et al.* (1998) High throughput assay for the simultaneous or separate detection of human immunodeficiency virus (HIV) and hepatitis type C virus (HCV). *Infusionstherapie und Transfusionsmedizin*, 25, 164–9.

Meng, Q., Wong, C., Rangachari, A., *et al.* (2001) Automated multiplex assay system for simultaneous detection of hepatitis B virus DNA, hepatitis C virus RNA, and human immunodeficiency virus type 1 RNA. *J Clin Microbiol*, 39, 2937–45.

Mine, H., Emura, H., Miyamoto, M., *et al.* (2003) High throughput screening of 16 million serologically negative blood donors for hepatitis B virus, hepatitis C virus and human immunodeficiency virus type-1 by nucleic acid amplification testing with specific and sensitive multiplex reagent in Japan. *J Virol Methods*, 112, 145–51.

Mortimer, J. (1997) Intersecting pools and their potential application in testing donated blood for viral genomes. *Vox Sanguinis*, 73, 93–6.

Mullis, K., Faloona, F., Scharf, S., *et al.* (1986) Specific enzymatic amplification of DNA in vitro: the polymerase chain reaction. *Cold Spring Harb Symp Quant Biol*, 51 Pt 1, 263–73.

Mullis, K.B. and Faloona, F.A. (1987) Specific synthesis of DNA in vitro via a polymerase-catalyzed chain reaction. *Methods Enzymol*, 155, 335–50.

Murakawa, G.J., Zaia, J.A., Spallone, P.A., *et al.* (1988) Direct detection of HIV-1 RNA from AIDS and ARC patient samples. *DNA*, 7, 287–95.

Najioullah, F., Barlet, V., Renaudier, P., *et al.* (2004) Failure and success of HIV tests for the prevention of HIV-1 transmission by blood and tissue donations. *J Med Virol*, 73, 347–9.

Ou, C.Y., Kwok, S., Mitchell, S.W., *et al.* (1988) DNA amplification for direct detection of HIV-1 in DNA of peripheral blood mononuclear cells. *Science*, 239, 295–7.

Prince, A.M. and Andrus, L. (1992) PCR: how to kill unwanted DNA. *Biotechniques*, 12, 358–60.

Roth, W.K., Weber, M. and Seifried, E. (1999) Feasibility and efficacy of routine PCR screening of blood donations for hepatitis C virus, hepatitis B virus, and HIV-1 in a blood-bank setting. *Lancet*, 353, 359–63.

Saiki, R.K., Gelfand, D.H., Stoffel, S., *et al.* (1988) Primer-directed enzymatic amplification of DNA with a thermostable DNA polymerase. *Science*, 239, 487–91.

Saiki, R.K., Scharf, S., Faloona, F., *et al.* (1985) Enzymatic amplification of beta-globin genomic sequences and restriction site analysis for diagnosis of sickle cell anemia. *Science*, 230, 1350–4.

Saldanha, J., Gerlich, W., Lelie, N., *et al.* (2001) An international collaborative study to establish a World Health Organization international standard for hepatitis B virus DNA nucleic acid amplification techniques. *Vox Sang*, 80, 63–71.

Saldanha, J., Heath, A., Lelie, N., *et al.* (2000) Calibration of HCV working reagents for NAT assays against the HCV international standard. The Collaborative Study Group. *Vox Sang*, 78, 217–24.

Saldanha, J., Heath, A., Lelie, N., *et al.* (2005) A World Health Organization international standard for hepatitis A virus RNA nucleic acid amplification technology assays. *Vox Sang*, 89, 52–8.

Saldanha, J., Lelie, N. and Heath, A. (1999) Establishment of the first international standard for nucleic acid amplification technology (NAT) assays for HCV RNA. WHO Collaborative Study Group. *Vox Sang*, 76, 149–58.

Saldanha, J., Lelie, N., Yu, M.W., *et al.* (2002) Establishment of the first World Health Organization international standard for human parvovirus B19 DNA nucleic acid amplification techniques. *Vox Sang*, 82, 24–31.

Sarkar, G. and Sommer, S.S. (1990) Shedding light on PCR contamination. *Nature*, 343, 27.

Schuttler, C.G., Caspari, G., Jursch, C.A., *et al.* (2000) Hepatitis C virus transmission by a blood donation negative in nucleic acid amplification tests for viral RNA (letter). *Lancet*, 355, 41–2.

Sun, R., Ku, J., Jayakar, H., *et al.* (1998) Ultrasensitive reverse transcription-PCR assay for quantitation of human immunodeficiency virus type 1 RNA in plasma. *J Clin Microbiol*, 36, 2964–9.

Sun, R., Schilling, W., Jayakar, H., *et al.* (1999) Simultaneous extraction of hepatitis C virus (HCV), hepatitis B virus, and HIV-1 from plasma and detection of HCV RNA by a reverse transcriptase-polymerase chain reaction assay designed for screening pooled units of donated blood. *Transfusion*, **39**, 1111–9.

Urdea, M. S. (1997) Synthesis and characterization of branched DNA (bDNA) for the direct and quantitative detection of CMV, HBV, HCV, and HIV. *Clin Chem*, **39**, 725–6.

Vrielink, H., Zaaijer, H. L., Cuypers, H. T., *et al.* (1997) Evaluation of a new HTLV-I/II polymerase chain reaction. *Vox Sang*, **72**, 144–7.

Wu, D. Y. and Wallace, R. B. (1989) The ligation amplification reaction (LAR) – amplification of specific DNA sequences using sequential rounds of template–dependent ligation. *Genomics*, **4**, 560–9.

Young, K. K., Resnick, R. M. and Myers, T. W. (1993) Detection of hepatitis C virus RNA by a combined reverse transcription-polymerase chain reaction assay. *J Clin Microbiol*, **31**, 882–6.

14 NUCLEIC ACID TESTING: GENERAL VIEW

W. Kurt Roth

Background

Despite thorough measures to select donors and sensitive EIA testing of blood donations, some transmissions of the most relevant transfusion-transmitted viruses, HCV, HIV and HBV, occurred. Even plasma products manufactured from large plasma pools that were additionally inactivated were not completely virus safe. In 1995, plasma fractionation companies were the first to introduce NAT of their plasma pools for fractionation prior to inactivation procedures (see Chapter 20). Although all donors were screened by antibody and antigen tests a high proportion of production pools consisting of several thousand litres of plasma were contaminated with HCV (Scheiblauer et al., 1996). Contamination by HIV and HBV was less frequent. However, those companies introduced NAT not only for HCV, but also for HIV and HBV, as an in-process quality control and to cover any potential failures in good manufacturing process. The quality requirements for HCV NAT were set at a detection limit of 100 IU/ml for pools of source plasma used for plasma-derived medicinal products. These requirements have been in force since 1 July 1999 (CPMP/BWP/390/1997; European Pharmacopoeia 2001). As soon as it was shown that NAT was feasible as a quality control measure in the plasma industry it fuelled discussions on whether these new techniques could also be applied to routine blood donor testing.

The plasma fractionation companies started to perform diagnostic testing on mini-pools of donor samples containing between 500 and 1000 individual samples, prior to carrying out pooling of several thousand donations for fractionation, to avoid the loss of whole pools of plasma in the event of a positive HCV RNA test. These mini-pools of donor samples were tested by NAT in most cases after enrichment of viruses by centrifugation, to concentrate any viruses which might be present, then compensate for the concentration effect. Reactive mini-pools were resolved by (sometimes) complex algorithms to identify the positive donation which could then be removed prior to pooling the plasma for fractionation. This led to a measurable decrease in viral risk of plasma products by reducing the viral load of production pools prior to inactivation. Inactivation procedures were no longer challenged by the occasional high viral loads associated with 'window-period (acute) infections'.

Although highly desirable, NAT could not be so readily applied to testing of blood components such as red cells and platelets. In contrast to plasma products, blood components have a shorter shelf life and must be freshly transfused. There is no possibility for a prolonged storage procedure during which labour intensive NAT and pool resolution procedures are performed. Since virus inactivation procedures cannot yet be applied to all cellular components it could be argued that it would not be appropriate to set a specific minimum threshold for viral detection, although in practice, most countries comply with a working standard. Sensitivity must be as high as possible, which argues in principle against pooled testing procedures and favours individual donor testing strategies. These considerations led to the general opinion in the mid-1990s that NAT for cellular components was technically not feasible and costs were not affordable. This opinion was also shared by the leading diagnostic companies including Roche and Chiron. It was stated at several meetings with the German Red Cross in 1996 that technology was not mature enough to introduce NAT either on individual donors or pooled samples in the near future. These companies were not prepared to accept the offer of the German Red Cross for a joint development of testing procedures for routine donor testing in blood bank settings. In Germany, despite the lack of support from the patent holders for HCV and PCR, blood transfusion services had already started to adapt NAT for screening of cellular components. The major criteria to be fulfilled in blood donor NAT can easily be summarized as having to achieve:

- The highest sensitivity
- The highest specificity
- The highest robustness
- The highest validity
- The highest throughput
- The highest speed possible.

HCV, HIV, HBV

It is well known that for the major relevant transfusion-transmissible viruses, HCV, HIV and HBV, minute amounts of viral particles are sufficient to infect a recipient after intravenous administration, for example by blood contaminated needlesticks. This clearly indicates that NAT cannot reduce viral transmission risk to zero. Sample volumes for NAT are presently restricted to <1 ml and usually range from 50–200 μl. The volumes of transfused components are at least 100-fold greater, resulting in a sufficient dose to cause infection even at a level of less than one virus particle/ml in the component. Therefore, reduction of the residual risk of transmission by NAT is strongly dependent on the specific biological and epidemiological characteristics of each individual virus tested for. It has been shown in several studies that the major residual transfusion risk arises from donations taken from recently infected donors in the pre-seroconversion ('window') phase of infection. The longer this diagnostic window lasts before detectable antibodies are present in the bloodstream,

Transfusion Microbiology, eds John A. J. Barbara, Fiona A. M. Regan and Marcela C. Contreras. Published by Cambridge University Press. © Cambridge University Press 2008.

the higher the residual risk for a specific virus. A second major determinant for this residual risk is the incidence of an infection which varies widely between viruses and countries according to the specific epidemiological situation. According to these parameters HCV and HBV present the highest risks, followed by HIV.

Moreover, additional criteria are relevant when considering the potential yield of NAT. The higher the viral load in the plasma, and the higher the replication rate of the virus, the easier it is for NAT to positively identify donors in the pre-seroconversion window phase and to shorten the window phase substantially, especially if testing pools of samples. During the window phase, the high viral titres of HCV of 10^6–10^9 particles/ml plasma and a rapid viral burst due to a viral doubling time of <1 day, as well as the long time to seroconversion (see Figure 14.1), made HCV the best candidate for application of NAT to identify the highest yield of contaminated donations, even when samples were pooled (Garcia-Retortillo *et al.*, 2002; Nubling *et al.*, 2002). Therefore, in many countries NAT started with HCV. Efficient, but nevertheless convenient detection limits for HCV were determined by investigating seroconversion panels which were usually derived from plasma donors who gave frequent donations during their pre-seroconversion

window period. Applying a sensitivity of 5000 IU/ml (10 000 geq/ml) was sufficient to reduce the window period on average by 40–60 days (see Figure 14.1). This moderate detection limit was first set by the Paul-Ehrlich-Institut, the German Authority for Blood Affairs (Paul-Ehrlich-Institut, 1998a). It is accepted worldwide and is sufficient to allow testing of pooled samples in minipools of a moderate size without specific enrichment procedures (Paul-Ehrlich-Institut, 1998b). Applying standard commercial HCV assays and extraction methods allows mini-pools to include up to 48 samples. For larger mini-pools, specific enrichment procedures are required, especially if additional viruses such as HIV or HBV are to be detected. These principles are reflected in the different pooling and testing strategies in different countries.

Pool size for NAT

German Transfusion Services (Roth and Siefried, 2002) were the first to introduce NAT for cellular components, rather than for final pool testing for fractionated products, utilizing pools of 96 donor samples and virus enrichment procedures which are still in place (see Figure 14.2). Pools of greater than 96 samples were used as early as 1995 (e.g. by Immuno Baxter). Other countries followed and most of them reduced the pool size to 48 or less in order to omit enrichment by centrifugation which is complicated and cannot be automated. Moreover, logistics are also easier and the blood supply is less affected in the event of reactive pools either due to truly positive samples or contamination.

However, the latter approach, which omits centrifugation, is more costly and does not allow the introduction of HIV and HBV testing as easily as if larger pools are tested after enrichment of viruses by centrifugation. Thus, in Germany, parallel testing of HCV, HIV and HBV was established from the very beginning and the feasibility and efficacy of this procedure was demonstrated (Roth *et al.*, 1999).

Without virus enrichment, pool size must be reduced further if NAT for HBV and HIV is to be established. Costs will increase and for bigger blood banks technical limits will quickly be reached. Present sensitivity limits suggested for HIV are 10 000 IU/ml of

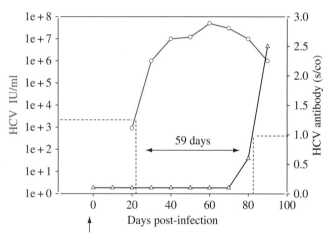

Figure 14.1 Diagnostic window period for hepatitis C.

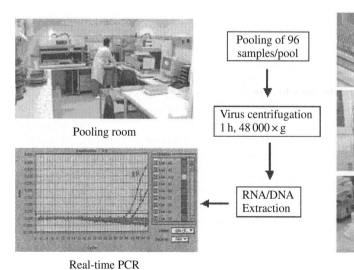

Pooling room

Real-time PCR

Pooling of 96 samples/pool

Virus centrifugation 1 h, 48 000 × g

RNA/DNA Extraction

Figure 14.2 Implementation of PCR in Frankfurt Transfusion Service. (See colour plate section).

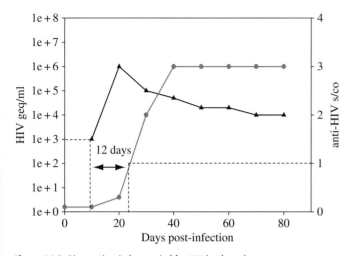

Figure 14.3 Diagnostic window period for HIV (real case).

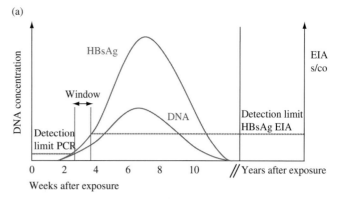

Figure 14.4 (a) Acute resolving HBV infection.

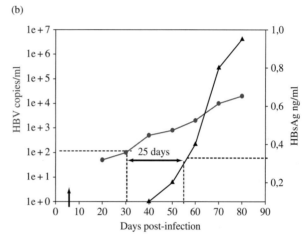

Figure 14.4 (b) Results of qPCR and HBeAg (Enr.-PCR) in a donor before seroconversion for hepatitis B.

individual donor plasma corresponding to 5,000 geq/ml (Paul-Ehrlich-Institut, 2003). This detection limit was shown to be sufficient to detect the majority of HIV pre-seroconverters. However, as shown recently in France and the USA, samples may be missed (Assal *et al.*, 2003; Delwart *et al.*, 2004) due to a copy number below the detection limit. Nevertheless, it was shown in the USA (FDA, 2001; Stramer, 2002) that NAT is superior to the p24 antigen test with respect to sensitivity. In Germany, only one HIV pre-seroconverting sample was missed by NAT of more than 20 million donations since 1997. Three additional transmissions of HIV by blood products have occurred in Germany since 1995; all were caused by donations that were not NAT tested. Retrospectively, it was shown that HIV NAT would have been detected in these donations had NAT been in place at the time. Therefore the Paul-Ehrlich-Institut (Paul-Ehrlich-Institut, 2001) mandated HIV NAT for Germany, starting from May 2004. One major reason for delaying mandatory HIV NAT in Germany was the already widespread voluntary introduction of HIV NAT and the low quality performance of most in-house procedures in proficiency testing.

In contrast to HCV, the window period for HIV is much shorter and the viral doubling rate, as well as viral load, is much lower during the window phase (see Figure 14.3). Therefore, more sensitive tests were required for HIV NAT and reliable commercial tests took time to develop.

For HBV the situation is even more difficult. In contrast to HCV and HIV, routine testing for HBV is based on HBsAg testing rather than detection of antibody. Due to the high sensitivity of HBsAg testing (as few as 1000 viral copies/ml (100–1000 IU) of plasma can be readily detected by the most sensitive assays) the gap between NAT and HBsAg detection of infection is short (see Figure 14.4a and b). This significantly decreases the yield of extra positives detected by NAT as long as NAT sensitivity is not substantially higher than that of antigen testing. The replication rate of HBV is very low, with a doubling time of 2.6 days and therefore it takes appreciable time for detectable levels of virus to be present in the plasma. However, components from low titre HBV positives are highly infectious since only a few particles are sufficient to induce infection. It could be shown that pooled PCR

in conjunction with virus enrichment is sensitive enough (as low as 300 geq/ml (50–100 IU/ml) of donor plasma) to detect a substantial number of donors in the pre-seroconversion phase, who were not detected by HBsAg testing (Biswas *et al.*, 2003; Roth *et al.*, 2002). Pre-seroconverters (e.g. HBsAg negative individuals were identified with short term peak viral loads of <2000 geq/ml who had very delayed seroconversion six months later (see Figure 14.5a and b). In addition, chronic low-level carriers were identified who were constantly HBsAg negative, anti-HBc positive with a viral load of as few as ten copies/ml donor plasma. Such donors who were anti-HBs negative could infect recipients, as demonstrated in look-back procedures. They were identified by pooled PCR only because of fluctuating viral levels, which incidentally reached the detection limit of pooled PCR at the time of donation (see Figure 14.6). There are also HBsAg negative, pooled PCR negative, anti-HBc positive and anti-HBs positive blood donors with a similar low viraemia of a maximum of 10 geq/ml. The infectivity of these donors is not yet established. Such low level viraemic donors would not be detectable even by highly sensitive single donation NAT (see Figure 14.6). Only if the individual sample size were increased to 1 ml and all the extracted nucleic acids introduced into the PCR would there be some

(a)

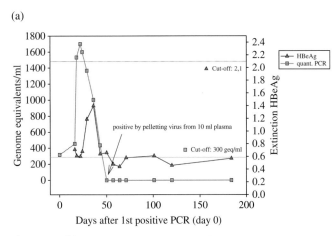

Figure 14.5 (a) HBV Pre-seroconverter qPCR + HBeAg.

(b)

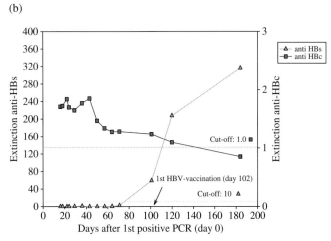

Figure 14.5 (b) HBV pre-seroconverter: anti-HBc + anti-HBs.

Donor	Mini-pool PCR	ID-PCR	Enr.-PCR	Anti HBs	Anti HBc
1	–	–	+ + + +	93.7	+
2	–	–	+ + + – –	213.1	+
3	–	–	+ + + –	>1000	+
4	–	–	+ + +	–	+
5	–	–	+ + +	>1000	+
6	–	–	+ + +	26	+
7	–	–	+ + +	11	+
8	–	–	+ + +	1000	+
9	–	–	+ + +	102	+
10	–	–	+ + +	7.3	+
11	–	–	+ + +	3.3	+
12	–	–	+ + +	26.7	+
13	–	–	+ + +	41	+
14	–	+	nd	–	+

1144 anti-HBc positive first-time donors were tested by pool, individual donation (ID) and 9.6 ml enrichment PCR.

Figure 14.6 HBsAg negative chronic (occult) carrier.

chance of detecting HBV in donors. Presently, we are far from establishing such testing scenarios, which would also require separate extraction and testing procedures for HBV in parallel with routine NAT for the other viruses. Although some additional yield could be expected, the tremendous cost would further reduce the benefit of NAT.

Hepatitis A (HAV) and parvovirus B19

Hepatitis A virus and parvovirus B19 are highly resistant to common inactivation procedures and frequently contaminate blood products manufactured from plasma pools. Therefore the plasma fractionation industry drove the introduction of routine HAV and parvovirus B19 NAT as an internal quality control measure. In addition, German Blood Transfusion Services were encouraged to test their blood donations for HAV and parvovirus B19 in order to avoid preparing and testing diagnostic mini-pools prior to pooling of the source plasma. Only the production pool itself need then be tested as an internal quality control measure.

The sensitivity required for HAV NAT is as high as possible, (Fields, 1996) because HAV viral load is low in plasma, reaching a maximum of 10^4 virus particles/ml donor plasma. Viraemia is short-lived and usually accompanied by an alanine amino transferase (ALT) elevation. Antibodies are neutralizing and induce lifelong immunity. Therefore, antibody testing offered no safety increment to blood transfusion services. In developed countries antibody prevalence increases with age and reaches 40–80% in blood donors (Mauser-Bunschoten et al., 1995; Prodinger, 1994; Thierfelder, 1999). In essence, there is no real necessity to screen blood components. Viral incidence is low in developed countries and was shown to be as low as 1 in 1 million for German blood donors after routine screening by NAT. Those identified by NAT also showed high ALT elevations. In countries where ALT and NAT are not performed, those donations would be missed. Detection limits of HAV NAT should lie below 1000 geq/ml (≈1,000 IU/ml) in order to reliably pick up positive donors. With NAT screening in place, ALT testing could definitely be discontinued as was decided recently for Germany (Arbeitskreis Blut, 2003). Alanine amino transferase as a surrogate marker would then not detect infections by hepatotropic viruses that are not detected by NAT.

In contrast to HAV, the incidence of parvovirus B19 is very high, reaching rates of 1 in 1000 among blood donors when applying sensitive NAT with detection limits of 1000 IU/ml of donor plasma (Roth et al., 2005). In intervals of 5–10 years, epidemics may occur where the incidence of NAT positives may rise to one in a few hundred (own observation) (see Figure 14.7b). It was shown that source plasma pools contaminated at a viral load of more than 10^4 geq/ml caused infection in recipients of plasma products such as clotting factor concentrates. Products manufactured from pools contaminated at a lower concentration did not transmit the virus to recipients. Calculating a fractionation pool size between 1000 and 10 000 litres of plasma, the concentration of an individual donor plasma entering a pool should not exceed 10^7 geq/ml in order to avoid break through of virus despite viral inactivation. Common inactivation procedures seem to have a

Sensitivty of NAT for B19	Pos./pools (%)	Pos./donation
10^3/ml	3470/34 661 (10.0)	1:564
10^5/ml	234/34 661 (0.68)	1:8361

Figure 14.7 (a) Parvo B19 positives over the past five years.

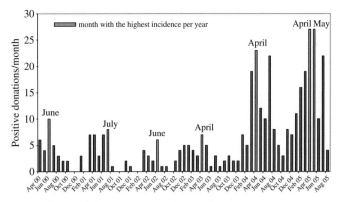

Figure 14.7 (b) Incidence of parvovirus B19 $> 10^5$ IU/ml per month.

limited capacity for parvovirus B19 inactivation of approximately four orders of magnitude in pooled plasma. To have some safety margin, German Blood Transfusion Services that introduced parvovirus B19 NAT for their donor population raised the threshold level to be detected in individual donor samples to 10^5 geq/ml. This relatively high threshold made testing and logistics much easier than a more stringent level of detection. The same pooling strategies as are established for HIV, HBV and HCV can also be applied to parvovirus B19 testing because only 1 in 5000–10 000 donors have a viral load of parvovirus B19 above the threshold of 10^5 geq/ml (see Figure 14.7a). Using pools of 96 samples approximately 1 in a 100 pools would be positive, whereas applying a sensitivity of 1000 geq/ml would result in one in ten pools testing positive (see Figure 14.7a). Large blood banks with more than 1000 donations per day would run into difficulties with respect to the blood supply because too many donations would be in 'inventory hold' until the individual positive donation could be identified.

Testing strategies

Please refer to Chapters 15 and 16.

Initial pool testing strategies, at least in Germany, were very cautious, because real incidence numbers were not available and legal aspects also had to be considered. Usually, transfusion services are not allowed, by regulation, to knowingly transfuse blood components contaminated by pathogenic organisms to susceptible recipients. This would be an infringement for which they could be sued. On the other hand, transfusion services have to guarantee sufficient supplies of blood for their patients and restricting supply of blood components due to parvovirus B19 contamination that is not usually pathogenic would also raise legal and ethical issues. A similar rationale applies in CMV testing where we have to transfuse CMV antibody positive donations due to the high rate of positive results among donors. The resolution of these constraints was to reduce the detection sensitivity of parvovirus B19 PCR to 10^5 copies/ml and to test blood donations used only for plasma products, but not for cellular components such as red cells and platelets. After NAT of mini-pools for HCV, HBV and HIV was completed, the remaining volume of nucleic acid extract was frozen. All platelet and red cell components relating to these pools were transfused. Extracts were thawed 45 days later and subjected to HAV and parvovirus B19 NAT. All plasma components testing positive for parvovirus B19 at a sensitivity of 10^5, or for HAV, were discarded after identification of the individual positive donation. This regimen was applied to plasma for fractionated products as well as to quarantined fresh frozen plasma (please refer to Chapter 20). The desensitized PCR with a detection limit of 10^5 geq/ml reduced the number of

positive pools to be resolved by a factor of 10, resulting in a reasonable workload. By this testing strategy, routine NAT screening of blood donors by HIV, HCV and HBV mini-pool NAT was not affected. However, parvovirus B19 is characterized by seasonal epidemics in late spring (Young et al., 2004) and early summer (see Figure 14.7b) which can result in an increase of positive donors by a factor of 5 to 10. However, this strategy led to an imbalance in safety procedures between plasma products and cellular components. Therefore, new approaches were considered.

Present strategies in place perform parvovirus B19 PCR and HAV PCR in parallel with HBV, HCV and HIV PCR without any delay (see Tables 14.1 and 14.2). Sensitivity has been enhanced and detection limits for both HAV and parvovirus B19 of less than 1000 copies/ml of donor plasma have been achieved. Parvovirus B19 PCR is a quantitative real-time PCR and quantitation standards are run on each plate. Only donations with a quantified viral load above 10^5 copies/ml of individual donor samples are identified and discarded. This procedure has been introduced in Germany by almost all Red Cross Blood Transfusion Services and is a significant improvement in safety for blood components because there is no longer transfusion of high titre infectious blood components that can reach virus loads up to 10^{14} geq/ml. If pools show viral loads for the individual donation contained in the pool between 10^5 and the detection limit of $<10^3$, the individual donation will not be identified and the pool will not be deconstructed. All samples of the pool will be labelled as 'weak positive', but donations will be released as if they were negative. For recipients at specific risk, for example women during the first three months of pregnancy, immunosuppressed patients and neonates, clinicians can specifically order parvovirus B19 negative components (e.g. below the detection limit of NAT). Implementing this new testing strategy at a blood transfusion service that tests up to 6000 samples/day in pools of 96 in conjunction with virus enrichment by centrifugation has led to a significantly increased workload. During epidemics, up to three pools have had to be resolved per day, which contained more than 10^5 copies/ml of parvovirus B19 per individual donor plasma. Transfusing known parvovirus B19 infected blood components to recipients may be ethically and legally disputable. However, preliminary data show that this threshold may be safe,

Table 14.1 Processing time for 'Frankfurt' PCR.

● Low-speed pre-centrifugation to remove debris	0.5 h
● Virus enrichment by medium-speed centrifugation	1.0 h
● Extraction of nucleic acids from virus pellets	1.5 h
● Pipetting extracted viral nucleic acids into HCV, HBV, HIV-1, HAV, PB19 PCR mixes	0.5 h
● TaqMan PCR	2.5 h
● Transfer of the data of the data management system	1.0 h
● **Release of blood components after**	**7.0 h**

Table 14.2 Example of workflow for 'Frankfurt' PCR.

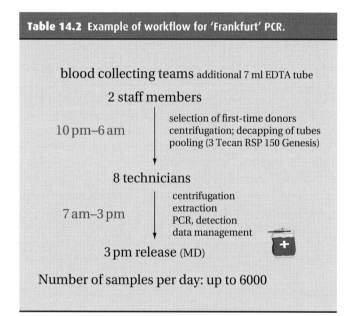

as most of these components already contain neutralizing antibodies. There have been preliminary clinical investigations which showed that parvovirus B19 negative recipients were not infected by weakly positive blood components (Roth *et al.*, 2005). Another factor is that 60–80 % of all blood donors have neutralizing antibodies and most recipients receive more than one component at a time. Moreover, recipients are infected at similar rates as blood donors and only immunosuppressed seronegative patients and children would be at significant risk and for these, parvovirus B19 negative components are provided as discussed earlier.

Alternative testing scenarios are under discussion. Donors could be screened at donation for antibodies by EIA tests and for the presence of viral particles by NAT. Units from donors who are antibody positive and negative for NAT at the highest possible sensitivity, could then be preferentially used for plasma fractionation and for patients at risk. After the initial screen, NAT and antibody screening could be discontinued in future for donors who are antibody positive and NAT negative, ie, immune. This strategy is based on the fact that antibodies are neutralizing and persist lifelong. A similar approach was adopted in the Netherlands (Groeneveld and van der Noordaa, 2003). Only those who are antibody negative and all first-time donors would subsequently require testing by EIA and NAT. Donors testing

positive by both antibody screening and NAT must be repeatedly tested by NAT until they become negative. Because of the high rate of repeat donors who are antibody positive and NAT negative this would significantly reduce costs and workload and would improve logistics.

Sensitivity and specificity

From the very beginning of NAT for blood donations, specificity was a burning issue. Even more than for EIA testing, specificity may decrease in NAT if attempting to increase sensitivity. More importantly, contamination of PCR with amplification products is of greater concern than specificity of primers and probes. The greatest risk in blood screening by NAT would be to overlook weak positives. Therefore, sensitivity needs to be enhanced to the lowest positive detection limits. In principle, one viral copy, when present in the PCR reaction mix, can be identified after amplification by PCR or transcription mediated amplification, or any other nucleic acid based amplification technology. This also implies that if there is only one molecule of amplification product transferred, for example by aerosols into a reaction tube, this would result in false-positives that will badly disrupt logistics. At the beginning of NAT in blood transfusion services, contamination was frequent and sometimes half of the pools were contaminated, resulting in transfusion of short-lived platelet concentrates without a valid NAT result. Therefore, transfusion services were some of the first to introduce closed tube systems such as TaqMan and other real-time-PCR technologies. They provide several advantages, one of which is that after amplification reaction tubes need not be opened for detection of the amplification products. Detection occurs online in a real-time mode through the closed tube.

It is also very important to have some certainty that negatives are true negatives. PCR and especially reverse transcriptase PCR (RT-PCR) for RNA viruses is a complex enzymatic exponential reaction that needs tight control. Therefore, multiplex PCRs were developed that include internal control sequences, preferably amplified by the same primers as the wild type virus sequences. If those internal controls give positive results, it indicates that wild type viruses would also have been amplified if they had been present in the reagent mix. If the control sequences are not amplified, some component of the reagent mix has failed and the PCR must be repeated until there is a valid result. Due to the competitive nature of internal controls (amplified with the same primers as wild type viruses) internal control sequences must be kept at low copy numbers in order not to reduce sensitivity for the wild type viruses through competition for the primers. It is also necessary to check with positive controls all other components of the whole procedure including pooling, centrifugation if applied, extraction, amplification and detection. Internal control sequence for PCR can also be used for controlling the extraction process when added to the lysis mix at the very beginning. To check for lysis efficiency, different spiking viruses or phage-packaged internal control sequences can be used (armoured RNA). Wild type spiking viruses are necessary to monitor the efficiency of the centrifugation process for each individual centrifuge run.

Wild type sequences also need to be amplified in a separate reaction on the same cycler in the same run with the same master mix to check for the integrity of the probes which are different for the virus and the internal control.

These new techniques have reduced the need for specific spatially separated laboratories and will in future probably even allow all steps of the NAT process to be performed in one room and, if automated, on one machine.

Throughput

Throughput capabilities depend on the number of donations to be tested at an individual site and also on pool size. For timely release of platelets that are tested by NAT, pooling needs to be started in most cases very soon after the donation. In many institutions it is done overnight in order to start early in the morning with extraction or, if enrichment is applied, to start with centrifugation of the pools followed by extraction and amplification. Strategies have been developed to perform NAT in parallel with EIA testing and to release blood products without any delay. To achieve this, the number of PCR and extraction procedures should be restricted to a minimum, which favours preparation of relatively large pools. However, large pools pose a risk that if they test positive a high number of donations that are urgently needed by patients might have to be held. Strategies were implemented to reduce the number of positive pools. Since first-time donors are at higher risk than repeat donors of being in the pre-seroconversion phase (as their incidence of infection is up to ten times higher than in repeat donors), their donations are often pooled separately from those of repeat donors. Cross-contamination must also be strictly avoided because this would also endanger the blood supply as discussed above. Experience has shown that pools of up to 96 samples are convenient for a high throughput, without significantly disturbing logistics and blood supply. However, due to the sensitivity requirements, centrifugation for enrichment of viruses is in our opinion, inevitable. Centrifugation has to be performed at sufficient centrifuge speed before enrichment in order to efficiently sediment viruses to the bottom of the centrifuge tube. With the appropriate centrifuge rotor, 48 000 g for one hour of centrifugation is sufficient to pellet viruses from a pool of 9.6 ml in total volume. In order to control centrifugation efficiency, each time a centrifuge run should incorporate a pool of negative samples spiked with all five viruses, with a concentration at 95% of the detection limit for each virus. By reducing the pool size down to 48 samples and below to avoid the need for centrifugation, HCV and HIV can be tested for very conveniently: otherwise, centrifugation would take at least one and a half hours and may reduce throughput. On the other hand, smaller pools mean more PCRs and a significant increase in costs. In addition, viruses which require a very high testing sensitivity, such as HBV and HAV, are not compatible with such strategies and need further reduction of pool size with further increase in costs and technical requirements. Enrichment of viruses from pools has the advantage that it is almost as sensitive as individual donation testing. However, input sample volume is restricted to a maximum of 100 μl using current technology. Nevertheless, this is sufficient for most viruses to achieve a sensitivity of <1000 geq/ml of

Table 14.3 Multicentre study of NAT among German Red Cross Transfusion Services: number of positive donations October 2004.

Virus	NAT only positive	Donations tested	Rate of positives	Incidence/ million
HBV	50	24.7 million	1:494 000	2.0
HCV	18	26.7 million	1:1.5 million	0.67
HIV-1	6	24.7 million	1:4.1 million	0.24

↑

Deduced residual risk before the introduction of PCR testing of unpaid donors

Table 14.4 Residual risk for transfused components in 2005.

Residual risk for Germany (Red Cross) after the introduction of NAT

• HCV	1:27 million
• HIV	1:25 million
• HBV	<1:1 million

individual donor sample and presently all five viruses, as discussed above, can be subjected to one pool preparation, one extraction procedure for all five viruses simultaneously, followed by diversion of the nucleic acid extract into five different PCRs. The extraction volume can be extended, depending on the required sensitivity for implementing NAT for further viruses (e.g. West Nile virus, SARS etc.). For viruses requiring high sensitivities, for example HBV and HIV, a higher volume of nucleic acid extract can be introduced into the PCR, whereas viruses like parvovirus B19 or HCV need only smaller volumes. To achieve a similar approach with pools that are not centrifuged, pool size should probably be reduced to <24 samples per pool. This latter approach is favoured by most countries, whereas in Germany pools of 96 in conjunction with centrifugation, are preferred, especially by the big Red Cross Transfusion Services who have several thousand samples per day. Results of PCR testing in German Red Cross Transfusion Services are shown in Tables 14.3 and 14.4.

Robustness

Since NAT has become a routine procedure for daily testing of a huge number of samples in complicated processes, it is essential to establish a robust procedure. This has now been achieved worldwide in countries with high HDIs by a tremendous increase in experience but also by establishing rigorous quality control measures for in-house methods.

Speed

Due to the short shelf life of platelets, many efforts were undertaken to make NAT as fast as EIA testing in order to release

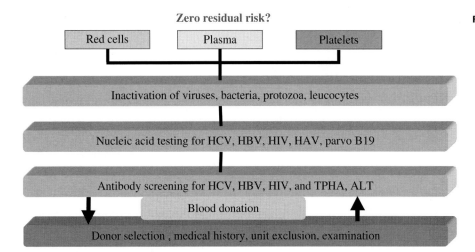

Figure 14.8 Layers of safety in transfusion.

platelets as early as possible after donation. Simultaneous detection during amplification by modern real-time PCR approaches such as TaqMan-PCR or LightCycler-PCR reduced analysis time significantly. Extraction procedures (mostly by chaotropic salts and silica columns) also allowed very rapid extraction and purification of nucleic acids prior to amplification. The use of automated pipetting for pooling and newly developed robotics for the extraction process will further reduce processing time and increase robustness. At present, many systems, and even those with virus enrichment by centrifugation, are faster than EIA testing of individual donations with respect to the total turnaround time. Procedures should ensure that if NAT is used in parallel with serological testing, the release of blood components, including platelets, is not delayed by NAT.

The future

There are two major approaches to NAT for viral screening for the future: automated NAT on pooled samples and automated NAT on individual donation. Diagnostic companies may have different interests from blood transfusion services, who need to constrain costs as much as possible, as well as enhance sensitivity and specificity. Irrespective of individual donation or pool testing, the predominantly manual extraction process of nucleic acid extraction would be the first target for automation. This will be followed by a fully automated process, including pooling, enrichment (if necessary) and PCR set-up. The whole process will be controlled by data management software and a fully barcoded procedure throughout. These systems will soon be available and reduce the costs significantly, primarily by reducing the numbers of operators and the hands-on time. Systems will be flexible enough to allow introduction of parallel testing of up to seven or more viruses on an individual NAT basis or even more by applying multiplex NAT systems. Automated systems will make NAT accessible to developing countries where the cost–benefit ratio for NAT will be much better than for Western countries, because of the higher incidence of viral infection. Developments are underway to extend NAT to bacteria and parasites also, providing a potential alternative to expensive inactivation procedures for cellular components (see Figure 14.8). Emerging unknown agents would not be covered by

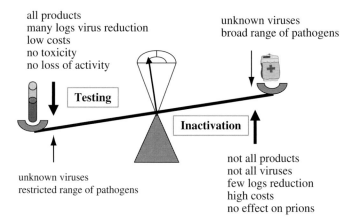

Figure 14.9 Testing versus pathogen inactivation.

NAT, whilst no sequence information on their nucleic acids is available. Enhanced testing versus pathogen inactivation is therefore still in the balance (see Figure 14.9). However, as experienced with West Nile virus and SARS, NAT tests became available shortly after these viruses emerged.

REFERENCES

Arbeitskreis Blut (2003) *Announcements of the Natl. Advisory Committee 'Blood' of the German Federal Ministry of Health and Social Security (Votum V30).* Abandoning the determination of alanine aminotransferase (ALT) levels as a criterion for release of blood components for transfusion and plasma for fractionation. Berlin, Springer Medizinverlag.

Assal, A., Caste J., Barlet V. *et al.* (2003) Application of molecular biology to blood transfusion safety: the nucleic acid testing. *Transfus Clin Biol*, **10** (3), 217–26.

Biswas, R., Tabor, E, Hsia, C. C., *et al.* (2003) Comparative sensitivity of HBV NATs and HBsAg assays for detection of acute HBV infection. *Transfusion*, **43** (6), 788–98.

Delwart, E. L, Kalmin, N. D., Jones, T. S., *et al.* (2004) First report of human immunodeficiency virus transmission via an RNA-screened blood donation. *Vox Sang*, **86** (3), 171–7.

European Pharmacopoeia Commission (2001) (Council of Europe). European Pharmacopocia 2001:0853. Human plasma for fractionation. Strasbourg.

Fields, B. N. (1996) *Virology*, 3rd edn, p. 759. Philadelphia, NY, US, Lippincott-Raven.

Food and Drugs Agency (2001) Application of nucelic acid testing to blood borne pathogenes and emerging technologies. Food and Drug Administration

Center for Biologics Evaluation and Research and Office of Blood Research and Review. 5 Dec 2001 Rockville, MD, Food and Drugs Agency.

Garcia-Retortillo, M., Forns, X., Feliu, A., *et al.* (2002) *Hepatology*, **35** (3), 680–7. Hepatitis C virus kinetics during and immediately after liver transplantation.

Groeneveld, K. and van der Noordaa, J. (2003) Blood products and parvovirus B19. *Neth J Med*, **61** (5), 154–6.

Mauser-Bunschoten, E. P., Zaaijer, H. L., van Drimmelen, A. A., *et al.* (1995) Risk of hepatitis A in Dutch hemophilia patients. *Thromb Haemost*, **74** (2), 616–8.

Nubling, C. M., Unger, G., Chudy, M., *et al.* (2002) Sensitivity of HCV core antigen and HCV RNA detection in the early infection phase. *Transfusion*, **42** (8), 1037–45.

Paul-Ehrlich-Institut (1998a) *BAnz. (Bundesanzeiger) Nr. 63 vom 04.04.1998, S4477.* Bekanntmachung vom 25.02.1998 über die Ergebnisse des Stufenplanverfahrens zur Verminderung des Risikos von Hepatitis-B, Hepatitis C und HIV-Infektionen bei Empfängern von Erythrozytenkonzentraten.

Paul-Ehrlich-Institut (1998b) *BAnz. (Bundesanzeiger) Nr. 53 vom 18.03.1998.* Bekanntmachung vom 05.06.1998. Abwehr von Arzneimittelrisiken Verminderung des Risikos von Hepatitis C Virus – Kontaminationen in Thrombozytenkonzentraten.

Paul-Ehrlich-Institut (2001) *BAnz. Nr. 90 vom 16.05.2001.* Bekanntmachung über die Zulassung und Registrierung von Arzneimitteln Anordnung der Testung auf HIV-1-RNA mit Nukleinsäure-Amplifikations-Techniken.

Paul-Ehrlich-Institut (2003) *BAnz. Nr. 103 vom 05.06.2003. S12269.* Bekanntmachung vom 06. Mai 2003 über die Zulassung und Registrierung von Arzneimitteln. Anordnung der Testung auf HIV-1-RNA mit Nukleinsäure-Amplifikations-Techniken.

Prodinger, W. M., Larcher, C., Sölder, B. M., *et al.* (1994) Hepatitis A in Western Austria – the epidemiological situation before the introduction of active immunization. *Infection*, **22** (1), 53–5.

Roth, W. K. and Seifried, E. (2002) The German experience with NAT. *Transfusion Medicine*, **12**, 255–8.

Roth, W. K., Weber, M., Petersen, D., *et al.* (2002) NAT for HBV and anti-HBc testing increase blood safety. *Transfusion*, **42**, 869–75.

Roth, W. K., Weber, M., Seifried, E., *et al.* (1999) Feasibility and efficacy of routine PCR screening of blood donations for hepatitis C virus, hepatitis B virus, and HIV-1 in a blood-bank setting. *Lancet*, **353** (30), 359–63.

Roth, W. K., Themann, A., Seifried, E., *et al.* (2005) NAT for Parvo B19 – five years of experience. *Abstract AABB 2005.*

Scheiblauer, H., Nübling, M., Willkommen, H., *et al.* (1996) Prevalence of hepatitis C virus in plasma pools and the effectiveness of cold ethanol fractionation. *Clin Ther*, **18** (Suppl. B), 59–70.

Stramer, S. L. (2002) US NAT yield: where are we after two years? *Transfus Med*, **12** (4), 243–53.

The Committee for Proprietary Medicinal Products (CPMP) (1998). CPMP/BWP390/97. The introduction of NAT for the detection of HCV RNA in plasma pools. London, The European Agency for the Evaluation of Medicinal Products.

Thierfelder, W., Meisel, H., Schreier, E., *et al.* (1999) Die Praevalenz von Antikörpern gegen Hepatitis-A-, Hepatitis-B- und Hepatitis-C-Viren in der deutschen Bevölkerung. *Gesundheitswesen*, **61**, 110–4.

Young, N. S. and Brown, K. E. (2004) Mechanisms of disease parvovirus B19. *N Engl J Med*, **350**, 586–97.

15 NUCLEIC ACID TESTING: THE US APPROACH

Susan L. Stramer

The central goal of blood centres is to provide a safe, adequate and effective blood supply. Towards that end, the focus on infectious disease testing has resulted in a high level of blood component safety. Today, in the developed world, the risk of transfusion-transmission of a major agent has been dramatically reduced by the introduction of next generation tests for antibodies and antigens, and with the introduction of nucleic acid testing (NAT). In the USA, with the introduction of NAT, the residual risk of HIV-1 and HCV has been reduced to approximately 1:2 000 000 donations screened (Dodd and Stramer, 2000). The yield of HIV-1 infected donors detected by NAT has been reported at 1:3.1 million and that for HCV (relative to third-generation antibody screening) at 1:270 000 (Stramer et al., 2004). The low frequency of these findings reinforces the safety of the blood supply today. In addition, the specificity of HIV-1 and HCV NAT relative to providing a false-positive result to a blood donor has been exceedingly high, with lower false-positive rates than any of the serological tests used in blood donor screening (e.g. 1:40 000 for NAT for the American Red Cross, ARC).

In addition to recipient safety, another aspect of the blood donation testing process is that it serves a public health function in identifying those individuals who are infected by a disease agent, particularly at the time shortly following exposure. Because donors identified by NAT that are antibody non-reactive are most likely in the early window period of infection, NAT for HIV-1 and HCV, for example, serves to identify early infection (in a very few cases, long-term immunosilent infections can also occur (Stramer et al., 2004)). While testing protects the safety of the blood supply, there is also a critical duty to correctly identify the donor as infected, communicate that result and provide encouragement to that individual to seek treatment and prevent secondary transmission. It is clear that multiple layers of testing for each of the current infectious disease agents, and the introduction of testing for new disease agents, not only increase the safety of the blood supply but also provide valuable diagnostic results for the tested donor.

Historically, confirmatory testing for infectious disease agents has been based on a variety of methods, including immunoblots containing viral or recombinant antigens, neutralization assays or immunofluorescence. There have been a number of limitations of each of these techniques, including false-positive and false-negative results (Dodd and Stramer, 2000), but most critical has been the large number of formally uninterpretable indeterminate findings. The introduction of NAT and integration of NAT results into routine blood donor serological testing results have provided a significant degree of improvement to the messages provided to blood donors.

Human immunodeficiency virus

Please refer back to Chapter 4.

Approximately 25.6 million donations were screened by the ARC from September 1999 to 30 June 2003, resulting in 17 090 HIV-repeat reactive blood donations (see Table 15.1). Only 4.8% of these donors (818) were Western blot positive, with approximately 90% (759) of those also being reactive by NAT. The concern regarding the remaining 10% of donors who are Western blot positive, but NAT non-reactive is whether their NAT non-reactive result is due to limitations in NAT sensitivity (false-negatives) in individuals who perhaps have HIV infection with low viral loads, or are due to false-positive, Western blot results (Kleinman, S., 1998). Upon further investigation of Western blot positive, NAT non-reactive results, they can be separated into two categories. First, are those donors who have very low signal to cut-off ratios on the screening EIAs, and have banding patterns on Western blot that are weak, in many cases having only envelope reactivity (one gene product), or if antibodies to multiple gene products are present, a band at p31 is lacking. Upon further testing, HIV-1 RNA cannot be demonstrated in these donors on index or follow-up testing. These donors represent Western blot, false-positive results (37 of 59 total Western blot positive, RNA negatives), which in the ARC blood donor population using the current test methods has an estimated frequency of 1:692 000 (previous rate reported at 1:173 000 to 1:379 000 (Kleinman et al., 1998)). Of those donors who are believed to be HIV infected, but NAT non-reactive in standard screening (i.e., the second category, or 22 of the 59 total), four did have low levels of virus that could be documented upon repeat testing (< 100–200 copies/ml).

Of the total number of anti-HIV EIA repeat reactive donors tested by Western blot, approximately 50% were indeterminate. When the Western blot results were combined with NAT screening results (which in some cases required additional NAT for clarification), only six samples of 8710 Western blot indeterminate and zero of 7562 Western blot negative samples were confirmed positive for RNA (1:4.27 million donations). The six NAT positive donors had viral loads of 9500 to 800 000 copies/ml. Therefore, combining the HIV-1 NAT results with the Western blot results demonstrates that fewer than 0.05% are truly infected with HIV-1. Of the anti-HIV EIA repeat reactive samples that tested NAT reactive, 99.6% of those that were Western blot positive also had a signal to cut-off ratio on the screening EIA of 15 or greater. In contrast, of those anti-HIV repeat reactive samples that tested NAT non-reactive, 98.5% of those that were Western blot negative or indeterminate had a signal to cut-off ratio of less than 15.

Transfusion Microbiology, eds John A. J. Barbara, Fiona A. M. Regan and Marcela C. Contreras. Published by Cambridge University Press. © Cambridge University Press 2008.

Table 15.1 Correlation of NAT with supplemental HIV serological data (17 791 RR donations of which 17 090 (96.1%) had EIA and WB data) 8 September 1999–30 June 2003.

| NAT result | Western blot result | | | Total |
	Pos.	Ind.	Neg.	
Reactive	**759** **(89.1%)**	56[a]	37[b]	852
		(10.9%)		
Non-reactive	59 (0.4%)	8654	7525	16 238
Total	**818** **(4.8%)**	8710	7562	17 090

[a] 6/56 (11%) dHIV and PCR reactive (9500–800 000 copies/ml)
[b] 0/37 (0%) dHIV and PCR reactive

Table 15.2 Correlation of NAT screening with supplemental HCV serological results (36 536 RR donations of which 34 656 (94.9%) had EIA and RIBA data) 8 September 1999–30 June 2003.

| NAT result | RIBA result | | | Total |
	Pos.	Ind.	Neg.	
Reactive	**13 182** (13 198[c]) **(80%)**	174[a] (159[c])	50[b]	13 407
		(1.7%)		
Non-reactive	3319	5967	11 963	21 249
Total	**16 502** (16 517[c]) **(48%)**	6141 (6126[c])	12 013	34 656

[a] 140/174 (80%) dHCV and PCR reactive (<100–48 000 000 copies/ml)
[b] 16/50 (32%) dHCV and PCR reactive (<100–24 000 000 copies/ml)
[c] 15 RIBA Ind due to ≥1 + hSOD (1:2310 in RR samples)

A more practical method to diagnose HIV infection is to simply rely on the results of NAT. A qualification study looking at a dual EIA algorithm in combination with NAT has been performed (Cyrus et al., 2002). In that study, two different FDA licensed EIA methods were used either as the first or second EIA in the algorithm. Of 7884 anti-HIV EIA repeat reactive samples tested, all Western blot positive, RNA positive samples were detected by both EIAs (317/317). The algorithm using Western blot only for those samples with discordant EIA values resulted in the elimination of 98.4% of the Western blot tests used, with a reduction of 98.6% in the number of indeterminate test results.

Hepatitis C virus

Please refer back to Chapter 1.

Testing the same population for HCV (approximately 25.6 million ARC donations from September 1999 to 30 June 2003) resulted in 34 656 anti-HCV repeat reactive results (see Table 15.2). Of those, 48% (16 502) were RIBA positive, with an additional 15 samples that should have been classified as RIBA positive. These 15 samples met the positive banding criteria, but also demonstrated reactivity to the HCV recombinant antigen carrier protein (hSOD) and according to the manufacturer's instructions were erroneously classified as indeterminate (Tobler et al., 2001). Eighty per cent of RIBA positive donors demonstrated NAT reactivity. Performing RIBA on HCV NAT reactive donations is unnecessary (CDC, 2003a) considering that over 98% of the NAT reactive donations were also RIBA positive. Of those RIBA positives without RNA, possible explanations, like those for HIV, include HCV positive donors with low viral loads, RIBA false-positive results, but also include those donors who resolved their HCV infection. NAT retesting was performed for 2255 of the 3319 RIBA positive, NAT non-reactive samples in this population of anti-HCV EIA repeat reactives. Regardless of whether the samples were originally tested in mini-pools of 16 or singly, 2.1% of the donation samples had a repeatable NAT reactive result. One half of these NAT reactive donors had viral loads of less than 100 copies/ml but others had viral loads of 1500 to 34 000 with one as high as 5.2 million copies/ml. Since the retested

samples had multiple freeze/thaw cycles and different handling from the blood donor samples undergoing screening (which were never frozen), one possible explanation for this discrepancy is viral aggregation and dissociation of aggregates with freeze/thaws.

Recombinant immunoblot assay indeterminate and negative donors represented 18% (6141) and 35% (12 031) of the anti-HCV repeat reactives. Ribonucleic acid positivity was confirmed for 80% (140/174) and 32% (16/50) of the RIBA indeterminate and negative samples that were initially reactive by NAT; viral loads in both groups range from less than 100 to 24–48 million copies/ml. Of the anti-HCV repeat reactive samples that tested NAT reactive, 98.9% of those that were RIBA positive also had a signal to cut-off ratio on the screening EIA of equal to or greater than 3.8 (a value validated by the CDC to use in place of RIBA or RNA testing (CDC, 2003a)). In contrast, of those anti-HCV repeat reactive samples that tested NAT non-reactive, 87.8% of those that were RIBA negative or indeterminate had a signal to cut-off ratio of less than 3.8. Overall, NAT results are likely to provide the donor with the most accurate information on the presence of active infection.

Hepatitis B virus

Hepatitis B virus NAT for routine use in screening of blood donors has not been adopted; indeed, the use of sensitive HBsAg assays coupled with anti-HBc testing has resulted in very low estimates of HBV residual risk of 1:205 000–1:488 000 (Dodd et al., 2002). These two measures together interdict the vast majority of HBV-infected individuals and reports of HBV transfusion-transmission in countries using both tests are virtually non-existent. Risk of HBV transmission will further decrease with the implementation (at least in the USA) of assays having HBsAg sensitivities of 0.1 ng/ml or better (Biswas et al., 2003). Studies have also been performed to define the HBV DNA frequencies and levels in those donations that test anti-HBc reactive. Rates of 0.24 to 0.63% were reported in two studies; these studies differ by time periods examined (1991–1995 versus 2001) and whether the rate was estimated or directly calculated (Kleinman *et al.*, 2003). In any event, the frequency is less than 1% and in all cases viral loads for the HBV DNA positives are extremely low (68% in the 2001 ARC study, with less than 100 copies/ml). The major advantage in coupling HBV DNA testing with anti-HBc testing is that donors may be counselled that, although HBsAg non-reactive, they nevertheless have evidence of active HBV infection. Other methods exist to improve the diagnostic message to anti-HBc repeat reactive donors, including repeat testing on another anti-HBc test; due to non-overlapping populations of non-specifics, most false-positives will not be reactive on the second test. Also, it is common for many blood centres that perform anti-HBc screening to perform anti-HBs testing to determine if the donor has been previously exposed to HBV; this is problematic in vaccinated individuals who might represent 30% or more of the population. This is even more problematic in areas where HBV is endemic; in those situations (e.g. Japan), high-titre anti-HBs coupled with low-titre anti-HBc may indicate immunity in the donor, especially if HBV DNA negative. The results of HBV DNA to detect early window-period donations (prior to the appearance of HBsAg) from US clinical trials have shown a frequency of positives of 1:269 000 (Pietrelli *et al.*, 2003). However, these studies were not performed against the HBsAg assays having the greatest sensitivities, so that this may represent a worst case figure.

West Nile virus (WNV)

Please refer back to Chapter 6.

Routine blood donation screening for WNV began in July 2003 in the USA in response to documented cases of transfusion-transmission in 2002 (Dodd, 2003; Pealer *et al.*, 2003). It is estimated that approximately 1000 WNV infected blood donors were identified in 2003 as a result of the implementation of testing under investigational protocols (versus over 9800 cases of clinical

disease reported to the CDC). During the 2003 WNV season, despite mini-pool screening in pools of 6 to 16 donations, there were two documented cases of transfusion-transmission from mini-pool screened blood (CDC, 2003b; 2003c). In both cases, the viral loads in the transmitting units were estimated to be very low, and both units lacked IgM. It has yet to be documented if a component containing detectable WNV RNA in the presence of antibody (IgM) is infectious via transfusion. In the WNV screening programmes, NAT reactive donors were informed of their test results and deferred until viral clearance and seroconversion (IgM) could be demonstrated. Because seroconversion eliminates virus, and is assumed to eliminate the possibility of transfusion-transmission, testing is only necessary to prevent transfusion of units in the short window period of infection. It is likely that this period is about 7.5 days, followed by a longer period of approximately 40 days in which decreasing amounts of virus and increasing amounts of antibody (IgM and then IgG) co-exist. Donor follow-up programmes (e.g. ARC) have been highly successful, with approximately 80% donor participation and reinstatement. In those individuals with confirmed WNV RNA reactivity that were followed, 96% seroconverted at a mean of 15 days from the calculated onset of circulating viraemia (including an approximate two- and five-day window period prior to the detection of virus by either mini-pool or single donation NAT). About one-quarter of the donors demonstrating seroconversion still remained viraemic at their first follow-up visit, with a small number demonstrating intermittent viraemia for approximately one month or longer. Figure 15.1 and Table 15.3 show the number of cases of WNV and clinical outcome throughout the USA in 2004; Figure 15.2 shows the number of viraemic blood donors identified on testing during 2004 (reproduced with permission from the CDC, USA). Two recent publications document the success of WNV NAT screening programs in the USA during the 2003 and 2004 WNV seasons (Busch *et al.*, 2005; Stramer *et al.*, 2005).

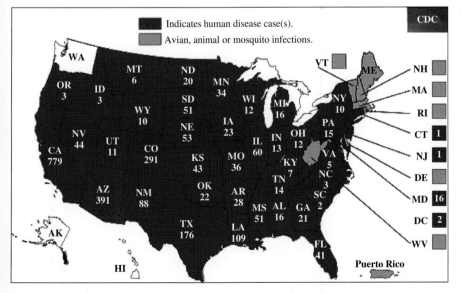

Figure 15.1 2004 West Nile virus activity in United States (reproduced with permission from CDC, USA).

Table 15.3 West Nile virus activity in the USA, 2004.

State	Neuro-invasive disease	Fever	Other clinical/ unspecified	Total human cases reported to CDC	Deaths
Arizona	214	160	17	391	16
Arkansas	17	10	1	28	0
California	289	395	95	779	28
Colorado	41	250	0	291	4
Connecticut	0	1	0	1	0
District of Columbia	1	1	0	2	0
Florida	33	8	0	41	2
Georgia	14	7	0	21	1
Idaho	1	2	0	3	0
Illinois	29	30	1	60	4
Indiana	8	2	3	13	1
Iowa	13	9	1	23	2
Kansas	18	25	0	43	2
Kentucky	1	6	0	7	0
Louisiana	85	24	0	109	7
Maryland	10	6	0	16	0
Michigan	13	3	0	16	0
Minnesota	13	21	0	34	2
Mississippi	31	18	2	51	4
Missouri	27	9	0	36	2
Montana	2	3	1	6	0
Nebraska	7	46	0	53	0
Nevada	25	19	0	44	0
New Jersey	1	0	0	1	0
New Mexico	31	53	4	88	4
New York	7	3	0	10	0
North Carolina	3	0	0	3	0
North Dakota	2	18	0	20	2
Ohio	11	1	0	12	2
Oklahoma	16	6	0	22	3
Oregon	0	3	0	3	0
Pennsylvania	9	5	1	15	2
South Carolina	0	2	0	2	0
South Dakota	6	45	0	51	1
Tennessee	13	1	0	14	0
Texas	119	57	0	176	8
Utah	6	5	0	11	0
Virginia	4	0	1	5	1
Wisconsin	5	7	0	12	2
Wyoming	2	7	1	10	0
Total	**1142**	**1269**	**128**	**2539**	**100**

Reproduced with permission from CDC, USA.

Parvovirus B19 and hepatitis A virus (HAV)

Please refer back to Chapter 5.

There is increasing discussion about selective screening of blood donations for parvovirus B19 and HAV. These two agents are of concern in relation to immunoglobulins, clotting factors and other manufactured plasma products such as albumin. Manufacturers of these products claim increased safety due to the removal of high levels of non-enveloped viruses that are not readily inactivated. Prevalence studies by the ARC for parvovirus B19 show that anywhere from 1:7000 to 1:10 000 donations contain DNA at levels greater than 1 million copies/ml. Although it is generally believed that parvovirus infection results in a short-lived, high-titre viraemia for seven to ten days, lower levels of

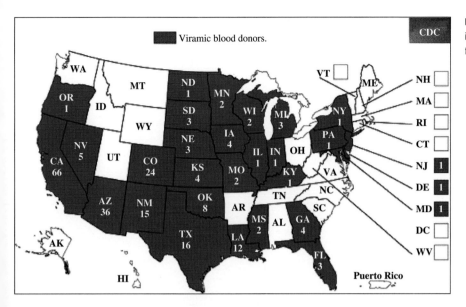

Figure 15.2 2004 West Nile virus blood donor activity in the United States (Reproduced with permission from CDC, USA).

virus of approximately 10 000 to 100 000 copies/ml may be present for several months in an infected individual prior to complete viral clearance (Young and Brown, 2004). The situation for HAV is comparable, with the exception that the level of viraemia in an infected individual is far lower with HAV (usually between 100 000 and 1 000 000 copies/ml). In one recent study (Bower *et al.*, 2000), longer duration of HAV viraemia was demonstrated, again corresponding to low levels of virus co-existing with antibody. The average duration of HAV viraemia in 13 infected humans in that study was 95 days (range of 36–391 days). If screening for either of these agents were to be considered, the significance of the donor counselling and public health message would require careful evaluation as high-level, or even potentially transmissible levels, of viraemia would have been cleared by the host's immunity by the time counselling could be conducted. Thus, the message may reduce to 'you were infected with this virus but are healthy'. This is a very different challenge from that previously discussed for HIV-1, HCV or HBV.

Conclusion

Although modern test methods have achieved a high degree of safety for blood components, they have also generated significant problems relating to diagnostic interpretations and counselling of seroreactive blood donors. However, careful use of data from NAT and creative use of confirmatory testing algorithms can greatly improve the accuracy of the overall testing process. The introduction of screening for additional agents requires validated diagnostic algorithms, as well as attention to all aspects of the counselling message given to donors.

REFERENCES

Biswas, R., Tabor, E., Hsia, C. C., *et al.* (2003) Comparative sensitivity of HBV NATs and HBsAg assays for detection of acute HBV infection. *Transfusion*, **43**, 788–98.

Bower, W. A., Nainan, O. V., Han, X., *et al.* (2000) Duration of viremia in hepatitis A infection. *J Infect Dis*, **182**, 12–7.

Busch, M. P., Caglioti, S., Robertson, E. F., *et al.* (2005) Screening the blood supply for West Nile virus RNA by nucleic acid amplification testing. *N Eng J Med*, **353**, 460–7.

Centers for Disease Control and Prevention (2003a) Guidelines for laboratory testing and result reporting of antibody to hepatitis C virus. *MMWR*, **52** (RR-3), 1–16.

Centers for Disease Control and Prevention (2003b) Update: detection of West Nile virus in blood donations – United States, 2003. *MMWR*, **52**, 916–9.

Centers for Disease Control and Prevention (2003c) Detection of West Nile virus in blood donations – United States, 2003. *MMWR*, **52**, 1160.

Cyrus, S., Robertson, G., Caglioti, S., *et al.* (2002) Evaluation of an alternate HIV confirmatory testing algorithm. *Transfusion*, **43** (9S), S131–040K.

Dodd, R. Y. (2003) Emerging infections, transfusion safety, and epidemiology. *N Eng J Med*, **349**, 1205–6.

Dodd, R. Y. and Stramer, S. L. (2000) Indeterminate results in blood donor testing: what you don't know can hurt you. *Transfus Med Rev*, **14**, 151–60.

Dodd, R. Y., Notari, E. P. and Stramer, S. L. (2002) Current prevalence and incidence of infectious disease markers and estimated window-period risk in the American Red Cross blood donor population. *Transfusion*, **42**, 975–9.

Kleinman, S., Busch, M. P., Hall, L., *et al.* (1998) False-positive HIV-1 test results in a low-risk screening setting of voluntary blood donation. *JAMA*, **280**, 1080–5.

Kleinman, S. H., Kuhns, M., Todd, D. S., *et al.* (2003) Frequency of HBV DNA detection in US blood donors testing positive for the presence of anti-HBc: implications for transfusion-transmission and donor screening. *Transfusion*, **43**, 696–704.

Pealer, L. N., Marfin, A. A., Petersen, L. R., *et al.* (2003) Transmission of West Nile virus through blood transfusion in the United States 2002. *N Eng J Med*, **349**, 1236–45.

Pietrelli, L., Gorlin, J., Holland, P., *et al.* (2003) A prospective study to evaluate the screening of plasma pools from volunteer blood donations for the presence of HBV DNA. *Transfusion*, **43** (9S), S86–040C.

Stramer, S. L., Fang, C. T., Foster, G. A., *et al.* (2005) West Nile virus among blood donors in the United States, 2003 and 2004. *N Eng J Med*, **353**, 451–9.

Stramer, S. L., Glynn, S. A., Kleinman, S. H., *et al.* (2004) Detection of HIV-1 and HCV infections among antibody-negative US blood donors by nucleic acid amplification testing. *N Eng J Med*, **351**, 760–8.

Tobler, L. H., Stramer, S. L., Kleinman, S. H., *et al.* (2001) Misclassification of HCV viremic blood donors as indeterminate by RIBA 3.0 because of human superoxide dismutase activity. *Transfusion*, **41**, 1625–6.

Young, N. S. and Brown, K. E. (2004) Parvovirus B19. *N Eng J Med*, **350**, 586–97.

16 NUCLEIC ACID TESTING: THE UK APPROACH

Roger Eglin

Background

The English National Blood Service (NBS) established a nucleic acid amplification technology (NAT) Steering Group in 1996 to produce a strategy in anticipation of a regulatory requirement for hepatitis C virus (HCV) RNA testing of manufacturing scale plasma fractionation pools. This subject was first raised in 1995 by the Committee for Proprietary Medicinal Products (CPMP) and the requirement was published in CPMP/BWP/390/971 (CPMP, 1998). The 'start pool' of plasma for fractionation had to be tested by NAT and shown to be negative for HCV RNA.

The implementation date for HCV NAT was 1 July 1999 for plasma fractionators. (Please refer to Chapter 20.) Hepatitis C virus RNA pre-testing of sub-pools (i.e. testing before pooling of all plasma takes place) was implemented in the National Blood Service to avoid the loss of large-scale plasma pools for fractionation as a result of contamination by HCV RNA. In addition, it was also important to prevent transmission of HCV via any other blood components from donors identified to be HCV RNA positive through testing of plasma pools for fractionation (please refer to Chapters 13 and 14). This inevitably led the blood services to introduce the requirement for real-time NAT to allow timely withdrawal of all labile blood components identified as HCV RNA positive. Nucleic acid testing for all labile components was introduced as soon as practicable and was completed by the NBS in July 2000. The steering group was commissioned in 1996 to establish a NAT system for NBS and Bio Products Laboratories (BPL), the plasma fractionators in England, to undertake HCV RNA testing on pools of 480 plasma samples which would meet the proposed CPMP requirements without potential wastage of any large start pools (final pools for fractionation). By making these small 'sub-pools' of plasma and then testing these for HCV RNA, the risk of contamination of the final pool for fractionation would be avoided.

The strategy

For the steering group originally commissioned in 1996 to oversee NAT of blood products, the initial strategy was to pool plasma samples, at NBS Testing Laboratories, and to undertake NAT of these pools, whilst minimizing wastage due to loss of large pools of plasma in the event of an HCV NAT positive result. Testing of pools was initially carried out at BPL, but this was later moved to blood centres, when European and USA requirements for HCV RNA testing of labile blood components in mid-1998 meant that HCV NAT results were required before the release of fresh frozen plasma (FFP) for clinical use and then subsequently for all labile components with a shelf life of greater than 48 hours. The move was also influenced by the decision of the Department of Health to cease using UK plasma for fractionation in 1998 (DoH, 1998), as a consequence of the perceived risk from vCJD in the donor population. The emphasis for NAT in the UK was therefore on testing of labile blood components and not plasma for fractionation. One resultant change strategy was the reduction in the size of the pools for testing from 480 to 96 donations. This was subsequently further reduced to pools of 48 donations to accommodate the release of shorter shelf-life components, for example platelets, once three NAT laboratories had been established for the NBS.

Second, the strategy for the location of NAT changed. NAT was introduced at three NBS centres in England, conveniently located in order to reduce the turnaround time for results (see Figure 16.1). This was essential for components with a short shelf life and is a contingency measure, against the risk of one testing site ceasing to function.

As part of its contingency planning, it was decided that one of the three NAT laboratories would continue to use the full Roche COBAS AMPLICOR system, which employed a manual extraction method. This was to cover the possibility of the simultaneous failure of the other two centres, which used the BioRobot automation methods. In addition, as part of the contingency planning each of the three sites has enough capacity to undertake the total national daily workload for NAT in the event of coincident failure of the other two sites.

As part of a review of the NAT system, it was also decided that in future more than one commercial provider of the NAT systems should be used. This decision was based on the NBS principle of always using more than one provider rather than being solely reliant on one, in case of any future problems. The outcome of the subsequent tender process was that the combined Qiagen-Roche Cobas system would continue to be used at Leeds and Birmingham Laboratories and the Chiron Procleix system for HCV was implemented at Brentwood in November 2003.

Use of the Procleix system, which simultaneously detects both HIV and HCV nucleic acid in the first assay with distinction between two viruses in the second assay, inevitably led to a reorganization of the operational NAT Laboratory at Brentwood. It remains the position for NBS that only HCV NAT is mandated by the Department of Health and that HIV NAT, although not required, offers additional bonuses in the region in which it is used. It is also the case that, as for HCV, donations which are HIV antibody positive are still tested by NAT, to give additional confirmation of the HIV infected donors.

A predictable bonus of the use of Procleix for HCV NAT was the detection of a late window-period HIV infection in a donor who

Transfusion Microbiology, eds John A. J. Barbara, Fiona A. M. Regan and Marcela C. Contreras. Published by Cambridge University Press. © Cambridge University Press 2008.

- NBS, Birmingham
- NBS, Brentwood
- NBS, Leeds

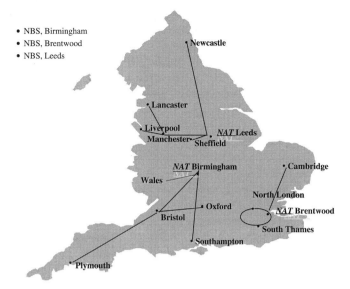

Figure 16.1 NAT: geographical laboratory locations.

could have been missed by serological testing. Following an interview with such a donor, it became clear that 18 days after sexual risk activity, the individual had donated blood. This donated unit was HIV NAT positive, HCV NAT negative, on Procleix and the unit was withdrawn from the system. On the following day (day 19) the donor phoned in to report feeling unwell, with a raised temperature, etc. Human immunodeficiency virus seroconversion illness was suspected and a further 14 days later, a blood sample was HIV antibody positive. It should be noted that, several HIV combined Ag/Ab assays were used to test the donated blood unit and only the Murex combined assay gave a positive result.

The performance of the Procleix assay was satisfactory with a 95% limit of detection (LOD) of 10.3 IU/ml HCV and 24.5 IU/ml HIV. This is a measure of the sensitivity of the system. As a result of the highly sensitive performance of this system for HCV it was decided to use a positive control for HIV with a $3 \times 95\%$ LOD, to demonstrate that the system was maintaining a consistently sensitive performance. It was felt that the extreme dilution required for $3 \times 95\%$ LOD for HCV internal control might lead to inaccuracies of dilution and therefore produce an inaccurate measure of the system's true performance.

Requirements of the assay and practical aspects

The test must be capable of the reliable detection of 5000 IU/ml HCV RNA, which is the level defined by the WHO international standard for HCV RNA testing (96/790) in the original donation, for compliance with Paul-Ehrlich-Institut (PEI) Directive 14 (98/79/EC). Although not a binding requirement for the UK, the PEI standard is the model which most European countries follow. In addition, it had to meet the NBS requirements for a high throughput automated assay, which are listed in Table 16.1. Experience of clinical diagnostic virology laboratories, which had been using NAT systems for virus identification and treatment monitoring for several years, identified that the sample to be tested should be:

Table 16.1 Requirements of a high throughput automated assay.

- Satisfying GMP requirements
- Fully automated
- Positive sample identification
- Automated data handling: IT links between all key instrument groups and core IT system
- Commercially available instrumentation and assays

- Plasma which is separated from a plastic collection tube containing EDTA as anticoagulant. This tube should be used only for NAT.
- On collection, the samples must be mixed with the EDTA in the tube and racked in an upright position.
- The whole unseparated sample is stable at room temperature for up to 12 h and at 4 °C for up to six days.
- Once separated, HCV RNA in plasma is stable for 120 h at 4 °C and must be stored at ≤ -20 °C.

These are National Blood Service operational requirements which were derived from validation work.

Pooling the samples

The system uses robotic samplers, with disposable tips, for preparation of the pooled samples and tracks the sample identities by means of barcoding. Each of the three pooling laboratories uses the Tecan Genesis RGP2000 sampling machine with its own pooling management software. Pools of 96 samples were replaced by pools of 48 samples at the time of introducing NAT for labile component release, by July 2001. Samples are centrifuged before pooling and a maximum of 480 suitable samples is loaded onto the Tecan sample handlers to produce ten pools. In addition to this pooling procedure, each sample is dispensed into individual wells of a deep microtitre plate (resolution plate) which is used for the identification of HCV RNA positive donations in pools found to be reactive. The resolution plates are sealed and stored at −20 °C for a minimum of three years.

The identification of HCV RNA positive samples in an initially reactive pool is undertaken using cross-pools produced from the resolution plate (see Figure 16.2) (please refer to Chapter 14). Any single sample from a viraemic donation will be identified by the intercept of a row and column mini-pool. All identified reactive samples are handled according to a standard algorithm which describes all appropriate actions.

Testing of the samples

The laboratory design for NAT follows the recommendations for good practice for PCR testing and employs a three area design with a 'clean to dirty' work flow. The 'clean' area is for reagent preparation; the 'semi-clean' area is for nucleic acid extraction and the 'dirty' area is for amplification and detection.

All the components of the testing system are commercially available. The combination of instruments used was not designed

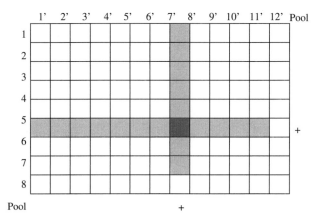

Figure 16.2 Pool resolution to identify a viraemic donation.

for this integrated purpose but they have been evaluated and validated by NBS and are also used as a linked system by several independent laboratories.

System at centres using automated extraction

Extraction of nucleic acid

This employs Qiagen Robotic 9604 extraction system to automate the extraction procedure. Nucleic acid is released by lysis procedures and then stabilized in the processing of 96 samples simultaneously. Originally, the viral extraction kit was used and this was changed to the total nucleic acid extraction kit by July 2001.

Reverse transcription, amplification and detection of AMPLICOR

Roche Cobas AMPLICOR instruments automate the stages leading to the specific detection of HCV RNA. Each Cobas machine has the capacity to process up to 24 samples per batch run. AMPLICOR kits were replaced by AmpliScreen kits in July 2001.

The differences, in both sensitivity of detection and robustness, in the performances of the two automated systems used, result from the improvements produced by the addition of heating and enzyme digestion steps into the Qiagen virus protocol, to improve its efficiency. The additional rounds of amplification in the AmpliScreen protocol, produce more amplicon and thus a greater signal.

System controls

An internal control (IC) comprising a naked HCV for Qiagen/ Roche and HIV for Procleix RNA, is added to each test sample prior to the extraction procedure. Optical density (OD) values of < 0.15 for the IC indicate that the test may have been faulty (sub-optimal). The required sensitivity of detection of the system is 50 IU/ml HCV RNA for pools of 96 samples and 100 IU/ml HCV RNA for pools of 48 samples (please refer to Table 16.2).

The 3.5 IU/ml working standard allows sensitive monitoring of changes in the system. It is expected to be positive in 33% of samples using AMPLICOR detection and 50% of samples using AmpliScreen detection. The 95% LOD for Qiagen viral extraction and AMPLICOR is 25.8 IU/ml (Grant *et al.*, 2002). The 95% LOD

Table 16.2 Controls used to monitor performance.

Controls	Purpose	OD	Frequency
P100	Go/no go for A ring	>0.15	1/A ring
P50	Target sensitivity		1/extraction run
P3.5	Poisson 1 hit sensitivity		1/A ring
Internal control	Go/no go for negatives	>0.5	Each sample

P50 dropped with move to pools of 48
P100 now used/pair of A rings per Cobas

Qiagen total nucleic acid extraction and AmpliScreen is 12.8 IU/ml, based on validation data produced by the National Blood Service. Procleix performance data is 95% LOD for HCV is 10.3 IU/ml, for HIV is 24.5 IU/ml.

Thus, the actual sensitivities of both systems used exceed the target of 5000 IU/ml of HCV RNA in the original sample, as required by the Paul-Ehrlich-Institut in 1998 (Directive 98/79/EC).

Data handling

All sample data and results generated during the NAT pooling and assay system are manipulated electronically by validated software, according to the Data Flow Chart (see Figure 16.3). Pulse Management Software (PMS) stores the location of each sample with the pools and gathers the results. It links the result to the donation for downloading to Pulse which is the NBS standard database. Pulse then manages the entire donor information and results of the testing. Qia Soft Plus operating system controls the extraction protocol and set up of the Cobas to track the location of all samples through the extraction procedure. The Cobas programme controls the instrument and collection of the test results. The AMPLILINK data is imported into Medusa 2000 (Sanguin Software), which uses set protocols to validate the test results. The results of the HCV NAT assay and the IC assay are assessed and an overall test result is assigned. These results are transferred to the PMS programme.

Performance monitoring

One of the NAT systems developed by NBS uses a combination of several different manufacturers' equipment and, as a result, NBS bears the responsibility for the robustness and continuity of the total system. It was therefore necessary to develop a performance monitoring system of the process which examined:
(1) The overall performance of the system, monitored by IC and 3.5 IU/ml working standard and turnaround time to issue of results (see Figures 16.4a, 16.4b, 16.4c and 16.5)
(2) The stage in the process at which failure occurred
(3) The failure rate of the system.

There is formal monthly review of these parameters and the charts illustrate the following points. The IC failure rate was followed using a six result rolling average, which highlights

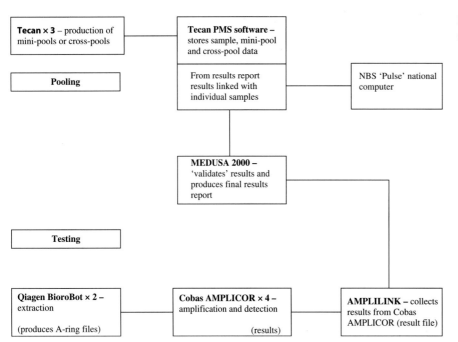

Figure 16.3 Data flow through the nucleic acid amplification technology (NAT) system.

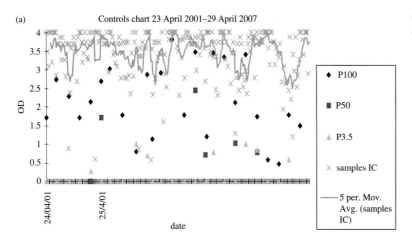

(a)

Figure 16.4(a) Controls used to monitor performance plots of ODs of controls with moving averages.

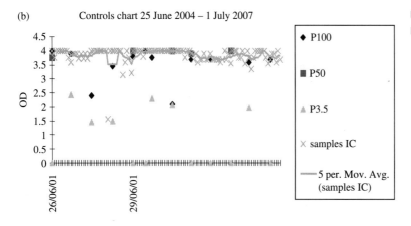

(b)

Figure 16.4(b) AmpliScreen/QiAmp virus extraction protocol performance.

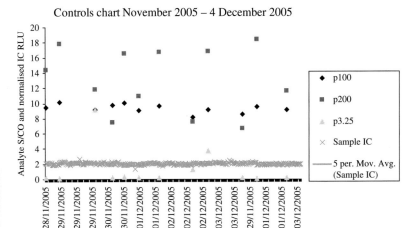

Controls chart November 2005 – 4 December 2005

Figure 16.4(c) Brentwood control charts (Procleix).

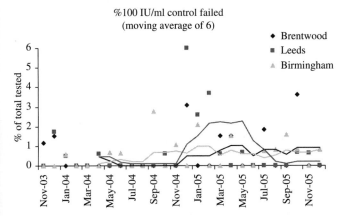

Figure 16.5 Internal control and 100 IU/ml control ('Go/No Go') monitoring.

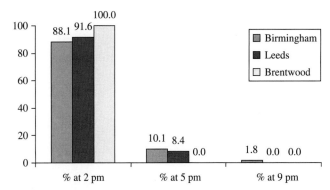

Figure 16.7 Monthly average of the percentage of donations released in the three NAT sites by 2 pm on day.

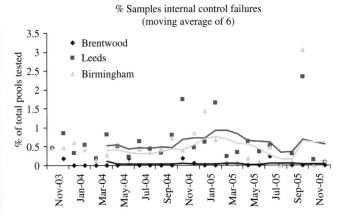

Figure 16.6 Internal control and 100 IU/ml control ('Go/No Go') monitoring.

performance failures. Monitoring of the 100 IU/ml and 3.5 IU/ml working standards (see Figure 16.6 and 16.7) is done to determine run failures (100 IU/ml) and variations in the overall sensitivity of detection of the system (3.5 IU/ml). Monitoring includes:

(1) Any failure to produce 90% results by the target time of 14.00 h on day 1 (day 0 being the day of sample collection), (see Figure 16.8).

(2) Identification of which element of the process was failing and the resultant delay in production of the results (see Figure 16.9 and Table 16.3), overall failure rate of the process (see Figure 16.10).

(3) Identification of those operators consistently failing to achieve a target of 33% positivity rate for the 3.5 IU/ml working standard and >95% positivity rate for the 100 IU/ml working standard, in order to offer retraining and identification of problems.

The percentage of invalid runs of the first system (viral RNA extraction and AMPLICOR) was 8–12% averaged over four-week periods. The percentage of invalid runs for the second system (total nucleic acid extraction and AmpliScreen) was 5% averaged in the first four weeks following the change over. The manual extraction system and AMPLICOR averaged a failure rate of 5% over four-week periods.

The differences in performance, regarding both sensitivity of detection and robustness, of the two automated systems used, result from the improvements produced by the addition of heating and enzyme digestion steps with the Qiagen virus protocol, to improve its efficacy and the additional rounds of amplification in the AmpliScreen protocol, which produces more amplicon and thus a greater signal.

Currently, the percentage of invalid runs for both the Procleix system and Qiagen and AmpliScreen is 0.1% for both HCV and

Table 16.3 Failures at a single site.

Stage failures	Number of runs/A-rings/ samples	Comment	Failure rate
Extraction	None		
Amplification and detection	2 A-rings	Samples lost owing to NATIF	2 of 323 A-rings = 0.6%
Meeting the validity criteria			
p100 failed	1 A-ring		1 of 323 A-rings = 0.3%
IC failed	14 samples		14 of 2859 samples = 0.5%
>2 IC failed	1 A-ring		1 of 323 A-rings = 0.3%
Positive mini-pools	4 mini-pools	1 Welsh	4 of 2859 samples = 0.14%

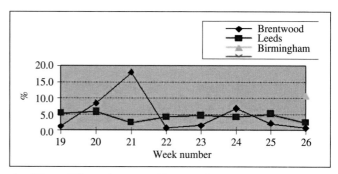

AmpliScreen/QiAmp virus protocol Brentwood and at Birmingham from week 25

Figure 16.10

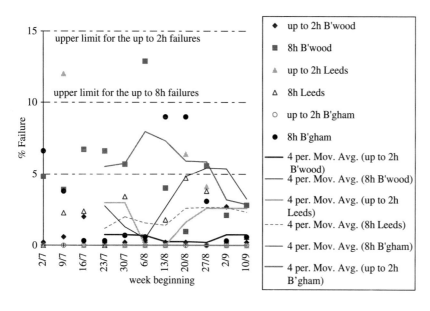

Figure 16.8 Failure chart corresponding to a time delay.

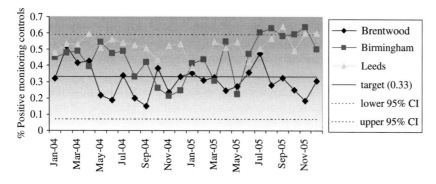

Figure 16.9 Monthly positivity rate for the monitoring control in the three NAT laboratories.

Table 16.4 Cumulative nucleic acid amplification technology (NAT) and serology results for England and Wales (1 April 1999–31 March 2006).

Number of acute-HCV tested	Anti-HCV positive			Anti-HCV negative	
	Total	NAT positive	NAT negative[a]	No result	NAT positive
17 254 628	944	695	202	47	11

[a] 50 of those tested by single donation NAT: 45 = negative, 5 = positive

Table 16.5 Hepatitis C virus nucleic acid testing window-period yield worldwide, 2004.

Country	Pool size	No. of units	NAT positive	Yield per million
Australia	24 or 1	3 527 000	9	2.55
Canada	24	3 506 000	1	0.28
France	8–24	2 600 000	2	0.49
Germany/Austria	96	3 615 000	6	0.69
Holland	24	4 050 000	2	0.25
Japan	50	6 806 000	25	4.20
USA	16–24	29 254 000	113	4.25
England and Wales	48	35 752 232	11	0.31

HIV. Thus, the NAT process has matured and settled to an acceptably low failure rate.

Hepatitis C virus ribonucleic acid testing screening results

The incidence of window-period HCV positive donors is 0.3 per million donations which is somewhat less than the predicted rate of 2 per million donations originally estimated.

It is NBS practice to test HCV antibody positive samples by NAT, as these samples act as a natural internal control of the system. This can give rise to complications in the resolution of the cross mini-pools, since there can be more than one intercept of positive findings on a resolution plate assay. Fortunately, the HCV antibody results are available by the time the resolution plate testing is completed. The findings of the cumulative NAT and serology results are shown in Table 16.4. Of the 897 HCV antibody positive samples tested, 77% are HCV RNA positive and 23% are HCV RNA negative. On single donation testing of the HCV antibody positive, pooled RNA negative samples by NAT 5 of 50 samples (10%) are HCV RNA positive. There have been no reported cases of HCV transmission by transfusion since NAT for HCV RNA was introduced into the NBS.

The HCV window-period yield by NAT in other countries shows, in Table 16.5, that only France, Holland and Canada approach NBS in the incidence of HCV NAT positive donors, with USA and Japan both detecting at least five times as many HCV NAT positive donors.

Conclusion

The experience of introducing HCV NAT has shown that, given the willingness to be adaptable both in the operational laboratories and with the commercial companies involved, a reasonably robust testing system can be produced without compromising the standards demanded of blood components for clinical use.

REFERENCES

CPMP (1998) The introduction of nucleic acid amplification technology (NAT) for the detection of hepatitis C virus RNA in plasma pools; CPMP/BWP/390/97, London, EMEA, Committee for Proprietary Medicinal Products.

Department of Health (1998) Further precautionary measures on blood products announced 1998; 98/076 London, Department of Health.

Grant, P. R., Sims, C. M., Krieg-Schneider, F., *et al.* (2002) Automated screening of blood donations for hepatitis C virus RNA using Qiagen Biorobot 9604 and the Roche COBAS HCV Amplicore assay. *Vox Sang*, **82**, 169–76.

17 QUALITY IN THE SCREENING OF DONATIONS FOR TRANSFUSION-TRANSMISSIBLE INFECTIONS

John A. J. Barbara and Alan D. Kitchen

Introduction

The field of transfusion microbiology has developed rapidly over the last 20 years. However, not only has the field developed in terms of the understanding of the biology and science of the infectious agents, the advent of automated mass screening systems, and the increased general focus on the microbial safety of blood and blood products, but importantly the overall quality – the reliability and effectiveness of screening has improved significantly. This quality improvement has come from a number of sources:

- The identification of those transmissible infectious agents of most concern for transfusion
- A more detailed and comprehensive understanding of the biology of transmissible agents
- The development of sensitive assays for transmissible agents
- The improvements in assay design, including the inclusion of specific features to monitor the step-by-step performance of the assay
- The introduction of quality management systems into blood transfusion services (BTSs)
- The development of appropriate automation
- The introduction of licensing/accreditation of BTSs
- The introduction of haemovigilance systems.

Overall, it is the amalgamation of the above elements into a single seamless system that has resulted in the current overall high level of safety of the blood supply in most countries with developed health care systems. Nonetheless, it must be understood that these systems are not always as robust as one would wish, and vigilance is necessary to ensure that quality standards are maintained. In addition, the potential threat of new, as yet unidentified, agents must not be forgotten.

This chapter considers those specific elements associated with blood screening for TTIs that help to ensure the overall safety of the blood supply. These include donor selection, screening strategies, assay design, assay evaluation, use of automated systems, validation of results, staff knowledge and skills, and haemovigilance. However, it must be remembered that these elements, although discussed as critical for the effective screening of donations for TTIs, are nonetheless part of the overall quality management system of any well organized national blood transfusion service. A major aspect of the quality assurance of donation screening is that of process control. In this context, process control can be defined as the control of all of those elements that contribute to the overall assurance that the laboratory screening performed and the results generated are accurate and reliable, and are also consistent from run to run and from laboratory to laboratory.

Process control clearly relates primarily to the laboratory screening processes themselves, the validation of all stages of assay performance and of the final results, and also validation of performance of automated systems. However, there is one important element that must be remembered when considering laboratory activities: that is the quality of the sample. When considering sample quality this includes the correct identity of the donor and correct linking of the donation number to the donor, the volume of sample collected, the type of sample (serum/plasma), the age of the sample and the storage conditions of the sample. It has to be assumed by the screening laboratory that all of the activities associated with the collection of the sample, which are outside the control of the laboratory, have been performed correctly. Thus, the laboratory accepts the sample with the assumption that it is the correct sample and has been stored correctly up to the point at which it is received in the laboratory. To ensure this, an effective and comprehensive quality management system is required which covers all of the activities of a BTS. The quality activities associated with the screening process are part of this overall quality system.

The donation screening process

The screening process can be considered to include all of the elements identified above:
- Donor selection
- Screening strategies
- Assay design
- Assay evaluation
- Lot release
- Use of automated systems
- QC samples and EQAS
- Validation and assessment of results and assay performance
- Identification of unsuitable donations
- Staff knowledge and skills
- Haemovigilance.

All of the above are critical to the whole process, but each also has their own unique role within the whole process. Although the donor selection process applies to the donor rather than the donation, nonetheless it is included here because of its unique place at the beginning of the whole process. Whilst this text will consider the elements individually, in reality the boundaries between them disappear, as all of them interact and cross-react with each other, and information generated by individual elements often feeds back into other elements. Figure 17.1 depicts the interaction of screening processes that result in the release of screened and safe products for clinical use.

Transfusion Microbiology, eds John A. J. Barbara, Fiona A. M. Regan and Marcela C. Contreras. Published by Cambridge University Press. © Cambridge University Press 2008.

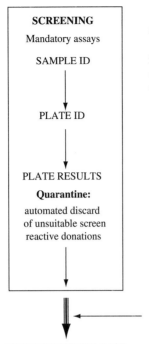

CONTRIBUTORY QUALITY INPUT	SCREENING Mandatory assays	REQUIRES Sample preparation
Training and competency assessment	SAMPLE ID	
Assay evaluation	↓	IN-PROCESS CONTROLS (in-well validation of critical steps) • sample addition monitor • colour coded reagents
Assay validation		
Lot release testing	PLATE ID	• incubation and wash control
	↓	
Equipment validation		• plate validation
Documentation	PLATE RESULTS	• 'go-no-go' standards
Change control and log	**Quarantine:**	• 'cut-off' decisions
Error and incident log	automated discard of unsuitable screen reactive donations	• validating correct retrieval of initial reactives • secure repeat testing
		• document archive • sample archive

Blood grouping →

INTEGRATED RELEASE

Figure 17.1 A quality framework for the microbiological screening of donations.

Donor selection

Please refer to Chapter 10.

Although laboratory screening is the ultimate determination of the status of a donation, it is not the first part of the overall screening process. Donor selection is the first screening step applied to the donor population, and serves to reduce the stresses on the laboratory by trying to exclude unsuitable donors prior to the collection of any donations. The selection/deferral process is clearly more subjective than the use of in vitro screening assays, and made more complicated as it has two major components, both of which have to be optimized to ensure the effectiveness and consistency of the process. First, donor suitability criteria and guidelines need to be developed, and second, these need to be applied comprehensively and consistently. Unfortunately, both parts of this process are not without their problems. The development of donor suitability criteria and guidelines is essentially a generic process, with certain core criteria that most would agree need to be applied globally, although there are some regional/country specific aspects that may need to be adopted locally. The guidelines must then be applied consistently to all potential donors. Whilst this would seem to be a relatively simple exercise, in reality it can be a complicated situation which requires the guidelines to be very comprehensive yet clear and simple. Collection staff should be well trained to deal with the wide range of potential donors coming forward. A further, and significant, complication is whether the same selection criteria and guidelines should be applied to donors of products such as tissues and stem cells. Here, the range of appropriate donors may be far more restricted, for example HLA matched unrelated stem cell

donors. The stringency of the selection criteria may need to be reviewed in the light of the risks to the recipient from not having a matched unrelated stem cell transplant.

In the context of blood donation, however, it must be remembered that the safest blood comes from the safest donors and the donor selection process is instrumental in trying to identify such donors at the outset before any donations are collected.

Screening strategies

The first stage of the laboratory screening process is to define the basic screening strategy. Whilst there are many factors that determine this, the overriding goal should be to maximize safety (sensitivity) and minimize waste (specificity). (Please refer to Chapter 11.) Although sensitivity and specificity are generally considered to be inherent characteristics of the assays themselves, they are parameters which can be used to help analyse the effectiveness of potential screening strategies to determine the most appropriate for any given situation. For donation screening it is clear that both sensitivity and specificity are important – safety balanced against sufficiency – and although there are different strategies that could be adopted, it is debatable whether there is actually more than one appropriate strategy. Whilst it is clear that any strategy is only as good as the assay used, at the same time a good assay used in a poor strategy is just as bad. The choice of strategy must reflect what is possible (availability of assays) and what is required (acceptable level of safety of the products). The most common situation that any blood transfusion service finds itself in is that where the screening performed generates reactive results. It is the action taken as a result of these that is important. (Please refer to Chapter 12.)

An effective strategy would be to retest all initial reactive samples, in duplicate, using the original assay, and determine the status of the donation only from the repeat results (two out of three strategy). This strategy does not reduce sensitivity – any initial reactive reflecting true infection would be repeatable (in at least one of the pair of repeat tests for very low level results) and therefore the donation would not be released for clinical use. This strategy may improve specificity – it is possible that any non-specific initial reactive results may not be repeatable and the donation could therefore be released for clinical use.

Finally, it is important that a strategy is developed to deal with those donors who are reactive in the screening assays. There are two issues to consider: the health of the donor – ensuring that any truly infected donor is identified and referred for clinical care; the sufficiency of the blood supply – as appropriate and depending upon any national legislation, the reinstatement of reactive but not truly infected donors. It is important to bear in mind that in a well selected, low-risk donor population, the expectation is that the majority of screen reactivity is due to non-specific rather than specific reactivity. Thus, a significant number of the reactive donors are not infected and may only have reacted in the screening assay on one particular occasion. To simply lose these donors is something that most services cannot afford. The confirmatory testing of screen reactive donors is therefore something that should be pursued wherever possible.

Assay design

Assay design can be considered in two parts: the design components that contribute to the scientific performance of the assay (sensitivity and specificity), and the design components that contribute to the operational performance of the assay (usability and process control features). Whilst the two parts are equally important, it is the operational performance that is significant as far as process control and assuring the quality of screening are concerned.

No matter how good the analytical sensitivity of any assay is reported to be, it is only a theoretical sensitivity unless it can be translated into actuality in the laboratory. The extent to which the actual sensitivity approaches the theoretical sensitivity depends upon the performance of the assay in the laboratory. The performance of the assay in the laboratory itself depends upon the type of assay, whether it is an open or closed system assay, the competence and ability of the staff (see later in this chapter) and the usability of the assay itself, that is, its usability and process control design features. No matter how good an assay is, if it is not performed correctly the results cannot be relied upon.

Engineering in both usability and process control features is something that most of the major international assay manufacturers have been doing for a number of years now. The relevant features are those considered under the heading of usability, which include appropriate sample volumes, incubation times and incubation temperatures, and those considered under process control – sample and reagent addition monitoring. These

features apply primarily to enzyme immunoassays (EIAs), which are the most commonly used antiglobulin assays in blood screening today. However, the existence of other assay formats must be acknowledged, and rapid/simple assays and particle agglutination assays must be considered. Rapid simple/assays are generally based on the standard EIA principles, but their presentation is generally that of a self-contained, single use, disposable cassette. These are single-use, single-test items that are not specifically designed for use for donation screening. Particle agglutination assays are relatively simple in their presentation, the format being that of a microplate EIA, using only sample diluent and the sensitized particles. These assays are used for blood screening, although in most countries this is restricted to syphilis screening. In both cases, however, whilst the scientific design of the assay is similar to that of an EIA, their format does not require or lend themselves to the same level of process control.

Usability

The usability of an assay is a measure of its 'user-friendliness'. The more user-friendly assay is in general easier to perform, and each assay run is more likely to be valid. The key elements in terms of usability centre around sample and reagent volumes, incubation times and temperatures and reagent presentation. However, the influence of each of these is very dependent upon whether the assay is an open system assay (microplate based and can be performed manually or on a range of open system instruments), or a closed system assay (can only be performed on a dedicated instrument).

Sample volumes

These need to be realistic: not too small, so that automated pipetting systems cannot pipette reliably and consistently, and not too large so that the available sample is used up too quickly. There is always a compromise, but most assays now utilize sample volumes in the range of 20–150 μl, depending upon the particular assay, which comfortably meet the above criteria. In addition, most well designed assays now incorporate a sample diluent containing a dye that changes colour in the presence of human serum or plasma which enables the positive confirmation of sample addition. Finally, the pre-dilution of samples is not appropriate for mass screening assays, adding another level of complexity with the consequent possibility of error. Most high quality assays used for donation screening do not require sample pre-dilution.

Reagent volumes

These also need to be realistic, although in general most reagent volumes are between 50–200 μl and these volumes can be pipetted easily and consistently both on automated systems and manually.

Reagent presentation

This is a further important factor in usability and, to a degree, process control. Ideally, ready-prepared reagents offer the highest level of usability, but not all reagents can be provided in that format. At the very least, reagents should be presented in a format which requires just the simple mixing of two components.

Incubation times/temperatures

These contribute to the overall usability of an assay, in most cases the times being more significant than temperature. Long incubation times are only problematical in that it takes longer to generate the final results. This may not be critical, but there are times when it is important to complete the screening as quickly as possible without compromising the quality of the results. Short incubation times can be very problematical, especially when using open automated systems to perform assays. Incubation times that are too short prevent the system generating proper time lines and may result in a situation where it takes longer to generate the final results as the individual plates are processed from start to finish one at a time (i.e. the next plate is started only when the preceding one has been finished and reported). Incubation temperature can be an issue when there is a room temperature stage but where the actual room temperature is outside the range stated by the manufacturer. This is very common in hot climates where there is no temperature control in the laboratory. In such situations the use of assays with all the incubation temperatures set at 37 °C is clearly beneficial.

The net benefit of these, and other, design features is to improve the overall control of the performance of the assay and thus the overall reliability and accuracy of the results generated.

Process control

The process control features in general are there to enable the user to provide evidence of the correct addition of sample and reagents at each stage of the assay. In general, the process control features are based upon a sample addition monitor (usually a colour change in the sample diluent upon addition of the sample), and the other reagents being coloured (Figure 17.2).

Sample addition monitors generally involve a chemical colour change using an indicator for a normal protein component of serum/plasma. The indicator is present in the sample diluent used in the assay and the colour change occurs upon addition of the sample to the diluent. In general, although the colour change is strongest when the correct amount of sample is added, it is not a quantitative change; it is a qualitative assessment only. Measurement of the optical density of the sample diluent after the addition of sample indicates whether or not the sample has been added. Similarly, the colouring of the other reagents, normally conjugate and substrate, also provides the means to detect, again by measurement of the optical density, whether the reagents have been added. The inclusion of a dye into assay reagents, except the substrate, is relatively straightforward. The inclusion of a dye into the substrate is clearly technically more complicated, but as long as the added dye absorbs light at a different wavelength from the activated substrate itself, it is very easy to distinguish the two by measuring the optical density at the appropriate wavelengths.

These assay features thus enable the addition of the sample and other reagents to be specifically monitored colourimetrically at each stage of the assay, and the data generated stored as part of the assay documentation. Such process control features may be found on both open system and closed system assays, and

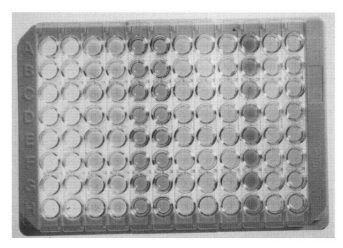

Figure 17.2 Colour monitoring of a microplate EIA using colour change and coloured reagents. (See colour plate section).

although they may function in very different ways, all provide documentable evidence of the correct addition of sample and reagents.

Assay evaluation

The selection of the most appropriate screening assays is central to ensuring product safety. The overall performance of the assays not only directly affects safety, but it also determines the effectiveness and appropriateness of the screening strategy.

The available assays should be evaluated and the 'most appropriate' assay selected for use. The issue here is how to decide which is the 'most appropriate' assay for any given situation, and to define exactly what 'most appropriate' actually means. In the donation screening situation 'most appropriate' means the assay that gives the best overall performance against the identified parameters, thus ensuring the highest quality of the screening results generated. These parameters include sensitivity and specificity, but also the usability in the routine screening environment and performance against the donor population from which the donations are collected. To ensure that the assays used are the most appropriate, it is essential that a formal evaluation process is set up and followed, all assays being evaluated through this process before any decisions are made about which assay should be used. This process should incorporate the scientific evaluation – sensitivity and specificity of the assays, and the operational evaluation – do the assays work to the expected standard in the laboratory?

The scientific evaluation is the part that most people are familiar with and includes all of the testing that is needed to ensure that the performance of the assay is sufficient to be used.

Specificity

This consists of testing a suitable number of screen-negative donation samples to determine how many non-specific reactives may be expected.

Sensitivity

Sensitivity is more involved, and to be properly effective, requires the use of panels of confirmed positive samples; strong, medium and low-level seroconversion panels; different genotypes; etc. Such samples are available commercially, but are expensive. In reality, these samples need to be collected over time, together with other samples that give interesting or unusual results. In some situations it is very hard to obtain not only reasonable numbers of samples for all of the markers being screened for, but also any low-level (naturally low titre) samples. Thus, it is virtually impossible to build suitable evaluation panels without purchasing the materials – which is again not an option for many BTSs. In such situations it is possible to perform 'paper' evaluations using sensitivity data from other sources. Manufacturers provide sensitivity data to support their claims for the assay. Many consider these data to be biased, but in reality they can be very useful. The data provided by the major manufacturers are generally accurate and sound to use, and should be incorporated into the evaluation process. More obviously independent sources of data are the published scientific evaluations performed by a number of national bodies. In Europe, such evaluations are performed by bodies such as the Health Protection Agency in the UK, the Agence de Medicament in France and the Paul-Ehrlich-Institut in Germany. In addition, the World Health Organization also commissions such evaluations for global dissemination. Once a 'paper' evaluation has been performed and the most appropriate assay selected, any locally generated confirmed positive samples available should be tested using the selected assay. This should help to finalize the selection.

Another factor in the evaluation process is that of usability. The assessment of usability is a parallel process to the scientific evaluation: no matter how scientifically good an assay is, if it is not very user friendly the reliability of the results cannot be guaranteed. Thus, the evaluation of usability needs to be carried out alongside the scientific evaluation. Indeed, in some cases it can be seen that an assay would not be useable (see earlier section above, page 218, the donation screening process for the parameters to be considered) even though its scientific performance was exceptional.

Finally, the evaluation process should be completed with a short operational validation – does the potential assay work as expected in the laboratory, under normal working conditions? This validation considers some aspects of usability, but goes further in that it considers the implementation of the assay into the daily routine. Does the assay run well on any automated or semi-automated systems, can staff perform it properly, are the results consistent with the current assay results? There are a number of elements to the operational validation, but all are associated with the routine use of the assay in the operational laboratory.

Once the evaluation process has been completed, documented fully and the final decisions made, the BTS will have a high degree of assurance that the assays selected, as long as they are performed correctly, will generate reliable and consistent results.

Some countries maintain formal 'approved lists' of assays that have been evaluated for donation screening and found to be suitable. Such an approach is very useful for the country, and also can be of value for any accreditation or licensing inspections. For example, in England the National Blood Service (NBS), has for over ten years had a formal kit evaluation group (KEG) (Barbara *et al.*, 2006). This group comprises experts in the field from both within the NBS and outside, and formally includes 'observers' from the Scottish, Welsh and Irish transfusion services. All screening assays used within the NBS must be evaluated and formally 'approved' for use for blood screening. The evaluation process is the standard approach, using a range of samples of known provenance which include low, medium and high titre seroconversion, and challenging or known problematical samples. The outcomes are then assessed in terms of blood screening needs rather than diagnostic testing. In addition, specificity and usability are also assessed by one of the ten NBS operational screening laboratories. In this way the performance characteristics of each assay, including compatibility with automated systems in use, are determined prior to use to ensure the reliability of the screening process.

Lot release

The checking of 'incoming goods' is fundamental to any quality system; therefore prior to the acceptance of any new manufacturer's lot of screening assay, the lot should be assessed to ensure that its performance is acceptable. Lot release testing is intended to give advance warning of any deterioration in assay performance prior to the acceptance of a new lot. However, it is not just any new 'lot' that should be assessed, each delivery of kits should also be assessed to ensure that the delivery conditions have not adversely affected the assay. Lot release must be performed in advance of the change to a new lot to ensure that there is time to complete the testing and deal with the outcomes before the new lot needs to be used.

There are different ways to perform lot release testing, but whatever approach is chosen, consideration must be given to the expected level of performance of the assay and how that can be assessed as reliably and objectively as possible, in a way that will identify any significant changes. Specifically designed lot release panels are probably the best approach, but do take considerable expertise, time and access to a wide range of materials in their construction and maintenance.

In general terms, lot release requires both sensitivity and specificity assessments, with predetermined acceptable/expected levels set. Ideally, the formal delivery of any new manufacturer's lot of kits would not be allowed until one kit had been received, assessed and approved for use. This is best performed by a centralized responsible laboratory, with the resources and expertise to undertake this type of work (Newham and Kitchen, 2006). Once the lot has been approved for use, the individual screening laboratories would only need to perform simple delivery checks to ensure there has not been significant deterioration of performance during transportation.

Finally, the action to be taken in the event of the failure of a new lot or an individual delivery should be considered. This may include action by the manufacturer/supplier as well as by the

NBTS. If a new lot fails the testing, a system must be in place to enable another lot to be assessed and a constructive dialogue to take place with the manufacturer/supplier. Importantly, there must be continuity of supply so that the screening programme is not compromised in any way.

Use of automated systems

The use of automated systems is a very specific way of standardizing the screening process and helping to ensure the overall quality of the products. Automating the whole screening process from end to end, from electronic read of sample ID and addition, through to result generation and possibly electronic transmission of the results to an IT system, ensures not only a consistency in the process, but also significantly reduces the risk of simple human errors.

As mentioned in the section above, page 219, on the donor screening process, assays basically exist as open system assays or closed system assays. Open system assays are generally in microplate format and can be performed on any microplate equipment. When using open systems, it is possible to use a range of assays from different manufacturers for the different screening markers. In addition, these assays can be performed manually (using the minimum of equipment). Closed system assays are specific dedicated assays that can only be used on the automated instrument that they were designed for; they cannot be performed manually.

The use of automated screening systems has obvious advantages to any laboratory. This is especially so in a routine screening environment where the focus is on a relatively small number of markers, but potentially screening large numbers of samples. The systems available are varied, either open or closed, but all function in broadly similar ways. As well as full systems, there are semi-automated systems (for example a system that processes an EIA plate but which does not add sample) and stand alone equipment (for example plate washers and readers).

Systems which perform the complete assay, from sample ID and pipetting to final reporting, are the ideal systems, but not always available to BTSs. The advantage of such systems is that 'positive ID' is maintained throughout the whole process. Positive ID is essentially the maintenance of a full audit trail, ideally electronically, for the performance of the screening from start to finish. The sample ID is read electronically, linked to a specific assay plate/well/carousel position, the processing of the assay is recorded at all stages, and the results are then tied up with the correct sample ID for either printing out or onward transmission via an IT system. Thus, the whole screening process has an electronic link running through it.

However, automation has pitfalls if not used and maintained correctly. No matter what the precise functionality of the equipment, the results generated as a result of using it are only as good as the equipment itself, which is dependent upon the maintenance and calibration performed on it. A comprehensive and effective maintenance and calibration programme must be developed for each item of equipment. For some items this will actually be very little work, whilst for others it may be more complex and involve reasonable amounts of work by both the user and supplier/

manufacturer. In most cases maintenance can be broken down into the daily, weekly and monthly activities required of the user, with the additional recommended periodic professional maintenance/servicing. Full records of the maintenance required, what was performed, when it was performed and who performed it must be kept. In addition, where calibration is required, a calibration schedule should be developed which ensures that the calibration required is identified, the expected ranges are defined and a suitable calibration period is defined to ensure that the equipment is always working within its required range(s). Again, full records of all calibration activities and who performed them must be kept.

Finally, all equipment in use should always be identified as having been serviced/calibrated, with the next due dates identified. Specific service/calibration labels should be used. In this way there is clear evidence that the equipment is being maintained and is safe to use.

The use of quality control samples and quality assessment schemes

The use of quality control (QC) samples and quality assessment (QA) schemes are important additional quality tools to help ensure and maintain quality within the screening process. Both can be further divided into internal and external sources: internal QC samples and QA Scheme being produced/provided by the laboratory itself; external QC and QAS being provided by external, expert laboratories that are often funded specifically to provide such services as part of their overall responsibilities.

Quality control samples

Quality control samples are generally provided by external expert laboratories and are used by laboratories to monitor their routine run-to-run and day-to-day assay performance (Ferguson, 1993). This may be by using the QC samples effectively as additional assay controls with specific performance criteria attached to them (go-no-go samples), or as simple monitoring tools. In general, QC samples are used in real-time by individual laboratories, and outside the laboratory itself further analysis of the results is not undertaken. However, in some cases the suppliers of the QC samples do request the results of testing of the samples from the laboratories, and retrospective evaluation of QC sample data from the different laboratories who use them is undertaken (see the next section below, page 223, quality assessment) (Hertzberg et al., 2006).

The samples are usually specifically manufactured low-level reacting material that is strong enough to give clear, consistent and thus comparable results, but at the same time weak enough to be able to indicate any changes in assay performance. Currently in the UK this is set at 0.2 IU/ml for HBsAg. Generally, it is considered that only changes that may result in a loss of overall performance are significant, but this is not true. Any increase in assay performance equally needs to be identified and understood. The samples cannot indicate the reasons for any such change, they simply indicate that a change has occurred and performance has changed. It is important that BTSs do include the appropriate QC samples in their screening programmes, and these samples can be most

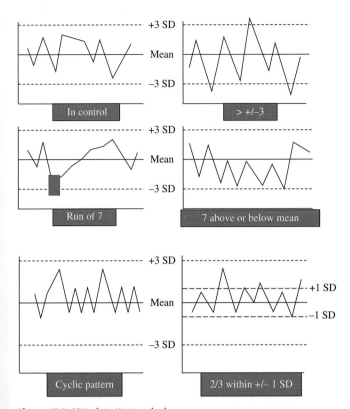

Figure 17.3 SPM plots, Westgard rules.

effectively used if they can be set as go-no-go samples. The QC sample is included as part of the overall validation criteria; for a run to be valid the QC sample must be within a specified range – normally the result must be reactive. If the QC result is not reactive the run would be considered invalid and have to be repeated.

As well as changes in performance due to the performance of the assay by the staff, QC results can also indicate changes in assay performance due to unnoticed manufacturing problems or changes. Probably the key value of the use of QC samples is that of using their results to provide the core data for statistical process monitoring (SPM) of the assay performance. SPM is used to monitor run/run and/or day/day performance, to ensure broad consistency in performance. The daily QC results are plotted on monitoring charts and the overall trends over time can be seen (see Figure 17.3).

Applying SPM rules such as the Westgard rules enables ongoing analysis of the results and early identification of any changes. The Westgard rules consist of a number of different decision criteria that can be used to determine if a screening run is in-control or out-of-control. In essence, the rules are used to identify specific trends in the data that fall outside the normal range of variation expected for the particular process. Importantly, they can be used to identify change early on, monitoring rather than controlling, before a process actually goes out of control and the results are considered invalid. The rules include such findings as:

- A specified number of consecutive control measurements show a trend in the same direction
- A specified number of consecutive control measurements fall on one side of the mean

- A number of consecutive control measurements exceed the mean plus/minus two standard deviations
- A cyclic pattern is seen.

An important issue is that the reason for the change cannot be identified, but the fact that a change has occurred is identified.

However, the QC samples used, whether internal or external, do need to be of a high quality if the results are to be relied upon. Thus, the provision of good QC samples is critical. Unfortunately, this can be problematical and it is essential that QC samples are evaluated properly before their formal adoption into the screening programme. The major issue is of stability. It is obviously essential that the QC materials can be totally relied upon to provide consistent results run after run. The only variation that should be seen is that due to the performance of the assay itself, not a change in performance of the QC sample due to deterioration/other changes in its composition/reactivity. In addition, the lot-to-lot variation also needs to be minimal so that once the basic parameters for a particular QC sample are set, they do not need to be changed every time a new lot of the material is received.

Quality assessment schemes

Quality assessment schemes (QAS) are another important aspect of ensuring quality in the laboratory. However, rather than just looking at assay performance, QAS are a means by which the whole screening process within the laboratory is monitored, from sample reception to result generation.

External quality assessment schemes (EQAS)

These are generally external schemes usually organized by an expert laboratory/institution. Laboratories choose to participate, although this is now more and more a regulatory/accreditation requirement, and receive a number of distributions each year (Health Protection Agency (HPA) Microbiology EQAS; National Serology Reference Laboratory (NSRL) Quality EQAS). Each distribution normally consists of a small set of samples of unknown status, but which cover one or more of the markers routinely screened for. These samples are then tested in the same way as, and alongside, the routine workload of the laboratory. The overall results generated are then returned to the organizing institution for analysis. The results generated not only assess the screening itself, they assess the whole of the process of the laboratory so that any weaknesses, which may not be anything to do with the performance of the assays themselves, can be identified. The results of the analysis of the distribution are then returned to each participating laboratory so that not only does each laboratory receive its score for the distribution, but it also receives the anonymous results of all of the other participating laboratories so that it can also determine how its overall performance compares with that of the other laboratories who also examined the samples. Overall involvement in EQAS is a very valuable tool for any donation screening laboratory. It has long been known that quality is not just assured through proper assay performance, it is the whole range of activities that take place within a laboratory that have an influence on the overall level of quality achieved. Major sources of error in most laboratories still involve human error. Because EQAS assess the whole process, these factors can more easily be assessed.

Internal quality assessment (IQA)

Although most laboratories are well aware of EQAS, internal QA is another important tool in assuring quality in the screening process. This is quite a different process in which the laboratory checks its own process by generating a 'new' sample by splitting a sample at random at the sample reception stage, allocating a separate sample ID to the 'new' sample and then processing normally both the original and the 'new' sample. The assessment process is to ensure that both samples have results generated at the same time and have the same final result. This is a very simple but effective means of continuously checking the overall laboratory process, and can be easily and very usefully performed on a monthly basis.

Validation and assessment of results and assay performance

Once the screening has been completed and the results obtained, specific validation of the results (run by run), and thus the screening process overall, is an important quality step. This individual assay run validation follows on from the in-process validation activities, discussed previously, that occur during the performance of the assay. The process control activities demonstrate that the assay has actually been performed within the acceptable limits, the result validation subsequently ensures that the results generated are also within the expected limits.

The quality system associated with the validation of the final results consists of a number of individual validation elements, all of which have to be considered and applied before the results can be considered valid. The application of individual evaluation elements is something that each BTS needs to consider, and is based upon the quality system in place, and what is practical and achievable. The following set of validation elements are presented to illustrate the levels of validation available (individual run, short- and long-term laboratory performance), the different approaches available, and how these all interact with each other to develop a structured, step-by-step validation process that includes the whole of the screening process from individual run to long-term performance.

Manufacturer's validation criteria

The initial level of individual run validation is that indicated by the manufacturer. For any assay run to be valid the assay controls must meet certain criteria. Generally, this would include the negative and positive (and cut-off if included) control results, which must be within the manufacturer's stated, expected ranges; this includes both the number of individual controls required to be valid as well as the individual results for the controls. If these criteria are met the assay run is considered to be valid, if they are not met it is considered to be invalid. An invalid run at this stage requires the whole run to be repeated.

User validation criteria

The second level of individual run validation includes any additional criteria that may be set by the BTS. For example, the application of any 'grey-zone', a maximum level of reactive results per run, or even a specific range within which all the negative sample results must lie. The use of 'grey-zones' is something that may be forced by the manufacturer, if a part of the overall result calculation. There is a lot of debate over the real value of such approaches. However, the easiest way to deal with 'grey-zones' where they have to be incorporated is to re-set the cut-off value at the lower end of the 'grey-zone' range, that is if the 'grey-zone' is set at $+/-10\%$ of the cut-off value, the cut-off should be re-calculated by multiplying by 0.9. Other criteria, such as limiting the number of reactives per run, can provide a very useful, if somewhat simplistic, additional validation criterion. As donor populations should be low risk and the screening assays selected should have good specificity, the expectation is that any test run would have very few, if any, reactive results. A reasonable limit on the number of reactive results would provide a useful quick validation check. There are a number of ways in which the result data generated can be further analysed to validate the run.

Quality control sample results

The final level of individual run validation considers the results of the QC samples included in the assay run. The use of 'go-no-go' (GNG) QC samples provides an independent (of the assay) evaluation of assay performance. The QC samples cannot only be used to determine run validity (GNG), but can also be used for more detailed ongoing performance monitoring looking for trends (please see section on automated systems above, page 222).

Quality assessment schemes

The value of QAS, especially EQAS must never be underestimated as it can provide high quality evidence of a laboratory's overall performance. As well as validating the individual run results, laboratory performance itself does need to be validated in some way. External quality assessment schemes validate performance both internally (the normal laboratory end-to-end process is validated) and externally (the overall results are compared to the results on the same panels of samples generated by other, broadly comparable, laboratories).

External review of quality control results

Although an activity performed retrospectively, the analysis of the QC sample results can provide useful additional data. Primarily, these data demonstrate inter-laboratory variability, but importantly, very often this is due more to differences in the performance of different assays rather than in laboratory performance. However, the retrospective analysis of large amounts of data can be used to examine the overall performance of a group of laboratories. The use of precision plots, etc. (see Figure 17.4) can give a

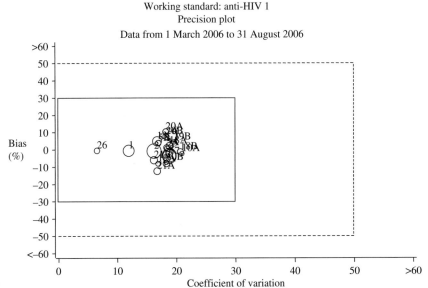

Working standard: anti-HIV 1
Precision plot
Data from 1 March 2006 to 31 August 2006

Figure 17.4 Precision plot, national QC sample.

very useful pictorial representation of the overall precision of the screening process for each marker of infection, but are independent of the assay used. Comparisons can be lab-to-lab, day-to-day, assay-to-assay, even operator-to-operator. Such data are very important in assuring the overall quality of not just each individual BTS, but of the national organization as a whole, whether the blood transfusion service activities are controlled through a formal national organization or whether the individual transfusion centres are autonomous bodies.

At the same time, care must be taken to ensure that such data are not over-analysed. In general, such data show what is happening, but cannot define why something is happening, that is, what is the root cause. The data should only be used to identify a change, to trigger an appropriate investigation, but not to pre-determine its outcome.

Identification of unsuitable donations

An often overlooked element of blood safety, and the quality system associated with screening, is that of ensuring that any donations that are identified as screen reactive or otherwise considered to be an infection risk, and therefore considered to be unsuitable for clinical use, are removed from inventory BEFORE the release of the screen negative donations.

The quarantining of all donations immediately after collection and until the required laboratory screening has been performed should be the standard procedure for all BTSs. Once all the screening has been completed and those donations unsuitable for clinical use have been identified, all of the donations, and any products prepared from them, must be actively retrieved and moved to a secure place before the formal checking and release of the suitable donations. This relatively simple action will prevent the release of those products and consequently contribute significantly to the overall safety of the products provided by the BTS.

Staff knowledge and skills

The overall ability and competence of the laboratory staff is a factor that can directly influence the quality of the screening and its outcomes. To ensure high quality screening the staff performing it must be well trained and educated, and, importantly, kept up to date at all times. Ensuring that there are sufficient, well-trained staff, and that there are the appropriate education and training systems in place is essential.

A fundamental message when developing quality systems is that of developing the culture of quality. The culture is something that is developed in staff, but the staff need to be able to both understand the message and act to fulfil the message. This is where it is important to have staff who have both the knowledge and skills to work in the laboratory, but who also have the understanding of the issues associated with work and the importance of ensuring a quality focused approach at all times.

Unfortunately, as automated systems increase in number and in reliability, especially closed systems, the demands upon the staff are decreasing. Automated systems provide a means of ensuring high quality results, but the need for staff intervention, especially with closed automated systems, is decreased to the point of very little being required from the staff running some systems beyond switching the machines on and off, loading samples and reagents, and performing basic user maintenance. This is a situation that gives rise to some concern as it means that laboratory staff risk becoming simply machine minders, and practical skills and expertise will quickly be lost. Those staff working in laboratories using open system assays generally have more involvement during the assay process, although as open systems develop further this, too, is likely to change.

It is hard to determine the best way forward in these situations. There is no doubt that the use of automated systems improves the overall quality of blood donation screening, but at the longer-term cost of gradually de-skilling laboratory staff. The real problem is that of being able to identify when things go wrong. Whilst most systems do run efficiently and effectively for > 90% of the time, there are times when things go wrong. Unfortunately, it is not the sudden breakdown of a system that needs considered intervention, it is the gradual change in performance that occurs over a period of time and which may not be immediately noticeable. Having staff with the knowledge and skills to recognize and deal with these more subtle changes and problems is essential. The problem is how to develop and maintain such skills in a laboratory which for most of the time does not need them.

It is therefore important to develop staff training programmes which cover both routine day-to-day activities as well as continued education and development, and which also provide the appropriate quality training. Very often training programmes look forward to new skills and knowledge, etc., without full consideration of the need to consolidate the training on current activities. This is especially true for quality training, which is very often completely overlooked in terms of providing specific, high quality training in the development and maintenance of quality systems in laboratories. Without the investment in the training of staff, the quality of the output of the laboratory cannot be assured.

Haemovigilance

Please refer to Chapter 21.

The final feedback system, which assesses the actual quality of the screening process, and other processes within a BTS, is that of the monitoring of patients post-transfusion/transplantation for any adverse events, that is, haemovigilance. This would embrace adverse events for any reason, including post-transfusion/transplantation infections.

National haemovigilance systems have been developed and implemented in many countries and do provide an effective means of gathering, collating and analysing information on the outcomes of transfusion/transplantation. The analysis of events

is essential, but to ensure that this is effective, the quality of the information supplied is critical. Organization is a key requirement of any effective haemovigilance system; definitions of adverse events should be provided, as should guidance on how to identify and how to report an adverse event. Standardization in reporting is essential to ensure that the right information is provided, and in the right format. Only then can events be analysed correctly and the proper comparisons made and conclusions drawn.

If any adverse event following the transfusion/transplantation of any blood/tissue products were to occur, it is critical that whatever happened is investigated fully, understood, and any appropriate measures put into place to prevent such an event happening again. Unfortunately, most of the haemovigilance systems are reactive rather than proactive, only reacting when recipients demonstrate signs and symptoms. Prospective monitoring of all recipients is not generally performed due to the high cost and complexity, but also because the overall safety of transfusion/transplantation in many countries is such that adverse events are not expected nor commonplace.

REFERENCES

Barbara, J., Ramskill, S., Perry, K., *et al.* (2006) The National Blood Service (England) approach to evaluation of kits for detecting infectious agents. *Transfus Med Rev*, **21**, 147–58.

Ferguson, M., Pipkin, P. A., Heath, A. B., *et al.* (1993) Working standards for hepatitis B surface antigen for use in the UK Blood Transfusion Service: results for a collaborative study. *Vox Sang.*, **65** (4), 303–8.

Hertzberg, M. S., Mammen, J., McCraw, A., *et al.* (2006) Achieving and maintaining quality in the laboratory. *Haemophilia*, **12** (Suppl. 3), 61–7.

HPA EQAS (available at: http://www.hpa.org.uk/cfi/quality/default.htm).

Newham, J. and Kitchen, A. D. (2006) Lot release of microbiology blood screening kits and HCV NAT in the English National Blood Service. *Vox Sang*, **91** (S3), 6 (Abs).

NSRL Quality Assurance Programme (available at: http://www.nrl.gov.au/dir185/nrl-pub.nsf/Structure/QualityAssuranceProgramme-JSOL-44Q9HG).

18 MICROBIOLOGICAL BLOOD TESTING AND NEW TECHNOLOGIES

Juraj Petrik

Current testing methods: brief technology background

Current microbiological testing is discussed in detail in Chapters 11 and 12. Preventive measures, inactivation and microbiology testing as performed, at least in developed countries, guarantee an extremely safe blood supply (Barbara, 1998). Recently, a technologically demanding and conceptually different type of testing, NAT (discussed in Chapter 14), has been implemented as a routine procedure. In countries with high development indices, residual risk estimates, especially for transfusion-transmitted viruses, are very low (Soldan et al., 2003) and not many other medical procedures (if any) can match them. Of course, there is always room for improvement on safety: a level of automation to limit operator-related errors, cost-efficiency, etc.

In order to compare the power of current testing techniques with the potential of newly developed candidate next generation testing techniques, a brief summary of current testing technologies follows.

Unique features of microbiological blood screening

Various aspects of microbiological blood screening make it a rather unique process when compared with other testing procedures for infectious agents (see Table 18.1). Under usual circumstances people are tested for infectious agents on the basis of symptoms at or after a visit to a primary care physician, or during a stay in hospital. In other words, the physician or hospital microbiology laboratory personnel know what range of tests to perform on the basis of the referral or a preliminary diagnosis. Consequently, a large proportion of tested samples will give a positive result for one or more tested pathogens. There is a significantly different situation with blood donors who are predominantly self-selected healthy individuals and the vast majority of samples (donations) test negative. However, because blood or blood components prepared from a donation are destined for recipients, the detection of each single infection or contamination with a transfusion-transmissible pathogen is an absolute priority. The sensitivity of the screening assays therefore needs to be extremely high, which may reduce specificity, so that repeat testing of reactives is part of the routine algorithm. To add to the demands on blood screening, there are time constraints on the testing procedures to allow timely blood processing and issue of components, especially those with a short shelf life, such as platelets. Furthermore, many blood centres might handle between 500–3000 donations a day and the testing procedures, especially those for individual sample testing, need to accommodate this

throughput. In summary, the requirements for each parameter of microbiological screening of blood donations are very demanding, due to the safety required for blood and components that will be intravenously transfused to patients.

Serology (antibody, antigen and combi assays)

Please refer to Chapter 11.

The power and simplicity of ligand assays developed during the 1950s revolutionized the whole diagnostic field. Immunoassays developed during the 1980s, using antibodies labelled with high specific activity non-radioisotope labels have taken these assays to a new, ultrasensitive level. The majority of currently used immunoassays represent variations on a non-competitive sandwich type assay (Ekins, 1998). The solid phase for immobilization of antigen (in antibody testing), antibody (in antigen testing) or both (combiassays) is usually the surface of a microplate well or a particle (bead or microsphere). Testing is based on the indirect antiglobulin test and after antibody-antigen interaction, labels can be attached to anti-human IgG, or in more elaborate multiple sandwich assays, to intermediate haptens such as biotin. Conjugated enzymes, most frequently horseradish peroxidase (HRP) or alkaline phosphatase (AP) convert the substrate into an optically measurable and quantifiable dye or chemiluminescence.

Antibody detection

The majority of currently used serological assays detect circulating antibodies developed against the infecting agent. In the majority of assays, IgG is detected, though a few detect both IgG and IgM. The residual window period with these assays varies between 20–80 days depending on the particular pathogen. Antibody tests are in most cases robust and reliable. The disadvantage is that they do not directly detect the pathogen, so that possible consequences are:

(1) Detection of antibodies in recovered individuals
(2) Detection of antibodies in vaccinated persons
(3) Failure to detect antibodies in immunosilent infections (immunosuppression or other causes).

For antibody detection, the infectious agent or, more frequently, its relevant components are immobilized on a solid phase. Since the development of recombinant DNA technologies in the 1980s, recombinant antigens are increasingly used. They are either complete proteins, truncated proteins (lacking certain regions which are not essential for, or which interfere with, antibody detection), or chimaeric proteins composed of regions from two or more antigens. Depending on the importance of post-translational modifications (e.g. glycosylation) for antigenicity

Transfusion Microbiology, eds John A. J. Barbara, Fiona A. M. Regan and Marcela C. Contreras. Published by Cambridge University Press. © Cambridge University Press 2008.

Table 18.1 Unique requirements for microbiological blood screening; comparison with other types of microbiology testing.

	Blood screening	Hospital diagnostic lab	Point of care testing
Population tested	Blood donors	Patients	General public
Frequency of positive sample	Very low (healthy population)	Very high (previous referral)	High (symptoms)
Throughput (no. of samples per assay)	$n \times 100$ to $n \times 1000$	$n \times 1$ to $n \times 10$	Individual samples
Turnaround time	<8 hrs	±24 hrs	<1 hr
Sensitivity required	Very high	High	Medium–high
Downstream application of tested material	Yes	No	No

the recombinant proteins can be produced in various systems: *Escherichia coli* or other bacterial systems, yeast, insect or mammalian cells using plasmids or engineered viral expression vectors. Various tags (cleavable or not) may be introduced to the molecule for an easy one-step purification of the recombinant products. In addition, synthetic peptides representing a region of the antigen containing a linear epitope(s) are often used.

Antigen detection

Antigen testing directly detects the presence of the infectious agent or its components. From this point of view it is the preferred way of testing. The drawback is usually the insufficient sensitivity of assays, generally or at particular stages of a pathogen's replication cycle. A successful example of antigen detection is hepatitis B surface antigen (HBsAg) due to extremely high circulating levels of this antigen. The immobilized capture agents are polyclonal or monoclonal antibodies. Alternatively, antibody fragments or in vitro produced single chain antibody fragments containing the variable portion (scFv), obtained by screening antibody phage libraries, may be used. With the advent of genomics, proteomics and metabolomics (see below) other alternatives may become available, such as any specifically interacting molecules or specifically induced host factors.

Antibody and antigen detection

Combi or 'fourth' generation assays contain both the antibody and the antigen immobilized on the solid surface and are measured in one assay. They have been developed mostly for HIV detection and those approaching the sensitivity of specialized antigen assays (1 – few pg/ml) can almost close the window-period gap on NAT assays (e.g. 2.75 days between HIV NAT and a combi-assay, Weber *et al.*, 2002). Recently a combi-assay for HCV has become commercially available.

Nucleic acid technology testing (NAT)

NAT is described in detail in other chapters of this book (see Chapter 14). For the purpose of this chapter it is important to stress that the introduction of NAT into routine blood screening operations represented a major change in blood screening practice. After decades dominated by serological assays which brought major improvements to blood safety, the 1990s saw a rather sudden push for embracing this new technology. The main reason lies in the exquisite sensitivity of techniques such as

polymerase chain reaction (PCR), transcription mediated amplification (TMA), nucleic acid sequence based amplification (NASBA) and a few other techniques based on target amplification. The target is the nucleic acid (usually genomic RNA or DNA). In PCR, a sequence flanked by specific primers is amplified up to a billion times in a space of 30–90 minutes. A few dozen molecules per ml are reproducibly detected. This sensitivity and the fact that it directly detects the pathogen component leads to a substantial shortening of the window period for selected viral pathogens.

Safety, complexity and cost-efficiency of current testing methods

As mentioned earlier, the microbiological safety of blood transfusion can hardly be matched by other medical procedures. (See Chapter 26.) Residual risk figures, especially those for blood-borne viruses tested for by NAT assays are in a range of one per few million donations (Soldan *et al.*, 2003). The implementation of conceptually different NAT assays into routine operation represented a major step for blood screening laboratories. Safety has been improved by detection of NAT-only-positive donations which could not have been detected by other means. (Please refer to Chapters 12 and 14.) Equally important is the fact that staff were trained in the use of new modern technology and became better prepared for future technological developments. At the same time it has transpired that NAT is perhaps less amenable to reliable multiplexing than originally thought and the cost-efficiency of NAT is questionable due to the lower than predicted numbers of NAT-only positives, especially in countries with low prevalence rates. In addition, NAT has not replaced other assays (perhaps with the exception of HIV-1 p24 testing), adding to the complexity of the existing testing algorithms (see section on 'Impact of new technologies on testing algorithms', below). It is hoped that the 'next generation' multianalyte microarray-based technologies can address much of the current complexity by providing one instrumental platform for testing each donation for a complete set of required markers (Petrik, 2001).

New developments: era of 'omics'

After the initial appearance of the term genomics in the 1980s we have since witnessed a whole series of 'omics'. The need for new disciplines was created by the change of approaches which focus on a comprehensive study of whole sets of genes or other molecules rather than single genes, proteins, small molecules, etc.

Genomics

One of the simplest definitions of genomics is the study of genes and their function. The change in the scale from individual genes to large sets of genes and complete genomes results from the technological developments such as highly parallel analysis provided by the microarray technology and huge information content provided by large sequencing programmes, especially the human genome project. Application of genomics and its tools to particular fields leads to more specialized disciplines such as pharmacogenomics for prediction of drug response, efficacy and toxicity due to the individual differences in targeted genes and gene products. In the course of sequencing projects, differences (mainly in the form of single nucleotide polymorphisms (SNP)), have revealed an average frequency of one change per 1000 base pairs. It is the cumulative effect of these polymorphisms which produces unique individual features.

Proteomics

The number of human genes as revealed by the human genome project was lower than originally predicted. Altogether we have around 26 000 genes. Huge variability comes mainly from gene products (i.e. proteins) and their interactions. Multiple forms of protein products can arise from the coding sequence of one gene. Apart from splicing variants, the variability at protein level is mostly the result of post-translational modifications such as glycosylation, phosphorylation, proteolytic cleavage, di- or multimerization, etc. Proteomics is the study of the full set of proteins (proteome) encoded by the genome. This includes various interactions and metabolic or signalling networks involving proteins. Proteomics is sometimes called functional genomics.

Metabolomics

The most current of 'omics' aims to measure the levels of small molecules, or metabolites. The metabolome represents the entire complement of all the small molecular weight metabolites, and metabolomics is the global analysis of these metabolites. In a sense, the direct measurement of a particular metabolite could be more informative than the measurement of a protein producing the metabolite or indeed, the gene transcript serving as a template for the synthesis of that protein.

Impact on diagnostics

Genomics, proteomics and metabolomics could all have a significant impact on development of diagnostic assays. Specific or group-specific pathogen expression patterns could be identified using expression profiling (Cummings and Relman, 2000). It is conceivable that the synthesis of certain molecules in response to the infecting agent, especially in the cells of the immune system, precedes the detectable synthesis of pathogen-specific structural or non-structural components. Detection of such molecules could lead to further shortening of the window period to the point of detection of the infecting agent. As at that stage, the dose of the infecting agent would most probably be insufficient for secondary transmission to the recipient, this would significantly increase the safety of transfusion. Even coinciding synthesis of the host agent-response specific molecules could strengthen the detection methods for certain pathogens. However, the successful detection of these new testing targets may require a different approach to sample preparation.

New diagnostic tools

The exquisite sensitivity and, in some cases, the higher precision of NAT compared with serology led to the development of numerous in-house and commercial assays, not only in microbiological testing but also in forward and reverse blood grouping assays. Assay sensitivity is undoubtedly an issue of primary importance. As mentioned earlier, reliable and robust NAT multiplexing is rather limited, although the recent development of automated triplex assays is encouraging. The question is, how flexible can these systems be, with respect to new and emerging testing targets? In each of the last few decades, testing for an additional transfusion-transmitted pathogen has been added (HCV, HIV, HTLV), accelerating more recently with the introduction of malaria and West Nile virus testing in some countries. The questionable cost-efficiency of NAT assays makes multiplexing the only viable option for the future. At the same time, the rigid constraints of the highly regulated field of blood screening makes swift addition of any new testing target to the existing multiplexed NAT assay rather problematical.

Serological assays are continually being improved and some of the recently developed assays (e.g. antigen/antibody combi) show impressive performance, almost matching the NAT assays in closing the window period. With the added bonus of easier multiplexing and improved detection limits by signal amplification methods, the serological methods seem to have entered into a new stage of development, especially in conjunction with miniaturization.

Simultaneous analysis of multiple analytes, with miniaturization, are the main features of microarray technology, originally developed to monitor the parallel expression of thousands of genes. It has quickly become clear that there is great potential for diagnostic use of this technology and diagnostics may indeed become the dominant application in the future. High throughput, however, comes at a price of insufficient sensitivity for some applications. While 'on-chip' NAT techniques have been developed, they require more complex chip design, potentially driving the cost too high and the throughput too low. Options for increased microarray sensitivity are discussed in the section on 'Microarray sensitivity', below.

Microarrays, biochips and biosensors

It is rather difficult to offer a simple definition of 'microarray' as there is a great variability in formats and systems developed in recent years. Perhaps the most frequent and accepted perception of microarray is a glass slide with surface modification allowing efficient robotic high-density spotting of numerous DNA probes at pre-programmed specific locations.

Multiple DNA probes derived, for example, from multiple genes, allow simultaneous investigation of transcription patterns through hybridization with fluorescently labelled RNA (cDNA) samples, and identification with a laser scanner (Brown and Botstein, 1999; Shalon *et al.*, 1996). Of course, there are other microarray applications utilizing arrayed proteins, carbohydrates, cells, tissues or small molecules (see the section on 'DNA, protein, cell, tissue, carbohydrate and small molecule microarrays', below, p232) and the term microarray is often used interchangeably with the term biochip (or DNA microarrays with DNA chip, protein microarray with protein chip, etc.). A common feature is highly parallel analysis providing a snapshot of the biological state of analysed molecules in the sample at a particular moment, detected by an extensive set of probes. If we consider a broad definition of biosensor as a biomolecular probe measuring the presence or concentration of biological molecules by translating biochemical interaction into a quantifiable physical signal, then microarrays and biochips represent a type of biosensor.

Microarrays resulted from technological rather than conceptual development of earlier techniques. We can consider the Northern and Western blots or dot blots on nitrocellulose, nylon or PVDF membranes as predecessors of current microarrays. Although DNA microarrays preceded the development of protein microarrays, studies on further miniaturization of immunoassays were initiated in the late 1980s (Ekins and Chu, 1991). However, to change a macroarray into a microarray, porous substrates had to be replaced with non-porous materials such as glass, silicon or plastic. This change allowed for a very significant reduction in the quantities of deposited probes and reaction volumes. Another change, apart from miniaturization, was the 'role reversal' for the probe and the sample. While the blots with deposited samples were addressed with the excess of labelled probes, in the microarray the probes are immobilized and the samples labelled. Only a small proportion of the probe spot will be occupied by the bound sample, allowing for a quantitative signal readout.

Multiple microarray formats and design features

The pace of development of new microarray materials, formats and applications is so high that it is difficult to provide a comprehensive list at any time. Table 18.2 provides examples of the main design features and of the companies developing particular approaches. Planar surfaces and microparticles in the form of beads or coated metal particles are two main substrate formats. The chemistry of surface modifications and probe attachment is similar in some cases but the probe immobilization to particles is carried out in solution, while different deposition techniques had to be developed for planar microarrays. When the performance was directly compared for detection of bacterial and viral proteins, both formats could provide sensitive multiplex assays, with the bead (Luminex) system more sensitive and planar microarray

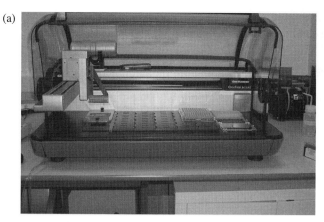

Figure 18.1 Contact printing equipment.
(a) An example of an automated Microarrayer.

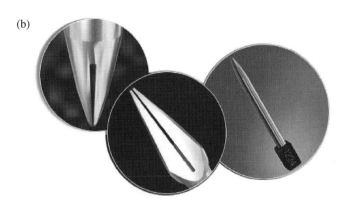

Figure 18.1 (b) A single split printing pin.

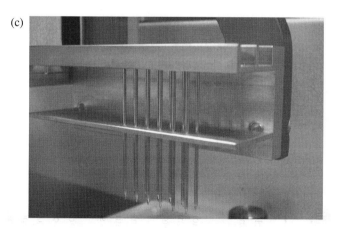

Figure 18.1 (c) Multiple pins in a printing head for contact printing.

more suitable for miniaturization (Rao *et al.*, 2004). Three principal deposition technologies were in situ synthesis of oligonucleotides (Fodor *et al.*, 1991), contact spotting of pre-synthesized cDNA or oligonucleotide molecules, pioneered by Pat Brown's group (Schena *et al.*, 1995), and contactless ink-jet printing of pre-synthesized molecules. (See Figure 18.1, Contact printing equipment.) Figure 18.1a shows an example of an automated Microarrayer (OmniGrid), Figure 18.1b, a single split printing pin and Figure 18.1c, multiple pins in a printing head for contact printing. The in situ synthesis has been used by Affymetrix to

Table 18.2 Main design features of microarrays/biochips.

Feature	Options	Example[a]	Company Website[a]
Substrate	Planar	Glass, silicon, plastic	various
	Microparticles	Beads, metal particles	various
Surface modification	Metal coating	Gold slides	www.eiresci.com
	Gel pads	Hydrogel slides	lifesciences.perkinelmer.com
	Membrane	Nitrocellulose (fast) slides	www.schleicher-schuell.com
	Derivatization: electrostatic absorption covalent attachment	Poly-L-lysine slides, silanized slides (GAPS)	www.corning.com
		Aldehyde, epoxy derivatized slides	arrayit.com
Probe deposition	In situ synthesis	Mask-guided sequential addition of nucleotides	www.affymetrix.com
		Maskless synthesis	www.nimblegen.com
	Contact printing	Quill, ring and pin, solid pin designs	arrayit.com
	Ink-jet printing	Contactless piezoelectric deposition	www.biorobotics.com
	Reaction in solution (beads)	Covalent or affinity attachment	www.packardinst.com
			various
Probe identification	Programmed deposition	Spotters, printers	various
	Particle encoding; beads	Different ratios of two dyes enclosed in particle	www.luminexcorp.com
	Particle encoding; nanobarcode particles	Barcode of metal strips	www.nanoplextech.com
	Random deposition and decoding; beads	Etched cores of optic fibres forming an array	www.illumina.com
Sample application	All probe sites simultaneously	Manual or automated hybridization, washing	www.amershambiosciences.com
	Individual probe sites (physically separated sites)	Microfluidics	www.agilent.com; www.caliperls.com
		Microfluidics + electronic addressing	www.nanogen.com
Detection method	Fluorescent methods	Fluorofore labelling; Confocal scanning; Flow cytometry based	various
	Resonance light scattering	Precious metal particles; signal depends on size, shape, composition	www.luminexcorp.com
			www.geniconsciences.com
	Surface plasmon resonance	Label-free; real-time; gold film	www.biacore.com; www.xantec.com
	Planar waveguide detection	Fluorofores; T_2O_5, TiO_2 film	www.zeptosens.com
	Mass spectrometry	Label-free; MALDI	www.sequenom.com
		SELDI	www.ciphergen.com

[a] Examples rather than a complete list.

develop GeneChip containing multiple 25-mer oligonucleotides per gene. Photomask-determined synthesis is used, in which a protected precursor is de-protected by exposure to light, controlled by an overlying mask, allowing addition only to the exposed positions. This process is repeated to build up an array of short nucleotides. For 25-mer oligonucleotides (Affymetrix chip) 100 different masks are needed (four bases for each of the 25 additions).The photomask-determined synthesis allows for an extremely high probe density and we are approaching a long-awaited era of one chip–one genome analysis. Contact spotting is the most widely used probe depositing technique, due to flexibility for the end user. Ink-jet printing will undoubtedly be used increasingly, with more instruments becoming available. All three techniques can usually be used for most of the surface modified slides as listed in Table 18.2. The difference between planar and microparticle systems is, however, in probe identification. While planar microarray deposition is pre-programmed and the identity of each spot recorded, microparticles carrying different probes have to be prepared separately as they are individually barcoded via different ratios of internal dyes or the sequence of metal strips. An exception is a random deposition of Illumina particles which are then identified in a series of quick hybridization steps (Michael *et al.*, 1998).

The sample is usually applied simultaneously to all sites on a planar microarray or to microparticles. There are, however, more sophisticated systems using microfluidics (e.g. Agilent) and additional features such as electronic addressing (Nanogen, Cheng *et al.*, 1998) to apply samples to individual sites and to effect sample movement and reaction kinetics. Additional features usually make chips rather complex and less suited for a high throughput, cost-efficient screening. Fluorescent detection is the most common detection technique using confocal scanning with laser scanners or charge-coupled device camera (CCD) for planar arrays, and variation on flow cytometry for beads. The sensitivity of the fluorescence signal can be increased by planar waveguide technology or using new materials as discussed in the next section. Resonance light scattering is an alternative sensitive detection for metal particles, while surface plasmon resonance (SPR) and mass spectrometry completely avoid sample labelling.

Microarray sensitivity

Insufficient sensitivity is probably the major obstacle of wider use of microarrays for diagnostic purposes. Fortunately, there are multiple approaches currently being developed to increase the detection limits.

Signal amplification methods probably provide the biggest gain in sensitivity. However, for the open plan microarrays they have to fulfil one basic requirement – the amplified signal needs to be localized, not soluble. Rolling circle amplification (RCA) (Schweitzer *et al.*, 2000) satisfies this requirement in one primer variant which can provide a signal amplification exceeding 8×10^3 (Nallur *et al.*, 2001). Another signal amplification method, tyramide signal amplification (TSA) has been developed for in situ detection of molecules in cells and tissues. Sometimes called CARD (Catalyzed Reporter Deposition), it is based on the catalytic activity of horseradish peroxidase (HRP) to generate high-density labelling of a target. TSA has been adapted to both DNA arrays (Karsten *et al.*, 2002) and protein arrays (Varnum *et al.*, 2004) reporting high sensitivity (at the sub-picogram/ml level).

New optical detection techniques are now being applied to microarrays. Resonance light scattering (RLS) uses a white-light source scanner to detect monochromatic, scattered light signals of metal (gold, silver, etc.) particles. The material, size and shape of particles determine the signal. The Genicon RLS System (developed by Genicon Sciences and now part of the Invitrogen Corporation), can achieve ten-fold greater sensitivity than with CyDyes. When RLS was directly compared with fluorescent detection of bacterial pathogens, the authors observed as high as a 50-fold more intense signal (Francois *et al.*, 2003).

Planar waveguide technology developed by Zeptosens (www.zeptosens.com) utilizes a special coating of T_2O_5 or TiO_2 to induce an evanescence field for efficient fluorescence detection (Pawlak *et al.*, 2002), at least ten times more sensitive than conventional fluorescence, if using the company's chips and a reader.

A different type of signal enhancement comes from new materials. Quantum dots or nanocrystals contain a cadmium-based semiconductor core enclosed in a shell and a polymer coat facilitating the attachment of probes. The brightness of the fluorescent signal is up to 1000 times that of the conventional flurophores, potentially increasing the assay sensitivity many times (Lian *et al.*, 2004). The technology is being developed by Quantum Dot Corporation (www.qdot.com).

Instead of using a linear probe, usually labelled with a single fluorophore, dendrimers or multiply-branched molecules provide the opportunity to introduce many dye molecules and to increase the signal generated. When used for DNA microarray human herpes virus diagnosis, the signal has been enhanced at least 30 times (Striebel *et al.*, 2004). Dendrimer technology is also being developed by Genisphere (www.genisphere.com).

Some of the approaches described can be further combined, leading to very sensitive assays, potentially approaching the sensitivity of nucleic acid amplification techniques. Combined with easier multiplexing, such assays could be well suited for high throughput blood screening in the future.

DNA, protein, cell, tissue, carbohydrate and small molecule microarrays

The main driving force behind the development of DNA microarrays was the possibility of analysing the expression patterns of many (and eventually all) genes at the same time under various stimuli and conditions. The expectation was that the expression patterns should tell us much about gene functions. Information content has been provided by the large sequencing projects. It did not take long after the initial exploratory experiments to realize the diagnostic potential of DNA microarrays, especially for complex multifactorial disease processes such as cancer (MacGregor and Squire, 2002). Single nucleotide polymorphisms (SNP) determining the individual differences were obvious targets for the pharmaceutical industry, among others (Shi, 2002). Infectious agents were a very useful subject of microarray studies for several reasons. They provided a simple model for whole genome expression studies, due to the limited number of genes, moving to microbe–host interactions and, of course multiplex diagnostics.

With the progress of the human genome project it was becoming increasingly obvious that the sequence information is insufficient to explain the gene function variability as seen at the protein interaction level. A lower than expected number of identified human genes only confirmed that proteomics rather than genomics should provide a number of missing answers. That stimulated the development of protein microarrays, which was delayed due to the more complex character of protein interactions. The first protein microarrays utilized porous membranes (Bussow et al., 1998; Wildt et al., 2000) but new techniques of DNA microarray preparation soon followed (Haab et al., 2001; MacBeath and Schreiber, 2000). A protein version of the expression profiling was developed using SELDI technology (Fung et al., 2001). In diagnostics, the difference between microplate EIA methods and its miniaturized microarray version was less dramatic than between nucleic acid amplification and DNA microarray analysis. Development of a microarray within microplate wells appropriately documented this trend (Mendoza et al., 1999). Selection of antigens and antibodies used in microbiological macroarray serological assays can facilitate transition to microarray, although the differences in solid phase used, the method of immobilization and the reaction kinetics may produce unexpected results. Increased multiplexing also requires a choice of reagents with limited cross-reactivity.

Cell microarrays represent another tool for functional genomic studies. Thousands of cell clusters on a microarray were transfected with DNAs, coding for various gene products, the effects of which could be investigated by a panel of assays (Wu et al., 2002).

Tissue microarrays proved to be extremely popular, mainly in the tumour biology field, as they greatly simplify analysis of hundreds of specimens from patients in different stages of disease. Sections from 1000 biopsies can be immobilized on a microarray in an ordered manner and addressed with the probes for parallel detection of DNA, RNA and proteins (Kononen et al., 1998).

Oligosaccharides from glycoproteins, glycolipids, proteoglycans, polysaccharides, extracted or chemically synthesized, were immobilized on a nitrocellulose array and used to investigate interactions with the carbohydrate recognizing proteins (Fukui et al., 2002).

Carbohydrates are exceptionally diverse, due to their composition, branching, ability to polymerize and association with other molecules such as proteins and lipids. Intriguingly, most pathogens possess unique surface carbohydrates. Wang et al. (2002) detected the carbohydrate-binding antibodies by investigating serum samples on nitrocellulose-coated glass slides spotted with glycans derived from the biological samples and semi-synthetic glycoconjugates.

Small molecule microarrays may prove useful for the identification of ligand binding to proteins and other targets in drug discovery and deciphering various signalling pathways. Kuruvilla et al. (2002) describe preparation and use of such arrays for the study of glucose signalling.

Microarrays in pathogen detection

Application of DNA microarrays is increasingly popular for the detection of multiple targets. In the majority of published papers the multiplexing power of microarray is combined with the sensitivity provided by the target amplification method, such as PCR. Table 18.3 shows examples of both DNA and protein arrays used for microbial detection. Polymerase chain reaction-microarray combination provides robust results, taking sensitivity down to 1–100 copies of adenovirus genomic DNA (Lin et al., 2004). One hundred viral copies per ml were detected by Foldes-Papp et al. (2004) for the detection of human herpes viruses, while Boriskin et al. (2004) described multiplex PCR-microarray detection of CNS viruses (echoviruses; HSV1,2; VZV, CMV, HHV 6A, 6B, HHV 7; polyoma BK, JC; mumps; measles) with a sensitivity of 93% of that for single virus PCR. At the same time, the discriminatory power can be as high as 45 human papillomavirus genotypes (Klaassen et al., 2004; Wallace et al., 2005). In relation to high throughput screening, however, this combination would represent the introduction of yet another step and instrument(s), making the screening even more complex. With NAT already successfully applied to blood screening, real-time PCR detection would of course be the preferred detection method. As mentioned earlier, a limited multiplexing potential of PCR, problematical addition of emerging testing targets and poor cost-efficiency are the main obstacles for a more widespread use of the technique for high throughput screening. Alternative options for pathogen nucleic acid detection are discussed in the next section.

There is no target amplification method available for antibody and antigen detection and the sensitivity of the best antigen assays is approximately 1 pg/ml or 8.4×10^6 molecules/ml for a 24 kilodalton protein. On the other hand, in a typical viral particle there are multiple (hundreds to thousands) copies of the major structural proteins per 1–2 genome molecules (Briggs et al., 2003). Even taking this ratio into account there is still a gap of sensitivity of some four orders of magnitude between PCR and serological assays, but development of new signal amplification and detection methods may significantly decrease or close this gap.

Options for pathogen nucleic acid blood screening

The multiplexing power of real-time PCR is limited not only by the interference of primer pairs (which is true also for the end-point PCR) but also by the interference of probes and a limited availability of suitable fluorophores and detection channels on the instruments. Otherwise it would undoubtedly be used more widely due to the extremely high sensitivity and simultaneous amplification and detection steps. Table 18.4 compares some parameters of real-time PCR with alternative nucleic acid

Table 18.3 Microarray based detection of infectious agents. Examples and parameters.

Ref.	Targeted sensitivity pathogens	Target amplification	Type of microarray	Probes	Detection method	Sensitivity or typing
(1)	Respiratory disease associated adenoviruses	PCR Degenerate primers	Derivatized glass slides	Oligos 60–70-mers	Fluorescently labelled PCR product	1–100 copies of genomic DNA
(2)	Human papilloma viruses	Multiplex PCR	Liquid bead microarray	Oligos 18-mers	Luminex flow cytometry based reader	45 genotypes
(3)	Human papilloma viruses	Multiplex PCR	Streptavidin coated slides	Oligos 19–20-mers	Immunohistochemical staining	45 types
(4)	HCV, HBV, HIV1,2; EBV, syphilis	NA	Semi-carbazide glass slides	Peptide, protein antigens	Immunofluorescence	
(5)	*Toxoplasma gondii*, Rubella, CMV, HSV1, 2	NA	Activated glass slides	Protein antigens	Fluorescently labelled secondary antibody	0.5 pg of bound IgM or IgG
(6)	Human rotavirus	RT – PCR	Silanized slides	Oligos 19–24-mers	Fluorescent dye incorporation during on chip primer extension	40 genotypes
(7)	Severe acute respiratory syndrome (SARS)	NA	Aldehyde slides	Antigens	Indirect fluorescence	86.1% positive rate

NA: not applicable

(1) Bacarese-Hamilton *et al.*, 2004 (2) Duburcq *et al.*, 2004 (3) Klaassen *et al.*, 2004 (4) Lin *et al.*, 2004 (5) Lovmar *et al.*, 2003 (6) Lu *et al.*, 2005 (7) Wallace *et al.*, 2005.

Table 18.4 Options for nucleic acid pathogen detection in blood screening.

	Specific target amplification		Non-specific target amplification	DNA microarray hybridization
	Real-time detection	Microarray hybridization	Microarray hybridization	Signal amplification (RCA)[a]
Amplification primers	Specific	Degenerate	Random hexa to nonamers	Universal (for signal amplification)
Probes	Specific	Specific (multiple)	Specific (multiple)	Specific (multiple)
Multiplexing	Limited (3–4)	Medium (n × 10)	Medium (n × 10)	High (n × 100)
Bias	High (>10^4)	Medium (10^2–10^3)	Low (2–20)	Low (2–20?)
Sensitivity	10^1	10^1–10^2	Single: 10^3–10^4 Tandem: 10^1–10^2	150 bound molecules
Throughput	Medium	Medium	Medium	High
Cost-efficiency	Poor	Moderate	Moderate	Moderate–Good
References	Mackay *et al.*, 2002	Lin *et al.*, 2004 Wallace *et al.*, 2005	Vora *et al.*, 2004	Nallur *et al.*, 2001

[a] RCA: Rolling circle amplification

Table 18.5 Options for antibody and antigen pathogen detection in blood screening.

	Microplate	Microparticles I	Microparticles II (encoded)	Microarray
Antigen probes	yes	yes	yes	yes
Antibody probes	yes	yes (combi)	yes	yes
Multiplexing	no	possible	yes	yes
Automation	yes	yes (full)	yes	partial
Throughput	medium	medium	high	medium–high
Reagent consumption	high	high	medium	low
Detection method	chromogenic	chemiluminescent	fluorescent (flow cytometry)	fluorescent; other (RLS[a], planar waveguide)
Company (example)	BioMérieux	Abbott	Luminex	Zeptosens, Biosite

Source: company literature, websites (www.bioMérieux.com; www.abbottdiagnsotics.com; www.luminexcorp.com; www. zeptosens.com; www.biosite.com)

[a] RLS: resonance light scattering

detection systems. Multiplex PCR with degenerate or group-specific primers and subsequent microarray detection/differentiation is the favoured option of current microarray based viral diagnostics as described earlier. This approach and the following approach using non-specific target amplification plus microarray detection would add another step to current testing algorithms. There are some advantages of these approaches, such as reduced amplification bias, preserved sensitivity and a potential to amplify unknown targets in the case of non-specific amplification. However, the cost-efficiency would be improved only by the increased multiplexing power and partially offset by the additional procedures. The last option involves signal (rather than target) amplification in the form of RCA, following microarray hybridization. As the RCA is performed 'on-chip', both procedures can be combined and automated. It remains to be shown using real samples how sensitive and robust this technique would be. However, as the section on 'Microarray sensitivity', above noted and Table 18.4, demonstrates, RCA can be combined with

other signal enhancing reagents such as dendrimer probes conjugated to multiple higher signal-producing labels in the form of quantum dots or RLS particles. A unique feature of RCA is its applicability to both DNA and protein microarrays, paving the way for a single testing platform (see below).

Options for antigen and antibody pathogen blood screening

Microplate and microparticle immunoassays are well established in blood-screening procedures. They provide reliable detection with a reasonable throughput and a high degree of automation at a relatively low cost (see Table 18.5). The sensitivity is being continuously improved. The main attraction of microarray technology would therefore be miniaturization, leading to reduced reagent consumption and perhaps to increased reaction kinetics. In addition, the easier multiplexing and new types of detection techniques would add further value to a new screening method.

The true benefit which microarray based screening could bring would be a unifying platform for a multitude of required tests, as discussed in the following section.

Impact of new technologies on testing algorithms

Potential benefits of single platform microarray testing

Current testing algorithms require the collection of at least three separate samples from each donation for microbiological serology, blood grouping and NAT. Testing is carried out on several instrumental platforms requiring dedicated reagents and trained staff (see Figure 18.2(1)). Microarray testing (see Figure 18.2(2)) could offer a single platform capable of combining not only nucleic acid and protein assays but probably microbiological and blood group testing, too. Potential benefits include reducing numbers of reagents and their consumption, also eliminating the need for multiple instruments. However, the most significant change would probably come from the transition from testing many samples in parallel sequentially for one or a few markers on different instruments, to testing each individual sample at the same time for all required markers on a single platform (instrument). This would greatly simplify the operational aspects of testing, not least the IT reconciliation of results before issuing blood and blood components. Because the incremental cost of additional probes on a microarray is low, an inclusion of multiple probes per target could eliminate repeat testing of initial reactives and reduce the confirmatory testing requirements.

Regulatory issues

One can imagine that in the highly regulated field of blood transfusion the licensing questions, validation and approval of multiplex multi-parameter assays would pose a major challenge and regulatory bodies would have to take a different approach to these processes. (Please refer to Chapter 27.) There are indications that these considerations are already being addressed. Further complications may arise from the miniaturization potential of microarray technology. If we accept the principle of 'one chip–one donation' where all required tests would be performed simultaneously on one (perhaps two) chip(s), this content would leave considerable space available on the chip. There would be a possibility of physically separating sub-arrays on the array and testing for multiple samples on one chip, bringing new logistical problems. A different approach has been suggested using ink-jet printing technology (Angenendt et al., 2003). The so-called 'multiple spotting technique' (MIST) allows, in the first step, immobilization of the capture reagents in pre-programmed positions and then spotting the second reagent (or sample) on top of the original spot. New technological improvements will undoubtedly emerge in the near future, adding to a perplexing array of possibilities.

Another related regulatory issue would then have to deal with the question of centralized or local testing as the miniaturization will most probably provide portable testing equipment. There are advantages and disadvantages to both testing approaches and the relative merits will have to emerge from extensive evaluation programmes.

In summary, the microarray and related technologies are quickly moving from the research and development phase into practical applications in many areas of medical practice, and

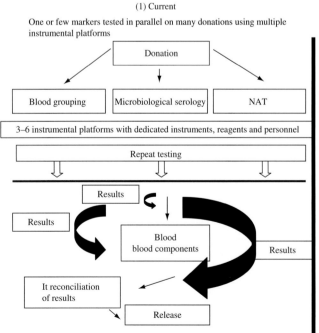
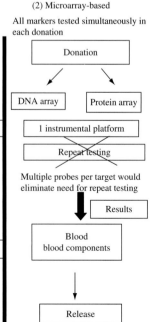

(1) Current

One or few markers tested in parallel on many donations using multiple instrumental platforms

(2) Microarray-based

All markers tested simultaneously in each donation

Figure 18.2 Testing algorithms.

blood services should prepare for another potential technological milestone, changing the face of transfusion medicine and blood diagnostics.

REFERENCES

Angenendt, P., Glokler, J., Konthur, Z., *et al.* (2003). 3D protein microarrays: performing multiplex immunoassays on a single chip. *Anal Chem*, **75**, 4368–72.

Bacarese-Hamilton, T., Messazoma, L., Ardizzoni, A., *et al.* (2004) Serodiagnosis of infectious diseases with antigen microarrays. *J Appl Microbiol*, **96**, 10–17.

Barbara, J. A. (1998) Prevention of infections transmissible by blood derivatives. *Transfus Sci*, **19**, 3–7.

Boriskin, Y. S., Rice, P. S., Stabler, R. A., *et al.* (2004). DNA microarrays for virus detection in cases of central nervous system infection. *J Clin Microbiol*, **42**, 5811–18.

Briggs, J. A. G., Wilk, T., Welker, R., *et al.* (2003) Structural organisation of authentic, mature HIV-1 virions and cores. *The EMBO Journal*, **22**, 1707–15.

Brown, P. O. and Botstein, D. (1999) Exploring the new world of the genome with DNA microarrays. *Nat Gen*, **21**, 33–7.

Bussow, K., Cahill, D., Nietfeld, W., *et al.* (1998) A method for global protein expression and antibody screening on high-density filters of an arrayed cDNA library. *Nucleic Acids Res*, **26**, 5007–8.

Cheng, J., Sheldon, E. L., Wu, L., *et al.* (1998) Preparation and hybridization analysis of DNA/RNA from *E. coli* on microfabricated bioelectronic chips. *Nat Biotechnol*, **16**, 541–6.

Cummings, A. and Relman, D. A. (2000) Using DNA microarrays to study host-microbe interactions. *Emerg Infect Dis*, **6**, 513–25.

Duburcq, X., Olivier, C., Malingue, F., *et al.* (2004) Peptide-protein microarrays for the simultaneous detection of pathogen infections. *Bioconjug Chem*, **15**, 307–16.

Ekins, R. P. (1998) Ligand assays: from electrophoresis to miniaturized microarrays. *Clin Chem*, **44**, 2015–30.

Ekins, R. P. and Chu, F. W. (1991) Multianalyte microspot immunoassay – microanalytical 'compact disk' of the future. *Clin Chem*, **37**, 1955–67.

Fodor, S. P. A., Read, J. L., Pirrung, M. C., *et al.* (1991) Light-directed, spatially addressable parallel chemical synthesis. *Science*, **251**, 767–73.

Foldes-Papp, Z., Egerer, R., Birch-Hirschfeld, E., *et al.* (2004) Detection of multiple human herpes viruses by DNA microarray technology. *Mol Diagn*, **8**, 1–9.

Francois, P., Bento, M., Vaudaux, P., *et al.* (2003) Comparison of fluorescence and resonance light scattering for highly sensitive microarray detection of bacterial pathogens. *J Microbiol Methods*, **55**, 755–62.

Fukui, S., Feizi, T., Galustian, C., *et al.* (2002) Oligosaccharide microarrays for high-throughput detection and specificity assignments of carbohydrate-protein interactions. *Nat Biotechnol*, **20**, 1011–7.

Fung, E. T., Thulasiraman, V., Weinberger, S. R., *et al.* (2001) Protein biochips for differential profiling. *Curr Opin Biotechnol*, **12**, 65–9.

Haab, B. B., Dunham, M. J. and Brown, P. O. (2001) Protein microarrays for highly parallel detection and quantitation of specific proteins and antibodies in complex solutions. *Genome Biol*, **2**, Research, 0004.

Karsten, S. L., Van Deerlin, V. M. D., Sabatti, C., *et al.* (2002) An evaluation of tyramide signal amplification and archived fixed and frozen tissue in microarray gene expression analysis. *Nucleic Acids Res*, **30**, e4.

Klaassen, C. H. W., Prinsen, C. F. M., de Valk, H. A., *et al.* (2004) DNA microarray format for detection and subtyping of human Papillomavirus. *J Clin Microbiol*, **42**, 2152–60.

Kononen, J., Bubendorf, L., Kallioniemi, A., *et al.* (1998) Tissue microarrays for high-throughput molecular profiling of tumor specimens. *Nat Med*, **4**, 844–7.

Kuruvilla, F. G., Shamji, A. F., Sternson, S. M., *et al.* (2002) Dissecting glucose signalling with diversity-oriented synthesis and small-molecule microarrays. *Nature*, **416**, 653–7.

Lian, W., Litherland, S. A., Badrane, H., *et al.* (2004) Ultrasensitive detection of biomolecules with fluorescent dye-doped nanoparticles. *Anal Biochem*, **334**, 135–44.

Lin, B., Vora, G. J., Thach, D., *et al.* (2004) Use of oligonucleotide microarrays for rapid detection and serotyping of acute respiratory disease-associated adenoviruses. *J Clin Microbiol*, **42**, 3232–9.

Lovmar, L., Fock, C., Espinoza, F., *et al.* (2003) Microarrays for genotyping human group A rotavirus by multiplex capture and type-specific primer extension. *J Clin Microbiol*, **41**, 5153–8.

Lu, D.-D., Chen, S.-H., Zhang, S.-M., *et al.* (2005) Screening of specific antigens for SARS clinical diagnosis using a protein microarray. *Analyst*, **130**, 474–82.

MacBeath, G. and Schreiber, S. L. (2000) Printing proteins as microarrays for high-throughput function determination. *Science*, **289**, 1760–3.

MacGregor, P. F. and Squire, J. A. (2002) Application of microarrays to the analysis of gene expression in cancer. *Clin Chem*, **48**, 1170–77.

Mackay, I. M., Arden, K. E. and Nitsche, A. (2002) Real time PCR in virology. *Nucleic Acids Res*, **30**, 1292–305.

Mendoza, L. G., McQuary, P., Mongan, A., *et al.* (1999) High-throughput microarray-based enzyme-linked immunosorbent assay (ELISA). *Biotechniques*, **27**, 782–6.

Michael, K. L., Taylor, L. C., Schultz, S. L., *et al.* (1998) Randomly ordered addressable high-density optical sensor arrays. *Anal Chem*, **70**, 1242–8.

Nallur, G., Luo, C., Fang, L., *et al.* (2001) Signal amplification by rolling circle amplification on DNA microarrays. *Nucleic Acids Res*, **29**, e118.

Pawlak, M., Schick, E., Bopp, M. A., *et al.* (2002) Zeptosens' protein microarrays: a novel high performance microarray platform for low abundance protein analysis. *Proteomics* **2**, 383–93.

Petrik, J. (2001) Microarray technology: the future of blood testing? *Vox Sang*, **80**, 1–11.

Rao, R. S., Visuri, S. R., McBride, M. T., *et al.* (2004) Comparison of multiplexed techniques for detection of bacterial and viral proteins. *J Proteome Res*, **3**, 736–42.

Schena, M., Shalon, D., Davis, R. W., *et al.*, (1995) Quantitative monitoring of gene expression patterns with a complementary DNA microarray. *Science*, **270**, 467–70.

Schweitzer, B., Wiltshire, S., Lambert, J., *et al.* (2000) Immunoassays with rolling circle DNA amplification: a versatile platform for ultrasensitive antigen detection. *Proceedings of the National Academy of Sciences*, **97**, 10113–9.

Shalon, D., Smith, S. J. and Brown, P. O. (1996) A DNA microarray system for analyzing complex DNA samples using two-color fluorescent probe hybridization. *Genome Methods*, **6**, 301–6.

Shi, M. M. (2002) Technologies for individual genotyping detection of genetic polymorphisms in drug targets and disease genes. *Am J Pharmacogenomics*, **2**, 197–205.

Soldan, K., Barbara, J. A. J., Ramsay, M., *et al.* (2003) Estimation of the risk of hepatitis B virus, hepatitis C virus and human immunodeficiency virus infectious donations entering the blood supply in England, 1993–2001. *Vox Sang*, **84**, 274–86.

Striebel, H. M., Birch-Hirschfeld, E., Egerer, R., *et al.* (2004) Enhancing sensitivity of human herpes virus diagnosis with DNA microarrays using dendrimers. *Exp Mol Pathol*, **77**, 89–97.

Varnum, S. M., Woodbury, R. L. and Zangar, R. C. (2004) A protein microarray ELISA for screening biological fluids. *Methods Mol Biol*, **264**, 161–72.

Vora, G. J., Meador, C. E., Stenger, D. A., *et al.* (2004) Nucleic acid amplification strategies for DNA microarray-based pathogen detection. *Appl Environ Microbiol*, **70**, 3047–54.

Wallace, J., Woda, B. A. and Pihan, G. (2005) Facile, comprehensive, high-throughput genotyping of human genital Papillomaviruses using spectrally addressable liquid bead microarrays. *J Mol Diagn*, **7**, 72–80.

Wang, D., Liu, S., Trummer, B. J., *et al.* (2002) Carbohydrate microarrays for the recognition of cross-reactive molecular markers of microbes and host cells. *Nat Biotechnol*, **20**, 275–81.

Weber, B., Gurtler, L., Thorstensson, R., *et al.* (2002) Multicenter evaluation of a new automated fourth-generation human immunodeficiency virus screening assay with a sensitive antigen detection module and high specificity. *J Clin Microbiol*, **40**, 1938–46.

Wildt, R. M. T. de, Mundy, C. R., Gorick, B. D., *et al.* (2000) Antibody arrays for high-throughput screening of antigen-antibody interactions. *Nat Biotechnol*, **18**, 989–94.

Wu, R. Z., Bailey, S. N. and Sabatini, D. M. (2002) Cell-biological applications of transfected-cell microarrays. *Trends Cell Biol*, **12**, 485–8.

19 PROCESSING AND COMPONENTS: LEUCODEPLETION AND PATHOGEN REDUCTION

Rebecca Cardigan, Chris Prowse and Lorna M. Williamson

Although donor selection and donation screening remain the critical elements of protection from transfusion-transmitted pathogens, there is increasing interest in achieving further safety enhancements by component modification. In the last five years, leucocyte depletion has moved from being a bedside procedure for specific patients to a universal and integral part of component processing. In this context, its potential for removal of leucocyte-associated viruses has been the subject of considerable debate. Over the same time period, techniques for pathogen reduction of fresh frozen plasma and platelets have been developed and, in some cases, licensed for routine use. Pathogen reduction for red cells is proving a more challenging prospect, but in time the current difficulties may be overcome. Such techniques present policy-makers with interesting decisions which must take into account cost-effectiveness, loss of functionality of components, potential toxicity, and the potential impact on current donor selection and screening policies.

Leucocyte depletion (LD)

Many countries now undertake universal LD of all components in blood centres within 1–2 days of collection. The reasons for this practice vary from country to country, but perceived benefits include reduced immunomodulation, fewer febrile reactions, and reduction of cytomegalovirus risk (reviewed in Williamson, 2000). In the UK, the main reason for implementation of universal LD was as a precaution against transmission of variant Creutzfeld-Jacob disease. Leucocyte depletion is achieved either by filtration of either whole blood or processed components, or by centrifugation/elutriation during platelet apheresis.

Precise specifications of LD vary between countries, but all reflect the ability of LD systems to remove $>4 \log_{10}$ of leucocytes, and the fact that only a sample of components produced can be subjected to leucocyte counting. In the UK, the LD specification is $<5 \times 10^6$ leucocytes/unit in 99% of components with 95% statistical confidence (Guidelines for the UK Transfusion Services, 2005), while the Council of Europe guidelines mandate $<1 \times 10^6$ leucocytes/unit, but in only 90% of components (Council of Europe, 2007). Because residual leucocyte counts generally follow a $\log_{10}$ normal distribution, these apparently disparate requirements are actually quite similar. Recent studies have shown $>3.8 \log_{10}$ removal of all leucocyte subtypes (granulocytes, monocytes and T and B lymphocytes) by whole blood filtration and $>3.1 \log_{10}$ by platelet filtration and apheresis using GAMBRO Spectra (Pennington et al., 2001). After whole blood filtration, most remaining cells appear to be neutrophils (Rider et al., 2000).

One concern regarding LD was the possibility that the LD processes themselves might disrupt cells, releasing either free virus or cellular microparticles which might carry pathogens such as prions. However, an extensive study of all LD processes in use in the UK showed overall net removal of cellular microparticles and a leucocyte membrane marker (Krailadsiri et al., 2002).

Table 19.1 shows the major transfusion-transmitted infections associated principally with leucocytes. In contrast to these purely cell-associated viruses, the human immunodeficiency virus (HIV) has CD4 + T helper lymphocytes as its primary target, but because carriers also have infectious titres of virus in plasma, LD is not considered relevant in reducing HIV risk by transfusion.

Cytomegalovirus (CMV)

Cytomegalovirus is a large DNA herpes virus, which is endemic in most societies. Primary infection, which can occur in adults as well as children, can be asymptomatic, or cause flu-like symptoms, and is then followed by co-existing seropositivity as well as low-level lifelong viral carriage. Blood monocytes are an important reservoir of CMV in the asymptomatic carrier, and transmission by cellular blood components is well documented (reviewed in Pamphilon et al., 1999). In an immunocompetent recipient, this can result in no clinical sequelae, or at worst, an acute self-limiting primary CMV infection. However, the importance of CMV in transfusion medicine lies in its capability to cause devastating and even fatal systemic infection in immunosuppressed individuals, including premature neonates. For some years, it has been standard practice to provide such recipients with cellular components (red cells and platelets) from unexposed CMV seronegative donors, but this places a perpetual strain on supplies of CMV seronegative platelets, particularly if HLA matching is also required. Transmissions from newly infected donors in the antibody negative 'window period' have also occurred (Williamson, personal observation). Furthermore, process control failures have more impact when the agent is highly prevalent, as with CMV.

Over the last ten years, a number of clinical studies have examined whether LD could provide an equivalent level of safety to that established for antibody testing. As shown in Table 19.2, most randomized studies of pre-storage leucocyte depletion have resulted in 100% protection of susceptible recipients. By contrast, a study using post-storage filtration at the bedside caused several transmissions, all of which resulted in CMV disease (Bowden et al., 1995). The failure of bedside filtration to provide reliable CMV protection is perhaps not too surprising, given that leucocytes disintegrate during storage, releasing free

Transfusion Microbiology, eds John A. J. Barbara, Fiona A. M. Regan and Marcela C. Contreras. Published by Cambridge University Press. © Cambridge University Press 2008.

Table 19.1 Transfusion-transmitted pathogens associated primarily or solely with leucocytes.

Pathogen	Leucocyte subtype
Viruses	
Cytomegalovirus	Mainly monocytes possibly small amount in granulocytes
Human T-cell leukaemia viruses I and II	T-lymphocytes
Human herpes virus 8	B-lymphocytes
Epstein-Barr virus	B-lymphocytes
Bacteria	
Yersinia enterocolitica	Granulocytes
Prions	
Leucocyte involvement	Unknown

CMV which is not susceptible to removal by filters (Sivakumaran *et al.*, 1993). However, a recent cohort study also showed an increase in CMV transmissions from 1.7% to 4%, associated with greater provision of LD apheresis platelets which were not CMV seronegative (Nichols *et al.*, 2003). It is unlikely that any further randomized controlled trials comparing LD with serological testing will be performed, due to the enormous numbers of patients required to demonstrate a difference.

Recent laboratory studies have therefore attempted to define the limitations of LD as a means of CMV removal. The low level of viral carriage precludes the use of quantitative PCR to examine this question, so spiking studies with monocytes infected in culture have been used (Table 19.3). In addition, an animal model of CMV showed that only transfused monocytes (but not granulocytes) were relevant for CMV transmission, and that the number of monocytes required (10^6) was far greater than that seen in an LD unit of blood (50 000) (Hillyer *et al.*, 2003).

Table 19.2 Incidence of CMV transmission (%) by seronegative and leucocyte-depleted components.

Study	Patient group	No. of patients	Seronegative components	LD components
(1)	BMT (auto and allo)	29	ND	0
(2)	Leukaemia	54	12–22	0
(3)	Leukaemia/lymphoma	59	ND	0
(4)	BMT-auto	24	23	0
(5)	BMT-allo	23	ND	0
(6)	BMT-auto	37	ND	0
(7)	BMT-auto and allo	60	ND	0
(8)	BMT-allo	62	ND	0
(9)	BMT-auto and allo	502	0.8[a]	1–2[a]
Ronghe *et al.*, 2002	BMT-allo children	93	ND	0
Nichols *et al.*, 2003[b]	BMT-auto and allo	807	1.7	4

Studies 1–9 are reviewed in Pamphilon *et al.*, 1999.

ND, not determined.

[a] Study 9 employed bedside filtration, so it is uncertain whether components fulfilled the criteria for leucocyte depleted.

[b] Compared filtered and apheresis platelets, which were transfused only if seronegative components were not available.

Table 19.3 Removal of CMV and HTLV I by whole blood and platelet LD by filtration, using spiking models (CMV and HTLV I) and natural carriers (HTLV I).

Viruses used to spike blood components	Virus removal by LD processes ($\log_{10}$)		Viral carriage in leucocytes		Relevant leucocyte subtype removal by LD processes ($\log_{10}$)	
	Whole blood filters	Platelet filters	Cell type	Cell marker	Whole blood filters	Platelet filters
Cytomegalovirus (Visconti *et al.*, 2003)	2.81	1.9	Monocytes	CD14	>4.1	>4.0
Human T-cell leukaemia virus I (Pennington *et al.*, 2002)	>3.6	2.7	T lymphocytes	CD3	>4.5	>3.6

A recent Consensus Conference concluded that while LD probably affords an acceptably high degree of protection if undertaken alone, it is probably premature to discontinue CMV serological testing of donors in the absence of prospective trials to demonstrate equivalent efficacy of screening and LD (Laupacis *et al.*, 2001). In practice, most countries practising universal LD also continue to CMV test donors.

Human T-cell leukaemia virus (HTLV) I and II

No clinical trials have been done to examine the degree of prevention of HTLV transmission by LD. Look-back studies in countries which have implemented HTLV screening have shown transmission rates of 20% and 45% from non-LD red cells and platelets respectively (reviewed in Williamson, 2000). No such data are yet available for LD components, but now that the UK is performing HTLV screening and conducting a look-back study, data on transmission frequency from both LD and non-LD components will be available.

One study has shown $>3 \log_{10}$ reduction of HTLV load by LD after spiking units with infected T-cells and in blood donated by chronic carriers (see Table 19.3, Pennington *et al.*, 2002). However, complete clearance was not achieved, particularly in donors with high levels of viral carriage. It remains to be seen whether the residual HTLV levels seen after LD are capable of transmission.

Bacteria

There is some evidence that bacteria entering blood units at the time of venepuncture are engulfed in the first few hours after collection by donor phagocytes. In theory, therefore, blood filtered after donated units are returned to the processing centre might have a reduced risk of bacterial contamination. Equally, there has been concern that apheresis platelets which are LD during collection might pose a greater risk since they will have had no opportunity to 'self-sterilize'. In practice, implementation of universal LD seems to have had little overall impact on the incidence of transmission of skin commensals. The situation is different with *Yersinia enterocolitica*, which circulates in granulocytes and which should be removed during LD, no matter how soon after collection it is performed. However, clinically apparent transfusion-transmitted Yersinia cases are rare, and it will take some years to show any clear benefit of universal LD (Gibb *et al.*, 1994).

Variant Creutzfeld-Jacob Disease (vCJD) and prion removal

This disease is believed to be caused by the same prion agent responsible for bovine spongiform encephalopathy (BSE) in cattle. A look-back study of blood donor and recipient vCJD cases has so far revealed three symptomatic cases possibly attributable to transfusion of non-leucocyte depleted red cells (Llewelyn *et al.*, 2004). In addition, a fourth asymptomatic recipient of non-leucocyte depleted red cells was found at post-mortem to have abnormal prion in spleen and one cervical lymph node, but not in either tonsil or brain (Peden *et al.*, 2004). This individual was unusual in being of PrP^c genotype met/val, as opposed to met/met found in all clinical cases so far. Unlike classical CJD, vCJD shows affinity for lymphoid tissue, with abnormal prion (PrPsc) demonstrated in the tonsils of affected individuals. Normal prion (PrPc) has been demonstrated on CD34 progenitor cells, red cells, lymphocytes and monocytes. It is also found on platelets, from which it is released on activation with physiological agonists, but its functional role remains unclear. PrP^c is also found in plasma; its source may be either platelets or endothelial cells. (Please refer back to Chapter 9.)

Experimental transmission studies in rodents and sheep suggest that in those species infectivity is present in blood, with both plasma and buffy coat able to transmit the infection (Brown *et al.*, 1998; 1999 (reviewed in Prowse and MacGregor, 2002); Cervenakova *et al.*, 2003). Thus, the possibility exists for transfusion-transmitted vCJD via leucocytes within blood components. Studies of leucocyte depletion processes have demonstrated consistent removal of normal prion protein (Krailadsiri *et al.*, 2006; Prowse *et al.*, 1999), and recent animal data suggest that the infectivity can also be reduced by LD filters, albeit by $<50\%$ (Gregori *et al.*, 2004). Pure platelets appear not to be infective (Holada *et al.*, 2002).

Recently, two commercial companies (Pall and PRDT) have developed filtration type technology to remove residual prions, using different chemical binding strategies. At present, both systems are designed to be applied to pre-processed red cells which have already been leucocyte depleted. In this scenario, $3–4 \log_{10}$ prion removal is claimed. These systems are currently under assessment by the UK Transfusion Services. As with any novel technology, the quality of the red cell product must be evaluated, and the possibility of formation of red cell neoantigens addressed. In addition, methods for real-time quality monitoring of the process by transfusion service production laboratories must be developed.

Effect of leucocyte depletion on quality of components

Leucocyte depletion of whole blood or plasma usually has a negligible effect on the coagulation factor content. However, this is dependent on the filter type used, with some resulting in a loss of up to 20% of certain individual coagulation factors (Cardigan *et al.*, 2001; Chabanel *et al.*, 2003). Studies examining platelet and red cell quality during storage have mainly shown a beneficial effect of LD, although some report no differences from standard components. Leucocyte depletion of cellular components also prevents the accumulation of leucocyte-derived cytokines and some proteases, which may explain why LD is effective in reducing febrile reactions to platelets (reviewed in Williamson, 2000; Yazer *et al.*, 2004). Since many red cell LD filters also remove a significant number of platelets, there are also lower levels of platelet-derived cytokines in such products (Wadhwa *et al.*, 2000).

Pathogen reduction overview

Specific virus inactivation technologies for protein concentrates prepared by plasma fractionation have been in routine use since the 1980s. However, pathogen reduction (PR) technologies for red cells, platelet and fresh frozen plasma for direct clinical use are a relatively recent innovation, in many cases only now reaching the clinics (Council of Europe, 2001; Epstein and Vostal, 2003; McCullough, 2003). The residual risk of transfusion-transmitted infection from those viruses that are routinely screened for in blood donations is miniscule, but there remain concerns about emerging infections, such as West Nile virus (WNV) and severe acute respiratory syndrome (SARS) virus, bacterial contamination (particularly for platelets, due to their storage at ambient temperatures), and, in some countries, protozoal diseases. The promise of the newer PR methods is that they might secure ongoing blood safety despite these emerging threats. However, there are also concerns common to all systems relating to toxicity, loss of component efficacy and value for money.

PR methods rely on two basic approaches: chemical inactivation and photo-inactivation (see Table 19.4). This is usually based on addition of heterocyclic compounds that have specific affinity for nucleic acids (both single and double stranded DNA and RNA), through interaction with the base groups of the linked nucleotides of nucleic acid. Subsequent excitation with UV or visible light results in an excited electronic state which may react directly with the nucleic acid (photochemical reaction, e.g. amotosalen, Corash, 2000; Lin *et al.*, 1997; Wollowitz, 2001) or result in secondary activation to form free oxygen radicals (type I) or reactive oxygen (type II) in a photodynamic reaction (e.g. methylene blue, Mohr *et al.*, 1997). The resulting cross-linking within or between strands of the nucleic acid results in inhibition of pathogen replication. As red cells and platelets are anuclear, and FFP is acellular, they do not require nucleic acid replication to function. It is worthy of note that this approach relies on the relatively high affinity of the added chemical for nucleic acids compared to other elements of the blood component. Side reactions may result in undesirable effects on blood cell membranes or coagulation factors if these are bound by the chemicals. A further characteristic of most PR systems is that they are designed to be carried out on single blood components.

An exception to these generalizations is the use of solvent/detergent (SD) treatment for PR of FFP. This relies on SD disruption of the lipid envelope of pathogens, but will also lyse any blood cells present. Hence, it has no effect on pathogens that do not possess a lipid envelope, and can only be applied to acellular products such as FFP (Horowitz *et al.*, 1992). In addition, the technology can only be applied to plasma pools, which usually contain 500–1000 plasma units.

As summarized in Table 19.4, such methods have been established using phenothiazine dyes, vitamins and tetrapyrrole compounds. The Springe Red Cross, now working with Macopharma, has established methylene blue treatment for the PR of FFP (Bachmann *et al.*, 1995; Lambrecht *et al.*, 1991; Mohr *et al.*, 1997) and are now developing thionine/UV for the PR of platelets (Mohr and Redecker-Klein, 2003). Gambro, through a subsidiary

company Navigant Biotechnologies, are developing a process that uses a combination of riboflavin and UV and visible light, initially for platelets but also for red cells (Corbin, 2002; Goodrich, 2000; Goodrich *et al.*, 2003; Kumar *et al.*, 2003a; 2003b). The Sylsens compounds from Photobiochem are at an earlier stage of development in Europe.

As shown in Table 19.4, many of the photo-inactivation methods require cellular components to be suspended in crystalloid additive solutions to avoid absorption of the UV or visible light by plasma proteins, and to promote good component function during storage. Most techniques also incorporate a post-illumination step to remove the residual added chemical sensitizers. This may involve washing of the cells, use of specific adsorption filters or incubation with a compound adsorption device. Due to the multiple steps carried out on individual donations and their derivatives, these methods are labour intensive both in terms of laboratory facilities and staff.

Photo-inactivation technologies are not well suited to the PR of red cell products since their high optical density makes it difficult to achieve UV or light penetration. Three of the four PR technologies in development for red cells use chemicals with high affinity for nucleic acid that react directly under physiological conditions of neutral pH. These are the S-303 compound developed by Cerus-Baxter (Corash, 2000) where the reactive group is a nitrogen mustard group; the Viperin compounds under development by Fresenius which rely on reactive heavy metals; and Inactine (PEN 110) an ethyleneimine derivative developed by Vitex. In the last case, binding of the compounds occurs via binding of imine groups to the backbone phosphates of the nucleic acid (Chapman, 2000; Goltsina *et al.*, 2003; Purmal *et al.*, 2002).

Extent of pathogen reduction

The conventional paradigm for transfusion-transmitted viruses is that of a high titre acute phase followed by low-level chronic carriage. This raises the possibility that a given pathogen reduction system could be inadequate to achieve complete viral clearance in the acute phase, at the very time when antibody-based screening tests may be negative. On the other hand, new agents (West Nile virus, for example) may demonstrate acute short-lived viraemia of low titre followed by complete viral clearance and seroconversion. For some of these new agents, pathogen reduction alone may be an adequate strategy, or as a minimum, buy time for measured development and full validation of genome tests before implementation.

To demonstrate that a particular technology can achieve clinically effective PR it is necessary to show that, for pathogens of concern (or suitable models for them), the technology is able to remove levels of the infectious agent that are greater than those likely to be found in an infected donation.

Figure 19.1 shows the estimated titres of virus (on a logarithmic scale in copies per ml) for a range of relevant viruses during acute infection and during later chronic carriage, where this occurs. Where nucleic acid testing (NAT) has been introduced to screen out infected donations, high titre donations will be removed from use prior to processing. From Figure 19.1 it can be seen that for

Table 19.4 Single component pathogen reduction technologies in use/under commercial development.

System	Manufacturer	Active compound	Treatment step	Removal step	Concentration of compound before/after removal	Development status
Platelets						
	Springe/Macopharma	None	UV-C 0.4 J/cm^2	None	None	Preclinical
Mirasol	Navigant/Gambro	Riboflavin[a]	6.2 J/cm^2 UV (8–10 min)	None	50 µmol/l	Licensed EU/phase III
Intercept	Cerus/Baxter	Amotosalen (s-59)[a]	3–4 J/cm^2 UV-A (4 min)	Adsorption device (6–16 hours)	150/0.2 µmol/l	Licensed EU
Plasma						
Mirasol	Navigant/Gambro	Riboflavin[a]	?	None	?	Preclinical
Intercept	Cerus/Baxter	Amotosalen (S-59)[a]	3 J/cm^2 UV-A (4 min)	Adsorption device (1 hour)	150/0.2 µmol/l	Licensed EU
Theraflex	Macopharma	Methylene blue[a]	180 J/cm^2 500nm (30 min)	Filtration (5–10 min)	1/ <0.1 µmol/l	Licensed EU
Red cells						
Mirasol	Navigant/Gambro	Riboflavin[a]	?	None	?	Preclinical
Inactine	Vitex	Pen110[b]	Incubation at room temperature 6 hours	Washing with 6L	0.1% (vol/vol)/ <50 ng/ml	Phase III (chronic transfusion trial suspended late 2003)
Intercept	Cerus/Baxter	S-303[b]	Incubation at room temperature 12–20 hours	Adsorption device (8 hours)	200 µmol/l/ <2 µmol/l	Phase II suspended late 2003

[a] = photochemical treatment
[b] = chemical treatment
L = litres

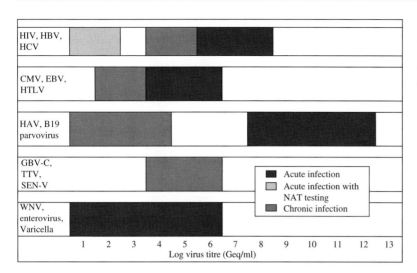

Figure 19.1 Levels of viraemia in blood. Viraemic titres (shown on a logarithmic scale) in genome equivalents per ml as determined by nucleic acid testing (NAT) of blood. For the specified pathogens, titre ranges are shown for acute infection (with and without exclusions of NAT reactive donations) and for chronic infection (after seroconversion).

the lipid-enveloped viruses of particular concern, titres between 100 000 and 100 000 000 (5 to 8 $\log_{10}$) are seen during acute infection, with even higher levels observed for some non-lipid enveloped viruses.

The ability of PR technologies to address such titres of microbes can usually be expressed as a reduction factor (RF): the ratio of total virus (titre $\times$ volume) before and after treatment, expressed on a logarithmic scale. Thus, a 6 $\log_{10}$ reduction factor denotes a process capable of reducing microbial load in a one litre unit containing 1000 infectious units (IU) per ml (1000 ml $\times$ 1000 IU/ml = 1 000 000 IU load) to a residual one IU in a one litre product.

The same principles apply to bacterial infection. At the time of donation the occasional donation containing bacteria rarely contains more than 100 bacteria per ml (up to 50 000 per unit). Although these may multiply rapidly during storage, inactivation close to the time of donation is achievable by many of the technologies in development.

As some of the pathogens of concern are difficult to grow in the laboratory, and because of safety concerns, most studies use more easily cultured and less pathogenic model agents. These are spiked (added) into the selected component, and assayed before and after treatment. The problem here is that stocks of model viruses may only be available in limited titres, such that all the available virus is inactivated. The RF can then only be expressed as greater than the titre of the stock, for example more than 6 $\log_{10}$, creating uncertainty as to whether the process is only just able to achieve 6 $\log_{10}$ inactivation, or whether it has a much larger reserve capacity. Kinetic studies, in which timed samples are taken and assayed during the course of treatment, can give additional data to help gauge overall PR capacity.

The Food and Drugs Agency, the regulatory body in the USA, have suggested a list of model pathogens to be used (Epstein and Vostal, 2003), and PR companies employ others in addition. These include a variety of viruses and bacteria, but also other pathogens such as malaria and the agent of Chagas' disease. As an example of the log RFs obtained for a variety of viral species, Figure 19.2 summarizes such data in graphical form for amotosalen-treated platelets in additive solution. Specific details on RFs for species are summarized in Table 19.5. More detail may be

obtained in publications from the companies involved (Corash, 2003; Edrich et al., 2003; Horowitz et al., 1992; Knutson et al., 2000; Lazo et al., 2002; 2003; Lin et al., 1997; Mather et al., 2003; O'Hagen et al., 2002; Zavizion et al., 2003a–c) and have been the subject of recent reviews (Ciaravino et al., 2003a; ICH, 1998). Generally, lipid-enveloped virus inactivation is in excess of 6 $\log_{10}$, with lesser or even minimal kill achieved for non-lipid enveloped viruses. West Nile virus is susceptible to killing by both methylene blue (Mohr et al., 2004) and amotosalen (Dupuis, 2003c). Recently, it has been proposed to use long-range PCR to assess qualitatively the effects of PR on viral reduction (Aytay et al., 2003).

Bacterial RFs are variable but probably sufficient to deal with the contamination levels mentioned above. In contrast, it is possible that the demonstrated level of inactivation may not be sufficient for some viral species except where high titre donations are excluded by prior screening. For other pathogens, such as malaria and mycoplasma, assays are less well established but data are now being accumulated (Dupuis & Alfonso, 2003a; 2003b; Rentas et al., 2003; Van Voorhuis, 2003; Zavizion et al., 2003b; 2003c). The value of PR for these agents obviously depends on the prevalence of infection, as well as the titre in those rare donations that are infected.

Prevention of transfusion-transmitted cytomegalovirus

There have been no clinical trials to establish the CMV safety of pathogen inactivated platelets or red cells. However, all pathogen reduction systems intended for cellular components have shown effectiveness against CMV, even though it is an almost entirely intracellular virus. In addition, as discussed above, the leucocyte depletion which is required in some pathogen reduction systems appears in itself to provide a very high degree of CMV safety. The combination of LD and specific pathogen reduction should remove the CMV risk to the point where consideration could be given to cessation of CMV testing. This would also help to offset costs of pathogen reduction, although CMV sero-testing is relatively low cost. The removal of the need to provide

Table 19.5 Summarized log reduction factors (RF) for selected pathogens for various pathogen reduction technologies. Data in bold indicates a log RF greater than the figure indicated.

Pathogen	Amotosalen platelets	Amotosalen plasma	S-303 red cells	Methylene blue plasma	Thionine platelets	Riboflavin platelets	Riboflavin red cells	Inactine red cells
HIV free	6.2	**5.9**	**6.5**	**5.5**	**5.7**	6.5	5.5	**5.6**
HIV cell active	**6.1**	6.4	**6.2**	**6.4**	—	5.9	3.4	**4**
HTLV-1	4.7	—	4.2	—	—	—	—	—
HTLV-II	**5.1**	—	5.1	—	—	—	—	—
Hepatitis B	**5.5**	4.5	—	—	—	—	—	—
Duck hepatitis B	**6.2**	**5.1**	**6.3**	3.9	—	—	—	**4.6**
Hepatitis C	**4.5**	**4.5**	—	—	—	—	—	—
BVDV (HCV model)	**6**	6	**7.3**	**5.4**	6	5.8	**6.0**	**6.95**
Vesicular stomatitis virus	—	—	—	**4.9**	**4.4**	**5.6**	5.0	**6.83**
Pseudorabies	5.1	—	—	**5.7**	—	3.0	5.0	**6.35**
Cytomegalovirus (free)	—	—	—	—	—	—	—	6
Cytomegalovirus (cell)	**5.9**	—	—	—	—	—	—	**4.6**
West Nile virus	6	—	—	**5.8**	—	**5.1**	**6.0**	**5.1**
Pig circovirus	5.2	—	—	—	—	—	—	2.5
Blue tongue virus	6.4	—	6	—	—	—	3.8	6.5
Porcine parvovirus	—	—	—	0	0	**5.0**	—	**6.3**
Human parvovirus B19	4	**3.5**	3.4	**5.9**	**5**	1.7	—	**7**
H-hepatitis A virus	1	—	—	0	**5**	1.7	1.7	**5**
Calicivirus	2.4	—	—	**3.9**	—	—	—	—
Staphylococcus aureus	6.6	—	**5.1**	—	**2**	**4**	—	—
Staphylococcus epidermidis	**6.6**	5.7	**6.9**	—	—	**4.2**	1.2	**2**
Bacillus cereus (incl. spores)	3.7	—	—	—	—	3.9	—	—
Bacillus cereus (vegetative)	**6**	—	**6.3**	—	—	—	—	—
Propionibacterium acnes	**6.7**	—	—	—	—	—	—	—
Clostridium perfringens	**7**	—	—	—	—	—	—	—
Yersinia enterocolitica	**5.9**	—	**7.4**	—	—	—	2.3	**2**
Pseudomonas fluorescens	—	—	5.7	—	—	—	—	2
Escherichia coli	**6.4**	—	**7.4**	—	**5**	—	—	—
Klebsiella pneumoniae	**5.6**	5.6	—	—	—	**3.8**	—	**2**
Serratia marcescens	**6.7**	4.9	4.1	—	—	—	—	**2**
Trypanosoma cruzi (Chagas')	**5.3**	4.9	6	—	—	—	—	**2**
Plasmodium falciparum (malaria)	**7**	8	6.8	—	—	—	**2.0**	**2**
Trep. pallidum (syphilis)	6.9	—	—	—	—	—	—	**2**
Borrelia burgdorfi	7.5	—	—	—	—	—	—	**2**
Mycobacter arthritidis	—	—	—	—	—	—	—	**8**
Mycobacter pneumoniae	—	—	—	—	—	—	—	**7**

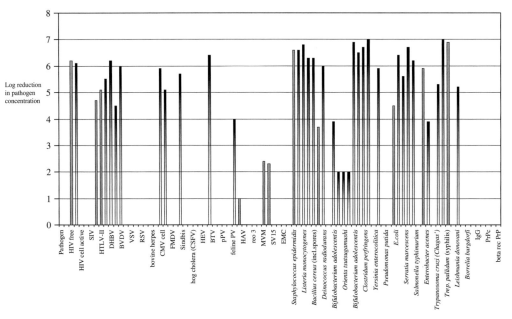

Figure 19.2 Log reduction in pathogen load by Amotosalen treatment of platelets. Shaded bars indicate no residual infectivity detectable, so the log reduction shown is at least equal to the maximum sensitivity of the detection system.

CMV-seronegative units for immunosuppressed patients would greatly simplify inventory management.

Toxicology

The viral safety of blood transfusion has never been greater, with improved methods of donor screening and testing options which include antibody, antigen and genome detection. In this scenario, there is less tolerance of pathogen reduction systems which carry any theoretical risk of short- or long-term toxicity. Chemicals that cause cell lysis and virus inactivation or modify genetic material are obviously toxic within those contexts. The technologies developed for PR address this in at least two ways. First, those methods that use photo-inactivation have an obvious advantage in that reaction in the dark or in ambient lighting is usually minimal. Second, nearly all PR technologies now incorporate a step to remove the added chemicals (see Table 19.4). In addition, concentrations of agent are chosen to minimize any potential risk to the patient.

Pathogen reduction companies are required to undertake pre-clinical studies to assess the margin of safety of the product. These usually involve tests on the treated product as well as the pure chemical used. Good recent reviews of this field have been published (Ciavarino *et al.*, 2003a, McCullough, 2003). The approach taken is based on that for pharmaceutical products, as laid down by the International Conference on Harmonization of Technical Requirements for Registration of Pharmaceuticals for Human Use (ICH, 1998). Table 19.6 summarizes the types of general and specific tests applied. This portfolio of tests has been developed over many decades and is generally regarded as being predictive of toxic effects in normal clinical use in man. The general tests involve observing animals for toxic effects after single (acute) and multiple doses, as well as studies on the distribution, half-life and breakdown in a range of animal species.

Table 19.6 Toxicology tests applied to PR compounds.

General	Specialized
Acute toxicity	Reproductive toxicity
Repeat dose toxicity (1 month)	Genotoxicity
Repeat dose toxicity (3 to 9 months)	Carcinogenicity
General pharmacology	
ADME *(absorption, distribution, metabolism, excretion)*	(Phototoxicity)
Neo-antigen tests	(Vein irritation)

See Ciavarino *et al.*, 2003a; ICH, 1998.

Nowadays, such studies emphasize the maximum tolerated dose or the minimum toxic dose, rather than the large studies undertaken in the past to determine doses causing death in 50% of animals (LD-50). The specific tests include assessment for effects on reproduction, genetic changes and induction of cancer as well as (where licensing agencies feel it appropriate) tests for phototoxicity and vein irritation. For PR treated components, the ability to undertake such studies can be limited by the volume of product it is possible to administer intravenously. Studies in which twice the plasma volume has been transfused intravenously every other day over a prolonged period have been reported. One way around this is to omit the usual removal step for added chemical and to test the resultant modified product containing higher levels of the compound.

The results of such studies are expressed in terms of a margin of safety, that is, the dose at which toxic effects are observed (or the maximum achievable dose used, even though this may have no effect) relative to the likely dose to be used clinically. The latter may be expressed as the maximum concentration of compound

Table 19.7 Examples of toxicity margins of safety for amotosalen[a].

Assessment	Treated 35% plasma	Pure psoralen
Acute toxicity		
Rat (death)	>1120 fold	250 000
Dog (CNS signs)		40 000
Repeat dose toxicity		
Rat (death)	>350	150 000
Dog (CNS signs)		30 000
Reproductive toxicity	>350	>75 000
Genotoxicity		
Ames test	≥2000	44 000
Mouse lymphoma	>167	7500
Hepatocyte UDS	>50	>34 000
Mouse micronucleus	>50	>66 000
Carcinogenicity (p53 +/− mice)	>350	>1000
Phototoxicity		
Dermal	>40	1000
Ocular		10 000

[a]Relative to an estimated clinical dose of 1 ug S-59/kg. Similar margins are estimated based on a final concentration of 1 ng/ml in the product, or if an average exposure of 14 platelet transfusions per patient is assumed.

seen in the blood after transfusion, as the dose given per kg or as the average number of units of component given clinically. For amotosalen treated platelets these are approximately 1 ng/ml, 1 ug/kg and 14 units of treated platelets. Table 19.7 lists the margin of safety for a selection of toxicity tests for both amotosalen and amotosalen-treated platelets.

For the PR technologies that have progressed to clinical assessment, such margins of safety for the full range of tests have been accepted by regulatory authorities as adequate, following expert toxicological input (Chapman et al., 2003a; 2003b; Ciavarino, 2001; Ciavarino et al., 2003b; 2003c). An additional level of reassurance can be provided by cumulative data on large numbers of treated patients. For methylene blue FFP and SD plasma, millions of units have been transfused without reports of an excessive number of side effects. For amotosalen-treated platelets and plasma, hundreds of patients and thousands of units have been transfused in trials undertaken over the last five years, but this remains a relatively small number, and the follow-up period is still relatively short. For other PR technologies clinical experience is much less extensive, where it has been undertaken at all. Only with large-scale implementation, and carefully designed long-term follow-up studies, can the question of possible late toxicity finally be answered.

Neoantigens

One area of particular concern is whether PR treated components induce new structures (neoantigens) specific to the chemical used. These can result in the patient mounting an undesirable immune alloantibody response to the product, which may result in rapid destruction of the transfused product. This field is complicated by at least three confounding factors. First, human blood components, with or without PR treatment, almost inevitably result in immune response in the animals used for toxicological studies. This may be overcome by use of animal blood components, but the use of such animal models is a very specialized field, in which experience is limited. Second, the available tests used in vitro to try and predict neoantigen formation are less well developed than other toxicity tests and are open to alternative interpretations. Last, many blood group antigens on blood cells and plasma proteins stimulate alloimmune reactions in patients receiving non-PR treated components. Laboratory studies can demonstrate lack of neoantigen formation in vitro (Mohr et al., 1992), but such concerns will only be definitively answered by acquisition of data from a large number of transfused patients.

The potential seriousness of immune responses to neoantigens is emphasized by the recent cessation of trials for two PR red cell products in the USA: Inactine (an ethylene diimine oligomer) and S-303 (a nitrogen mustard derivative). Trials for both these products followed successful studies in volunteers (AuBuchon et al., 2002; Greenwalt et al., 1999; Snyder et al., 2001), and protocols agreed with the US regulator. Trials involved assessment of acute transfusions in surgical patients (unlikely to have been previously transfused) and of chronic transfusion in haemoglobinopathy patients, who receive regular red cell transfusion throughout life and who are frequently sensitized to multiple red cell antigens. In trials of both compounds, antibodies were detected at an early stage in patients in the chronic transfusion arms of the trials. These antibodies reacted with red cells after, but not before, PR treatment. This has resulted in the suspension of chronic transfusion trials for both technologies. For other PR technologies, the extensive clinical experience with methylene blue and SD plasma provides reassurance that the possibility of antibody formation to neoantigens is remote. The lesser experience with amotosalen products, so far administered to about 12000 trial patients, is encouraging (Rhenen et al., 2003), but more data are needed.

Pathogen reduction: individual methods

Many systems are in development in the commercial sector, but as there are as yet no licensed systems suitable for red cells, the day when a national blood supply can be totally pathogen inactivated has not yet arrived. However, this is a rapidly changing field, and further developments can be expected in the next few years. Table 19.4 summarizes the different systems and their progress through development.

Pathogen reduction systems for platelets

Amotosalen (S59) and ultraviolet A (UVA)

This technology, developed by Cerus and Baxter, utilizes amotosalen (S59), a synthetic psoralen designed to achieve maximum

Table 19.8 Platelet increments and transfusion requirements in two randomized trials of amotosalen-treated platelets.

	EuroSPRITE (buffy coat platelets; Rhenen *et al.*, 2003)		SPRINT (apheresis platelets; McCullough *et al.*, 2004)	
	S59	Control	S59	Control
Patients	52	51	318	327
Mean platelet dose/transfusion ($\times 10^{11}$)	3.9[a]	4.3	3.7[a]	4.0
Mean 1 hour corrected count increment (CCI, $\times 10^3$)	13.1	14.9	11.1[a]	16.0
Mean no. platelet transfusions	7.5[a]	5.6	8.4[a]	6.2
Mean inter-transfusion interval (days)	3.0	4.3	1.9[a]	2.4

[a] Statistically significant $p < 0.05$.

penetration into organisms and cells, which by virtue of being a small three-ringed planar molecule, can intercalate within the helices of both single and double stranded DNA and RNA. When activated by long wave UVA (320–400 nm), the amotosalen molecules form permanent adducts approximately every 100 base pairs between and within nucleic acid strands, thus preventing replication and also transcription. This means that a wide range of viruses, bacteria and leucocytes are susceptible to the treatment. However, prions, since they have no nucleic acid, are not.

For the commercial integral blood bag system, recently licensed in Europe, the manufacturers have recommended that for platelet concentrates (PC) to be amotosalen-treated they must be suspended in an additive solution (Intersol, PASIII) with 32–47% residual plasma, in a volume of 300–390 ml, with a platelet content of 2.5–5.0 $\times 10^{11}$ per unit and red cell contamination of $<4 \times 10^6$ per unit. A set volume of amotosalen is added to the PC, resulting in a final concentration of approximately 150 µmol/l, followed by exposure to 3–4 J/cm^2 of UV-A in an illumination device for approximately four minutes. Amotosalen and its photodegradation products are removed by agitating the PC with a compound adsorption device (CAD) for 6–16 hours, leaving residual levels of amotosalen in the order of 0.2 µmol/l.

Several in vitro studies have shown that amotosalen treatment does not have a significant impact on the following variables in PC during storage for 5–7 days: platelet count, pH, bicarbonate, morphology score, glucose consumption, platelet aggregation to ADP and collagen, extent of shape change (ESC), hypotonic shock response (HSR) and ATP (Knutson *et al.*, 2000; Lin *et al.*, 1997; Rhenen *et al.*, 2000). However, van Rhenen showed that the loss in platelet number during storage was greater in treated platelets (8–11%) compared with controls (0–5%). This was also associated with higher levels of platelet lysis (15% compared with 5%). As well as possibly potentiating any loss in platelet number during storage, amotosalen treatment results in a 7–15% loss of platelets in the component due to the extra processing steps required. Amotosalen treatment of PC prevents the increase in the leucocyte derived cytokines IL-8 and IL-1 seen during storage of non-LD PC (Hei *et al.*, 1999), but there are no data on platelet derived cytokines. In a primate model, recovery and survival of platelets was unaffected by treatment with amotosalen, but platelets were only stored for 24 hours and in 100% plasma (Lin *et al.*, 1997).

In human volunteers, recovery and survival of ^{111}In-labelled S59 treated platelets were slightly reduced compared to controls, with recovery of 42.5% (50.3% in controls) and survival of 114.5 hours (145 hours for controls, Corash *et al.*, 1997). This may be due to the 10–20% increase in the expression of CD62P (P-selectin) in amotosalen-treated platelets compared with controls when stored for 5–7 days (Knutson *et al.*, 2000; Lin *et al.*, 1997; Rhenen *et al.*, 2000). These volunteer studies were followed by two phase III randomized trials in thrombocytopenic haemato-oncology patients, one in Europe using buffy coat pooled platelets (EuroSPRITE), and a larger trial of single donor apheresis platelets (Baxter Amicus) in the USA (SPRINT). EuroSPRITE involved 103 patients in five sites, and used platelet count increment (CI) over the first eight platelet transfusions as the primary endpoint. Since platelets exposed to amotosalen treatment contained a lower infused platelet dose, corrected count increments (CCI) were also used. The overall conclusions were that although there was no statistically significant difference in CCI between the two study arms, patients in the amotosalen arm received significantly more platelet transfusions during the course of their treatment (see Table 19.8), because the inter-transfusion interval was reduced from 4.3 to 3 days. There was no difference in haemorrhagic events, refractoriness or adverse events between the two arms of the study (Rhenen *et al.*, 2003).

SPRINT involved 645 patients at 12 sites, and used World Health Organization grade 2 bleeding as the primary endpoint. Although there was no difference between the study arms in grade 2 or any other severity of haemorrhage, or in the number of red cell transfusions required, there was again a significant difference in inter-transfusion interval and total number of platelet transfusions received (McCullough *et al.*, 2004). This appears to relate to platelet dose, since these differences disappeared when only transfusions containing $>3 \times 10^{11}$ platelets were analysed (Murphy *et al.*, 2003). Recipients of amotosalen-treated platelets experienced fewer reactions, with the biggest difference being in urticarial type effects, probably due to the platelet additive solution as well as leucocyte inhibition (Lopez-Plaza *et al.*, 2003).

It is unclear why the difference in one hour CCIs between S59 platelets and controls was so much more pronounced with apheresis than buffy coat platelets. However, the trial evidence suggests that if amotosalen-treated platelets manufactured by either method were introduced routinely, greater production through-put would be required to treat the same number of patients, and donor exposure could increase significantly. It could be argued that increased donor exposure is less important with a pathogen treated product, but there could be a concomitant increase in hazards not prevented by amotosalen treatment, such as transfusion errors and transfusion-related acute lung injury. The extra platelet production required also needs to be taken into account in cost-effectiveness analyses.

The amotosalen/UVA system is currently licensed in Europe for buffy coat derived PC and those collected by Baxter apheresis technology. Studies are underway to extend this to include PC collected by other apheresis technologies that are in use internationally. The main problem has been establishing how apheresis PC can easily be prepared in the required additive solution (Intersol). It is possible that differences in how PC are collected and processed prior to amotosalen treatment will influence the quality of treated platelets during storage. The in vitro data suggest that platelet function is relatively well maintained during storage of amotosalen-treated PC to day seven. Clinical studies to date have used a five-day shelf life, but more recent studies have permitted the CE mark to be extended to 7 day storage PC.

Thionine

This technique is only in preclinical study, so the variables relating to how the system would operate routinely have not yet been established. Preliminary studies suggest that treatment would involve a two-step procedure: illumination under yellow light at $200 \, J/cm^2$ in the presence of $1 \, \mu mol/l$ thionine for 30 minutes followed by exposure to UV-B at $1.2–1.8 \, J/cm^2$ for 4–6 minutes. Data on platelet function are limited and have been obtained using PC stored in plasma, whereas pathogen reduction is greater in PC stored in additive solution. Platelet concentrate treated with thionine and $1.8 \, J/cm^2$ UV-B shows a 25–30% decrease in HSR and aggregation in response to collagen compared with controls, although platelet swirling and pH are well maintained (Mohr and Redecker-Klein, 2003). The effect on platelet function is dependent upon the amount of UV-B exposure. Indeed, it is the UV-B step that mainly contributes to the loss of platelet functionality. Interestingly, the latest iteration of this system involves exposure of platelets to UV-C light alone, without the use of photosensitising chemicals.

Riboflavin

The riboflavin process for platelets has now commenced clinical trial, but it is likely that the system would involve the addition of $30 \, ml$ of $500 \, \mu mol/l$ riboflavin in sodium chloride to give an approximate final concentration of $50 \, \mu mol/l$, and exposure in an illuminator to $6.2 \, J/cm^2$ light (265–370 nm) for 8–10 minutes. Neither riboflavin nor its photoproducts are removed prior to storage or transfusion of the component.

Data to day five of storage suggest that the treatment results in an increase in glycolysis compared with controls, as shown by increased consumption of O_2 and glucose and production of lactate, with a reduction in pH (Li et al., 2004; Ruane et al., 2004). There appears to be little effect on the platelet morphology score, hypotonic shock response, or platelet swirling. However, platelet expression of CD62P is 100% higher in treated platelets, suggesting that the process results in platelet activation. It is not clear what the clinical consequences of increased activation are; any impact on platelet recovery and survival can only be assessed following phase I clinical studies.

Fresh frozen plasma

Systems for pathogen reduction in fresh frozen plasma have been available for the longest time, with methylene blue (MB) photo-inactivation and solvent/detergent (SD) treatment reaching wide clinical use in a number of countries. The amotosalen/UVA system developed for platelets has been modified for plasma use, and this system is now licensed in the EU.

Solvent detergent FFP

Solvent detergent treatment can be applied only to pools of several hundred ABO-identical units, so requires industrial scale plant for production (Hellstern et al., 1992). As the treatment destroys the lipid envelope of red cells, no RhD matching is required. In the Octapharma process the plasma pool is incubated with a solvent (tri-n-butyl phosphate) and a detergent. These reagents are then removed by oil extraction and chromatography before plasma is filtered and frozen. The number of plasma donations per pool and the exact nature of the process varies depending on the manufacturer. Exposure to SD destroys the lipid envelope of the human immunodeficiency virus (HIV) and hepatitis B and C viruses, and no such transmissions have been reported. Non-lipid-coated viruses such as parvovirus B19 and hepatitis A (HAV) are not specifically inactivated, but their titre may be reduced in downstream processing. In addition, plasma pools with high genomic titres of these viruses are rejected, and pools must contain specified levels of viral antibodies, which may be at least partially protective. No increase in clinical cases of HAV or parvovirus B19 in SD FFP recipients is evident, although there were some B19 transmissions documented in volunteers with the US product. A 'universal FFP', produced by neutralization of anti-A and anti-B by A and B substances present in plasma, is in development for potential administration to patients of any ABO group (Solheim et al., 2002).

Methylene blue fresh frozen plasma

Methylene blue (MB) treatment of plasma was developed in the early 1990s by the Springe group in Germany. The original system used an initial freeze thaw step to disrupt intact leucocytes, then a variable amount of MB solution was added to achieve the same MB concentration in every pack ($1 \mu mol/l$). Later systems were developed by Baxter and Macopharma for small-scale use in blood centres, involving sterile connection of the plasma pack (before or after freezing), to a pack with a leucocyte depletion filter upstream of a liquid pouch or a dry pellet containing

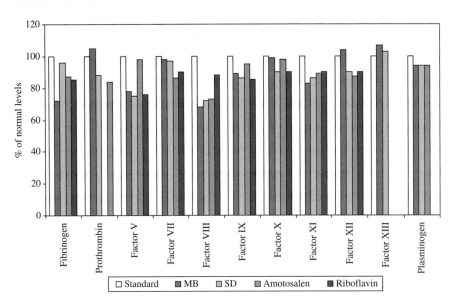

Figure 19.3 Coagulation factors in standard and PR FFP.

85–95 µg of MB. To achieve the desired final MB concentration of 1µM, the input plasma volume has to be within a 200–300 ml range. In both the Springe and commercial systems, the MBFFP packs are then exposed to visible wavelengths of light to activate the MB (usually for about 30 minutes). Finally, MB removal filters are now available to reduce residual MB to <0.1µmol/l prior to plasma storage. The system has been in routine use in several European countries and has recently gained approval from the Paul Erlich Institut in Germany.

Amotosalen fresh frozen plasma

The amotosalen system for plasma treatment is identical to that for platelets except that the compound removal step is achieved by plasma filtration, so is considerably shortened. Clinical studies have now been completed, and the product is licensed in the EU.

Effect of amotosalen, solvent detergent and methylene blue on coagulation proteins

A summary of the effect of amotosalen, SD and MB treatment of plasma on coagulation proteins is shown in Figure 19.3.

Clotting factor levels

For SD plasma, manufacturers can guarantee that each batch of plasma contains >0.50 U/ml of all clotting factors since each batch is a large pool and can be tested for many coagulation parameters (Doyle *et al.*, 2003; Leebeek *et al.*, 1999). However, SD plasma is known to have different characteristics in terms of residual levels of coagulation factors and their activation status, depending on how the plasma has been processed. Compared with SD plasma produced in Europe, SD plasma from the USA contains around half the amount of citrate, protein S, $\alpha_2$antiplasmin, $\alpha_1$antitrypsin and plasminogen activator inhibitor 1 (PAI-1)

(Heiden *et al.*, 2003; Solheim and Hellstern, 2003). These studies also showed higher levels of activated FXII in the US product, but not levels of activated FVII or markers of thrombin generation. Therefore SD-treated plasma produced by different manufacturers cannot be assumed to be of the same composition.

Due to individual donor variability, there is less consistency of content in PR plasma produced by single donation methods. Methylene blue treatment of plasma affects the functional activity of various coagulation proteins and inhibitors, with differences in processing methods between studies possibly accounting for some of the variability in results seen in different reports (Figures 19.3 and 19.4). The proteins most severely affected by MB treatment of plasma are factor VIII and fibrinogen, where activity is reduced by 20–35% (Aznar *et al.*, 1999). The decrease in fibrinogen is seen when assayed by the method of Clauss, but not in antigenic assays (Zeiler *et al.*, 1994), suggesting that MB treatment affects the biological activity but not concentration of fibrinogen. This is possibly due to the photo-oxidation of fibrinogen inhibiting polymerization of fibrin monomers (Inada *et al.*, 1978). Methylene blue treatment using red light has been shown to influence fibrin polymerization and gelation (Suontataka *et al.*, 2003). However, fibrinogen isolated from MB-treated plasma retains normal ability to bind to GPIIb/IIIa receptors on platelets (Lorenz *et al.*, 1998), an important mechanism in platelet activation and aggregation. Changes in coagulation proteins induced by MB removal filters appear to be negligible compared to the effect of the MB process itself (Garwood *et al.*, 2003).

In general, the loss of coagulation factors is less using amotosalen treatment than MB (Pinkoski *et al.*, 2001a; 2001b; 2002a; 2002b). This is especially true for fibrinogen, where the loss is 13% for amotosalen and 25–40% for MB.

Clotting factor activation

Ratios of FVIIC:FVIIag, FIXC:FIXag and levels of FXa are not affected by SD treatment, suggesting that these factors do not become activated during the process (Piquet *et al.*, 1992).

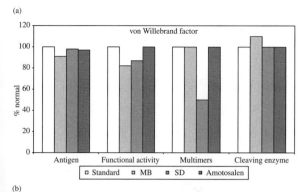

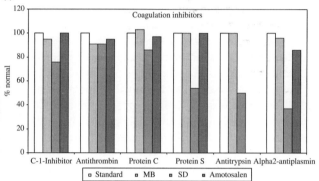

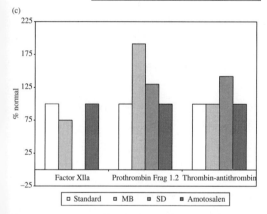

Figure 19.4 Functional levels of von Willebrand factor, inhibitors of coagulation and markers of activation of coagulation in standard and pathogen reduced FFP.

However, when measured directly, levels of activated FVII are higher following treatment (166 compared with 58 mU/ml, Beeck and Hellstern, 1998) and compared with standard FFP (Nifong *et al.*, 2002). Levels of thrombin-antithrombin complexes are not elevated in MB, SD or amotosalen-treated plasma, indicating that any coagulation factor activation during treatment is not associated with excessive thrombin generation. However, prothrombin fragment $1 + 2$, another marker of thrombin generation, appears to be increased in MB and SD plasma. The clinical significance of this is unclear.

Inhibitors of coagulation and fibrinolytic pathway

Functional measurements of the naturally occurring anticoagulant proteins C and S and antithrombin appear to be relatively unaltered by either MB or amotosalen treatment. Both treatments

also have little effect on levels of plasminogen, plasminogen activator inhibitor-1 (PAI-1, the main inhibitor of plasminogen activator) α_2-antiplasmin (the main inhibitor of plasmin), fibrin monomer and D-dimers, suggesting that the use of either is unlikely to enhance fibrinolysis.

In contrast, protein S activity in SD plasma is reduced to 40–60% of normal, and protein C and antithrombin activity are reduced by 10%. In addition, >90% of α_2-antiplasmin is in a latent or polymerized form that lacks activity (Mast *et al.*, 1999). Concerns have therefore been expressed in the USA that SDFFP might be associated with either increased thrombotic risk or increased risk of hyperfibrinolysis, depending on the clinical situation. This resulted in a manufacturer's warning on the product data sheet, and eventually the product was withdrawn from manufacture in the USA. These complications have not been prominent in recipients of SDFFP manufactured by the European method, although a recent study from the UK has raised concerns regarding a possibly increased risk of deep vein thrombosis in patients treated with SDFFP during plasma exchange procedures for thrombotic thrombocytopenic purpura (Yarranton *et al.*, 2003a).

Clinical studies of SDFFP, MBFFP and amotosalen-treated FFP

Solvent/detergent treated fresh frozen plasma

Solvent/detergent treated fresh frozen plasma has been evaluated for efficacy and tolerability in a number of non-randomized studies in patients with congenital single clotting factor deficiencies (Horowitz & Penta, 1998; Inbal *et al.*, 1993); undergoing cardiac surgery (Solheim *et al.*, 1993); with a long prothrombin time (Lerner *et al.*, 2000); and in intensive care (Hellstern *et al.*, 1993). In addition, randomized studies have been performed against normal FFP in routine use (Beck *et al.*, 2000); in liver disease and transplantation (Williamson *et al.*, 1999); and in cardiac surgery (Haubelt *et al.*, 2002). In addition, a comparison with MBFFP has also been performed (Wieding *et al.*, 1999). In all of these studies, the safety profile and overall efficacy of SDFFP has been excellent, with the possible thrombotic risk of the US product identified as the only problem.

Methylene blue fresh frozen plasma

Because this technology was licensed as a device rather than a drug, the clinical trial data on this product are rather limited. Following transfusion of MB treated plasma to healthy adults, there was no significant difference from baseline pre-infusion values in Activated Partial Thromboplastin Time (APTT), Prothrombin Time (PT), Thrombin Time (TT), FVIII, FXI, Clauss fibrinogen, fibrin degradation products, or platelet aggregation induced by collagen or ADP, suggesting no major influence on coagulation or fibrinolytic systems (Simonsen & Sorensen, 1999). Most studies in patients have been small, and/or have used laboratory rather than clinical endpoints. Despite usage of >1 million units in Europe, there have been no full reports of large, randomized trials of MBFFP using relevant endpoints such as blood loss or exposure to other blood components. Early studies described successful use of MBFFP in either single or small groups of patients with deficiencies of factors V or XI, thrombotic thrombocytopenic purpura, and exchange transfusion in neonates (Pohl *et al.*, 1995a; 1995b). One study of 71 patients compared MBFFP with solvent/detergent treated FFP in cardiac surgery and showed better replacement of protein S and alpha 2-antiplasmin with MBFFP, but no difference in blood loss (Wieding *et al.*, 1999). However, one hospital in Spain has reported that following a total switch to MBFFP, FFP demand rose by 56%, with a two- to threefold increase in demand for cryoprecipitate, which was not MB treated (Atance *et al.*, 2001). The authors suggest that the increase in demand, particularly for cryoprecipitate, may have been required to offset the reduced fibrinogen level in the product. However, longer term data suggests that MBFFP is not associated with increased usage of FFP (Solheim *et al.*, 2006). Indeed, following orthopaedic surgery, transfusion of MBFFP has been associated with increased reptilase clotting times and ratio of immunological to functional measured fibrinogen (Taborski *et al.*, 2000), suggesting that MB may interfere with fibrin polymerization in vivo.

No problems with MBFFP treated infants requiring phototherapy have been reported in Europe, and glucose 6 phosphate dehydrogenase deficiency is not a contraindication to its use (Walker, written communication, 2002). Similarly, digital capillary measurement of oxygen saturation by colorimetric means is not affected by infusion of MBFFP.

Amotosalen fresh frozen plasma

In a phase 1 randomized dose escalation study, 15 volunteers received up to 1000 ml of amotosalen-treated or control autologous fresh frozen plasma. No side effects were noted. This was followed by a further study in volunteers to examine reversal of four days' warfarin treatment by either amotosalen-treated or control autologous plasma. Twenty-four hours after plasma infusion, the warfarin was definitively reversed with vitamin K, so kinetic studies were possible only for factor VII, which has the shortest half-life. The results were similar after infusion of either product, with a measurable increase in factor VII present only for eight hours (Hambleton *et al.*, 2002).

These data allowed three phase III clinical studies to be carried out. The first study was in 34 patients with a variety of single congenital coagulation factor deficiencies treated in a non-randomized way with 15–20 ml/kg of amotosalen-treated FFP. This allowed recovery and half-life studies of each clotting factor to be performed, albeit in a small number of patients for each factor. Recoveries were > 90% for factors V, X, XI, XIII and, importantly, also for protein C, protein S and antithrombin. However, losses of fibrinogen and factor V were 15–20%, and there was 20–25% loss of factor VIII. Half-lives of factors V, VII, X, XI and protein C were as expected, but for factors I, II and XIII, which in any case have the longest half-lives, the terminal half-lives were longer than expected (Alarcon *et al.* 2003). The clinical significance of these findings for the types of patient who commonly receive FFP was then examined in a randomized study of 121 patients with acquired multiple coagulation deficiencies. The single largest group in the study was liver transplant patients (Mintz *et al.*, 2002). No differences between the two groups in correction

of PT or APPT were noted, nor in clinical haemostasis or side effects. Hepatic artery thrombosis was noted after liver transplant in both groups.

Suitability for production of cryoprecipitate

There have been relatively few studies examining cryoprecipitate produced from pathogen inactivated plasma, but production from FFP treated by any of the three PR methods described above is feasible. Since most cryoprecipitate use in the UK nowadays is for fibrinogen replacement, functional fibrinogen is a particularly important endpoint, but content of FVIII and von Willebrand factor are also important. In cryoprecipitate produced from SDFFP, there are reductions in levels of FVIII (40%), fibrinogen (25%) and vWF activity (65%) (Keeling *et al.*, 1997). This is partly due to reduced levels in the plasma used as starting material, and partly due to altered precipitation, and suggests that this component would not be suitable for treatment of von Willebrand's disease. In cryoprecipitate produced from MB-treated plasma, levels of FVIII and fibrinogen activity are 20–40% lower than untreated units, but remain within Council of Europe Guidelines (Aznar *et al.*, 2000; Hornsey *et al.*, 2000). This reduction can be overcome by modifications to the production method (Hornsey *et al.*, 2004). vWF activity in MB cryoprecipitate is relatively unaltered. In an unpaired study, FVIII, vWF and fibrinogen concentrations and content were not significantly different in cryoprecipitate produced from amotosalen-treated plasma compared with untreated (Wages *et al.*, 2000).

Suitability for plasma exchange for thrombotic thrombocytopenic purpura

The laboratory features usually examined to assess suitability of FFP or cryosupernatant for the treatment of TTP are the pattern of vWF multimers and levels of vWF cleaving protease (ADAMTS 13). Many TTP patients have tended to have unusually large vWF multimers, which can promote platelet aggregation (Chow *et al.*, 1998). There is thus a theoretical advantage in using a product lacking high MW multimers. This applies to cryosupernatant produced from standard, MB or amotosalen-treated plasma (Aznar *et al.*, 2000; Yarranton *et al.*, 2003b), and also to SDFFP, which has been used successfully in TTP (Evans *et al.*, 1999; Moake *et al.*, 1994), even when resistant to other forms of treatment (Harrison *et al.*, 1996). The importance of vWF cleaving protease in TTP has now been demonstrated, with low levels in many patients (Allford *et al.*, 2000; Furlan *et al.*, 1998). Levels of vWF cleaving protease are normal in MBFFP (Cardigan *et al.*, 2002), and in both amotosalen-treated plasma (Hillyer *et al.*, 2001) and the cryosupernatant produced from it (Yarranton *et al.*, 2003b), but have not yet been measured in MB cryosupernatant. However, one study of two small cohorts of patients (13 treated with FFP and 7 with MBFFP) reported an increase in the number of plasma exchange procedures and days in hospital in the MBFFP group (De la Rubia *et al.*, 2001). This is of concern, although the small patient numbers make it difficult to draw conclusions; clearly larger studies are required to establish the role of MBFFP in TTP.

Given that levels of vWF cleaving protease appear to be relatively unaltered in MB plasma, it is likely they would be within the normal range in MB treated cryosupernatant. It would therefore appear that MB or amotosalen-treated cryosupernatant would be suitable for the treatment of TTP, but neither has yet been manufactured for clinical use.

Pathogen inactivation systems for red cells

The challenge for pathogen reduction in red cells is that the absorption spectrum of haemoglobin hinders the use of visible or ultraviolet light as a chemical activator.

S-303

S-303 is a 3-moiety molecule, with anchor, linker and effector elements. The molecular mechanism of action is similar to that of amotosalen, but activation is achieved via a change in pH. Extracellular reactions are minimized by the inclusion of the quencher molecule glutathione in the system. S-303 enters cells and pathogens rapidly, but the molecule is designed to degrade under physiological conditions via a frangible ester bond. This generates S300, which has reduced affinity for nucleic acids. The starting product is LD red cell concentrate which must be in a purpose-designed additive solution. Solutions of S-303 (0.2 mM), dextrose and glutathione are added and incubated at room temperature for 12–20 hours. There is then a further eight-hour incubation in a separate container with the compound removal device, which eliminates >90% of the S300.

S-303 treatment does not appear to affect haemolysis, extracellular potassium, glucose, lactate, 2,3 DPG or ATP levels (Cook *et al.*, 1997). In mouse and canine models, S-303 treatment had no effect on red cell recovery 24 hours following transfusion (Cook *et al.*, 1997; 1998). When red cells are put under oxidative stress by the addition of methylene blue, prior treatment with S-303 does not appear to reduce their ability to recover (Clark *et al.*, 2003).

Phase I studies using autologous ^{51}Cr-labelled S-303 treated red cells in volunteers revealed acceptable >80% recovery up to 35 days of storage. No neoantigens were observed in vitro, and despite the fact that no S-303 removal was employed, no erythrocyte antibodies were seen, even after either repeated exposure or after an entire red cell unit was infused (Greenwalt *et al.*, 1999). As mentioned above, a phase III acute study in cardiac surgery patients and a chronic transfusion study in sickle cell anaemia patients commenced. However, all clinical trials of this compound were voluntarily halted by the company in late 2003 because of the development of erythrocyte alloantibodies in patients in the chronic study.

Inactine (PEN110)

This agent is a proprietary mixture of ethyleneimine oligomers, which, being water soluble, can easily enter cells and pathogens. The compounds interact with nucleic acids to prevent replication, with the positively charged Inactine molecules attaching to the negatively charged phosphate backbone of DNA and RNA, leading to the modification of guanine residues. The opening of the imidazole ring structure leads to loss of bases and strand breakages, effectively acting to block nucleic acid strand replication. No photo-inactivation is required.

The commercial system requires incubation of LD red cells with PEN110 to a final concentration of 0.1% v/v for 6–24 hours at room temperature, followed by extensive automated washing in a closed system with up to six litres of 5% dextrose in normal saline to reduce the residual PEN110 concentration to <50 ng/ml. It is possible that the washing stage could be less rigorous pending results of toxicology studies.

In human red cells, PEN110 treatment is reported to have no effect on red cell haemolysis or intracellular potassium at day 42 of storage, but ATP levels were 25% lower (Purmal *et al.*, 2002). However, in this study the control group were also washed in the same manner as treated cells which is not a normal process for red cell components and may have some effect in itself. The differences observed in vitro were not, however, seen in baboon blood used as a model, in which PEN110 treatment resulted in a small but significant reduction in red cell post-transfusion survival (but not recovery) when stored for 28 days. There were no apparent differences after 42 days (Purmal *et al.*, 2002). AuBuchon *et al.*, (2002) compared PEN110 treated cells with standard red cells in additive solution that had not been washed. The washing step resulted in a 20% loss of red cells (likely to be less if optimized), a 50% loss of 2,3 DPG, and no effect on ATP. In fact, 2,3 DPG is almost entirely lost in red cell components by two weeks of storage, but the reduction at the beginning of storage might have clinical implications for oxygen delivery where fresh RCC are mandated, for example for exchange transfusion. AuBuchon *et al.*, showed that lactate production was double and glucose consumption 30% higher in control units. Supernatant potassium levels were lower in the treated group due to washing, but the rate of increase during storage was similar for both groups. At day 42 of storage haemolysis was about three-fold higher in the treated units, but remained <1% in all units. The ATP levels were 38% lower in treated units by day 42.

Phase I studies in human volunteers showed comparable recovery of control and PEN110 treated autologous radio-labelled red cells when treated for six hours and stored for 28 days (AuBuchon *et al.*, 2002). Phase 2 studies used 24 hours of treatment and both 35 and 42 day storage (Snyder *et al.*, 2001). Although 24-hour recovery was comparable to controls, survival of 42-day stored red cells was shorter. In these studies, none of 60 subjects developed antibodies to red cells. On the basis of these findings, phase III randomized controlled trials began in cardiac surgery and transfusion-dependent patients, but the latter trial was brought to a close in late 2003 due to development of erythrocyte alloantibodies.

Riboflavin

Studies to date have mainly used 500 μmol/l riboflavin and visible light in red cells diluted to a haematocrit of 37%. This may imply the need to re-centrifuge the treated red cells to the usual haematocrit for red cell concentrates. The process will probably be optimized further prior to clinical studies. There are no published data to date on red cell quality.

Pathogen reduction: additional considerations

Prevention of transfusion-associated graft-versus-host disease

Since this condition is mediated via donor T-lymphocytes, studies of amotosalen, S-303 and PEN110 have examined T-lymphocyte inactivation in laboratory and animal studies. All three technologies have demonstrated several logs of T-cell inactivation and prevention of TA-GVHD in animal models (Ciaravino, 2001; Corash and Lin, 2004; Fast *et al.*, 2002a; 2002b; 2004; Grass *et al.*, 1998). Given that the T-lymphocyte load can also be reduced by >3 logs by upstream leucocyte depletion, there can be a high degree of confidence that these systems can substitute for gamma irradiation. It seems likely that most if not all DNA interactive PR methods will be effective in TA-GVHD prevention. This would simplify production and help reduce costs. Equally, there do not seem to be disastrous effects on platelets if they are also gamma irradiated as well. Removal of the requirement for gamma irradiation would certainly offset some of the costs, but until systems are also available for red cells and granulocytes, the costs of purchase and maintenance of gamma irradiators cannot yet be totally avoided. If PR is accepted to supplement LD in the prevention of both CMV and TA-GVHD, then inventory management becomes greatly simplified, with a single red cell and platelet component suitable for all recipients. However, reliance on a single step for so many patient safety issues makes it especially important that the process is carried out to high standards of good manufacturing practice.

Inactivation of parasites

In tropical areas, there would clearly be huge benefits to health from systems which could inactivate malaria and trypanosomes in blood components. Where tested, parasites do appear to be susceptible to both S-303 and PEN110 (see Table 19.5). In the developed world, many donors are deferred because of travel to tropical areas, so there is potential for significantly reduced donation wastage (Leiby, 2004).

Health and safety of staff

Some pathogen reduction compounds are toxic to skin and eyes in the concentrations provided before dilution in the blood component. Although they are designed to be employed in closed blood bag systems, appropriate measures must be taken to ensure no potential for staff exposure to the agents should there be bag breakages or leaks. No special monitoring of staff is considered necessary.

Quality assurance and process control

In addition to standard leucocyte depletion methodology, pathogen reduction systems involve addition and removal of potentially toxic agents, and in some cases, exposure to light of particular wavelengths at predetermined intensity for specified periods of time. There are no simple measures analogous to gamma irradiation-sensitive labels which can prove that a given blood unit received an adequate dose of chemicals and light exposure. Tight process control is required to ensure that all units go through the process as intended. Computer links between light box and blood centre mainframe can provide a permanent record of exposure dose.

These systems also raise interesting issues concerning the requirement for and feasibility of blood centres to monitor the levels of residual chemicals, both the initial additive and its photodegradation products. The complex chemical assays such as high pressure liquid chromatography required to measure low levels of such mixtures are likely to be outside the expertise of most blood establishments and may have to be performed by the manufacturers or a third party.

Cost-effectiveness

This is one of the most difficult issues surrounding pathogen inactivation. In the developed world, the risk of viral transmission is now so low that all pathogen reduction systems will almost certainly fail conventional health care cost-effectiveness criteria. This has already been shown for solvent/detergent fresh frozen plasma, for example (Jackson *et al.*, 1999; Pereira, 1999; Riedler *et al.*, 2003). However, no government has categorically decreed what is a reasonable sum to spend on blood safety, and many current testing strategies, such as HCV genome testing, also require heavy expenditure to prevent only the occasional transmission. In the developing world, where organizational and laboratory infrastructure is often lacking and there are multiple pathogens, for example HIV, hepatitis B and C, malaria and trypanosomes, there would be real benefits from implementation of pathogen reduction, particularly for red cells. Unfortunately, these are the very economies for whom the cost of pathogen reduction is likely to prove prohibitive. These issues continue to be debated as the scientific aspects of the technology are developed.

Could universal pathogen reduction allow relaxation of donor selection and/or testing schedules?

Inevitably, the advent of pathogen reduction systems has triggered a debate regarding the requirement to maintain certain donor deferral criteria and viral screening tests which together have already achieved a high level of blood safety. For example, deferral of donors after body piercing and travel to malarious areas both cause loss of many thousands of donations per year. In addition, screening for new agents will add to donation loss through false-positive reactions. Careful risk assessment will be required, however, before any relaxation to donor selection or screening could be contemplated.

Conclusion

Alteration of blood components by leucocyte depletion and/or pathogen reduction can potentially result in further reductions in the already low risk of pathogen transmission. However, these benefits need to be balanced against possible disadvantages of loss of component quality, neoantigenicity, toxicity and cost. For most agents, including new viruses, genome and other tests have high sensitivity and, as was seen with West Nile virus, such tests can be developed rapidly for new agents. The place of pathogen reduction in an overall strategy for transfusion safety is likely to emerge over the next few years.

Addendum

Since the manuscript was submitted it is noteworthy that:

- In November 2005 new Blood Quality and Safety Regulations came into force in the UK which enact a European Directive (2004/33/EC) and includes specifications for many blood components.
- There is an interesting recent editorial by Drew & Roback, 2007, providing an update of CMV transmission by transfusion.
- Cerus have revised their process for red cell pathogen reduction and have restarted clinical work for this product. They have also published a trial on the use of Intercept plasma in treatment of TTP (Mintz et al., 2006). The Intercept process is now CE marked also for plasma and for apheresis platelets. There is a further report of the reduced efficacy of MB plasma in TTP (Alvarez- Larrán et al., 2004).
- Macopharma's work on platelet pathogen reduction is now utilising UV treatment alone, without the addition of thionine. Experience in Greece has not shown the increased demand for MB plasma ascribed to reduced potency in Spain mentioned above (Politis et al., 2007).
- There have now been two additional cases of vCJD transmission by non-leucoreduced red cells.
- There is an Irish report of three fatalities following use of OctaPlas during liver transplantation (Magner et al., 2007).
- There was a recent consensus conference on pathogen reduction which is summarised in Klein et al., 2007.

REFERENCES

Alarcon, P. de, Benjam, R. J., Shopnick, R., et al. (2003) Patients with congenital coagulation factor deficiencies demonstrate consistent therapeutic responses to repeated transfusions of plasma prepared with pathogen inactivation treatment (INTERCEPT plasma). Blood, 102(11), 815a.

Allford, S. L., Harrison, P., Lawrie, A. S., et al. (2000) von Willebrand factor-cleaving protease activity in congenital thrombotic thrombocytopenic purpura. Br J Haematol, 111, 1215–22.

Alvarez-Larrán, A., Del Rio, J., Ramirez, C., et al., (2004) Methylene blue-photoinactivated plasma vs. fresh-frozen plasma as replacement fluid for plasma exchange in thrombotic thrombocytopenic purpura. Vox Sang, 86, 246–51.

Atance, R., Pereira, A. and Ramirez, B. (2001) Tranfusing methylene blue-photoinactivated plasma instead of FFP is associated with an increased demand for plasma and cryoprecipitate. Transfusion, 41, 1548–52.

AuBuchon, J. P., Pickard, C. A., Herschel, L. H., et al. (2002) Production of pathogen-inactivated RBC concentrates using PEN110 chemistry: a phase I clinical study. Transfusion, 42(2), 146–52.

Aytay, A., Ohagen, A., Busch, M., et al. (2003) Development of a sensitive long-range PCR system to demonstrate viral nucleic acid inactivation. Transfusion, 43(Suppl. 8A), S26–030E.

Aznar, J. A., Bonand, S., Montoro, J. M., et al. (2000) Influence of methylene blue photoinactivation treatment on coagulation factors from fresh frozen plasma, cryoprecipitates and cryosupernatants. Vox Sang, 79, 56–160.

Aznar, J. A., Molina, R. and Montoro, J. M. (1999) Factor VIII/von Willebrand factor complex in methylene blue-treated fresh plasma. Transfusion, 39, 748–50.

Bachmann, B., Knuver-Hopf, J., Lambrecht, B., et al. (1995) Target structures for HIV-1 inactivation by methylene blue and light. J Med Virol, 47(2), 172–8.

Beck, K. H., Mortelsmans, Y., Kretschmer, V. V., et al. (2000) Comparison of solvent/detergent-inactivated plasma and fresh frozen plasma under routine clinical conditions. Infusionstherapie und Transfusionsmedizin, 27, 144–8.

Beeck, H. and Hellstern, P. (1998) In vitro characterisation of solvent/detergent-treated human plasma and of quarantine fresh-frozen plasma. Vox Sang, 74(Suppl. 1), 219–23.

Bowden, R. A., Slichter, S. J., Sayers, M., et al. (1995) A comparison of filtered leukocyte-reduced and cytomegalovirus (CMV) seronegative blood products for the prevention of transfusion-associated CMV infection after marrow transplant. Blood, 86, 3598–603.

Brown, P., Cervenakova, L., McShane, L. M., et al. (1999) Further studies of blood infectivity in an experimental model of transmissible spongiform encephalopathy, with an explanation of why blood components do not transmit Creutzfeldt-Jakob disease in humans. Transfusion. 39, 1169–78.

Brown, P., Rohwer, R. G., Dunstan, B. C., et al. (1998) The distribution of infectivity in blood components and plasma derivatives in experimental models of transmissible spongiform encephalopathy. Transfusion, 38(9), 810–6.

Cardigan, R., Allford, S. and Williamson, L. M. (2002) Levels of von Willebrand factor cleaving protease are normal in methylene blue treated fresh frozen plasma. Br J Haematol, 117, 253–4.

Cardigan, R., Sutherland, J., Garwood, M., et al. (2001) The effect of leucocyte depletion on the quality of fresh frozen plasma (FFP). Br J Haematol, 114, 233–40.

Cervenakova, L., Yakovleva, O., McKenzie, C., et al. (2003) Similar levels of infectivity in the blood of mice infected with human-derived vCJD and GSS strains of transmissible spongiform encephalopathy. Transfusion, 43, 1687–94.

Chabanel, A., Sensebe, I., Masse, M., et al. (2003) Quality assessment of seven types of fresh frozen plasma leucoreduced by specific plasma filtration. Vox Sang, 84, 308–17.

Chapman, J. (2000) Progress in improving the pathogen safety of red cell concentrates. Vox Sang, 78 (Suppl. 2), 203–4.

Chapman, J., Moore, K. and Alford, B. (2003b) Whole body autoradioluminography of the pathogen reduction compound INACTINE™ PEN110. Transfusion, 43(Suppl. 86A), SP–150.

Chapman, J. R., Moore, K. and Butterworth, B. E. (2003a) Pathogen inactivation of RBCs: PEN110 reproductive toxicology studies. Transfusion, 43, 1386–93.

Chow, T. W., Turner, N. A., Chintagumpala, M., et al. (1998) Increased von Willebrand factor binding to platelets in single episode and recurrent types of thrombotic thrombocytopenic purpura. Am J Hematol, 57(4), 292–302.

Ciaravino, V. (2001) Preclinical safety of a nucleic acid-targeted Helinx compound: a clinical perspective. Seminars in Hematology, Oct, 38(4 Suppl. 11), 12–19.

Ciaravino, V., McCullough, T. and Cimino, G. (2003a) The role of toxicology assessment in transfusion medicine. Transfusion, 43, 1481–92.

Ciaravino, V., McCullough, T., Cimino, G., et al. (2003b) Preclinical safety profile of plasma prepared using the INTERCEPT Blood System. Vox Sang, 85, 171–82.

Ciavarino, V., Sullivan, T. and McCullough, T. (2003c) The absence of reproductive toxicity demonstrated by the INTERCEPT™ blood system for platelets. Transfusion, 43(Suppl. 84A), SP–143.

Clark, B., Castro, G. and Stassinopoulos, A. (2003) Treatment with Helinx® technology does not affect the ability of red blood cells to overcome oxidative stress. Transfusion, 43(Suppl.), S30–030E.

Cook, D., Stassinopoulos, A., Merritt, J., et al. (1997) Inactivation of pathogens in packed red blood cell (PRBC) concentrates using S-303. Blood, 90(Suppl. 1), 409a.

Cook, D., Stassinopoulos, A., Wollowitz, S., *et al.* (1998) In vivo analysis of packed red blood cells treated with S-303 to inactivate pathogens. *Blood,* **92**(Suppl. 1), 503a.

Corash, L. (2000) Inactivation of viruses, bacteria, protozoa and leukocytes in platelet and red cell concentrates. *Vox Sang,* **78**(Suppl. 2), 205–10.

Corash, L. (2003) Pathogen reduction technology: methods, status of clinical trials, and future prospects. *Current Hematology Reports,* **2**, 495–502.

Corash, L. and Lin, L. (2004) Novel processes for inactivation of leukocytes to prevent transfusion-associated graft-versus-host disease. *Bone Marrow Transplantation,* **33**, 1–7.

Corash, L., Behrman, B., Rheinschmidt, M., *et al.* (1997) Post-transfusion viability and tolerability of photochemically treated platelet concentrates (PC). *Blood,* **90**(10), S1, 267a.

Corbin, F. (2002) Pathogen inactivation of blood components: current status and introduction of an approach using riboflavin as a photo-sensitizer. *Internat J Hematol,* **76**(Suppl. 2), 253–7.

Council of Europe (2001) Council of Europe expert committee in blood transfusion study group on pathogen inactivation of labile blood components. Pathogen inactivation of labile blood products. *Transfus Med,* **11**(3), 149–75.

Council of Europe (2007) *Council of Europe Guide to the Preparation, Use and Quality Assurance of Blood Components.* 13th edn, 2007, Strasbourg. Council of Europe Publishing.

De la Rubia, J., Arriaga, F., Linares, D., *et al.* (2001) Role of methylene blue treated or fresh frozen plasma in the response to plasma exchange in patients with thrombotic thrombocytopenic purpura. *Br J Haematol,* **114**, 721–3.

Doyle, S., O'Brien, P., Murphy, K., *et al.* (2003) Coagulation factor content of solvent detergent plasma compared with fresh frozen plasma. *Blood Coag Fibrinolysis,* **14**, 283–7.

Drew, W.L. and Roback, J.D. (2007) Prevention of transfusion-transmitted cytomegalovirus: reactivation of the debate? *Transfusion,* **47**, 1955–8.

Dupuis, K.W. (2003c) West Nile virus is inactivated by the Helinx® technology in human platelet concentrates. *Transfusion,* **43**(Suppl. 82A), SP–135.

Dupuis, K.W. and Alfonso, R. (2003a) Helinx® technology inactivates *Trypanosoma cruzi* in human red blood cells. *Transfusion,* **43**(Suppl. 83A), SP–139.

Dupuis, K.W. and Alfonso, R. (2003b) Helinx® technology inactivates intra-erythrocytic *Plasmodium falciparum* in human red blood cells. *Transfusion,* **43**(Suppl. 83A), SP–140.

Edrich, R., Benford, L., Urioste, M., *et al.* (2003) Bacterial decontamination of apheresis platelets using a photochemical treatment process with riboflavin. *Transfusion,* **43**(Suppl. 79A), SP–125.

Epstein, J.S. and Vostal, J.G. (2003) FDA approach to evaluation of pathogen reduction technology. *Transfusion,* **43**, 1347–50.

Evans, G., Llewelyn, C., Luddington, R., *et al.* (1999) Solvent/detergent fresh frozen plasma as primary treatment of acute thrombotic thrombocytopenic purpura. *Clin Lab Haematol,* **21**, 119–23.

Fast, L.D., DiLeone, G., Edson, C.M., *et al.* (2002a) PEN110 treatment functionally inactivates the PBMNCs present in RBC units: comparison to the effects of exposure to gamma irradiation. *Transfusion,* **42**, 1318–25.

Fast, L.D., DiLeone, G., Edson, C.M., *et al.* (2002b) Inhibition of murine GVHD by PEN110 treatment. *Transfusion,* **42**, 1326–32.

Fast, L.D., Semple, J.W., DiLeone, G., *et al.* (2004) Inhibition of xenogeneic GvHD by PEN 110 treatment of donor human PBMNCs. *Transfusion,* **44**(2), 282–5.

Furlan, M., Robles, R., Galbusera, M., *et al.* (1998) Von Willebrand factor-cleaving protease in thrombotic thrombocytopenic purpura and the hemolytic-uremic syndrome. *N Eng J Med,* **339**, 1578–84.

Garwood, M., Cardigan, R., Hornsey, V., *et al.* (2003) The effect of methylene blue photoinactivation and removal on the quality of fresh-frozen plasma (FFP). *Transfusion,* **43**, 1238–47.

Gibb, A.P., Martin, K.M., Davidson, G.A., *et al.* (1994) Modelling the growth of *Yersinia enterocolitica* in donated blood. *Transfusion,* **34**, 304–310.

Goltsina, H., Chapman, J. and Purmal, A. (2003) Chemical interaction of INACTINE ™ PEN110 with nucleic acids. *Transfusion,* **43**(Suppl. 85A), SP–145.

Goodrich, R.P. (2000) The use of riboflavin for the inactivation of pathogens in blood products. *Vox Sang,* **78**(Suppl. 2), 211–5.

Goodrich, R.P., Janssens, M., Ghielli, M., *et al.* (2003) Correlation of in vitro parameters and in vivo recovery and survival for PRT treated platelets in normal human donors. *Transfusion,* **43**(Suppl. 79A), SP–126.

Grass, J.A., Hei, D.J., Metchette, K., *et al.* (1998) Inactivation of leukocytes in platelet concentrates by photochemical treatment with psoralen plus UVA. *Blood,* **91**, 2180–8.

Greenwalt, T.J., Hambleton, J., Wages, D., *et al.* (1999) Viability of red blood cells treated with a novel pathogen inactivation system. *Transfusion,* **39**, S497.

Gregori, L., McCombie, N., Palmer, D., *et al.* (2004) Effectiveness of leucoreduction for removal of infectivity of transmissible spongiform encephalopathies from blood. *Lancet,* **364**, 529–31.

Guidelines for the Blood Transfusion Services in the United Kingdom. 7th edn, 2005. London, Stationery Office.

Hambleton, J., Wages, D., Radu-Radulescu, L., *et al.* (2002) Pharmacokinetic study of FFP photochemically treated with amotosalen (S-59) and UV light compared to FFP in healthy volunteers anticoagulated with warfarin. *Transfusion,* **42**, 1302–7.

Harrison, C.N., Lawrie, A.S., Iqbal, A., *et al.* (1996) Plasma exchange with solvent/detergent-treated plasma of resistant thrombotic thrombocytopenic purpura. *Br J Haematol,* **94**, 756–8.

Haubelt, H., Blome, M., Kiessling, A.H., *et al.* (2002) Effects of solvent/detergent-treated plasma and fresh-frozen plasma on haemostasis and fibrinolysis in complex coagulopathy following open-heart surgery. *Vox Sang,* **82**, 9–14.

Hei, D.J., Grass, J., Lin, L., Corash, L. and Cimino, C. (1999) Elimination of cytokine production in stored platelet concentrate aliquots by photochemical treatment with psoralen plus ultraviolet A light. *Transfusion,* **39**, 239–48.

Heiden, M., Salge, U., Breitner-Ruddock, S., *et al.* (2003) Significant difference between S/D plasma qualities of different origin. *Transfusion,* **43**(Suppl. 56A), SP–47.

Hellstern, P., Larbig, E., Walz, G.A., *et al.* (1993) Prospective study on efficacy and tolerability of solvent/detergent-treated plasma in intensive care unit patients. *Infusther Transfusmed,* **20** (Suppl. 2), 16–18.

Hellstern, P., Sachse, H., Schwinn, H., *et al.* (1992) Manufacture and in vitro characterization of a solvent/detergent-treated human plasma. *Vox Sang,* **63**, 178–85.

Hillyer, C.D., Roback, J.D., Saakadze, N., *et al.* (2003) Transfusion-transmitted cytomegalovirus (CMV) infection: elucidation of role and dose of monocytes in a murine model. *Blood,* **102**(11), 57a.

Hillyer, K.L., Kelly, V.A., Roush, K.S., *et al.* (2001) Von Willebrand factor-cleaving protease (VWF-CP) activity in S-59 treated donor plasma. *Blood,* **98**(Suppl. 1), 539a.

Holada, K., Vostal, J.G., Theisen, P.W., *et al.* (2002) Scrapie infectivity in hamster blood is not associated with platelets. *J Virol,* **76**, 4649–50.

Hornsey, V.S., Krailadsiri, P., MacDonald, S., *et al.* (2000) Coagulation factor content of cryoprecipitate prepared from methylene blue plus light virus-inactivated plasma. *Br J Haematol,* **109**, 665–70.

Hornsey, V.S., Young, D.A., Docherty, A., *et al.* (2004) Cryoprecipitate prepared from plasma treated with methylene blue plus light: increasing the fibrinogen concentration. *Transfus Med,* **14**, 369–74.

Horowitz, B., Bonomo, R., Prince, A.M., *et al.* (1992) Solvent/detergent-treated plasma: a virus-inactivated substitute for fresh frozen plasma. *Blood,* **79**, 826–31.

Horowitz, M.S. and Pehta, J.C. (1998) SD plasma in TTP and coagulation factor deficiences for which no concentrates are available. *Vox Sang,* **74** (Suppl. 1), 231–5.

ICH (International Conference on Harmonisation of Technical Requirements for Registration of Pharmaceuticals for Human Use) (1998) downloadable files (available from: www.ich.org) under guidelines/safety topics (see also Fed. Reg., 1997, 62, 62922).

Inada, Y., Hessel, B. and Blomback, B. (1978) Photo-oxidation of fibrinogen in the presence of methylene blue and its effect on polymerization. *Biochim Biophys Acta*, **25**(532), 161–70.

Inbal, A., Epstein, O., Blickstein, D., *et al.* (1993) Evaluation of solvent/detergent treated plasma in the management of patients with hereditary and acquired coagulation disorders. *Blood Coag Fibrinolysis*, **4**, 599–604.

Jackson, B. R., AuBuchon, J. P. and Birkmeyer, J. D. (1999) Update of cost-effectiveness analysis for solvent-detergent treated plasma. *J Am Med Assoc*, **282**, 329–30.

Keeling, D. M., Luddington, R., Allain, J.-P., *et al.* (1997) Cryoprecipitate prepared from plasma virally inactivated by the solvent detergent method. *Br J Haematol*, **96**, 94–197.

Klein, H. G,, Anderson, D., Bernardi, M. J., *et al.* (2007) Pathogen inactivation: making decisions about new technologies – preliminary report of a consensus conference. *Vox Sang*, **93**, 179–82.

Knutson, F., Alfonso, R., Dupuis, K., *et al.* (2000) Photochemical inactivation of bacteria and HIV in buffy-coat-derived platelet concentrates under conditions that preserve in vitro platelet function. *Vox Sang*, **78**, 209–16.

Krailadsiri, P., Seghatchian, J., Macgregor, I., *et al.* (2006). The effects of leuko-depletion on the generation and removal of microvesicles and prion protien in blood components *Transfusion*, **46**, 407–17.

Kumar, V., McLean, R., Keil, S., *et al.* (2003b) Mirasol™ pathogen reduction technology for blood products using riboflavin and UV illumination: mode of action of riboflavin on pathogen nucleic acid chemistry. *Transfusion*, **43**(Suppl. 79A), SP-124.

Kumar, V., Motheral, T., Luzniak, G., *et al.* (2003a) Mirasol™ plasma pathogen reduction technology: riboflavin-based process conserves protein C, protein S and antithrombin activities. *Transfusion*, **43**(Suppl. 80A), SP-128.

Lambrecht, B., Mohr, H., Knuver-Hopf, J., *et al.* (1991) Photoinactivation of viruses in human fresh plasma by phenothiazine dyes in combination with visible light. *Vox Sang*, **60**, 207–13.

Laupacis, A., Brown, J., Costello, B., *et al.* (2001) Prevention of post-transfusion CMV in the era of universal WBC reduction: a consensus statement. *Transfusion*, **41**, 560–69.

Lazo, A., Tassello, J., Jayarama, V., *et al.* (2002) Broad-spectrum virus reduction in red cell concentrates using INACTINE PEN110 chemistry. *Vox Sang*, **83**, 313–23.

Lazo, A., Tassello, J., Ohagen, A., *et al.* (2003) Inactivation of human parvovirus B19 by INACTINE™ PEN110. *Transfusion*, **43**(Suppl. 86A), SP-147.

Leebeek, F. W. G., Schipperus, M. R. and van Vliet, H. H. D. M. (1999) Coagulation factor levels in solvent/detergent-treated plasma. *Transfusion*, **39**, 1150–51.

Leiby, D. A. (2004) Threats to blood safety posed by emerging protozoan pathogens. *Vox Sang*, **87** (Suppl. 2), 120–2.

Lerner, R. G., Nelson, J., Scorcia, E., *et al.* (2000) Evaluation of solvent/detergent-treated plasma in patients with a prolonged prothrombin time. *Vox Sang*, **79**, 161–7.

Li, J., de Korte, D., Woolum, M. D., *et al.* (2004) Pathogen reduction of buffy coat platelet concentrates using riboflavin and light: comparisons with pathogen-reduction technology-treated apheresis platelet products. *Vox Sang*, **87**, 82–90.

Lin, L., Cook, D. N., Wiesehahn, G. P., *et al.* (1997) Photochemical inactivation of viruses and bacteria in platelet concentrates by use of a novel psoralen and long-wavelength ultraviolet light. *Transfusion*, **37**, 423–35.

Llewelyn, C. A., Hewitt, P. E., Knight, R. S. G., *et al.* (2004) Possible transmission of variant Creutzfeld-Jacob disease by blood transfusion. *Lancet*, **363**, 417–21.

Lopez-Plaza, I., Snyder, E., Goodnough, L. T., *et al.* for the *SPRINT* Study Group. (2003) INTERCEPT platelet transfusions are associated with fewer transfusion reactions than conventional platelet transfusions prepared by apheresis with process leukoreduction. *Transfusion*, **43** (9S) 84A.

Lorenz, M., Muller, M., Jablonka, B., *et al.* (1998) High doses of methylene blue/light treatment crosslink the A-alpha-sub-unit of fibrinogen: influence of this photo-oxidization on fibrinogen binding to platelets. *Haemostasis*, **28**, 17–24.

Magner, J. J., Crowley, K. J. and Boylan, J. F. (2007) Fatal fibrinolysis during orthotopic liver transplantation in patients receiving solvent/detergent-treated plasma (Octaplas). *J Cardiothorac Vasc Anesth*, **21**, 410–3.

Mast, A. E., Stadanlick, J. E., Lockett, J. M., *et al.* (1999) Solvent/detergent-treated plasma has decreased antitrypsin activity and absent antiplasmin activity. *Blood*, **94**, 3922–7.

Mather, T., Takeda, T., Tassello, J., *et al.* (2003) West Nile virus in blood: stability, distribution and susceptibility to PEN110 inactivation. *Transfusion*, **43**, 1029–37.

McCullough, J. (2003) Progress toward a pathogen-free blood supply. *Clin Infect Dis*, **37**, 88–95.

McCullough, J., Vesole, D. H., Benjamin, R. J., *et al.* (2004) Therapeutic efficacy and safety of platelets treated with a photochemical process for pathogen inactivation: the SPRINT trial. *Blood*, **104**, 1534–41.

Mintz, P., Steadman, R., Blackall, D. *et al.* (2002) Pathogen inactivation of plasma using S-59 and UVA light is efficacious and well tolerated in the treatment of end-stage liver disease patients – the STEP AC trial. *Transfusion*, **42**(Suppl.), 15S.

Mintz, P. D., Neff, A., MacKenzie, M. *et al.* (2006) A randomized, controlled Pase III trial of therapeutic plasma exchange with fresh-frozen plasma (FFP) prepared with amotosalen and ultraviolet A light compared to untreated FFP in thrombotic thrombocytopenic purpura. *Transfusion*, **46**, 1693–704.

Moake, J., Chintagumpala, M., Turner, N., *et al.* (1994) Solvent/detergent-treated plasma suppresses shear-induced platelet aggregation and prevents episodes of thrombotic thrombocytopenic purpura. *Blood*, **84**, 490–7.

Mohr, H. and Redecker-Klein, A. (2003) Inactivation of pathogens in platelet concentrates by using a two-step procedure. *Vox Sang*, **84**, 96–104.

Mohr, H., Bachmann, B., Klein-Struckmeier, A., *et al.* (1997) Virus inactivation of blood products by phenothiazine dyes and light. *Photochem Photobiol Sci*, **65**, 441–5.

Mohr, H., Knuver-Hopf, J., Gravemann, U., *et al.* (2004) West Nile virus in plasma is highly sensitive to methylene blue/light treatment. *Transfusion*, **44**, 886–90.

Mohr, H., Knuver-Hopf, J., Lambrecht, B., *et al.* (1992) No evidence for neoantigens in human plasma after photochemical virus inactivation. *Ann of Hematol*, **65**, 224–8.

Murphy, S., Snyder, E., Cable, R., *et al.* (2003) Transfusion of INTERCEPT platelets vs. reference platelets at doses $\geq 3 \times 10^{11}$ results in comparable haemostasis and platelet and RBC transfusion requirements: results of the SPRINT trial. *Blood*, **102**(11), 815a.

Nichols, W. G., Price, T. H., Gooley, T., *et al.* (2003) Transfusion-transmitted cytomegalovirus infection after receipt of leukoreduced blood products. *Blood*, **101**, 4195–200.

Nifong, T. P., Light, J., Wenl, R. E. (2002) Coagulant stability and sterility of thawed solvent-detergent-treated plasma. *Transfusion*, **42**, 1581–4.

O'Hagen, A., Gibaja, V., Aytay, S., *et al.* (2002) Inactivation of HIV in blood. *Transfusion*, **42**, 1308–17.

Pamphilon, D. H., Rider, J. R., Barbara, J. A. J., *et al.* (1999) Prevention of transfusion-transmitted cytomegalovirus infection. *Transfus Med*, **9**, 115–23.

Peden, A. H., Head, M. W., Ritchie, D. L., *et al.* (2004) Preclinical vCJD after blood transfusion in a PRNP codon 129 heterozygous patient. *Lancet*, **364**, 527–9.

Peirera, A. (1999) Cost-effectiveness of transfusing virus-inactivated plasma instead of standard plasma. *Transfusion*, **39**, 479–87.

Pennington, J., Garner, S. F., Sutherland, J., *et al.* (2001) Residual subset population analysis in leucocyte depleted blood components using real-time quantitative RT-PCR. *Transfusion*, **41**, 1591–600.

Pennington, J., Taylor, G. P., Sutherland, J., *et al.* (2002) Persistence of HTLV in blood donations after leucocyte depletion. *Blood*, **100**, 677–81.

Pinkoski, L., Amir, S., Smyers, J., *et al.* (2001a) Photochemically treated plasma retains protein C, protein S and antithrombin activities. *Transfusion Clinique et Biologique*, **8**(Suppl. 1), 101.

Pinkoski, L., Corash, L., Ramies, D., *et al.* (2002a) The INTERCEPT Plasma System: Helinx™ pathogen inactivation technology does not activate thrombin, complement, or the contact system of coagulation. *Vox Sang*, **83**(Suppl. 2), 574.

Pinkoski, L., Ramies, D., Wiesehahn, G., *et al.* (2002b) The INTERCEPT blood system for plasma conserves key proteins necessary for effective transfusion support of hemostasis. *Transfusion*, **42**(Suppl.), 575.

Pinkoski, L., Smyers, J., Corash, L., *et al.* (2001b) Pathogen inactivation of plasma using Helinx technology conserves the activity of coagulation, anticoagulation and fibrinolytic proteins. *Blood*, **98**, 541a.

Piquet, Y., Janvier, G., Selosse, P., *et al.* (1992) Virus inactivation of fresh frozen plasma by a solvent detergent procedure: biological results. *Vox Sang*, **63**, 251–6.

Pohl, U., Becker, M., Papstein, C., *et al.* (1995b) Methylene blue virus inactivated plasma in the treatment of patients with thrombotic thrombocytopenic purpura. ISBT 5th Regional (European) Congress, Venice.

Pohl, U., Wieding, J. U., Kirchmaier C. M., *et al.* (1995a) Treatment of patients with severe congenital coagulation factor V or XI deficiency with methylene blue virus inactivated plasma. ISBT 5th Regional (European) Congress, Venice.

Politis, C., Kavallierou, L., Hantziara, S., *et al.* (2007) Quality and safety of fresh-frozen plasma inactivated and leucoreduced with the Theraflex methylene blue system including the Blueflex filter: 5 years' experience. *Vox Sang*, **92**, 319–26.

Prowse, C. V., Hornsey, V. S., Drummond, O., *et al.* (1999) Preliminary assessment of whole-blood, red-cell and platelet-leucodepleting filters for possible induction of prion release by leucocyte fragmentation during room temperature processing. *Br J Haematol*, **106**, 240–7.

Prowse, C. V. and MacGregor, I. R. (2002) Mad cows and Englishmen: an update on blood and vCJD. *Vox Sang*, **83**(Suppl. 1), 341–9.

Purmal, A., Valeri, C. R., Dzik, W., *et al.* (2002) Process for the preparation of pathogen-inactivated RBC concentrates by using PEN110 chemistry: preclinical studies. *Transfusion*, **42**, 139–45.

Reidler, G. F., Haycox, A. R., Duggan, A. K., *et al.* (2003) Cost-effectiveness of solvent/detergent-treated fresh-frozen plasma. *Vox Sang*, **85**, 88–95.

Rentas, F. J., Lippert, L., Harman, R., *et al.* (2003) Inactivation of Orientia tsutsugamuchi (scrub typhus) in an animal model using the INTERCEPT™ blood system for human platelets. *Transfusion*, **43**(Suppl. 84A), SP-141.

Rhenen, D. van, Gulliksson, H., Cazenave, J. P., *et al.* and EuroSPRITE trial (2003) Transfusion of pooled buffy coat platelet components prepared with photochemical pathogen inactivation treatment: the euroSPRITE trial. *Blood*, **101**, 2426–33.

Rhenen, D. J. van, Vermeij, J., Mayaudon, V., *et al.* (2000) Functional characteristics of S-59 photochemically treated platelet concentrates derived from buffy coats. *Vox Sang*, **79**(4), 206–14.

Rider, J. R., Want, E. J., Winter, M. A., *et al.* (2000) Differential leucocyte subpopulation analysis of leucodepleted red cell products. *Transfus Med*, **10**, 49–58.

Ronghe, M. D., Foot, A. B. M., Cornish, J. M., *et al.* (2002) The impact of transfusion of leucodepleted platelet concentrates on cytomegalovirus disease after allogeneic stem cell transplantation. *Br J Haematol*, **118**, 1124–7.

Ruane, P. H., Edrich, R., Gampp, D., *et al.* (2004) Photochemical inactivation of selected viruses and bacteria in platelet concentrates using riboflavin and light. *Transfusion*, **44**, 877–85.

Simonsen, A. C. and Sorensen, H. (1999) Clinical tolerance of methylene blue virus-inactivated plasma: a randomized crossover trial in 12 healthy human volunteers. *Vox Sang*, **77**, 210–7.

Sivakumaran, M., Hutchinson, R. M., Wood, J. K., *et al.* (1993) Removal of cytomegalovirus (CMV) infected leucocytes from CMV positive blood units by bedside blood filtration. *Br J Haematol*, **85**, 232–4.

Snyder, E., Mintz, P., Burks, S. *et al.* (2001) Pathogen inactivated red blood cells using INACTINE technology demonstrate 24 hour post-transfusion recovery equal to untreated red cells after 42 days of storage. *Blood*, **98**, 709a.

Solheim, B., Tollofsrud, S., Noddeland, H., *et al.* (2002) Universal solvent/detergent treated plasma. *Vox Sanguinis*, **83**, 111.

Solheim, B. G. and Hellstern, P. (2003) Composition and efficacy and safety of solvent-detergent treated plasma. *Transfusion*, **43**, 1176–8.

Solheim B. G., Svennevig, J. L., Mohr, B., *et al.* (1993) The use of Octaplas in patients undergoing open heart surgery. In *DIC: Pathogenesis, Diagnosis and Therapy of Disseminated Intravascular Fibrin Formation*, ed. G. Muller-Berghaus, pp. 253–62. Amsterdam, Elsevier.

Solheim, B. G., Cid, J. and Osselaer, J. C. (2006) Pathogen Reduction Technologies. Global Perspectives in Transfusion Medicine (ed. by M. Lozano, M. Contreras, & M. A. Blajchman), pp. 103–148. AABB Press, Bethesda.

Suontataka, A. M., Blomback, M. and Chapman, J. (2003) Changes in functional activities of plasma fibrinogen after treatment with methylene blue and red light. *Transfusion*, **43**(5), 568–575.

Taborski, U., Oprean, N., Tessmann, R., *et al.* (2000) Methylene blue/light-treated plasma and the disturbance of fibrin polymerization in vitro and in vivo: a randomized, double-blind clinical trial. *Vox Sang*, **78**, 546.

Van Voorhuis, W. C., Barrett, L. K., Eastman, R. T., *et al.* (2003) *Trypanosoma cruzi* inactivation in human platelet concentrates and plasma by a psoralen (amotosalen HCl) and long-wavelength UV. *Antimicrob Agents and Chemother*, **47**, 475–9.

Visconti, M. R., Pennington, J., Garner, S. F., *et al.* (2003) Assessment of removal of human cytomegalovirus from blood components by leucocyte depletion filters using real-time quantitative PCR. *Blood*, **103**, 1137–9.

Wadhwa, M., Seghatchian, M. J., Dilger, P., *et al.* (2000) Cytokine accumulation in stored red cell concentrates: effect of buffy coat removal and leucoreduction. *Transfus Sci*, **23**(1), 7–16.

Wages, D., Eden, P., Smyders, J., *et al.* (2000) Preparation of cryoprecipitate from photochemically treated fresh frozen plasma. *Transfusion*, **40** (Suppl.), 63S.

Wieding, J. U., Rathgeber, J., Zenker, D., *et al.* (1999) Prospective randomized and controlled study on solvent/detergent versus methylene blue/light virus-inactivated plasma. *Transfusion*, **39** (Suppl.), 23S.

Williamson, L. M. (2000) Leucocyte depletion of the blood supply – how will patients benefit? *Br J Haematol*, **110**, 256–72.

Williamson, L. M., Llewelyn, C. A., Fisher, N. C., *et al.* (1999) A randomised trial of solvent/detergent and standard fresh frozen plasma in the coagulopathy of liver disease and liver transplantation. *Transfusion*, **39**, 1227–34.

Wollowitz, S. (2001) Fundamentals of the psoralen-based Helinx technology for inactivation of infectious pathogens and leukocytes in platelets and plasma. *Semin Hematol*, **38**(Suppl. 11), 4–11.

Yarranton, H., Cohen, H., Pavord, S. R., *et al.* (2003a) Venous thromboembolism associated with the management of acute thrombotic thrombocytopenic purpura. *Br J Haematol*, **121**, 778–85.

Yarranton, H., Lawrie, A., Mackie, I., *et al.* (2003b) Coagulation factor levels in cryosupernatant treated with amotosalen hydrochloride (S-59) and UVA light – A suitable plasma replacement in thrombotic thrombocytopenic purpura. *Blood*, **102**(11), 817a.

Yazer, M. H., Podlosky, L., Clarke, G., *et al.* (2004) The effect of prestorage WBC reduction on the rates of febrile non-hemolytic transfusion reactions to platelet concentrates and RBC. *Transfusion*, **44**, 10–5.

Zavizion, B., Purmal, A. and Chapman, J. (2003b) Inactivation of Mycoplasma species in blood by INACTINE™ PEN110. *Transfusion*, **43**(Suppl. 86A), SP-149.

Zavizion, B., Purmal, A., Serebryanik, D., *et al.* (2003c) Inactivation of anaerobic bacteria in red cell concentrates using INACTINE™ process. *Transfusion*, **43**(Suppl. 86A), SP-148.

Zavizion, B., Serebryanik, D., Serebryanik, I., *et al.* (2003a) Prevention of *Yersinia enterocolitica*, *Pseudomonas fluorescens*, and *Pseudomonas putida* outgrowth in deliberately inoculated blood by a novel pathogen-reduction process. *Transfusion*, **43**, 135–42.

Zeiler, T., Riess, H., Wittmann, G., *et al.* (1994) The effect of methylene blue phototreatment on plasma proteins and in vitro coagulation capability of single-donor fresh-frozen plasma. *Transfusion*, **34**, 685–9.

20 FRACTIONATED PRODUCTS

Peter R. Foster and Carol Bienek

Fractionated products are plasma proteins that have been extracted from pooled human plasma and manufactured into stable pharmaceuticals in dose forms suitable for clinical administration (Foster, 2005). The major categories of fractionated products are immunoglobulins for the treatment of disorders of immunity, the prevention of specific infections and the prevention of RhD immunization, albumin for volume and protein replacement and coagulation factors for haemostasis. The annual requirement for fractioned plasma products in the UK includes over 2000 kg of intravenous immunoglobulin (IGIV) for the treatment of more than 1800 patients with primary immune deficiency; 120 000 doses of anti-D immunoglobulin to prevent haemolytic disease of the newborn in about 65 000 pregnancies; over 5000 kg of albumin for tens of thousands of patients treated for burns, shock and major trauma. In addition, over 500 000 doses of factor VIII concentrate, recombinant or plasma-derived, are required to treat about 6000 people with haemophilia A. In the USA it is estimated that as many as 1 million patients are treated each year with products derived from human plasma, with over 400 000 recipients of albumin and more than 20 000 recipients of IGIV. Worldwide, some 25 million litres of human plasma are fractionated each year, providing over 500 metric tonnes of human protein for therapeutic use (see Table 20.1).

Blood-borne infections which exist naturally in the human population present a particular threat to recipients of fractionated products because each batch of product may be prepared from many thousands of donations and because some patients may be treated repeatedly throughout their lives, thereby considerably increasing their probability of exposure to a batch associated with an infected donation (Lynch et al., 1996). Pooling of plasma is necessary to provide uniformity of products, to obtain a suitable range of specificities in each batch of normal immunoglobulin; to provide samples for in-process and final product testing necessary to comply with good pharmaceutical manufacturing practice (GMP) and to achieve the volume throughput required to meet patient needs. In the USA, large-volume plasma pools have been restricted to 60 000 donors (Tabor, 1999), but some product batches manufactured prior to 1999 were obtained from several hundred thousand donors after pooling of intermediates and the use of albumin as an excipient are taken into account. The challenge facing the fractionation industry is to manufacture safe and efficacious products from pooled plasma against an estimated world background prevalence of 360 million people chronically infected with hepatitis B virus (HBV) (Shepard et al., 2006), 170 million infected with hepatitis C virus (HCV) (Butt, 2006) and almost 40 million infected with human immunodeficiency virus (HIV) (Centers for Disease Control, 2006).

The first human plasma products to be developed were albumin and normal (polyvalent) immunoglobulin, both of which were extracted from plasma using fractionation processes devised in the early 1940s under the leadership of Edwin J. Cohn (Surgenor, 2002). Processing was designed to distribute selected proteins into different precipitate fractions by exploiting differences in solubility behaviour in the presence of cold-ethanol (Cohn et al., 1946; Oncley et al., 1949; Strong, 1948). In 1945, albumin was re-formulated to allow the introduction of pasteurization to prevent bacterial spoilage (Edsall, 1984; Scatchard et al., 1945). Subsequently, human albumin (pasteurized) and human immunoglobulin, prepared by the cold-ethanol method, were found to be safe from hepatitis transmission, even when prepared from plasma known to be highly infectious (Murray and Ratner, 1953; Murray et al., 1955a). By contrast, Cohn Fraction I was found to transmit hepatitis (Janeway, 1948), a risk that continued to be associated with coagulation factor concentrates for many years (Gerety and Aronson, 1982).

When the epidemic of Acquired Immunodeficiency Syndrome (AIDS) emerged in the early 1980s, neither human albumin nor human immunoglobulin transmitted human immunodeficiency virus (HIV), whereas many recipients of coagulation factor concentrates were infected (Evatt, 2006). Other infectious agents known to have been transmitted clinically by plasma products are listed in Table 20.2.

Today, all fractioned plasma products are essentially safe with respect to HIV, HBV and HCV when manufactured correctly. This has been achieved by advances in the testing and selection of donors and by the development of technologies suitable for the elimination of viruses from labile proteins. In addition, more stringent systems of quality control and regulation provide a greater assurance of product safety. Nevertheless, concerns remain over the possible continued transmission of small, non-enveloped heat resistant viruses, such as human parvovirus B19 (B19) and the possibility that new or unknown infectious agents, such as agents of prion diseases, might be transmitted in this manner.

Plasma fractionation

Plasma for fractionation

Plasma for fractionation is obtained from whole blood donations (recovered plasma) and by plasmapheresis (source plasma); the former, from unpaid donors, being about 250 mL per donation and the latter, mainly from paid donors, contains approximately 825 mL per donation with up to two donations per week allowed

Transfusion Microbiology, eds John A. J. Barbara, Fiona A. M. Regan and Marcela C. Contreras. Published by Cambridge University Press. © Cambridge University Press 2008.

Table 20.1 Principal plasma products, their medical applications and an estimate of the quantities used worldwide in 2005.

Plasma product	Primary clinical applications	Quantity used worldwide (2005, estimate)
Albumin	Restoration of plasma volume in shock, burns, trauma and surgery; protein replacement.	457 000 kg protein
Immunoglobulin (polyvalent)	Treatment of immune deficiencies and immune disorders; passive immunization for hepatitis A and measles.	62 000 kg protein
Immunoglobulin (anti-D)	Prevention of RhD immunization in RhD negative women.	6500 million IU
Immunoglobulin (other specificities)	Prevention and treatment of specific infections, for example tetanus, hepatitis B, varicella/zoster, rabies, cytomegalovirus (CMV), vaccinia.	4000 million IU
Factor VIII concentrate (plasma-derived)	Treatment of haemophilia A	2200 million IU VIII:C
Factor VIII concentrate (recombinant)	Treatment of haemophilia A	2200 million IU VIII:C
Factor IX concentrate (plasma-derived)	Treatment of haemophilia B	450 million IU IX:C
Factor IX concentrate (recombinant)	Treatment of haemophilia B	330 million IU IX:C
Fibrin sealant (fibrinogen + thrombin)	Haemostasis	2.5 million doses
Prothrombin complex concentrate (PCC)	Reversal of coumarin (warfarin) anti-coagulant therapy	180 million IU IX:C
Alpha 1 antitrypsin	Treatment of emphysema	390 kg protein
Antithrombin III	Treatment of antithrombin III deficiency and thromboembolism	530 million IU

Table 20.2 Viruses transmitted clinically by human plasma derivatives.

Virus	Envelope/genome	Size nm	Products implicated
HIV-1	yes/ssRNA	80–100	Coagulation factors, prior to the development of effective virus inactivation (VI) technology.
Hepatitis A virus	no/ssRNA	27–32	High purity coagulation factors with SD treatment as the only VI technology.
Hepatitis B virus	yes/dsDNA	42	Coagulation factors prior to the development of effective VI technology. Immunoglobulin, i.m. (very rarely) prior to development of effective VI technology. Plasma protein fraction (very rarely) due to inadequate pasteurization.
Hepatitis C virus	yes/ssRNA	40–50	Coagulation factors, prior to the development of effective VI technology. Immunoglobulin, i.v. (occasionally) prior to the introduction of effective VI technology.
Hepatitis D virus	yes/ssRNA	35	Coagulation factors (rarely) prior to the development of effective VI technology.
GB virus C (hepatitis G virus)	yes/ssRNA	50	Coagulation factors prior to the development of effective VI technology.
Human parvovirus B19 (human erythrovirus)	no/ssDNA	18–26	Coagulation factors, immunoglobulin (rarely).
TT virus	no/ssDNA	32	Coagulation factors, immunoglobulin, albumin.

in the USA. Although the World Health Organization recommends that plasma products be derived from unpaid donors (WHO, 2005), over 1 million paid USA donors provide almost 70% of the world's plasma needs (Foster, 2005). The fractionation of plasma from UK unpaid volunteer donors has been banned since 1998 as a precaution against the possibility that variant Creutzfeldt-Jakob disease (vCJD) is transmissible by plasma products (DoH, 1998). Plasma for fractionation by the NHS is currently obtained predominantly from USA paid donors (DoH, 2002), with NHS products supplemented by imported commercial products also derived predominantly from US paid-donor plasma.

Plasma testing

There are many factors required by regulatory bodies which contribute to the viral safety of plasma products, the first of which is performed prior to collection of blood, by acceptance of donations only from healthy donors from regions with acceptable epidemiology for HIV, HCV, HBV and vCJD. Once the donor fulfils these criteria, all individual plasma donations are tested for anti-HIV-1, anti-HIV-2 and anti-HCV antibody and for hepatitis B virus surface antigen (HBsAg) and in some countries HIV antigen (e.g. in antigen/antibody combinations), HCV antigen (e.g. in antigen/antibody combinations), antigen for B19 (in Japan), HIV,

MAINSTREAM PROCESS	INTERMEDIATES (FROZEN)	FURTHER PROCESSING (Purification, pathogen elimination, formulation and stabilization)	PRODUCTS

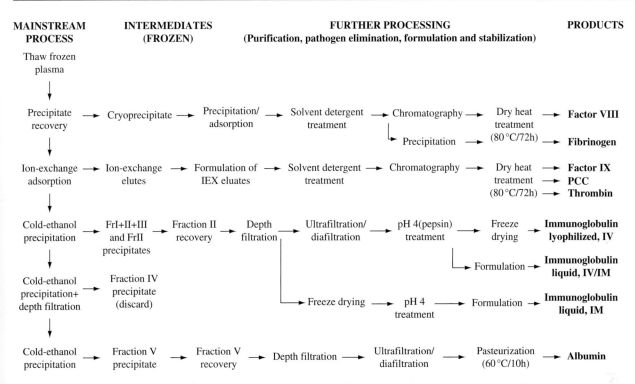

Figure 20.1 Process flow-sheet for plasma fractionation (based on processes employed at SNBTS Protein Fractionation Centre).

HBV and West Nile virus (WNV) (in North America) by nucleic acid amplification technology (NAT). Positive samples are retested and repeat-reactive donations for any test are excluded from the plasma pool. Plasma is also tested for HCV RNA by NAT testing of mini-pools (Committee for Proprietary Medicinal Products, 1998), for example mini-pools of 96 donations are tested and any positive mini-pool can then be dissected into the individual donations on a 96 well plate to identify and eliminate the positive donation. Once the plasma is pooled for manufacturing, it is again tested for the same viral markers as the individual donations, and HCV RNA by NAT (European Pharmacopoeia, 2004) in order to eliminate potential testing errors. A requirement has also been introduced recently that plasma used in the preparation of anti-D immunoglobulin must be screened by NAT for B19 DNA (Committee for Medicinal Products for Human Use, 2006).

Some manufacturers go beyond these minimum regulatory requirements and perform additional testing such as mini-pool and/or plasma pool testing for other viral markers, for example NAT for HIV, HBV, HAV, WNV and/or B19. (See Chapters 14–16.) All such assays must be validated to determine, amongst other things, the detection limit of the assay to the agent in question (Committee for Proprietary Medicinal Products, 1995a). Although the detection limit of NAT assays means that the virus can be detected at the very early stages of infection, there remains a short period of time during which the marker is below the limit of detection of the assay, that is, the window period, which varies depending on the virus and detection method. Although extremely rare, such 'window-period' donations may enter the pool undetected. Most manufacturers now delay processing of plasma for 60 days or more to provide time for infected donors

to be identified by testing positive on a subsequent donation. Despite these precautions, virus elimination steps contained within the manufacturing process are essential to ensure the safety of final products, not only against 'window-period' donations but also contamination by viruses that are not screened for, for example emerging viruses, or failures in GMP such as testing errors.

Fractionation processes

The objective of plasma fractionation is to extract a number of clinically useful proteins from plasma and to manufacture each of them into a suitably purified and concentrated pharmaceutical dose form. A typical set of processes for this purpose is illustrated schematically in Figure 20.1. At first, a number of semi-purified, intermediate, fractions are isolated sequentially from the plasma stream, mostly by exploiting differences in protein solubility (Cohn et al., 1946; Foster, 1994). Precipitates are recovered either by centrifugation or by filtration, with supernatants being clarified by depth filtration. Intermediates from a number of batches are combined and subjected to further concentration and purification by precipitation and often by ion exchange or affinity chromatography. Products may also be concentrated by ultra-filtration, with dia-filtration against a suitable buffer to remove undesirable solutes and to achieve a suitable product formulation. Procedures for virus inactivation are integrated into each product stream and can involve treatment at an intermediate position in the process or treatment in the final sealed container. Solvent detergent treatment is the most common example of the former, whilst pasteurization of albumin is the most common example of the latter. All products are filtered

Table 20.3 Early reports of hepatitis transmission by pooled human blood plasma or serum[a].

Product	No. infected/no. treated	% infected	No. deaths	Location	Reference
Serum, anti-measles	37/109	33.9	8	UK	MacNalty, 1938; Propert, 1938
Serum, anti-measles	29/172	16.8	1	UK	Ministry of Health, 1943
Plasma or serum	9/50	18.0	n/a	UK	Morgan and Williamson, 1943
Plasma or blood	7/n/a	n/a	0	USA	Beeson, 1943
Plasma, anti-mumps	119/266	44.7	n/a	UK	Beeson, et al., 1944
Serum	42/73	57.5	0	UK	Bradley, et al. 1944
Plasma or serum	77/1054	7.3	0	UK	Spurling, et al. 1946
Plasma	8/n/a	n/a	1	USA	Grossman and Saward, 1946
Plasma	11/n/a	n/a	4	USA	Scheinberg, et al., 1947
Plasma, dried	30/650	4.6	4	USA	Brightman and Korns, 1947
Plasma, large pool	54/453	11.9	3	UK	Lehane, et al., 1949
Plasma, small pool	5/396	1.7	0	UK	Lehane, et al., 1949
Plasma, dried	7/10	70.0	3	UK	Cockburn, et al., 1951

[a] Modified from Paine and Janeway, 1952.

to 0.2 μm to remove bacteria and must be stable over their intended shelf-life, with some being freeze dried for this purpose (Foster, 2005).

History

Viral hepatitis – early iatrogenic transmissions

The first report of iatrogenic transmission of hepatitis concerns an incident in Bremen, Germany, in which hepatitis developed in 191 of 1339 recipients of a vaccine against smallpox containing pooled human lymph derived from cases of vaccinia (Lürman, 1885; Zuckerman, 1975). Transmission of hepatitis was also associated with vaccines that were stabilized with human plasma or serum. There were a number of outbreaks in Brazil in the period 1937–1941 following vaccination against yellow fever, in which up to 30% of recipients were infected with hepatitis (Findlay et al., 1939; Fox et al., 1942; Soper and Smith, 1938). Similarly in 1939, in southern Russia, 92 of 350 recipients of a vaccine against pappataci (sand-fly) fever developed hepatitis (Sergiev et al., 1940), with the implicated batch of virus-containing serum confirmed as being responsible by transmission experiments in patients in a Moscow psychiatric hospital (Sawyer et al., 1944). In the largest episode of vaccine-transmitted hepatitis, over 26 000 USA troops were infected in 1941–1942 following vaccination against yellow fever, with 62 fatalities. Serum used in the preparation of the vaccine had been donated by 970 volunteers; 367 were available for questioning, 23 of whom were found to have a history of jaundice (Sawyer et al., 1944). Shortly after this incident, a report of transfusion-transmitted hepatitis by Beeson (1943) led the US National Research Council Subcommittee on Blood Substitutes to suggest that people with symptoms of jaundice within the last six months should be rejected as blood donors (Surgenor, 2002).

Transmissions of hepatitis by pooled plasma or serum were the subject of numerous reports during this period (see Table 20.3)

leading Scheinberg et al. (1947) to advise that 'fractionation products' be used 'in preference to pooled plasma' as 'the products of plasma fractionation do not seem to transmit the icterogenic agent.' Although human albumin and immunoglobulin appeared free from hepatitis transmission (Janeway, 1948), the production of fibrin foam was discontinued because thrombin, used during the application of the foam, carried a risk of hepatitis transmission (Palmer, 1976).

Fractionation products associated with hepatitis transmission are listed in Table 20.4. Clinical use of Cohn fraction IV was abandoned as a result of hepatitis being transmitted to 4 of 16 children treated in a clinical study (Hsia et al., 1953). In the USA, prior to the testing of donors for hepatitis B, hepatitis B surface antigen (HBsAg) was detected in 25% of factor VIII batches, 4% of fibrinogen batches, 24% of albumin batches and 0.8% of immunoglobulin batches. Following the introduction of donor screening, 11% of factor VIII batches and 24% of albumin batches remained HBsAg positive (Hoofnagle et al., 1976). Although HBsAg was no longer detectable in batches of fibrinogen, licences for human fibrinogen were revoked by the Food and Drug Administration (FDA) in December 1977 because the risk of hepatitis transmission was higher than from cryoprecipitate derived from single units of plasma (Hile, 1978).

Viral hepatitis – infectious agents and their transmission

During the 1940s, two types of hepatitis were recognized: one, with an incubation period of 20–40 days, transmitted by the faecal-oral route, termed 'infectious hepatitis', the other, with an incubation period of 60–180 days was transmissible via blood serum and therefore termed 'serum hepatitis' (Editorial, 1947). MacCallum (Editorial, 1947; Zuckerman, 1975) suggested the designations hepatitis A and hepatitis B respectively. However, it was 20 years before the virus responsible for hepatitis B was identified when Blumberg et al. (1967) associated viral hepatitis

Table 20.4 Initial reports of hepatitis transmissions by fractionated plasma products.

Product	Initial reports of hepatitis transmission
Cohn fraction I	Janeway, 1948.
Thrombin	Kekwick and MacKay, 1954; Lesses and Hamolsky, 1951; Paine and Janeway, 1952; Porter et al., 1953
Immunoglobulin	Cockburn et al., 1951; Pennell, 1957; Petrilli et al., 1977.
Cohn fraction IV	Hsia et al., 1953.
Fibrinogen	Anderson et al., 1966; Anderson and Gibson, 1957; Cronberg et al., 1963; Mainwaring and Brueckner, 1966; Phillips, 1965; Skinner, 1957.
Cryoprecipitate	Del Duca and Eppes, 1966; Fitzpatrick and Kennedy, 1969; Lewis, 1970; Whittaker and Brown, 1969.
Factor VIII concentrate	Kasper and Kipnis, 1972; Lewis, 1970; Maycock, 1964; Maycock et al., 1963.
Factor IX concentrate	Boklan, 1971; Breen and Tullis, 1969; Hellerstein and Deykin, 1971; Kasper and Kipnis, 1972; Kingdon, 1970.

with an antigen from an Australian aborigine which had cross-reacted with sera from a multiply-transfused American haemophiliac (Blumberg, 1964). This discovery paved the way for serological testing for infection with hepatitis B (Levene and Blumberg, 1969) and the isolation of the whole hepatitis B virus (Dane et al., 1970).

The availability of a serological assay confirmed that many recipients of coagulation factor concentrates had been exposed to HBV (Burrell et al., 1978; Craske et al., 1975; 1978; Hoofnagle et al., 1975; Lewis et al., 1974) including patients treated repeatedly with cryoprecipitate (Counts, 1977; Stirling et al., 1983). Coinfection with the delta agent (HDV), a defective virus that can replicate only in the presence of HBV (Rizzetto et al., 1977; 1980), was also observed in people with haemophilia (Jacobson et al., 1985; Lee et al., 1985; Rizzetto et al., 1982; Rosina et al., 1985).

The virus responsible for hepatitis A was isolated in 1973 (Feinstone et al., 1973). Transmission of hepatitis, which was not accounted for by HAV or HBV, continued to be observed via blood transfusion (Feinstone et al. 1975; Prince et al., 1974) and by coagulation factor concentrates (Craske et al., 1975; Mannucci et al., 1975), leading to the conclusion that an unknown virus (or viruses), termed non-A, non-B hepatitis (NANBH) must be responsible.

Some 20 years after the discovery of HBV, the agent responsible for NANBH was identified by molecular cloning (Choo et al., 1989) and a serological assay suitable for testing blood donors and patients was developed (Kuo et al., 1989). It was soon apparent that most people with haemophilia who had been treated prior to the development of effective virus inactivation technologies had been exposed to the virus, now termed HCV (Brettler

et al., 1990; Esteban et al., 1989; Ludlam et al., 1989; Noel et al., 1989; Roggendorf et al., 1989; Rumi et al., 1989), some as early as 1965 (Lee, 1995). The newly identified agent was also found to have been responsible for virtually 90% of post-transfusion hepatitis in the USA (Alter, 2000). Hepatitis A virus was subsequently transmitted by some solvent/detergent (SD) treated highly purified coagulation factor concentrates. These incidents are described below under the development of SD treatment.

Another virus associated with hepatitis, the so-called hepatitis G virus (HGV), more correctly referred to as GB virus C (GBV-C), was discovered in 1996 (Leary et al., 1996; Linnen et al., 1996). Antibodies to GBV-C have been detected in recipients of coagulation factor concentrates (Garcia et al., 1996; Gerolami et al., 1997; Hanley et al., 1998; Mauser et al., 1998; Yamada-Osaki et al., 1998) and a moist heat-treated concentrate of C1 Inhibitor (De Filippi et al., 1998). Hepatitis G virus-C RNA has been detected in IGIV, but not in recipients (Farshid et al., 1997; Nubling et al., 1998).

Acquired immune deficiency syndrome (AIDS)

The emerging epidemic of AIDS first became apparent in late 1980 amongst gay men in Los Angeles (Centers for Disease Control, 1981a) and New York (Centers for Disease Control, 1981b). Reports of AIDS in a number of people with haemophilia (Centers for Disease Control, 1982a; 1982b), together with an apparent transmission via a blood transfusion (Centers for Disease Control, 1982c), lent credence to the hypothesis that the syndrome was caused by a blood-borne infectious agent (Centers for Disease Control, 1983).

Discovery of HIV, the agent responsible, was originally attributed to Gallo et al. (1984). However, it is now known that the retrovirus described in Gallo et al. (1984) had been isolated from a gay French student in June 1983 and delivered to Gallo's home in July 1983 by Montagnier of the Institute Pasteur (Crewdson, 2002; Wain-Hobson et al., 1991; Wong-Staal et al., 1985). It is now also known that an earlier isolate from the Institute Pasteur, derived from a homosexual fashion designer in January 1983, formed the basis of the first description of HIV (Barré-Sinoussi et al., 1983; Crewdson, 2002), although this was not appreciated at the time.

The isolation and culture of the virus responsible for AIDS enabled serological testing to be developed (Sarngadharan et al., 1984) and the sensitivity of the virus to potential methods of inactivation determined (Spire et al., 1985). From experiments in which HIV was added to factor VIII, it was discovered that HIV was relatively heat sensitive and could be inactivated by heating conditions that freeze dried coagulation factor concentrates could tolerate (Centers for Disease Control, 1984; Evatt, 2006; Levy et al., 1985; McDougal et al., 1985).

A US patent for a serological test was granted to Gallo et al. (1985), despite applications from the Institute Pasteur having been filed earlier (Montagnier et al., 1983). Joint inventorship was eventually assigned to both groups (Torchin, 1987). In the UK, a screening test developed by Weiss (Cheinsong-Popov et al., 1984) using materials supplied by Gallo, was not authorized for routine screening of blood donors, as licences had already been awarded to a number of companies in the USA (Crewdson, 2002). Of the companies licensed to market the Gallo test, Abbott Laboratories were first to be granted an FDA licence in March 1985, but were unable to supply enough test kits to meet demand in the USA or in Europe until autumn 1985 (Crewdson, 2002). Genetic Systems, who had licensed the Institute Pasteur test, received FDA approval in February 1986 (Crewdson, 2002).

Most developed countries began formal testing of donors for antibodies to HIV between March 1985 and January 1986 (Glied, 1999) enabling infected donations to be screened out (Gunson and Rawlinson, 1991). Testing of patients revealed that many people with haemophilia had been infected prior to the development of donor screening and the introduction of heat treated concentrates (Aymard et al., 1985; Cheinsong-Popov et al., 1984; Evatt et al., 1985; Jason et al., 1985; Lederman et al., 1985; Ludlam et al., 1985; McGrath et al., 1985; Machin et al., 1985; Madhok et al., 1985; Melbye et al., 1984; Mortimer et al., 1985; Ramsay et al., 1984; Rouzioux et al., 1985; Zanetti et al., 1985).

Other viral transmissions by plasma products

Human parvovirus B19

Human parvovirus B19 (B19) was discovered by chance in a serum sample from a healthy donor that had been included in a panel of samples (panel B, serum 19) that had given anomalous results in different screening tests for HBsAg (Cossart et al., 1975). Infection is often acquired in childhood, with over 60% of adults having evidence of infection (Cohen, 1995). Transmissions have been described by coagulation factor concentrates prior to the introduction of virus inactivation procedures (Bartolomi Corsi et al., 1988; Grosse-Bley et al., 1994; Mortimer et al., 1983; Williams et al., 1990b) and by concentrates which had been subjected to pasteurization (Azzi et al., 1992; Grosse-Bley et al., 1994), moist heat treatment (Bartolomi Corsi et al., 1988) and dry heat treatment (Bartolomi Corsi et al., 1988). As B19 is non-enveloped (see Table 20.2) it should not be inactivated by solvent/detergent treatment, and transmission by solvent-detergent treated concentrates has been described (Azzi et al., 1992; Grosse-Bley et al., 1994; Laurian et al., 1994), including concentrates purified by immunoaffinity chromatography (Matsui et al., 1999; Wu et al., 2005). Despite the introduction of virus inactivation technologies, B19 DNA was detected in 13 different products examined, with 42% of batches being positive (Schneider et al., 2004). In addition, B19 has been reported to have been transmitted by fibrin sealant (Enoki et al., 2002; Hino et al., 1999; 2000; Kawamura et al., 2002).

Although B19 infection is rarely a serious problem clinically, infection during pregnancy can be dangerous, with a risk of abortion, fetal death or congenital anaemia after birth. Transmission of B19 by IGIV (Hayakawa et al., 2002) has increased concern that B19 might be transmitted to pregnant women by anti-D immunoglobulin and a requirement has therefore been introduced that plasma pools used in the preparation of anti-D should contain no more than 10^4 IU/ml of B19 DNA (Committee for Medicinal Products for Human Use, 2006).

The TT virus

The TT virus (TTV), a small, blood-borne, non-enveloped virus (see Table 20.2) was identified in 1997 (Nishizawa et al., 1997) and was found to be prevalent in blood donors worldwide (Chen et al., 1999; Prescott and Simmonds, 1998). The TTV infection has been reported in recipients of coagulation factor concentrates (Gerolami et al., 1998; Simmonds et al., 1998; Sumazaki et al., 1998).

Safety of human albumin

Human albumin has a long history of viral safety due both to the method of purification and to pasteurization of the final product at $60\,°C$ for ten hours. Human albumin, without pasteurization, was first trialled clinically in May 1941 and approved for use by the US armed forces following successful treatment of casualties at the US naval base at Pearl Harbor (Coates and McFetridge, 1964; Palmer, 1976). The development of pasteurization has its origins in the choice of dose form in April 1941. Cohn had recommended a highly purified crystalline preparation, but Dr Milton Veldee, of the National Institute of Health (NIH), preferred a 25% (250 g protein/l) solution, an option prepared by Cohn because a 100 ml dose was equivalent osmotically to 500 ml of citrated plasma (Coates and McFetridge, 1964; Cohn 1948; Strong 1948). In order to avoid spoilage in tropical locations, the US Navy specified that the solution should be stable at $45\,°C$ for 'protracted periods', causing Cohn to establish a test of heat stability whereby samples from each batch were examined for turbidity after heating at $50\,°C$ for 12 days (Cohn, 1948). In order to pass this test reproducibly, the ethanol fractionation process had to be refined and the sodium chloride concentration of the product increased from 0.15 M (isotonic) to 0.30 M. Subsequently, a preparation of albumin containing acetate, used to adjust pH during fractionation, was sent to Dr Murray Luck at Stanford University for research purposes. Luck observed that the acetate ion conferred greater thermal stability than chloride, leading to a systematic investigation of organic anions and the discovery that certain anions with attached non-polar groups, such as phenylacetate and mandelate, provided a high degree of thermal stability (Boyer et al., 1946; Edsall, 1984).

There was concern that a mercury preservative, added to the original product at the insistence of the NIH, might be responsible for adverse reactions and that the high sodium chloride concentration was restricting clinical use. With sodium acetyl phenylalanine as stabilizer, the sodium chloride concentration could be returned to isotonic. George Scatchard, at the Massachusetts Institute of Technology, suggested that stabilized albumin could be pasteurized to destroy bacteria, eliminating the need to add the mercury preservative (Edsall 1984; Scatchard et al. 1945). Consequently, in mid-1945, pasteurized albumin, known as 'human albumin, salt-poor' replaced the non-pasteurized, high-salt formulation, with a recommendation from Cohn that studies be undertaken to determine the heating conditions needed to destroy the agent responsible for hepatitis (Coates and McFetridge, 1964).

Two studies were performed to address this question, both of which used prison volunteers as experimental subjects. In the first, an aliquot of infectious plasma was added to human albumin which was then pasteurized for ten hours at either 60 °C or 64 °C. A total of 15 volunteers received either pasteurized material or the unheated control; no hepatitis was observed in those given pasteurized material whereas three of five recipients of the unheated control developed hepatitis (Gellis et al., 1948). A second, more substantive study led by Dr Roderick Murray, involved the preparation of albumin by method 6 of Cohn (Cohn et al., 1946) from an infectious pool of plasma. Pasteurized (60 °C/ 10 h) albumin was administered to a total of 20 volunteers, none of whom developed hepatitis; by contrast hepatitis was observed in two of ten volunteers who had received 100 ml of unheated albumin intravenously (Murray et al., 1955a). Similarly, in a separate experiment, hepatitis was observed in two of five volunteers who had been given unpasteurized albumin (Pennell, 1957; Tabor, 1999) prepared by method 12 of Cohn (Cohn et al., 1950), in which zinc had been used to precipitate proteins rather than cold-ethanol.

Following the development of serological testing for hepatitis B, serum samples retained from the prison-volunteer studies of Murray et al. were tested for hepatitis B surface antigen (HBsAg), including samples from volunteers who had been given infected plasma at different dilutions in order to measure dose response (Barker and Murray, 1972). From the results, the infectious plasma pool was estimated to have contained 7.5 $\log_{10}$ infectious doses per ml (ID_{50}/ml) with the cold-ethanol fractionation process being responsible for a 5–6 $\log_{10}$ reduction in HBV titre and pasteurization responsible for inactivating the remaining infectivity (Hoofnagle and Barker, 1976).

Although the safety of albumin is usually ascribed to its having been pasteurized, it is important to appreciate that from this analysis most hepatitis infectivity was removed by the cold-ethanol fractionation process. Indeed, in experiments involving pasteurization of serum containing HBV, pasteurized material transmitted hepatitis to human volunteers (Soulier et al., 1972) and to chimpanzees (Shikata et al., 1978). Nevertheless, the importance of pasteurization was emphasized when, in 1973, transmission of hepatitis was associated with batches of albumin, in the form of plasma protein fraction, that had been manufactured by Armour Pharmaceutical Company (Centers for Disease Control, 1974) using method 6 of Cohn. Pasteurization had been carried out in a bulk-tank prior to bottling and the subsequent investigation discovered that, because of the tank design, 50 ml of solution might not have been adequately mixed and therefore not subjected to the complete heating cycle (Pattison et al., 1976). This incident led to a requirement that pasteurization of all types of albumin be performed in the sealed final container, a procedure employed by Armour for its 25% solution of human albumin which had not been not associated with any hepatitis transmissions.

Albumin has not been implicated in the transmission of HIV, even when prepared from plasma collected before the screening of donors (Tabor, 1999). Pasteurization at 60 °C for ten hours has been shown to be highly effective in inactivating

HIV (Cuthbertson et al., 1987a; Hilfenhaus et al., 1990) and cold-ethanol fractionation has also been shown capable of removing HIV during the preparation of albumin (Cai et al., 2005).

There have been no reports of HAV transmission by human albumin and pasteurization has been shown to inactivate 4.4 and ≥ 3.9 $\log_{10}$ of HAV infectivity in 5% and 20% solutions of human albumin respectively (Adcock et al., 1998). Inactivation of ≥ 4 $\log_{10}$ of B19 parvovirus has been observed after ten minutes at 60 °C in 5%, 20% and 25% solutions of albumin (Blümel et al., 2002).

Safety of human immunoglobulin

History

Research by Cohn to discover a means of pasteurizing immunoglobulin was not successful and was abandoned (Surgenor, 2002), but despite the absence of a defined virus inactivation step the product appeared not to transmit hepatitis (Janeway, 1948; Stokes et al., 1948). The prison-volunteer studies undertaken by Murray in the early 1950s included the investigation of preparations of immunoglobulin which, like albumin, had been prepared from pools of infectious plasma. No hepatitis was observed in ten recipients of immunoglobulin following subcutaneous administration of 2 ml of a 16% solution (Murray and Ratner, 1953) prepared by cold-ethanol methods 6 and 9 (Cohn et al., 1946; Oncley et al., 1949). By contrast, all five recipients of immunoglobulin prepared by method 12 (Cohn et al., 1950) developed hepatitis after intravenous administration of 4 ml of an 8% solution (Pennell, 1957). Whether infection was due to the method of preparation or to the route of administration was not clear. At this time, immunoglobulin was not normally given intravenously as this route of administration had frequently resulted in adverse reactions (Cohn, 1948). The evidence that immunoglobulin remained safe even when prepared from infectious plasma (Murray and Ratner, 1953) led Experts of the World Health Organization to recommend that human immunoglobulin, including anti-D (World Health Organization, 1971), should be prepared by either the cold-ethanol procedure of Cohn, the ether technique of Kekwick and MacKay (1954) or ammonium sulphate precipitation, as these methods were considered to provide products free from known virus contamination (World Health Organization, 1966). It was noted that the cold-ethanol technique was by far the most widely used and that ion exchange chromatography was 'yet to be proved free from infective virus.' (World Health Organization, 1966).

Other than the experimental transmission performed by Murray, there are few recorded instances of hepatitis being transmitted by intramuscular immunoglobulin. In the UK, 1 of 43 recipients developed hepatitis from immunoglobulin that had been prepared by ether fractionation from a pool of plasma subsequently found to be infectious (Cockburn, et al., 1951). Petrilli et al. (1977) described transmission of hepatitis B to over 100 recipients of a drug prepared in Italy, which contained immunoglobulin that had been imported from the USA. An HBsAg subtype that was relatively rare in Italy was detected both in infected recipients and the immunoglobulin, demonstrating that the immunoglobulin was the most likely source of infection (Petrilli *et al.*, 1977). Transmission of hepatitis B by immunoglobulin has also been described in South America (Morgado and da Fonte, 1979; Silva *et al.*, 1977) and in India (John *et al.*, 1979). Infectivity of a batch of immunoglobulin manufactured in the USA and implicated in an outbreak of hepatitis B was confirmed by transmission in chimpanzees (Tabor and Gerety, 1979).

Despite these occasional transmissions, immunoglobulin products were regarded as essentially safe from hepatitis transmission until NANBH was observed in 12 recipients of a new preparation of IGIV prepared at the UK Blood Products Laboratory (BPL) (Lane, 1983; Lever *et al.*, 1984). The product had been prepared using ethanol fractionation and it was initially suggested that the batch may have remained infective because of the omission of a freeze drying step (Lane, 1983). However, contamination from a multi-purpose chromatography column, used for additional purification, could not be discounted (Gerety, 1985; Yap, 1996). Transmission of NANBH by two pilot batches of IGIV prepared via ethanol fractionation by Baxter (Ochs *et al.*, 1985; 1986) led to a suggestion that immunoglobulin products should be subjected to a defined virus inactivation procedure, even when prepared using ethanol fractionation (Cuthbertson *et al.*, 1987b).

Detection of antibodies to HIV in batches of immunoglobulin (Aiuti *et al.*, 1986; Gocke *et al.*, 1986; Piszkiewicz *et al.*, 1986b; Tedder *et al.*, 1985) and isolation of HIV from two recipients of IGIV (Webster *et al.*, 1986) led to concern that HIV might have been transmitted via immunoglobulin products. However, in further studies, no evidence of HIV transmission by immunoglobulin was found (Bremard-Ourcy *et al.*, 1986; Centers for Disease Control, 1986; Lee *et al.*, 1987). Although HIV was detected in the sera of patients following treatment with IGIV it was concluded that this was a result of passive antibody administration, not infection (Benveniste *et al.*, 1986; Ikeda *et al.*, 1986).

Transmission of hepatitis C by anti-D

Major episodes of HCV transmission by anti-D immunoglobulin have occurred in Eastern Germany and in the Republic of Ireland, both of which involved products prepared by ion exchange purification of IgG from plasma according to the method of Hoppe (Hoppe *et al.*, 1967; 1973).

In East Germany, 2533 recipients treated between August 1978 and March 1979 were infected from 14 contaminated batches of anti-D immunoglobulin (Meisel *et al.*, 1995; Wiese *et al.*, 2005). It was subsequently discovered that two hyperimmune plasma donors had been immunized with red blood cells from an anti-D positive individual who was suffering from inapparent hepatitis (Dittmann *et al.*, 1991).

In Ireland, an observation that a disproportionate number of anti-HCV positive blood donors were rhesus-negative women who had received anti-D (Power *et al.*, 1994) led to national screening of over 62 000 women, 704 of whom had evidence of infection (Fanning, 2002; Kenny-Walsh *et al.*, 1999) from batches of anti-D produced from May 1977–November 1978 using plasma

from a donor who had experienced jaundice after a therapeutic plasma exchange (Finlay, 1997). Further infections were associated with anti-D prepared from 1991–1994 and involved a different hepatitis C genotype (Smith *et al.*, 1999). Over 1600 women were infected in total.

The anti-D products implicated in both Germany and in Ireland were prepared from small pools of plasma by ion exchange chromatography, despite cold-ethanol fractionation being recommended (WHO, 1966). In both countries, an ethanol precipitation step was applied to the IgG solution after ion exchange purification (Cunningham, 1980; Dittmann *et al.*, 1991), possibly in the belief that this would eliminate viruses in a manner comparable to cold-ethanol fractionation.

At the time of these transmissions, there were some 70 manufacturers of immunoglobulin worldwide, including 30 manufacturers of anti-D (Foster *et al.*, 1995). Virtually all of these products were manufactured using ethanol fractionation and were generally regarded as safe, despite the absence of donor-screening for hepatitis C. However, recipients of anti-D are not normally monitored for markers of infection; raising the possibility that hepatitis infection from anti-D may have been more widespread. This question was addressed in Austria by a study of 520 women who had received anti-D from 1968–1992 (Kirchebner *et al.*, 1994) and in the USA by an analysis of the rhesus-status of HCV positive blood donors (Watanabe *et al.*, 2000), both studies confirming the general safety of anti-D immunoglobulin.

Transmission of hepatitis C by intravenous immunoglobulin

During 1993–1994, hepatitis C was transmitted to 200 recipients of Gammagard, an IGIV manufactured in the USA by Baxter Healthcare Corporation. Although the product had been in use since 1986, it was withdrawn in February 1994 and replaced by a solvent/detergent-treated version, Gammagard SD, for which a licence application, submitted in August 1992, was approved by the FDA in May 1994 (Gomperts, 1994). Transmissions had occurred in the USA (Bresee *et al.*, 1996; Centers for Disease Control, 1994; Gomperts, 1996), the UK (Christie *et al.*, 1997), France (Lefrere *et al.*, 1996), Scandinavia (Widell *et al.*, 1997), Italy (Rossi *et al.*, 1997), Spain (Cabrera Chaves *et al.*, 1996; Echevarria *et al.*, 1996) and Germany (Berger *et al.*, 1997).

These transmissions coincided with the introduction of serological testing of blood and plasma donors for hepatitis C, a measure which was somewhat controversial as the acknowledged safety of immunoglobulin products was thought to be dependent on the presence of neutralizing antibodies and it was thought the exclusion of anti-HCV positive donations might compromise product safety (Finlayson and Tankersley, 1990). Testing of plasma donors in the USA was delayed until this issue was resolved by a study in chimpanzees, which concluded that the safety of IGIV would not be compromised by withholding anti-HCV positive donations (Biswas *et al.*, 1994). Following transmission of hepatitis C by Gammagard, a small-scale simulation of the ethanol fractionation process was performed and HCV RNA was detected in the IgG fraction (fraction II) (Yei *et al.*, 1992) leading to the conclusion that exclusion of anti-HCV reactive donations had altered the partitioning behaviour of HCV (Yu, 1996; Yu *et al.*, 1995). The idea that HCV was now partitioning into fraction II and that an infected donation(s) had not been detected using second-generation anti-HCV testing (Healey *et al.*, 1996) led regulatory authorities to decide that IGIV products manufactured without a virus inactivation step should be prepared from plasma pools which were negative for HCV RNA by NAT (Nubling *et al.*, 1995). The detection of HCV RNA in intramuscular immunoglobulin, including specific immunoglobulin products, as well as IGIV (Yu *et al.*, 1994) led to this decision being extended to intramuscular immunoglobulin (Committee for Proprietary Medicinal Products, 1995b) which, because of its long history of safety, was normally prepared without a defined virus inactivation step. This extension to intramuscular immunoglobulin made the requirement to test plasma pools for HCV RNA universal, encompassing products prepared from recovered plasma as well as from source plasma. The notion that a higher standard of testing was being applied to plasma products than to blood components derived from the same donor, resulted in testing for HCV RNA then being extended to all blood donations (Nubling *et al.*, 1999).

In a recent study, antibodies that were neutralizing and protective against HCV were found in Gammagard which had been prepared from untested plasma and which did not transmit HCV, but not in batches of Gammagard prepared from anti-HCV-screened plasma that did transmit HCV (Yu *et al.*, 2004), supporting the original concern of Finlayson and Tankersley (1990) that donor screening might compromise the safety of immunoglobulin. Prior to the transmissions of HCV by Gammagard in 1993–1994, transmission of NANBH was associated with two pilot batches (Ochs *et al.*, 1985; 1986) and, although possible explanations for this were identified, the cause was never established (Yap, 1996). Transmissions of NANBH were also associated with an IGIV manufactured in Sweden by Kabi, using essentially the same manufacturing method as Baxter Healthcare Corporation (Björkander *et al.*, 1988; Bjøro *et al.*, 1994; Iwarson *et al.*, 1987; Weiland *et al.*, 1986).

The desirability of treating IGIV products with a defined virus inactivation step had been noted long before the Gammagard incident (Cuthbertson *et al.*, 1987a; Welch *et al.*, 1983b) and many IGIV products were already being treated in this manner. Given the uncertainty over the cause of NANBH transmission by pilot batches of Gammagard, the transmission of NANBH by a comparable product in Sweden and concern that anti-HCV testing might compromise the safety of IGIV, it is disappointing that it was not until after the Gammagard incident that regulatory authorities required a suitable virus inactivation step to be incorporated into the manufacture of all preparations of IGIV.

Treatment of haemophilia

Without treatment, most children with haemophilia died before the age of 14 (Forbes and Prentice, 1977) and those who survived faced crippling disability. A large number of empirical treatments were attempted before the cause of the condition was known, some bizarre, others lethal (Biggs and McFarlane, 1957). Lane

(1840) is credited with the first successful use of blood transfusion, but it was not until the work of Emile-Weil (1906) that the value of blood transfusion came to be appreciated. Transfusion of fresh plasma (Feissley, 1924; Payne and Steen, 1929) was found to be more suitable than whole blood, but the volume of blood or plasma needed to achieve haemostatis in severe haemophilia was so large that it was considered that 'concentrated preparations of A. H. G. seem to provide the only practical form of therapy.' (Biggs and MacFarlane, 1957).

A finding by Patek and Taylor (1937) that a euglobulin fraction of normal plasma could shorten the clotting time of haemophilic blood led to a collaboration with Cohn's group in which various 'Cohn fractions' were tested for their effect on haemophilic blood. The anti-haemophilic factor (AHF), later termed factor VIII, was found to be especially high in fraction I, which was therefore supplied for clinical trial (Cohn, 1948). At first, intravenous injections gave prompt haemostasis (Minot *et al.*, 1945; Taylor *et al.*, 1945) but in some haemophiliacs who had responded previously, results were not always satisfactory, especially in patients with internal bleeding (Cohn, 1948). In 6 of 52 cases there was no response at all, causing Minot and Taylor (1947) to comment that haemophilia may not always be due to a deficiency of a single factor. Biggs *et al.* (1952) confirmed this, by distinguishing two forms of haemophila; one, a deficiency of AHF (factor VIII) and another, a deficiency of Factor IX, initially termed Christmas disease (haemophilia B). This discovery led to the development of coagulation factor concentrates specifically for the treatment of haemophilia B (Biggs *et al.* 1961; Didisheim *et al.*, 1959; Hoag *et al.*, 1969).

Despite encouraging results (Cumming *et al.*, 1965; Kekwick and Wolf, 1957; McMillan *et al.*, 1961; Maycock *et al.*, 1963; Nilsson *et al.*, 1962), large-scale supplies of early factor VIII concentrates, such as Cohn fraction I, were not widely available. A chance observation by Pool and Robinson (1959) that the last residue of thawed plasma left after transfusion was rich in factor VIII, led to the discovery of cryoprecipitate and its introduction by blood transfusion services for the treatment of haemophilia A (Pool and Shannon, 1965). Nevertheless, in the UK, there was no reduction in mortality in haemophilia during the period 1955–1972, despite the use of cryoprecipitate from 1966 onwards (Forbes and Prentice, 1977); the average age at death in the period 1969–1974 being 42.3 years (Biggs, 1977). Recovery of cryoprecipitate at industrial-scale (Pool *et al.*, 1964) and its further purification (Brinkhous *et al.*, 1968; Hershgold *et al.*, 1966; Johnson *et al.*, 1967; Newman *et al.*, 1971; Wagner *et al.*, 1968) led to the introduction of intermediate-purity factor VIII concentrates, with commercial products (Webster *et al.*, 1965) being licensed in the USA from 1966 (Kasper *et al.*, 1993; Wagner, 1967).

Cohn fraction I and factor VIII concentrates were both associated with a risk of hepatitis, as was fibrinogen (see Table 20.4), the major constituent of intermediate-purity factor VIII concentrates. The importance of studying the incidence of hepatitis in recipients of factor VIII was stressed (Wagner, 1967) and statements warning of a risk of hepatitis infection were included in product literature. The following extracts from product inserts

Table 20.5 Batches of heat treated SNBTS factor VIII concentrate that did not transmit HIV and which were found retrospectively to have been manufactured from plasma pools containing an HIV positive donation[a].

FVIII batch	Dry heat conditions	Date plasma fractionated	Date batch heat treated	Date batch issued
A	68 °C/2 h	April 1984	November 1984	December 1984
B	68 °C/2 h	July 1984	November 1984	December 1984
C	68 °C/2 h	April 1984	February 1985	March 1985
D	68 °C/2 h	November 1984	January 1985	March 1985
E	68 °C/24 h	February 1985	May 1985	August 1985
F	68 °C/24 h	March 1985	June 1985	September 1985

[a] Absence of HIV transmission by two of these batches was reported by Cuthbert et al., 1988.

illustrate the warnings issued with early commercial factor VIII concentrates:

Caution ... This concentrate is prepared from large pools of fresh human plasma. Such plasma may contain the causative agents of viral hepatitis.... The concentrate should, therefore, be used when its expected effect is needed in spite of the unknown hepatitis risk associated with its use. Special consideration should be given to the use of this concentrate in newborns and infants where a higher morbidity and mortality may be associated with hepatitis. (Hyland, 1975)

Warning Koate® concentrate is a purified dried fraction of pooled plasma obtained from many paid donors. The presence of hepatitis virus should be assumed and the hazard of administering Koate concentrate should be weighed against the medical consequences of withholding it, particularly in persons with few previous transfusions of blood and plasma products. (Cutter Biological, 1978)

By 1972, there was sufficient factor VIII concentrate available in the USA to treat all patients with acute haemorrhage (Aronson, 1990). In the UK, most patients continued to be treated with cryoprecipitate, with commercial concentrate accounting for only 13% of the factor VIII used in 1974 (Biggs, 1977). It was pointed out that 90% of UK patients were receiving sub-optimal treatment and that failure to purchase commercial factor VIII concentrates, licensed in the UK since 1973, was unethical as patients were in dire need of this material (Biggs, 1974), an opinion shared by haemophilia doctors (Blackburn, 1974; Dormandy, 1974; Ingram, 1974; Jones, 1974; Mannucci, 1974) and by the UK Haemophilia Society (Prothero, 1974). Thereafter, the quantity of factor VIII used to treat haemophilia in the UK increased substantially, with concentrate replacing cryoprecipitate and use of commercial factor VIII exceeding that of NHS concentrates (Rizza et al., 2001).

A preparation of heat treated factor VIII was first licensed in the USA in 1983 (Kasper et al., 1993) but the product, dry heat treated at 60 °C for 72 hours, continued to transmit NANBH (Colombo et al., 1985). Failure to inactivate the agent(s) responsible for NANBH and concern that neo-antigens might induce inhibitors to factor VIII, resulted in a continued preference for unheated factor VIII (Evatt, 2006). This assessment changed when preliminary data demonstrated that HIV could be inactivated by heating conditions which factor VIII concentrates could tolerate (Centers for Disease Control, 1984), with a 4 $\log_{10}$ inactivation of HIV after one hour of dry heat treatment of factor VIII at 68 °C (Jason, 1984). Although this information resulted in many countries deciding to switch to heated concentrates, the time required to manufacture and distribute new concentrates meant that unheated products continued to be used well into 1985 in most countries (Glied, 1999) including the USA (Crewdson, 2002) and the UK (Bloom et al., 1985).

Within the UK, the Scottish National Blood Transfusion Service (SNBTS) began to dry heat factor VIII concentrate in November 1984, heating its 12-month stock of factor VIII at 68 °C for two hours, thereby heat treating batches that had been derived from donations collected as early as October 1983. This enabled heat-treated factor VIII to be supplied for all patients in Scotland during December 1984 and allowed unheated stock to be recalled. A modification to the product formulation in January 1985 enabled the period of heating to be increased to 24 hours. Following the introduction of donor screening, it was later discovered that some of the first batches that were heat treated at 68 °C had been prepared from plasma pools containing an HIV-positive donation (see Table 20.5). None of these batches transmitted HIV, supporting the effectiveness of the heat treatment. In England, factor VIII concentrate dry heat treated at 80 °C for 72 hours (8Y) was issued routinely by BPL from September 1985. Absence of HIV transmission by heated concentrates was demonstrated in a number of clinical studies (Rouzioux et al., 1985; Mösseler et al., 1985; Felding et al., 1985; Meer et al., 1986). In the USA, no haemophiliac born since 1984 has tested positive for HIV-1 (Soucie et al., 2001) confirming the effectiveness of heat treatment and other virus inactivation procedures implemented at the time.

Human immunodeficiency virus was heat-inactivated more easily than HCV and further advances were required to eliminate hepatitis transmission. Prior to the discovery of HCV, it was necessary to determine the degree of safety from NANBH by monitoring susceptible patients using liver function tests, as results obtained in animal studies had not been replicated in humans (see Table 20.6). Protocols for this purpose, based on Colombo et al. (1985) were drawn up by the International Society of Thrombosis and Haemostasis (Mannucci and Colombo, 1989; Schimpf et al., 1987). Results from such studies were subsequently confirmed by testing recipients for antibodies to HCV (see Table 20.7). The success of these developments

Table 20.6 Failure of studies in chimpanzees to predict hepatitis safety in humans of treated coagulation factor concentrates.

Method of virus elimination (manufacturer)	Subject	No. infected/no. treated	Infection	Reference
Dry heat treatment, 60 °C/30 h (Armour Pharma)	chimpanzee	0/3	NANBH	Purcell et al., 1985
	human	2/2	NANBH	Preston et al., 1985
Dry heat treatment, 60 °C/72 h (Baxter)	chimpanzee	0/4	NANBH	Hollinger et al., 1984
	human	11/13	NANBH	Colombo et al., 1985
Heat treatment of dry powder in organic solvent (n-heptane) suspension, 60 °C/24 h (Alpha Pharma)	chimpanzee	0/4	NANBH	Heldebrandt et al., 1985
	human	5/18	NANBH	Kernoff et al., 1987
Hydrophobic chromatography (Kabi)	chimpanzee	0/2	NANBH	Einarsson et al., 1985
	chimpanzee	0/2	Hepatitis B	Iwarson et al., 1987
	human	4/n/a	Hepatitis	Mannucci and Columbo 1988

Table 20.7 Absence of infection in susceptible patients treated with virus inactivated coagulation factor concentrates[a].

Method of virus inactivation	Manufacturer	No. patients infected / No. treated				References
		HIV	HBV	HCV	NANBH	
Pasteurization (60 °C/10h)	Behringwerke, Germany	0/26	0/10	n/a	0/26	Schimpf et al., 1987
		0/155	n/a	n/a	n/a	Schimpf et al., 1989
		0/29	0/15	0/29	0/29	Mannucci et al., 1990
		n/a	n/a	0/98	0/98	Kreuz et al., 1992
		0/36	n/a	0/36	0/26	Pollmann and Richter, 1994
	Armour Pharma, USA	0/13	n/a	n/a	0/12	Mauser-Bunschoten et al., 1993
Dry Heat (80 °C/72h)	Bio-Products Laboratory, UK	0/32	0/16	n/a	0/32	Colvin et al., 1988
		n/a	n/a	0/27	n/a	Colvin, 1990
		n/a	n/a	0/18	0/18	Pasi et al., 1990
		0/27	0/6	0/27	0/27	Rizza et al., 1993
	Protein Fractionation Centre, UK	0/13	n/a	n/a	0/13	Bennett et al., 1993
Solvent/detergent	New York Blood Center, USA[b]	0/14	n/a	n/a	0/14	Horowitz et al., 1988
	Biotransfusion, France[b]	0/10	n/a	n/a	0/10	Gazengel et al., 1988
		n/a	n/a	0/16	n/a	Noel et al., 1989
		0/55	0/4	0/55	n/a	Guérois et al., 1993
	Santa Caterina, Brazil[b]	0/20	0/14		0/20	Gonzaga and Bonecker, 1990
	Baxter, USA[c]	0/41	n/a	0/21	0/28	Addiego et al., 1992
	AIMA, Italy[b]	0/31	0/14	0/31	0/30	Mariani et al., 1993
	Alpha Therapeutics, USA[b]	0/10	n/a	0/10	0/10	Becton et al., 1994

[a] Adapted from Foster et al., 1997a.

[b] Tri-n-butyl phosphate, 0.3% (TNBP) + polysorbate-80, 1% at 25 °C /6 h (Horowitz, 1989).

[c] TNBP, 0.3% + Triton X-100 at room temperature for 15 minutes (Griffin, 1991).

(Mannucci, 1993; Morfini et al., 1994) is illustrated by the fact that no haemophiliac born in the USA has tested positive for HCV since 1992, nor positive for HBV since 1993 (Soucie et al., 2001).

Following the introduction of virus inactivated factor concentrates, an enhanced incidence of inhibitors to factor VIII was associated with pasteurized factor VIII concentrates from two manufacturers (Laub et al., 1997; Peerlinck et al., 1993; 1997; Rosendaal et al., 1993), indicating that concern that

heat treatment might generate neo-antigens (Bird et al., 1985; Chandra and Brummelhuis, 1981; Evatt, 2006; C. A. Ludlam, personal communication, 1983; Mannucci, 2003) was not misplaced.

Although transmission of the major pathogens, HIV, HBV and HCV by coagulation factor concentrates was essentially eliminated over 15 years ago, continued fear of pathogen transmission by plasma-derived therapies has led to recombinant coagulation factors being preferred by clinicians and by patient representatives, despite the higher cost and greater incidence of inhibitors (Ettingshausen and Kreuz, 2006; Goudemand et al., 2006a; 2006b).

Virus inactivation processes and their development

Background

A growing appreciation of the risk of hepatitis associated with pooled plasma (see Table 20.3) and plasma derivatives (see Table 20.4) together with the discovery that albumin could be pasteurized led to numerous investigations into potential methods of virus inactivation. Measles convalescent serum, treated with a mixture of phenol and ether, had transmitted hepatitis (Ministry of Health, 1943; Sawyer et al., 1944). Plasma that had been pasteurized for four hours at 60 °C also continued to transmit hepatitis (Murray and Deifenbach, 1953). Allen proposed storage of plasma at 30–32 °C for six months (Allen et al., 1954) but factor VIII activity was destroyed by the procedure (J. Garrott Allen, personal communication, 1983) and hepatitis transmission was observed in 10% of recipients (Murray et al., 1954; Redeker et al., 1968).

Considerable work was undertaken on the irradiation of plasma by ultraviolet (UV) light (Blanchard et al., 1948; Oliphant and Hollaender, 1946; Wolf et al., 1947). However, UV treated plasma continued to transmit hepatitis (Murphy and Workman, 1953; Murray et al., 1955b; Rosenthal et al., 1950). From studies in human volunteers, it was found that infected plasma was not sterilized at a dose of UV three times greater than that used commercially, nor at all practical levels of irradiation (Murray, 1955). Three of the prison volunteers involved in these studies died from hepatitis, leading to the suicide of Dr Oliphant who had pioneered the UV treatment (Tabor, 1999). Ultraviolet-irradiation was also used to treat Cohn fraction I and fibrinogen (McCall et al., 1957) but the resultant products continued to be associated with hepatitis transmissions (Anderson and Gibson, 1957; Mainwaring and Brueckner, 1966). Treatment of fibrinogen with 2% nitrogen mustard was also attempted (Pennell, 1957).

Other procedures investigated included cathode ray irradiation (Trump and Wright, 1957) and gamma radiation (Jordan and Kempe, 1957). Hartman et al. (1955) evaluated 550 chemicals for their ability to inactivate viruses; of these only β-propiolactone and nitrogen mustard (HN_2) inactivated two or more viruses in 90% whole blood, but complete haemolysis occurred at minimal virucidial concentrations. Nitrogen mustard failed to inactivate hepatitis in whole blood when tested in human volunteers (Drake et al. 1952), but a combination of β-propiolactone and UV-irradiation was found to be synergistic and was considered the most promising option (Hartman et al., 1956; LoGrippo and Rupe, 1957), eventually leading to the procedure being applied by Biotest Pharma in Germany. β-propiolactone/UV treated serum and the resultant prothrombin (factor IX) complex concentrate were introduced in 1968 and 1975 respectively (Stephan, 1989) and a β-propiolactone-treated IGIV was developed subsequently

(Dichtelmuller et al., 1993; Mondorf et al., 1981; Scheidler et al., 1998; Stephan, 1975). Transmission of HIV to ten recipients of β-propiolactone-UV treated factor IX concentrate (Karcher, 1991; Kleim et al., 1990; Kupfer et al., 1995) resulted in the method being discontinued for coagulation factors. A more recent study of the virucidal action of β-propiolactone alone found only a 2–4 log_{10} reduction of HIV in IgG and concluded that β-propiolactone had a limited capacity to inactivate viruses (Scheidler et al., 1998). The procedure has not been adopted elsewhere because of its limited applicability and concern over the carcinogenic nature of β-propiolactone.

The labile nature of coagulation factors and evidence that the agent(s) responsible for serum hepatitis was relatively resistant to inactivation caused investigators to consider instead methods that might be able to remove viruses physically (see methods of virus removal below). Other limitations included an inability to culture hepatitis viruses, unavailability of pedigree strains of HBV and NANBH until 1976 and 1979 respectively, limited availability of naive chimpanzees, long incubation periods required for monitoring experiments in animals, ethical issues surrounding experiments in chimpanzees and in human volunteers, uncertainty over the nature of the agent(s) responsible for NANBH and absence of serological markers for HIV and HCV until 1984 and 1989 respectively.

By the late 1970s, knowledge and expertise in the manufacture of factor VIII concentrates had advanced considerably and developments in methods of analysis of factor VIII provided a means of studying both the coagulation activity and antigenic activity during processing (Foster et al., 1980b; Prowse et al., 1981). Continued concern over hepatitis transmission and evidence that factor VIII might withstand heat treatment caused manufacturers to reconsider this approach, resulting in a number of different heat treatment procedures being applied by different manufacturers (Kasper et al., 1993). Of these, only two, pasteurization at 60 °C for ten hours and dry heat treatment at 80 °C for 72 hours, were shown to be effective against NANBH and HCV (see Table 20.7). Knowledge that HIV was lipid-enveloped stimulated the development of chemical inactivation of enveloped viruses, with a solvent/detergent mixture developed at the New York Blood Center shown to be effective against NANBH and HCV as well as HIV (see Table 20.7).

Pasteurization of labile proteins

The pasteurization of albumin set a standard that proved difficult to extrapolate to other products (Edsall, 1984), particularly after Cohn had abandoned his attempts at pasteurizing immunoglobulin (Surgenor, 2002). It was not until the late 1970s that investigators at two companies independently discovered that factor VIII could be stabilized by a combination of glycine and sucrose, enabling heating in solution for ten hours at 60 °C to be tolerated.

At Behringwerke in Germany, Dr Horst Schwinn, a research biochemist, was assigned the task of increasing the purity of factor VIII. In order to achieve this it was necessary to discover a method of separating factor VIII from fibrinogen, as this constituted up to 60% of the total protein present. After many failed attempts, Schwinn decided, as a last resort, to see if fibrinogen could be removed by heating at 56 °C for 30 minutes, conditions under which fibrinogen was known to be denatured. This approach had been attempted previously but had resulted in too high a loss of factor VIII activity (Bidwell, 1955; A. J. Johnson, personal communication, 1999). Schwinn was not successful at first, but, after studying earlier work (Blombäck and Blombäck, 1956), he decided to explore the use of glycine as a possible stabilizer. This proved successful, enabling him to devise a 'heat shock' method for fibrinogen removal and encouraging the exploration for other substances which in combination with glycine might enable the heating conditions to be extended (Schwinn, 1996). It was eventually found that 50% of the factor VIII activity could be retained following pasteurization for ten hours at 60 °C in the presence of high concentrations of sucrose and glycine (Heimburger et al., 1981b; Schwinn et al., 1981) and the resultant pasteurized factor VIII concentrate was licensed in Germany in 1981. However, as the overall yield was only 8% (Heimburger et al., 1981a) few patients were treated, reimbursement was restricted to patients who tested negative for hepatitis B, and most factor VIII was issued unheated until mid-1985 (Schwinn, 1996). Subsequently, further stabilization was obtained by addition of calcium (Foster et al., 1983b) and precipitation of factor VIII to remove sucrose and glycine was replaced by ion exchange adsorption (Heimburger et al., 1986), advances in processing that would be expected to increase yield, but which required new safety studies to be performed (Mannucci et al., 1990).

At Bayer in the USA in the late 1970s, research scientist Dr Pete Fernandes was assigned the task of discovering how to prevent a precipitate forming in IGIV during aseptic dispensing. Heating samples at 57 °C for four hours was routinely employed as an accelerated test of stability. Using this test, Fernandes investigated the possibility that dextrose might prevent the precipitate forming, as he had noted that this was present as an excipient in immunoglobulin produced by Immuno AG in Austria. One day, he forgot to turn off the 57 °C water-bath on going home and was surprised to find the next day that the IgG solution was only slightly opalescent. He then began to explore the possibility of heating to 60°C for ten hours and chose to add glycine, an amino acid commonly used to stabilize immunoglobulin. Success with a mixture of glycine and dextrose encouraged him to test samples of other plasma products present in the research laboratory, including factor VIII concentrate. He was eventually to discover that factor VIII batches with a low fibrinogen content that were stabilized in this manner could also tolerate pasteurization (Fernandes, 1997). The resultant product (Fernandes and Lundblad, 1984), Koate HS, although licensed in the USA in 1986, was discontinued in 1991 following the development of a solvent/detergent-treated product (Kasper et al., 1993) which was higher yielding and more highly purified.

A high concentration of carbohydrate, with either an amino acid or neutral salt (Feldman et al., 1989; Hrindra et al., 1990), was found to stabilize proteins in general and has enabled pasteurization to be applied to a wide range of plasma proteins,

including factor IX, fibrinogen and immunoglobulins (Nowak et al., 1992; Welch et al., 1983b) in addition to factor VIII. Although the heating conditions of ten hours at 60 °C are the same as those used with albumin, it was appreciated at the outset that the safety record of albumin could not be extrapolated to products stabilized in this manner (Schwinn, 1996). Indeed, experimental studies have shown a much lower degree of virus inactivation than with albumin (Hilfenhaus et al., 1986; MacLeod et al., 1984; Ng and Dobkin, 1985). Nevertheless, transmission of hepatitis was not observed in safety studies in animals (Heimburger et al., 1980) nor in humans (see Table 20.7) and HIV was found to be readily inactivated (Hilfenhaus et al., 1986; Nowak et al., 1993). Although HAV was substantially inactivated, residual infectious HAV was detected after ten hours pasteurization (Hilfenhaus and Nowak, 1994). A small number of isolated cases of HCV transmission have been reported in routine use (Gerritzen et al., 1992a; Schulman et al., 1992).

Many people with haemophilia have been vaccinated against hepatitis B, therefore safety from HBV is more difficult to establish by surveillance of haemophilic patients (see Table 20.7). Hepatitis B infection has been reported in two recipients of pasteurized factor VIII, Haemate HS (Brackmann and Egli, 1988). In addition, pasteurized factor IX concentrate Beriplex HS was associated with HBV infection in over 30 non-haemophilic patients (Jantsch-Plunger et al., 1995). As a result of this incident, the German regulatory authority concluded that the effectiveness of the Behringwerke method of pasteurization was subject to fluctuation and decided that an additional virus inactivation step should be included and that overall processes should have at least a 10 $\log_{10}$ capacity for reduction of enveloped viruses (Paul-Ehrlich-Institut, 1994).

Subsequently, an enhanced incidence of inhibitors was observed in recipients of pasteurized factor VIII concentrates manufactured by the Netherlands Red Cross (Peerlinck et al., 1993; Rosendaal et al., 1993) and by Octapharma (Laub et al., 1997; Peerlinck et al., 1997) with the first incident being linked to activation of factor VIII (Barrowcliffe, 1993) and the latter to exposure of a phospholipid binding site on the factor VIII molecule (Raut et al., 1998).

Dry heat treatment

Background

The labile nature of coagulation factors makes freeze drying necessary to obtain a suitably stable final product. Heat treatment of freeze dried fibrinogen for ten hours at 60 °C was investigated as a means of inactivating the virus responsible for Botkin's hepatitis, hepatitis A (Rosenberg et al., 1971) using experimental preparations of fibrinogen containing Cocksakie virus and adenovirus as marker viruses. Application of the technique to early factor VIII concentrates was unsuccessful (A. J. Johnson, personal communication, 1999), but later, freeze dried concentrates from different manufacturers were found to be capable of withstanding heating from 60 °C to 68 °C for up to 72 hours (Kasper et al., 1993; Rubinstein, 1984; Rubinstein and Dodds, 1982). Why these products were able to tolerate dry heat treatment better than early concentrates is not clear, but it may have been due to improved collection and storage of plasma and to incremental advances in processing aimed at increasing product solubility.

Although dried products heat treated under these conditions continued to transmit NANBH (Colombo *et al.*, 1985; Preston *et al.*, 1985), this degree of heating was effective against HIV (Evatt, 2006). Nevertheless, HIV was transmitted by factor VIII (Factorate® H. T.) manufactured in the USA by Armour Pharmaceuticals and dry heat-treated at 60 °C for 30 hours (Dietrich *et al.*, 1990; Remis *et al.*, 1990; Williams *et al.*, 1990a; Wolfs *et al.*, 1988). There were also a small number of reports of HIV transmission with dry heated concentrates in which the product implicated was not disclosed (Berg *et al.*, 1986; Weisser, 1988; White *et al.*, 1986).

Development of dry heat treatment at 80 °C

During 1984, researchers led by Dr James K. Smith at the Plasma Fractionation Laboratory (PFL) Oxford, a pilot plant for the Blood Products Laboratory (BPL) Elstree, found that a particular experimental preparation of factor VIII was able to withstand dry heat treatment at 80 °C for 72 hours. The process was developed and transferred to BPL, from where the result product, 8Y, was issued routinely from September 1985, with sufficient available to meet 25–30% of the factor VIII requirement of England and Wales. No transmissions of NANBH or HCV were observed in clinical studies (see Table 20.7), demonstrating the effectiveness of the heat treatment. Although such severe heating of factor VIII 'was viewed with some astonishment by other fractionators at the time' (Lindsay, 2002, p. 93), similar products were introduced by SNBTS Protein Fractionation Centre (PFC) in 1987 and by CSL in Australia in 1990 (Australian Senate, 2004).

The development of 8Y began with an experiment using zinc/heparin precipitation to increase factor VIII purity (Foster *et al.*, 1983b). More heparin was added than intended (L. Winkelman, personal communication, 1985), resulting in a higher degree of purification and a preparation that could withstand heating at 80 °C after freeze drying (Winkelman, 1988; Winkelman *et al.*, 1985; 1989). The features that enabled heating to be tolerated to this degree included the addition of calcium for factor VIII stabilization and the presence of a freeze dried plug with an amorphous crystal structure. This particular crystal structure had formed because the solution had super-cooled and frozen instantaneously, a situation which had occurred naturally given the freezing procedure employed, the solution composition and the dose form. The critical importance of the crystal structure of the dried plug was identified by McIntosh and co-workers who discovered that, with an amorphous plug, dry heating of less purified factor VIII concentrates could be extended to 80 °C for 72 hours. This observation led to the design of a freezing procedure that would achieve the necessary crystal structure uniformly in every vial on every occasion (McIntosh *et al.*, 1987; 1990).

When dry heat treatment was applied to established factor IX concentrates, a small amount of thrombin was generated. The material failed to comply with European Pharmacopoeia specifications and highlighted concerns that heated factor IX

concentrates might be more thrombogenic than unheated concentrates. The generation of thrombin was prevented by the addition of anti-thrombin III and products formulated in this manner were able to withstand dry heat treatment at 80 °C for 72 hours. Safety studies were undertaken in animals and confirmed freedom from thrombogenicity (Littlewood *et al.*, 1987) resulting in 80 °C/72 h dry heat treated factor IX concentrates being issued in the UK by both BPL and PFC from October 1985.

Dry heat treatment at 80 °C for 72 hours has also been reported to inactivated $\geq$4.3 $\log_{10}$ HAV (Hart *et al.*, 1994b) and 3.4 $\log_{10}$ and 4.1 $\log_{10}$ of a model virus for hepatitis B and an animal parvovirus respectively (Ristol *et al.*, 1996). In a study using B19, Roberts *et al.* (2006) obtained a $\geq$4.7 $\log_{10}$ inactivation and observed that both bovine parvovirus and porcine parvovirus were more resistant than B19 to dry heat inactivation. A similar observation has been made for dry heat treatment of fibrinogen at 100 °C (Prikhod'ko, 2005).

Solvent/detergent (SD) treatment

Development of solvent/detergent treatment

Prior to the discovery of HCV in 1989, there was limited knowledge concerning the properties and characteristics of the agent or agents responsible for NANBH. Lipid-enveloped viruses were known to be sensitive to treatment with organic solvents such as ethyl ether (Andrewes and Horstmann, 1949) or tri-n-butyl phosphate (TNBP) (Neurath *et al.*, 1972), and by detergents (Theiler, 1957) or by a combination of solvent + detergent (Mussgay, 1964). Evidence that there could be more than one agent responsible for NANBH (Shimizu *et al.*, 1979) was supported in late 1982 by Bradley, who reported the transmission in chimpanzees of at least two agents from a coagulation factor concentrate known to be infectious in humans (Bradley and Maynard, 1983). One of these was resistant to treatment with chloroform, but the other was sensitive, implying that one of these agents was lipid-enveloped and the other non-enveloped. Somewhat different results were obtained by Feinstone *et al.* (1983) who reported that viruses responsible for hepatitis B and for NANBH were inactivated by chloroform. Subsequently, Prince and co-workers at the New York Blood Center (NYBC) found that a pedigree strain of NANBH was sensitive to treatment with the detergent Tween-80 (polysorbate-80) and the organic solvent ether combined (Prince *et al.*, 1984) indicating that this particular strain was lipid-enveloped. With this procedure, it is believed that detergent makes the virus more accessible to the organic solvent which is then able to disrupt the lipid-envelope (Horowitz *et al.*, 1985). Encouraged by these findings, the group at NYBC went on to develop the procedure for application to coagulation factor concentrates. It was decided that ethyl ether was undesirable because of its explosive properties and it was replaced by TNBP, which had been used in the preparation of vaccines and was non-volatile and non-flammable. Sodium cholate was also used initially as the detergent instead of Tween-80, as it could be removed completely using gel filtation (Horowitz *et al.*, 1985).

Table 20.8 Transmission of hepatitis A by coagulation factors treated with solvent/detergent and chromatographically purified.

Product	Manufacturer	No. infected	Location	Reference
Factor VIII concentrate:				
Emclot, Octa VI	AIMA	52	Italy	Mariani *et al.*, 1991; Mannucci, 1992; Mannucci *et al.*, 1994.
Octa VI	Octapharma	13	Germany	Gerritzen *et al.*, 1992b.
		17	Rep. of Ireland	Temperley *et al.*, 1992; Johnson *et al.*, 1995.
		6	Belgium	Peerlinck and Vermylen, 1993.
		6	Germany	Chudy *et al.*, 1999.
Factor VIII	Natal Bioproducts	7	South Africa	Cohn *et al.*, 1994.
Alphanate	Alpha Therapeutics	3	USA	Centers for Disease Control, 1996.
Factor IX concentrate:				
Alphanine SD	Alpha Therapeutics	1	USA	Centers for Disease Control, 1996.

A major issue facing the NYBC investigators was the extent to which the chemicals employed had to be removed to avoid potential toxicity in recipients, bearing in mind that a person with severe haemophilia A might be expected to receive about 2000 IU of factor VIII an average of 30 times per annum, throughout their life. These considerations resulted in limits for the final products being set at less than 10 ppm for TNBP (Horowitz, 1991) and less than 100 ppm for polysorbate-80 (B. Horowitz, personal communication, 1988). In the original method, a precipitation process was used to separate factor VIII from the SD reagents. However, polysorbate-80 could not be removed to the required limit by this method and was substituted by sodium cholate, which could be removed to the level required using gel filtration (Horowitz *et al.*, 1985). There were a number of limitations with the process at this time; the degree of virus inactivation was reduced by the use of sodium cholate instead of Tween-80, factor VIII losses were higher and the process was difficult to scale-up for industrial application. Nevertheless, the possibility that the SD treatment could enhance the safety of coagulation factor concentrates was illustrated in laboratory experiments using marker viruses (Horowitz *et al.*, 1985) and in hepatitis transmission studies carried out in chimpanzees (Prince *et al.*, 1986). The possibility that AIDS might be caused by a lipid-enveloped retrovirus (Barré-Sinoussi *et al.*, 1983) provided a strong impetus and the ability of the procedure to inactivate HIV was studied as soon as possible, with Prince *et al.* (1985) finding that HIV in factor VIII concentrate could be inactivated by SD treatment.

At this time, factor VIII concentrates were not highly purified, as the labile nature of factor VIII activity and lack of knowledge of its molecular properties had made the development of industrial-scale purification technology difficult. A discovery that loss of factor VIII activity during processing could be prevented by the control of ionized calcium (Foster *et al.*, 1983b; 1988a) together with advances in the manufacture of reagents and equipment for large-scale chromatography led to further purification of factor VIII being developed at an industrial scale (Aronson, 1990). Although an SD treated factor VIII concentrate prepared by NYBC was licensed in the USA in 1985, the introduction of affinity or ion exchange chromatography to remove SD reagents enabled a return to the superior detergents such as Tween-80 or Triton

X-100 (see Table 20.7) and more widespread adoption of the SD treatment procedure (Burnouf *et al.*, 1991; Kasper *et al.*, 1993; Michalski *et al.*, 1988). Solvent/detergent treatment has been applied to other plasma products, including immunoglobulins (Edwards *et al.*, 1987; Horowitz, 1989), and has proven highly effective against the lipid-enveloped viruses HIV, HBV and HCV, (Horowitz and Ben-Hur, 2000). Nevertheless HCV (Evensen *et al.*, 1995) and HIV (Cho *et al.*, 2007) have been transmitted by SD-treated products. The more complex lipid-enveloped virus, vaccinia, has been found to be partly resistant to inactivation by SD treatment (Hart *et al.*, 1995; Roberts, 2000) raising the possibility that other enveloped viruses with complex structures might also be more resistant.

Hepatitis A transmission by solvent/detergent treated products

As the SD method targets lipid-enveloped viruses, it is not effective against non-enveloped viruses. When the method was developed, B19 parvovirus was the only non-enveloped virus known to be have been transmitted by fractionated plasma products. Another non-enveloped virus, hepatitis A, had been transmitted by blood components (Azimi *et al.*, 1986; Barbara *et al.*, 1982; Hollinger *et al.*, 1983; Noble *et al.*, 1984; Seeberg *et al.*, 1981; Sherertz *et al.*, 1984; Skidmore *et al.*, 1982) but not by plasma products. It was therefore unexpected when transmission of hepatitis A by factor VIII concentrates occurred in a number of European countries shortly after the introduction of SD treatment (see Table 20.8). Hepatitis A virus transmissions also occurred in the UK, but were not published (Chudy *et al.*, 1999).

The reason for these transmissions lies in the greater degree of purification which resulted from the extra processing required to remove the SD reagents, something that was welcomed by clinicians (UK Regional Haemophilia Centre Directors, 1992) who were concerned that immunological abnormalities in patients were due to extraneous proteins present in intermediate-purity concentrates (Seremetis *et al.*, 1993: Watson and Ludlam, 1992) rather than to viral infection (Berntorp, 1996; Funk *et al.*, 1993). However, the earlier generation of factor VIII concentrates had contained a significant amount of immunoglobulin (Allain, 1984) which may have either neutralized HAV in the product (Hart *et al.*,

1994a) or have provided patients with passive immunity (Peerlinck *et al.*, 1994).

Treatment with solvent/detergent, followed by heat treatment

Following the outbreak of HAV transmissions by factor VIII concentrates (see Table 20.8), European regulatory authorities decided to recommend that two complementary virus inactivation steps should be included in the manufacture of products considered to be at high risk, such as coagulation factor concentrates (Committee for Proprietary Medicinal Products, 1996b). Progress towards this goal has been mixed. Dry heat treatment has been combined successfully with SD treated, purified factor VIII (Hart *et al.*, 1994b; Powell *et al.*, 2000; Ristol *et al.*, 1996; Smith *et al.*, 1997). By contrast, an SD treated, purified factor VIII pasteurized at 63 °C for ten hours (Biesert *et al.*, 1995) was associated with an abnormal incidence of inhibitors (Peerlinck *et al.*, 1997; Laub *et al.*, 1997) and was withdrawn in 1995. Some SD treated factor VIII concentrates, purified by immuno-affinity chromatography, have been unable to tolerate dry heat treatment, possibly because of instability associated with the factor VIII activity (Hubbard *et al.*, 2002). Although products from only a small number of manufacturers were implicated in HAV transmission (see Table 20.8), it is conceivable that vaccination of haemophilia patients against hepatitis A may have prevented infection being more widespread.

Low pH treatment

Treatment at low pH (e.g. pH 4) is widely used in the manufacture of immunoglobulin products and, although it is comparable to SD treatment in being particularly effective at inactivating lipid-enveloped viruses (Hart *et al.*, 1995), it was not initially introduced for this purpose. Its origin lies in the development of immunoglobulin suitable for intravenous administration. Immunoglobulin obtained via cold-ethanol fractionation (Enders, 1944; Oncley *et al.*, 1949) was found to be unsuitable for intravenous use (Cohn, 1948). In studying intolerance of patients to immunoglobulin given intravenously, Barundun *et al.* (1962) detected a decrease in total complement in all patients, something which did not occur when immunoglobulin was administered by the intramuscular route. It was well known that preparations of immunoglobulin would fix complement in vitro (Enders, 1944) and Barundun and colleagues discovered that this anti-complementary (AC) property was associated with aggregates of immunoglobulin. They therefore investigated how this material could be removed, studying chemical disaggregation and digestion using proteolytic enzymes. Papain digestion had already been used for the preparation of antibody fragments (Porter, 1960) and Barundun *et al.* found that all AC activity could be removed by treatment with pepsin, using a pepsin/globulin ratio of 1:100. Hydrolytic enzymes such as pepsin are only active at low pH, therefore incubation with pepsin was performed at pH 4.0, a suitably low pH which immunoglobulin could tolerate. Further studies were carried out in which the pepsin/globulin

ratio was varied and AC activity was removed at even the highest dilution examined. It was then observed that the control tube, incubated at pH 4.0 for 17 hours, without pepsin, was also free of AC activity (Barundun *et al.*, 1962).

A further 20 years were to pass before vasoactive substances, such as prekallikrien activator, were also associated with adverse reactions to immunoglobulin administered intravenously (Alving *et al.*, 1980), a finding which, together with the work of Barundun, underpinned the widespread development of IGIV during the 1980s (Welch, 1983a). Low pH treatment is used in the manufacture of IGIV by a number of manufacturers, either with or without traces of pepsin. Following the transmission of NANBH by a preparation of IGIV in which aggregates had been removed by chromatography (Lane, 1983), it was suggested that pH 4.0/pepsin treatment may contribute to the viral safety of IGIV (Welch *et al.*, 1983b), given the well established sensitivity of flaviviruses to low pH (Horzinek, 1981). This was supported by experimental studies using marker viruses (Biesert, 1996; Bos *et al.*, 1998; Hamalainen *et al.*, 1992; Kempf *et al.*, 1991; Omar *et al.*, 1996; Reid *et al.*, 1988) and by safety studies in patients (Atrah, *et al.*, 1985; Imbach *et al.*, 1991; Leen *et al.*, 1986). Incubation at pH 4 for two hours has also been shown to inactivate ≥ 6 $\log_{10}$ of HIV (Kempf *et al.*, 1991) and ≥ 5 $\log_{10}$ of B19 (Boschetti *et al.*, 2004). A treatment at pH 4.25, applied to IGIV in its final formulation, has been shown to inactivate HIV (Mitra *et al.*, 1986) and a marker virus for HCV (Louie *et al.*, 1994).

Transmission of NANBH has been associated with one batch of pH 4.0/pepsin-treated IGIV (Williams *et al.*, 1989). This was an isolated event which occurred prior to testing of donors for hepatitis C and is believed to have been due to re-contamination of the process after pH 4.0/pepsin treatment had been completed (Foster *et al.*, 1997b).

Antibody mediated neutralization of viruses

Immunoglobulin preparations normally contain a wide range of bacterial and viral antibodies (Hooper, 1997) representative of the antibody specificities present in the donor population from which a product is prepared. A finding that HBsAg, present in intramuscular immunoglobulin, was coated with anti-HBs antibody (Hoofnagle and Wagoner, 1980) led to a requirement that all batches of immunoglobulin must contain at least 0.5 IU of anti-HBs antibody per g immunoglobulin. Similarly, normal intramuscular immunoglobulin must contain at least 100 IU of anti-hepatitis A antibody per ml (British Pharmacopoeia, 2005).

IGIV has been found to contain neutralizing antibody to B19 parvovirus (Callet-Fauquet *et al.*, 2004; Takahashi *et al.*, 1991) and has been used to treat B19 infection (Kumar *et al.*, 2005; McGhee *et al.*, 2005). The formation of complexes between B19 and anti-B19 antibodies has enabled the virus to be removed from immunoglobulin solutions by nanofiltration (Kreil *et al.*, 2006). Immune neutralization in IGIV has also been described for HAV, coxsackievirus-B6, polio-virus-1, herpes simplex virus type-1 (Biesert, 1996) respiratory syncytial virus types A and B, parainfluenza-3 and cytomegalovirus (Hooper, 1997).

Physical removal of viruses

Background

The relative resistance of HBV to physical and chemical methods of inactivation led investigators to search for methods that might physically separate viruses from plasma products, especially labile coagulation factors. Methods examined included precipitation with polyethylene glycol (PEG) (Johnson et al., 1976) and adsorption using either insoluble silicic acid (Hedlund, 1973), affinity chromatography (Charm and Wong, 1974), solid-phase polyelectrolytes (Johnson et al., 1978) or hydrophobic interaction chromatography (Einarsson et al., 1981).

PEG precipitation was not suitable for the removal of viruses from the factor VIII von Willebrand factor complex, but application to factor IX concentrate was progressed using HBsAg as a marker. However, tests in chimpanzees demonstrated that HBV had not been removed completely (Johnson et al., 1976). Precipitation conditions were revised (Foster et al., 1980a), but the earlier transmission in chimpanzees, plus concern that the product might be thrombogenic in high doses (Cash et al., 1975), resulted in the approach being superseded by advances in heat treatment.

A method for purifying plasma products via semi-specific adsorption to solid-phase poly-electrolytes was also devised by Johnson et al. (1978), with the prospect that viruses could be removed (Galpin et al., 1984; Harris et al., 1979). Unfortunately the method utilized specialist reagents available only for research and was overtaken by developments in heat treatment whilst fractionators sought assurances over the long-term availability of the adsorbents. The procedure was employed in the purification of human factor VIII from cryoprecipitate for the development of recombinant factor VIII (Rotblat et al., 1985).

Removal of hepatitis viruses from a factor IX concentrate was also attempted using hydrophobic interaction chromatography (Einarsson et al., 1981). Despite encouraging results from studies in chimpanzees (Einarsson et al., 1985; Iwarson et al., 1987), hepatitis and HIV were transmitted by the product (Mannucci and Columbo, 1988).

Although none of these procedures became established, processes used to separate plasma proteins offer the possibility that viruses might be removed adventitiously during fractionation. This has been the subject of a number of experimental studies.

Precipitation

Studies concerning removal of viruses during ethanol fractionation were first undertaken by Bird, Enders and Boyd, who added vaccinia, tobacco mosaic virus and mouse encephalomyelitis (EMC) to plasma and recovered viable virus in all fractions (Pennell, 1957). Similar studies were performed by Hampil, Spizizen and Pennell using T_6 bacteriophage and EMC, with most virus being removed in the early fractions but with viable virus being detectable in fraction II (immunoglobulin) and fraction V (albumin) (Pennell, 1957).

Following the discovery of the virus responsible for hepatitis B, experiments were undertaken to determine how HBsAg partitioned during the ethanol fractionation process of Cohn (Crovari et al., 1975; Schroeder and Mozen, 1970), a modification of the Cohn method (Berg et al., 1972) and during the Kistler and Nitschmann (1962) method of ethanol fractionation (Trepo et al., 1978). Fraction IV was found to contain most HBsAg, with partitioning also into fraction III and fraction I. Little or no HBsAg was found in fraction II (from which immunoglobulin is prepared), whereas fraction V (from which albumin is prepared) contained a small amount of detectable HBsAg in all studies.

Yei et al. (1992) examined the partitioning of HCV RNA in a small-scale simulation of the Cohn-Oncley process used to prepare immunoglobulin. Although $4.7 \log_{10}$ of HCV RNA was eliminated by cold-ethanol fractionation, the resultant fraction II contained detectable HCV RNA. However, in other studies, bovine viral diarrhoea virus (BVDV) and Sindbis, used as markers for HCV infectivity, were removed to a high degree over ethanol fractionation (Cai et al., 2005; Hooper, 1997; Louie et al., 1994). A $\geq 2.6 \log_{10}$ reduction of BVDV was also observed by Bos et al. (1998), but Dichtelmuller et al. (1993) reported only a $0.9 \log_{10}$ reduction, perhaps indicating a lack of robustness in the procedure.

Similar studies have been performed to determine the distribution of HIV infectivity. Wells et al. (1986) examined partitioning across each step separately, finding that virtually all added infectivity partitioned into the precipitate at cryoprecipitation, fraction I precipitation and fraction III precipitation, but with only 0.1% of added infectivity being recovered in fraction II. One study has reported an HIV reduction of $3.0 \log_{10}$ by ethanol fractionation of IgG (Bos et al., 1998) whereas, in experiments undertaken by Biesert (1996), Henin et al. (1988), Hilfenhaus et al. (1987), Mitra et al. (1989), Piszkiewicz et al. (1986a), and Uemura et al. (1994), HIV infectivity was not detected in the fraction II precipitate from which immunoglobulin is derived.

In separations involving protein precipitation, the phase equilibria are determined by a number of parameters, including various characteristics of the macromolecules and particular properties of the aqueous environment (Foster, 1994). Although these features may be reproduced relatively accurately in small-scale experiments, separation of the precipitate phase by centrifugation or by filtration at industrial scale is more difficult to simulate. Solid/liquid separation is influenced by the size and density of the particles formed during precipitation and by the type of centrifuge used. Differences in design between laboratory and industrial centrifuges make equivalent centrifugal forces difficult to obtain. In addition, shear forces within the entry region of centrifuges can reduce the particle size and must be taken into consideration if industrial performance is to be simulated accurately (Boychyn et al., 2004).

Adsorption

Depth filtration

Depth filtration is used to clarify immunoglobulin and albumin solutions following key ethanol precipitation steps and after re-suspension of the fraction II and fraction V precipitates. Asbestos pads were used originally for this purpose (Cohn et al., 1946) but were replaced during the 1980s with filters containing

Table 20.9 Removal of viruses from immunoglobulin and albumin by depth filtration.

Type of virus	Virus used	Virus reduction index ($\log_{10}$)	
		IgG, pH 5.4[a] Cuno Zeta Plus®	Albumin, pH 6.9[b] Seitz KS80
Retrovirus	Human immunodeficiency virus, HIV	Not done	3.5
Enveloped, RNA	Bovine viral diarrhoea virus, BVDV	0.9	2.4
Enveloped, DNA	Pseudorabies virus, PRV	$\geq$3.8	4.5
Non-enveloped, RNA	Hepatitis A virus, HAV	$\geq$4.0	0.6
	Reovirus type 3, Reo	$\geq$4.5	not done
Non-enveloped, DNA	Porcine parvovirus, PPV	$\geq$4.7	0.4
	Bovine parvovirus, BPV	$\geq$2.7	not done

[a] Savage and Hinskens, 1997.
[b] SNBTS Protein Fractionation Centre, unpublished results.

diatomaceous earth, which remove particles and dissolved substances by electrokinetic capture as well as by mechanical sieving (Fiore *et al.*, 1980). There is little information available on the extent to which viruses might be removed by standard depth filtration processes and this is probably why most studies of virus removal by cold-ethanol fractionation have tended to omit these steps. Nevertheless, some studies have been performed which suggest that depth filtration may contribute to viral safety (see Table 20.9). Although different filters and protein solutions were used, both examples demonstrate a good reduction of a large enveloped DNA virus. A significant reduction of HIV and BVDV (a model for HCV) was obtained in albumin with the Seitz KS80 filter, whereas good removal of non-enveloped viruses from IGIV was observed with the Cuno ZetaPlus® filter, possibly because of formation of virus-antibody complexes in IgG solutions.

Chromatography

Solid-phase adsorbents are used in the purification of factor VIII concentrates by ion exchange chromatography (Burnouf *et al.*, 1991) and by immunoaffinity chromatography (Griffin, 1991; Hrindra *et al.*, 1990). Similarly, ion exchange chromatography (Dike *et al.*, 1972; Heystek *et al.*, 1973; Middleton *et al.*, 1973), affinity chromatography (Burnouf *et al.*, 1989; Herring *et al.*, 1993) and immunoaffinity chromatography (Hrindra *et al.*, 1991) are used in the preparation of factor IX concentrates. Chromatographic purification may also be used in the further purification of IGIV (Hooper, 1997; Hooper *et al.*, 1988; Roussell and McCue, 1991) and albumin (More and Harvey, 1991), following ethanol fractionation.

Chromatographic purification of albumin and immunoglobulin has also been used instead of ethanol fractionation (Adcock *et al.*, 1998a). Anion exchange chromatography removed 4.2 $\log_{10}$ and 5.3 $\log_{10}$ of HAV with different matrices (Adcock *et al.*, 1998a), but only 1.5 $\log_{10}$ of HBsAg over a combination of three chromatographic steps (Adcock *et al.*, 1998b). A reduction of 2 $\log_{10}$ of B19 was observed by Schwarz *et al.* (1991) using anion exchange chromatography.

Affinity chromatography has been reported to remove 1.6 $\log_{10}$ of HAV (Johnston *et al.*, 2000) and 2 $\log_{10}$ of HIV and 7.6 $\log_{10}$ of a model virus for HBV (Ristol *et al.*, 1996). Human immunodeficiency virus infectivity has been shown to be reduced by 3–4 $\log_{10}$ by immunoaffinity chromatography used in the purification of factor VIII (Piszkiewicz *et al.*, 1989; Schreiber *et al.*, 1989). However, there have been at least three cases of HCV transmission by immunoaffinity purified factor VIII, two described by Shopnick *et al.* (1996) and one unpublished (J. Lusher, personal communication, 1991).

Many parameters determine the chromatographic behaviour of viruses, some of which are poorly understood (Burnouf, 1993). In order to control the process, it is necessary to establish the mechanism by which a virus is separated from the protein of interest. In the experimental studies reported, it is often not clear if the virus was unbound and removed by washing prior to product elution or if it was adsorbed to the matrix more strongly than the product. In the latter situation, a suitable procedure for decontaminating the matrix between each use is necessary to avoid potential contamination of subsequent product batches.

Nanofiltration

Developments in the manufacture of microporous membranes have resulted in membrane filtration technology being used for the removal of viruses from protein solutions, with the objective of retaining viruses whilst allowing the protein to pass through the membrane. As separation is based on size difference, the size of relevant proteins and viruses is critical (see Figure 20.2). The first applications of nanofiltration targeted removal of HIV (DiLeo and Allegrezza, 1991; Hamamoto *et al.*, 1989), a relatively large virus in comparison to most plasma proteins. Today, the principle objective is to eliminate viruses which may survive established methods of virus inactivation, in particular the non-enveloped viruses B19, HAV, TTV and similar viruses (Welch *et al.*, 2006).

Nanofiltration membranes are specified according to pore size, and are available with mean pore diameters ranging from 75 nm

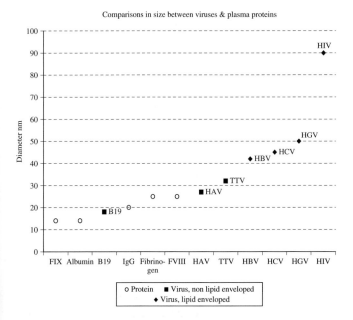

Comparisons in size between viruses & plasma proteins

Figure 20.2 Comparisons in size between viruses and plasma proteins.

to 15 nm, operating in either a cross-flow or a dead-end mode (Burnouf and Radosevich, 2003). However, it is the mean pore diameter that is specified, not the pore size-distribution, nor the diameter of the largest pore. This may explain why RNA from HCV (40–50 nm diameter) passed through a nominal 35 nm filter, although the filter complied with all pre- and post-filter integrity tests recommended by the manufacturer (Eibl *et al.*, 1996).

Nanofiltration has been applied to high-purity factor IX concentrates using membranes with a mean pore size from 35 nm to 15 nm (Burnouf-Radosevich *et al.*, 1994; Feldman and Roberts, 1998; Johnston *et al.*, 2000) with one manufacturer employing two 15 nm filters in series to ensure complete removal of a parvovirus (Over, 1998). Concentrates of prothrombin complex (PCC) contain proteins which are larger than factor IX and are consequently more difficult to filter (Burnouf and Radosevich, 2003). It is therefore not surprising that transmission of B19 has been reported (Lubetsky *et al.*, 2004) from a PCC that was nanofiltered using a 50 nm membrane (Josic *et al.*, 2000).

Immunoglobulins have also been subjected to nanofiltration, with most manufacturers using 35 nm filters (Dichtelmuller *et al.*, 1998; Holten *et al.*, 2002; Troccoli *et al.*, 1998). In order to use filters below 35 nm, it is necessary to remove aggregates and dimers from IgG (Troccoli, *et al.*, 1998) and some products have been processed to allow filtration at either 20 nm or 15 nm (Ireland *et al.*, 2004; Omar and Kempf, 2002; Stucki *et al.*, 1997; Terpstra *et al.*, 2006). In a study of process robustness, Terpstra *et al.* (2006) found pH to be the dominant process parameter, implying that virus retention may be influenced by charge interactions or small changes in protein solubility, both of which are pH dependent.

In some experimental studies, parvoviruses were surprisingly removed using a 35 nm filter. This behaviour may have been due to virus particles aggregating in the presence of amino acids (Yokoyama *et al.*, 2004) or to the formation of antibody-virus complexes (Kreil *et al.*, 2006). Viruses may adsorb to membranes

by charge or other interactions or may be retained by the polarized layer of concentrated protein which forms at membrane surfaces. All of these features must be simulated in down-scaled validation studies and must be controlled in routine manufacture to ensure that the expected degree of virus removal is achieved in routine practice.

Virus removal and inactivation at full scale

Virus removal is invariably measured in small-volume experiments which aim to simulate a manufacturing procedure. In addition to the difficulty of achieving accurate down-scaling using laboratory equipment, the complexity of overall manufacturing processes means that process operations tend to be studied individually rather than as the combined series of steps that make up a complete process. Even where scale-down is accurate, questions may remain over the validity of adding together results from steps studied individually.

Human parvovirus B19 DNA is present in most plasma pools at up to 10^8 to 10^9 genome equivalent/ml (Saldanha and Minor, 1996; Schmidt *et al.* 2001), a situation which provides an opportunity to determine how B19 partitions over a complete, full-scale, routine, manufacturing process. Hart *et al.* (1996) examined the distribution of B19 DNA in the manufacture of three batches of an ion-exchange purified factor VIII concentrate (Liberate®) using plasma collected in Scotland during a seasonal period of B19 infection. The mean volume of the plasma pools was 2800 litres, with the B19 DNA content of the pools estimated to be 1.5×10^7 copies/ml. The $\log_{10}$ reduction indices are shown for each of the main process steps in Table 20.10. Removal of B19 DNA over the complete process ranged from $\geq 4.2 \log_{10}$ to $\geq 6.4 \log_{10}$, with a mean reduction index of $\geq 5.5 \log_{10}$.

Freeze drying and heat treatment of Liberate® at 80 °C for 72 hours have been shown to inactivate 4.7 $\log_{10}$ of bovine parvovirus (BPV) (Roberts and Hart, 2000). Recently, Roberts *et al.* (2006) have found BPV more resistant to dry heat inactivation than B19, with $\geq 4.7 \log_{10}$ of B19 inactivated over freeze drying and 80 °C/72 h heat treatment of intermediate-purity factor VIII (8Y). If it can be assumed that B19 inactivation in dry heat treated Liberate® would be at least comparable with BPV inactivation, then combining the worst case physical removal of B19 DNA with an estimate of inactivation by dry heating, gives an overall B19 reduction for the complete Liberate®HT process of the order of $\geq 8.9 \log_{10}$.

Virus validation studies

Regulatory requirements

Although pasteurization was introduced for albumin in 1945, the development of effective physical or chemical treatments for virus inactivation of coagulation factors was not established until the 1980s. In 1987, the USA Food and Drug Administration (FDA) issued points to consider concerning the production of monoclonal antibodies, which touched upon the validation of processes for virus removal (Office of Biologics Research and Review, 1987). However, it was in 1991 that the EEC

Table 20.10 Removal of human parvovirus B19 DNA in full-scale manufacture of SNBTS high purity Factor VIII concentrate (Liberate®)[a].

Stage in FVIII process	Volume of process (L)[b]	B19 DNA (copies/mL)[b]	Reduction index ($\log_{10}$) for B19 DNA at each process stage			
			Batch A	Batch B	Batch C	Mean
Plasma	$2\,806 \pm 576$	$15 \pm 14 \ (\times 10^6)^c$				
Washed cryoprecipitate	96 ± 24	$92 \pm 112 \ (\times 10^6)$	1.1	1.5	0.6	1.1
Purified cryoprecipitate	112 ± 27	$1.7 \pm 1.2 \ (\times 10^6)$	1.9	1.9	2.9	2.3
SD treated, ion exchange eluate	16.6 ± 2.1	$\geq 2.5 \ (\times 10^3)^d$	≥ 2.8	≥ 0.8	≥ 3.0	≥ 2.2
Overall process			≥ 5.8	≥ 4.2	≥ 6.4	≥ 5.5

[a] Presented by Hart *et al.*, 1996.

[b] Mean and standard deviation from three production batches of SNBTS Factor VIII (Liberate®). NAT for B19 DNA performed by S. Graham and F. Davidson under the guidance of P. Simmonds and P. L. Yap.

[c] B19 DNA content of plasma pools estimated by addition of values measured for cryoprecipitate and cryosupernatant.

[d] Limit of detection.

Committee for Proprietary Medicinal Products (CPMP) issued guidance specifically on virus removal and inactivation procedures (Committee for Proprietary Medicinal Products, 1991), which specified how virus validation procedures should be performed and interpreted, with further guidance in 1992 for products derived from human plasma (Committee for Proprietary Medicinal Products, 1992).

In October 1993, the Federal Health Office in Germany discovered that plasma was being tested incorrectly for HIV by the company UB Plasma (Gedye, 1993), an event which resulted in the closure of the Federal Health Office and the transfer, in July 1994, of responsibility for the regulation of blood and blood products in Germany to the Paul-Ehrlich-Institut (PEI). At the same time there were transmissions in Germany of HBV by pasteurized factor IX concentrate from Behringwerke (Jantsch-Plunger *et al.*, 1995), HIV by β-propiolactone/UV treated factor IX concentrate from Biotest (Kupfer *et al.*, 1995), HAV by SD treated factor VIII concentrate from Octapharma (Gerritzen *et al.*, 1992b) and HCV by IGIV from Baxter (Berger *et al.*, 1997). In response, the PEI announced, in August 1994, that plasma products must achieve at least a 10 $\log_{10}$ reduction for enveloped viruses and a 6 $\log_{10}$ reduction for non-enveloped viruses, with each manufacturing procedure containing two steps capable of reducing enveloped viruses by 4 $\log_{10}$ each, and with at least one step that reduces non-enveloped viruses by 4 $\log_{10}$ (Paul-Ehrlich-Institut, 1994). The European regulatory authority accepted the main principles introduced by the PEI and revised its policy to include the guidance that: 'It will be desirable in many cases to incorporate two distinct effective steps which complement each other in their mode of action such that any virus surviving the first step would be effectively inactivated/removed by the second. At least one of the steps should be effective against non-enveloped viruses.' (Committee for Proprietary Medicinal Products, 1996b).

Current European regulations relevant to the plasma fractionation industry are contained within two documents, namely, *Note for Guidance on Plasma-derived Medicinal Products* (Committee for Proprietary Medicinal Products, 2001) and *Note for Guidance on Virus Validation Studies: the Design, Contribution and Interpretation of Studies Validating the Inactivation and Removal of Viruses* (Committee for Proprietary Medicinal Products, 1996a). Virus validation studies are performed following these guidance documents in order to estimate the potential of a particular step within a manufacturing process to remove or inactivate viruses. These studies are conducted using representative 'scale-down' version of the manufacturing process by deliberately spiking with high titre virus prior to the virus elimination step, followed by processing of the virus containing material, and measuring the virus remaining afterwards. The logarithmic values of the virus present at the end of the process step compared with that at the start provide a measure of its potential to eliminate the virus under test. Guidance in CPMP (2001) outlines the types of manufacturing process steps during the manufacture of plasma products that can contribute to virus elimination, the process variables and in-process limit considerations for virus removal, and the choice of viruses to be used in these studies, whereas CPMP (1996a) is a generic guidance document for virus validation studies of biologicals. Table 20.11 lists the viruses that are recommended for use in virus validation studies on plasma-derived products, except that West Nile virus is not required by CPMP.

Design of virus validation studies

Virus validation studies are normally performed separately, on each individual step in a manufacturing process and the reduction factors for each step added together, so long as the steps eliminate the virus by independent means, and the level of virus inactivation or removal for the step is more than 1 $\log_{10}$. When validating a process step for virus elimination the step may either be one already incorporated into the manufacturing process, for example precipitation as part of the protein purification process, or a treatment such a solvent/detergent (SD) treatment, specifically included in the process for virus inactivation. Alternatively, the step may be one that has been added to an existing process, such as terminal dry heat treatment or nanofiltration in order to complement virus elimination step(s) already present. In each

Table 20.11 Viral agents of concern in plasma products and viruses for use in validation studies.

Virus	Family	Genome	Lipid envelope	Size (nm)	Model	Relevance	Resistance of relevant/model viruses to physicochemical treatments
Human immunodeficiency virus (HIV-1 and HIV-2)	Retroviridae	ssRNA	Yes	80–100	HIV-1	Relevant virus	Low
Hepatitis A virus (HAV)	Picornaviridae	ssRNA	No	27–32	HAV EMC[a]	HAV – relevant virus EMC – model virus	High
Hepatitis B virus (HBV)	Hepadna viridae	Partly dsDNA	Yes	42	None[b]	PRV recommended as a model virus	Low
Hepatitis C virus (HCV)	Flaviviridae	ssRNA	Yes	40–50	BVDV[c] Sindbis	Model viruses	Low
B19	Parvoviridae	ssDNA	No	18–26	CPV[d] BPV PPV MVM B19[e]	Model viruses	Very high
West Nile virus (WNV)	Flaviviridae	ssRNA	Yes	40–50	WNV	Relevant virus	High Low

[a] EMC – encephalomyocarditis virus; this may be used in validation studies for immunoglobulin processes where neutralizing effects of the product may overestimate the potential of the process to inactivate/remove virus.

[b] Although there is no practical model virus for HBV, guidelines (CPMP, 1996a) recommend inclusion of a herpesvirus such as PRV (pseudorabies virus) to represent enveloped DNA viruses.

[c] BVDV – bovine viral diarrhoea virus.

[d] CPV – canine parvovirus; BPV – bovine parvovirus; PPV – porcine parvovirus; MVM – minute virus of mice.

[e] Although not a regulatory requirement, some studies have been performed with B19 using plasma containing high titre parvovirus B19 and assayed on an erythroid based cell line susceptible to B19 infection (Blümel et al., 2002; Boschetti et al., 2004; Prikhod'ko, 2005; Roberts et al., 2006).

case, process variables will exist that are either fixed within already defined ranges, for example temperature during SD treatment, or which may need to be defined or adjusted following the results of virus elimination studies, for example residual moisture limits during dry heat treatment. When designing the study, these process variables will be validated for virus elimination including how the process limits influence virus elimination. This approach becomes very complex and expensive when a process has several parameters that can vary simultaneously, and the combined effect of each variable may not be predictable for any of the viruses being validated. In such circumstances, a matrix approach using two or more levels (e.g. high, low and standard), normally of three or more parameters, can be taken. An alternative approach, where the limits of process parameters may be predicted as 'worst case' conditions for virus contamination, such as lower temperature limits, pH farthest from neutral, can be taken together with standard conditions. However, depending on the results, further studies may be required.

Once the parameters to be examined in a study have been selected, further details of the study design are made. These include selection of sampling time points, which is particularly relevant for virus inactivation steps, in order to demonstrate the rate at which the virus is killed (kinetics of inactivation) and whether this rate varies during the process, in order to support claims of effectiveness. In addition, it may be necessary to perform the study in duplicate, as reproducibility of the ability of a process to remove/inactivate viruses provides assurance of the reliability of the data. Reproducibility of the data is of greater importance for processes that do not completely eliminate viruses and/or are sensitive to small variations in process parameters, for example during precipitation steps.

Guidance on sampling time-points can either be gained from the literature or be based on experience. For example, treatment at low pH can be highly effective for inactivation of some enveloped viruses with all detectable virus inactivated during the first few minutes under standard processing conditions. In these circumstances, samples should be taken at several early time-points in addition to later time-point(s) when the virus has been inactivated to below the limit of assay detection. Enveloped virus inactivation by SD treatment is often so rapid that little or no infectious virus remains immediately following treatment under normal manufacturing conditions; therefore the virus inactivation kinetics can be difficult to measure. Under such circumstances, regulatory guidance from CPMP (1996a) requires other studies be performed to demonstrate that the virus is indeed inactivated using process parameters that are at the manufacturing limits that would represent a 'worst case' for virus inactivation, for example low temperature, low SD concentrations, high protein/lipid concentrations, or even beyond the limits that would be experienced within the manufacturing process. Other processes may inactivate the virus more slowly, such as dry heat treatment at 80 °C of material spiked with parvovirus models; therefore samples can be taken at time intervals separated by several hours (Hart *et al.*, 1994b; Roberts and Hart, 2000; Savage *et al.*, 1998).

Where a process eliminates a virus either partly or wholly by removal it should be shown, wherever possible, where the virus

partitions and whether virus removal from one area of the process can be balanced by its concentration in another part of the process, for example during precipitation steps both supernatant and precipitate fractions should be assayed even if only one of these materials remains in the product stream and the other is discarded.

Selection of virus

Selection of which virus(es) to use in studies is generally straightforward. The panel of viruses currently recommended for virus validation of plasma products (CPMP, 2001) is presented in Table 20.11, which also includes West Nile virus that is not required by CPMP (2001). However, there are some processes for which only certain viruses need be selected, or where some model viruses may represent a greater challenge to the virus elimination process. For example, it is well established that SD treatment is highly effective for enveloped viruses but not for non-enveloped viruses; therefore validation of such processes need only be performed on the enveloped viruses, HIV, an enveloped DNA virus such as pseudorabies virus and a hepatitis C virus model. Regulations require manufacturing processes to include at least one step that is effective against non-enveloped virus (CPMP, 2001); therefore when a manufacturing process introduces a virus elimination step to complement one that is effective only for inactivation of enveloped viruses, this step should be validated for non-enveloped viruses of concern in plasma (HAV and parvovirus). It may also be validated for its effectiveness for enveloped viruses to provide further evidence that the manufacturing process can eliminate these agents. In such circumstances, the extent to which the validation of the non-enveloped viruses is performed may be more detailed than for enveloped viruses, for example robustness studies examining variation on process parameters would normally only be performed using the non-enveloped virus offering the greater challenge to the virus elimination procedure. In summary, virus validation data for plasma products should be gained for all five virus models listed in Table 20.11 for at least one step that is effective against that virus, with process parameters varied for the virus(es) most resistant to elimination by that step.

Where a cell culture system does not exist for the relevant virus, as is the case for HCV, there is a choice of several model viruses including BVDV, Sindbis (SIN) and Semiliki Forest virus (SFV), all of which have been used by plasma fractionators to provide data in support of their processes. However, considerable variation exists between these model viruses in their susceptibility to treatment at low pH (pH 4). Figure 20.3 illustrates the virus inactivation kinetics of BVDV and Sindbis in the low pH incubation step of the SNBTS liquid immunoglobulin process. This clearly illustrates that the BVDV strain used in this study (NADL) is more resistant to low pH inactivation than Sindbis. Others have also reported incomplete inactivation of the NADL strain of BVDV with low pH (Bos *et al.*, 1998). However, an alternative strain of BVDV, Oregon C24 V, was rapidly and completely inactivated at pH 4 (Omar *et al.*, 1996). Therefore, not only the choice of model virus but also the particular strain of virus may influence how effective a step appears to be.

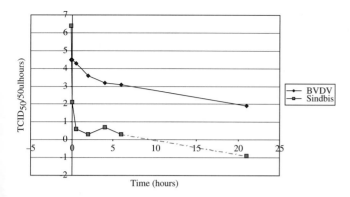

Figure 20.3 Inactivation of HCV model viruses in SNBTS Liquid Immunoglobulin at pH 4.1 and 34–35°C. The dashed indicates viruses beyond this point were below the limit of assay detection.

Recently, data have become available for the inactivation of human parvovirus B19, owing to the availability of erythroid based cell lines that support the replication of this virus (Miyagawa *et al.*, 1999). Results demonstrate that B19 is more sensitive to virus inactivation by pH 4, pasteurization and dry heat treatment than parvovirus models commonly used (Blümel *et al.*, 2002; Boschetti *et al.*, 2004; Kaserman *et al.*, 2004; Roberts *et al.*, 2006). Therefore, validation data generated using parvovirus model viruses may underestimate the ability of a process to inactivate B19 parvovirus. However, the animal parvovirus models, such as porcine parvovirus (PPV), bovine parvovirus (BPV), canine parvovirus (CPV) and minute virus of mice (MVM) remain useful as, not only do they offer a relatively easy cell culture assay system, they also challenge the process with an agent more resistant to inactivation by physicochemical means and therefore test a process for its potential to inactivate viruses more resistant than B19.

Establishing a down-scaled process

Virus validation studies involve the deliberate addition of virus to in-process material followed by sampling at various points during the process. Therefore, such studies are performed in laboratories that are specialized in virology methodologies and are separate to the manufacturing facility. In order to provide a reliable measure of the potential of the process to eliminate virus, the processing used in the laboratory, that is, the 'scale-down process' must represent the manufacturing process as closely as possible. For some virus elimination steps, such as terminal pasteurization or dry heat treatment, 'scale-down' is relatively straightforward because the spiked material can be processed with the same volume, containers and critical parameters (e.g. pH and temperature) used in manufacturing. For other processes involving much larger volumes at manufacturing scale, such as precipitation or chromatography, demonstration that the scale-down is representative of full-scale is more complex. Comparisons of various process characteristics such as pH, temperature, protein concentration, yield, etc., will be required and must be shown to be equivalent. Once a scaled-down model has been established, its use in virus spiking studies may also be altered

by the presence of the spike itself. For this reason, the volume of virus added to a process should be less than 10% and for some processes may need to be significantly less, for example during nanofiltration studies the proportion of virus is normally of the order of ≤1% so that the filtration rate is not affected greatly. In any event, critical process parameters that may be affected by the presence of the virus spike, such as pH, can be adjusted after spiking to help minimize the influence of the virus on processing. The influence of the spike can further be assessed, either prior to the virus spiking study, or in parallel with it, by performing the scale-down process in the presence of a 'dummy' spike (i.e. the virus-free medium representative as close as possible to that in which the virus spike is prepared) so that critical process parameters, that cannot be easily measured if virus is present in the sample, such as moisture content and product yield, can be assessed in non-virology laboratories. If the dummy spike is found to influence the scale-down process sufficiently, to the extent that it is no longer a valid representation of the manufacturing process, it would be necessary to modify the spiking procedure, for example reduce the proportion of virus added or use a more purified preparation of the virus.

Performing a virus validation study

It is a regulatory requirement that virus validation studies used to support the licensing of a plasma product are performed to the principles of good laboratory practice (GLP). Therefore, laboratories performing such studies must comply with GLP as defined by their national monitoring authority (Department of Health, 1999). In practical terms the facility conducting the study must have the correct systems for planning, performing, monitoring, recording and reporting the study. Part of the measures taken to ensure GLP compliance of a regulatory study are that a 'study plan', detailing the procedures to be followed, and a 'study director' (i.e. an individual responsible for the GLP compliance of the study) are provided for each study before the study begins.

In conducting a virus elimination study, it is recommended that minimal manipulation of samples is made prior to quantitation of the virus, that is, samples are best assayed for virus concentration immediately following sampling rather than storing them frozen or concentrating by ultracentrifugation or dialysis because the effects of such procedures on individual samples may be difficult to control. It is therefore necessary to assess whether the material into which virus is being spiked has any cytotoxic effect on the cell line(s) used for virus quantitiation, and whether it may also interfere with detection of the virus prior to initiating the virus spiking part of the study. In addition, it may be necessary to determine whether the material has any neutralizing antibodies that may affect interpretation of the data. Such cytotoxicity/interference/neutralization studies are therefore conducted using material(s) representative of those that will be used and generated during the study. These material(s) are tested in various dilutions on the relevant cell lines to identify a non-cytotoxic dilution, and additionally will be spiked with known quantities of virus to identify dilutions of material where any interfering or neutralizing effects on virus will be removed. The study plan therefore includes such preliminary testing of the in-process material so that when the virus spiking, processing and sampling is performed, samples can be diluted immediately upon collection to the non-cytotoxic, non-interfering/neutralizing level and assayed for virus titres.

Interpreting results of a virus validation

Virus quantitation is routinely performed either by quantal methods, such as $TCID_{50}$ (tissue culture infectious dose when 50% of the cultures are affected), or quantitative, such as tissue culture plaque assays, where one plaque represents one infectious particle. In either case, the quantity of virus present in samples is expressed as log_{10} per unit volume inoculated and the capacity of the process step to eliminate virus (the 'reduction factor') is calculated by subtracting the logarithmic value of virus present in the processed material from that in the spiked material prior to processing, taking into account any volume changes that may have occurred during processing (CPMP, 1996a). Where the process results in no virus being detected after treatment, the minimum detectable limit of the assay can be calculated and the reduction factor expressed as a '≥' value (CPMP, 1997). When a process is anticipated to eliminate large amounts of a particular virus, the reduction factor can be maximized by assaying as much processed material as is practical. Processes that generate reduction factors around 4 log_{10} or greater can be considered to have a 'clear effect' for that particular virus tested. However, other considerations, such as whether the most appropriate model virus was used, whether the scale-down used during the virus validation was comparable to the manufacturing process, whether the reduction factor is influenced by variations in key process parameters, and the kinetics of inactivation (if appropriate) should also be taken into account before the process can be concluded as effective. Reduction factors that are less than 4 log_{10} (but greater than 1 log_{10}) may not be as effective but, assuming they are robust and the scale-down is comparable to manufacturing scale, can be considered to contribute to the overall virus reduction of the process. The overall reduction factor for a manufacturing process for each of the viruses of concern should have a target of $\geq 6 \log_{10}$. This can be achieved for some viruses in a single process such as inactivation of enveloped viruses by SD treatment, or may require summing of reduction factors from more than one distinct virus elimination step, or may require the introduction of an additional step specifically to remove/inactivate viruses, for example nanofiltration.

Features illustrated in virus validation studies

Treatment with solvent/detergent

In SD treatment, HIV-1 and model viruses such as BVDV, Sindbis and PRV are inactivated rapidly, indicating that measured reduction factors considerably underestimate the potential of the process to inactivate these viruses (Biesert, 1996; Biesert and Suhartono, 1998; Horowitz et al., 1998; Roberts, 2000).

Treatment at low pH

Incubation at pH 4.0–4.4 has proven effective against lipid-enveloped viruses such as HIV, PRV, Sindbis and Semiliki Forest virus (SFV) (Bos et al., 1998; Cai et al., 2005; Hamalainen et al., 1992; Kempf et al., 1991; Omar et al., 1996; Reid et al., 1988), but the rate of inactivation can vary according to the virus used. Sindbis is inactivated more rapidly than HIV and inactivation of BVDV was incomplete in one study (Bos et al., 1998) but not in another (Omar et al., 1996). The non-enveloped viruses polio and CPV are unaffected by pH 4 treatment (SNBTS unpublished results) but a $\geq 5 \log_{10}$ reduction of B19 infectivity has been observed at pH 4 (Boschetti et al., 2004) and a 2.6 log_{10} reduction of EMC, a model for HAV, at pH 4.25 (Bos et al., 1998). These variations in susceptibility to low pH demonstrate that choice of virus is important and that data from model virus studies may not necessarily represent the true virus inactivation potential of a manufacturing process.

Dry heat treatment

Heat treatment of the dried product is normally undertaken in the final sealed container and, unlike other virus elimination procedures, carries no risk of re-contamination. Heating at 80 °C or greater has proven to be effective against HIV, HAV, HBV and HCV. Effectiveness against parvovirus B19 has been demonstrated recently (Roberts et al., 2006). However, studies with model viruses have shown that both the kinetics and degree of inactivation can be influenced by the residual moisture content of the freeze dried plug (Savage et al., 1998; Snape, 1987; SNBTS, unpublished data) and by the product formulation (Chandra et al., 2002; SNBTS, unpublished data) indicating that operating limits for these parameters are essential (McIntosh et al., 1996).

Operational considerations

Freedom from infectious agents cannot be established by end-product testing and is therefore critically dependent on suitable pathogen elimination procedures being performed correctly on every occasion and on the avoidance of any re-contamination following their completion (Foster et al., 1988b).

In order to ensure that a process is performed correctly it is necessary to know the mechanisms and the parameters that determine the outcome and to establish suitable limits for all influential parameters (see Table 20.12). Where chemicals are added, it is necessary to confirm that the correct quantities have been added by weight or volume reconciliation and by chemical analysis of samples. Temperature and mixing profiles should be determined for each type of vessel used, with control of selected parameters throughout the process using separate sensors for monitoring and control. A continuous record of temperatures and of mixer operation should be obtained throughout the treatment. For in-process treatments, such as SD treatment, it is desirable to perform the process in two stages, with a period of treatment in one sealed vessel followed by aseptic transfer to a second sealed vessel situated within a contained 'virus-free' area.

A number of virus inactivation procedures are performed at an intermediate stage of processing, including SD treatment, low pH

Table 20.12 Examples of virus elimination procedures and the process parameters to be considered.

Virus elimination step	Key process parameter	Process values/limit[a]
Solvent/detergent treatment	pH	Product dependent
	Solvent concentration	0.3% (w/w)/0.24–0.36%
	Detergent concentration	1.0% (w/w)/0.8–1.2%
	Temperature	$25 \pm 1\,°C$
	Duration	>6 hours
	Protein concentration	Product dependent
	Lipid concentration	Product dependent
pH4/pepsin treatment	pH	4.0 ± 0.1
	Temperature	$35 \pm 1\,°C$
	Duration	>21 hours
	Protein concentration	Product dependent
	Stabilizer (e.g. sugar/amino acid) concentration	Product dependent
Dry heat treatment	Temperature	$80.25 \pm 0.75\,°C$
	Duration	>72 hours
	Protein concentration	Product dependent
	Stabilizer (e.g. sugar/amino acid) concentration	Product dependent
	Residual moisture content	Product dependent, for example 0.2–2% (w/w)
Pasteurization	Temperature	$60 \pm 0.5\,°C$
	Duration	>10 hours
	Protein concentration	45–200 g/l
Cohn fractionation	pH and ionic strength	Varies dependent on fractionation step
	Ethanol concentration	
	Temperature	
	Duration in ethanol	
	Centrifugation conditions	
Nanofiltration	pH and ionic strength	Product dependent
	Protein concentration	
	Pressure	
	Flow rate and flux	

[a]The values given are those used for products prepared at the SNBTS Protein Fractionation Centre.

treatment and pasteurization processes involving carbohydrate stabilization. In these circumstances, recontamination following virus inactivation must be avoided to ensure product safety. Strict containment is required to achieve this, involving control of facilities, equipment and procedures. This was more difficult to achieve prior to the screening of donors for hepatitis C, when virtually all plasma pools contained infectious material, and isolated incidents of virus transmission may well have been a result of a cross-contamination rather than the failure of the virus inactivation procedure. These considerations apply equally to processes used for the physical removal of pathogens, but are more difficult to achieve in practice because of the closely integrated nature of many of the fractionation procedures.

Risk assessments

It is now also a regulatory requirement that risk assessments of viral contamination should be undertaken for plasma-derived medicinal products (Committee for Medicinal Products for Human Use, 2004a). These guidelines outline the various factors that should be considered in estimating the potential input of viruses against the potential of the process to eliminate viruses. Factors contributing to the the virus input are the likelihood of viraemic donations entering the plasma pool (influenced by factors such as the prevalence of disease in the donor population, length of window period) and the titre of the virus that could enter the plasma pool (determined by the sensitivity of detection tests, the volume tested, the volume of donation, and the number of donors contributing to the plasma pool). Once the theoretical viral load in the plasma pool has been estimated, the overall potential of the fractionation process to remove virus, using virus validation data, can be incorporated, together with the number of final product vials produced from the pool, so that the theoretical level of virus in a final product vial can be calculated. The calculation can be summarized by the equation: $N = c \times V \div R$, where N is the number of virus particles per vial of product, c is the concentration of virus in the plasma pool, V is the volume of plasma to produce one vial of product and R is the overall reduction factor obtained from virus validation studies (Committee for Medicinal Products for Human Use, 2004a).

Table 20.13 HCV risk assessments for IVIG and Factor VIII concentrate.

(a) Estimated HCV load in a manufacturing pool of German plasma

Product	IVIG (5 g)	FVIII (500 IU)
Pool size (donations)	10 000	14 000
Residual risk of an infectious donation entering the plasma pool after testing[a]	2.27×10^{-7}	2.27×10^{-7}
Potential number of infected donors per plasma pool	2.27×10^{-3}	3.18×10^{-3}
Titre per donation (geq/ml)[b]	≤ 6105	≤ 6105
Total virus in production pool (geq)[c]	≤ 3469	≤ 3469

(b) Estimated HCV load in a final product dose manufactured from German plasma

Product	IVIG (5 g)	FVIII (500 IU)
Pool size (donations)	10 000	14 000
No. doses of final product	1 400	600
Quantity of virus per dose (geq)[d]	$\leq 10^{0.4}$	$\leq 10^{0.9}$
Virus inactivation during processing ($\log_{10}$)	$\geq 6.5^{e}$	$\geq 4.4^{f}$
		$\geq 3.7^{g}$
Total quantity of virus per vial (geq)	$\leq 10^{-6.1}$	$\leq 10^{-7.2}$

[a] From Offergeld et al., 2005. HCV incidence = 1:4 400 000 with NAT testing and a window period of ten days.

[b] Value based on 95% confidence limits for HCV PCR in mini-pools (29geq. x 96 = 2784 geq.).

[c] Titre per ml × donation volume (300 ml) × potential number of infected donations in the pool.

[d] Total quantity of virus in production pool ÷ no. of vials of final product obtained from the plasma pool.

[e] Low pH treatment, using Sindbis as the marker virus for HCV.

[f] Solvent/detergent treatment, using BVDV as the marker virus for HCV.

[g] Dry heat treatment (80 °C/72h), using BVDV as the marker virus for HCV.

Neutralizing antibody may also be considered as a virus elimination step. However, the true contribution made by antibodies is difficult to demonstrate. Whilst incorporating virus elimination data it is important to use data that satisfy criteria set out in regulatory guidelines (CPMP, 1996a; 2001), for example only results from steps that eliminate the virus by independent means can be added together.

An example of a risk assessment for HCV is given in Table 20.13 for IGIV and factor VIII concentrate prepared by SNBTS. In this assessment, several 'worst case' assumptions have been made, for example a potentially infected donation only fractionates into the product in question, all window-period donations are infective and for NAT tests the viraemic titre equals the 95% cut-off sensitivity. The estimated potential contamination in each final product vial is therefore likely to be a significant over-estimate. The regulatory guidelines do not specify what constitutes a safe limit.

Emerging viruses

Please refer back to Chapter 6.

Although plasma products manufactured today are extremely safe and the risk of transmission of a life-threatening virus is highly controlled, newly emergent viruses may challenge plasma product manufacturing processes and reinforce the need for robust procedures, capable of eliminating a range of known and unknown viral contaminants. Recent blood-borne viral pathogens that have been of concern include West Nile virus (WNV) and severe acute respiratory syndrome coronavirus (SARS-CoV). Although WNV infections are normally mild or asymptomatic, occasionally the virus can cause severe meningoencephalitis which can be fatal, particularly in the elderly. Outbreaks have been described in various countries in the last century. However, an epidemic in the USA in 2002 raised concerns over the safety of blood products. Although WNV transmission occurred through organ transplant and blood components, no transmissions have been described through plasma products. The safety of plasma products against WNV transmission is primarily due to the fact that WNV belongs to the same family as HCV, that is Flaviviridae, and steps directed at the elimination of HCV should also be effective for WNV. Studies performed since the 2002 USA outbreak have shown WNV to be sensitive to pasteurization, SD treatment and low pH treatment (Jakubik et al., 2004; Kasermann et al., 2004; Kreil, 2004; Kreil et al., 2003; Remington et al., 2004). Similarly, no transmissions of SARS-CoV have been described through plasma products, and studies performed on this virus, which is also enveloped, have demonstrated it to be inactivated effectively by established virus inactivation processes including pasteurization (Yunoki et al., 2004) and by SD treatment (Darnell and Taylor, 2006). It is fortuitous that these recent outbreaks of viral infection involved enveloped viruses which, like the other major viruses of concern, HIV, HBV and HCV, are inactivated by virus inactivation methods already established in plasma fractionation.

Although non-enveloped viruses have been described in the recent past that could potentially be transmitted by plasma products, namely small anelloviruses including torquetenovirus (TTV), these viruses have not been associated with disease. Such small non-enveloped viruses present a considerable challenge to the plasma fractionation process as they are resistant to methods directed at the viral envelope, and their small size (around 30 nm or less) may leave removal by nanofiltration incomplete. Recent model virus inactivation studies using chick anaemia virus, which is similar in size to TTV and has similarities in its genomic layout, and porcine circovirus (17 nm) have demonstrated a high level of resistance to pasteurization and dry heat treatment (Welch et al., 2006). Although plasma products manufactured today are much safer than they have ever been, the development of a generic virus inactivation process, that would eliminate small non-enveloped virus of this type, remains a challenge to the plasma fractionation industry.

Recombinant coagulation factor concentrates

Concern over potential pathogen transmission by plasma-derived coagulation factors has resulted in recombinant-derived concentrates of factor VIII and factor IX being used preferentially for the treatment of haemophilia A and B, respectively. Despite the view that recombinant products are safer theoretically, recombinant coagulation factors are manufactured using a number of substances of animal origin, each of which could harbour infectious agents. Human albumin may be used to support cell culture and to stabilize the product, although this latter application is now being phased out.

Rodent cell lines

Recombinant coagulation factors are obtained by the culture of genetically engineered Chinese hamster ovary (CHO) or baby hamster kidney (BHK) cells and the resultant cell lines must be screened for a wide range of viruses (Committee for Proprietary Medicinal Products, 1997). Monoclonal antibodies used for immunopurification must also comply with these guidelines. Although screening of the master cell bank provides a degree of assurance that products will be free from infection, viruses which are present below the limit of detection, known viruses which are not included in the screening, unknown viruses and new viruses will not be detected.

Growth media

A number of biological substances may be used to support cell culture, including bovine serum, insulin and human albumin. Although advances are being made in the development of protein-free media, it is likely that the culture of seed stocks will continue to require the use of protein-containing media. Fetal bovine serum (FBS) is believed to have been the source of the bovine viral diarrhoea virus (BVDV) which contaminated a recombinant interferon (Harasawa and Sasaki, 1995) and the

epizootic haemorrhagic disease virus (EHDV) which was detected during the production of a recombinant product from CHO cells (Rabenau et al., 1993). Bovine polyomavirus (BPyV), a small non-enveloped virus, has been detected in 70% of batches of commercial FBS produced in Europe, North America and New Zealand (Kappeler et al., 1996; Schuurman et al., 1991; Wang et al., 2004) and BPyV DNA has been detected in veterinary vaccines (Kappeler et al., 1996). It is commercial practice to test FBS for viruses only after pooling; consequently, low prevalence contaminants may escape detection. One example concerns the Cache valley virus (CVV), which can cause serious disease in humans (Sexton et al., 1997) and which has been implicated in three major production incidents concerning the manufacture of biotechnology products (Onions, 2004).

Virus elimination

The first generation of recombinant coagulation factor concentrates depended on chromatographic purification for the elimination of viruses. This is no longer viewed as adequate and all products are now expected to be subjected to a defined virus inactivation or removal process. However, as with plasma products, further advances are required to ensure elimination of small non-enveloped viruses, such as BPyV.

Transmission of viruses

The possible transmission of animal viruses to patients treated with recombinant coagulation factor concentrates does not appear to have been investigated. However, studies have been performed concerning the transmission of human viruses. Antibodies to human parvovirus B19 (Aygoren-Pursun and Scharrer, 1997; Gaboulaud et al., 2002) and to TTV (Azzi et al., 2001) have been detected in patients following treatment with recombinant concentrates, with human albumin, present as an excipient, being regarded as responsible. However, the relative sensitivity of B19 to inactivation by pasteurization (Blümel et al., 2002) suggests that B19 infection may have been community acquired or due to an animal parvovirus producing antibodies similar to those of B19.

Prion agents

Please refer back to Chapter 9.

Background

The possibility that human prion diseases might be transmissible by blood products was first raised (Preece, 1986) after sporadic Creutzfeldt-Jakob disease (sCJD) had been transmitted to patients being treated with human growth hormone. Although no good evidence was found to support this hypothesis (Foster, 2000) the discovery of variant CJD (vCJD) and its association with the epidemic of bovine spongiform encephalopathy (BSE) in the UK (Will et al., 1996) subsequently raised concern that vCJD might be transmissible via plasma products (Ludlam, 1997). As a result of these concerns, a number of precautionary measures were introduced

(Foster, 2000), including a ban on the use of UK donor plasma for fractionation (Department of Health, 1998) and the purchase of a paid-donor plasma collection company in the USA by the UK government (Department of Health, 2002). There is evidence of transfusion-transmitted vCJD infection to four UK patients following transfusion of red cells (Llewelyn *et al.*, 2004; Peden *et al.*, 2004; Wroe *et al.*, 2006) but, as of October 2007, no cases of vCJD had been associated with the administration of plasma products.

Currently, 204 cases of vCJD have been diagnosed worldwide, with 166 in the UK, 22 in France, 4 in Ireland and 3 in the USA. Although 97% of known cases of BSE have been found in the UK, infected animals have been diagnosed in 26 different countries. In the absence of suitable diagnostic screening, neither the number of animals infected with BSE nor the prevalence of vCJD infection in the human population is known. Given the high resistance of prion agents to inactivation (Taylor, 2003), attention has focused on their removal by separation technologies compatible with plasma products. Manufacturers are encouraged to undertake product-specific investigational studies (Committee for Medicinal Products for Human Use, 2004b) and to critically evaluate their manufacturing processes in light of published data (Committee for Medicinal Products for Human Use, 2004c).

Investigational fractionation studies

A number of studies have been undertaken to determine the extent to which prion agents may be removed by processes used in the preparation of plasma products. Most experiments have been carried out by adding high titre prion infectivity to a small volume of solution and processing this in a manner intended to simulate full-scale manufacturing, with the distribution of prion agent determined immunochemically, by Western blotting or a conformation dependent immunoassay (CDI) (Vey *et al.*, 2002), or by a rodent bioassay designed to measure infectious dose, 50 (ID_{50}). High titre materials for 'spiking' starting solutions have been extracted from infected brain in the form of either brain homogenate (BH), a microsomal fraction (MF), caveola-like domains (CLD) or semi-purified fibrils (PrP^{Sc}). Prion agents employed have included hamster-passaged scrapie (strains 263 K and Sc237), murine-passaged scrapie (strain ME7) and murine-passaged BSE (strain 301 V).

Processes have also been examined using infected rodent blood, with the distribution of prion agent determined by bioassay using the method of limiting dilution titration (Brown *et al.*, 1999). The prion agents employed in these studies include murine-passaged Gerstmann-Sträussler-Scheinker (GSS) syndrome (Fukuoka-1 strain), hamster-passaged scrapie (strain 263K) and murine-passaged BSE (strain 301 V).

Most prion removal studies have examined the performance of process operations individually. Unit operations studied include various precipitation steps, depth filtration processes, adsorption chromatography and nanofiltration. In some studies, the performance of a number of process operations has been examined in sequence or in combination. Technologies examined in this manner include multiple precipitation steps (Brown *et al.*, 1998; 1999; Cai *et al.*, 2002; Thyer *et al.*, 2006a), precipitation

followed by depth filtration (Reichl *et al.*, 2002), precipitation with filter aid (Gregori *et al.*, 2004; Morgenthaler *et al.*, 2002), two different depth filtration processes (Reichl *et al.*, 2002), and two ion exchange steps used in the chromatographic purification of IgG and albumin (Thyer *et al.*, 2006a).

Ideally, investigational studies should examine prion removal over a complete process as well as at individual steps (Pocchiari, 1991). The degree to which a prion agent is removed is described by a reduction factor (RF) expressed in logarithmic form. Reduction factors of $<1 \log_{10}$ are regarded as not significant due to the degree of error associated with the assay of prion agents. The interpretation of RF data may be misleading if an apparently high RF value reflects a high titre present in a spiking material rather than a high degree of partitioning.

Removal of prions by precipitation

Prion agents have generally been found to partition predominantly into the solid phase in protein precipitation processes. A number of cold-ethanol precipitation steps have been found to have significant reduction factors in individual spiking experiments, precipitation of fraction (I) + II + III and fraction IV in the preparation of human albumin and precipitation of fraction (I) + III in the preparation of human immunoglobulin being of particular importance (see Table 20.14).

Where successive precipitation steps have been studied in combination, a progressive reduction of prion agent by precipitation into successive precipitate fractions has been generally observed, both in experiments using brain-derived material for spiking (Brown *et al.*, 1998; Cai *et al.*, 2002; Thyer *et al.*, 2006a) and in experiments in which infected rodent plasma was processed (Brown *et al.*, 1998; Brown *et al.*, 1999). However, the substantial difference in the titre of prion agent processed and differences in the way results are expressed make quantitative comparisons between endogenous and exogenous experiments difficult.

Removal of prions by depth filtration

Depth filtration processes are employed in the manufacture of human immunogloblin and human albumin to clarify solutions following both precipitation and re-suspension of precipitates. Many of the procedures currently in use exhibit a high degree of prion removal (Table 20.15). In contrast to results obtained with solutions of IgG and albumin that were relatively highly purified, Vey *et al.*, (2002) found no prion removal when a mixture of proteins (Supernatant I) was depth filtered. This suggests that protein present in Supernatant I adsorbs preferentially to the filter matrix, thereby preventing the prion agent from being removed from the solution.

Removal of prions by chromatography

Prion agents tend to adsorb readily to chromatographic materials (Foster, 1999) and Prion reduction by the order of $3 \log_{10}$ or more has been observed with both anion and cation matrices (Foster

Table 20.14 Removal of prion agents by precipitation in ethanol fractionation[a].

Precipitation step	Resultant product	Prion agent	Prion spike	Prion assay	Reduction factor ($\log_{10}$)	Reference
Fraction (I) + II + III	Albumin	263 K	BH	W blot	≥ 4.7	Lee et al., 2000
		263 K	BH	bioassay	6.0	Lee et al., 2001
		Sc237	BH/MF/CLD/PrP^{Sc}	CDI	3.6/3.1/3.1/4.0	Vey et al., 2002
		263 K	MF	W blot	≥ 2.8	Flan and Aubin, 2005
Fraction (I) + III	IgG	263 K	MF	W blot	≥ 3.7	Foster et al., 2000
		263 K	BH	W blot	≥ 4.3	Lee et al., 2000
		263 K	BH	bioassay	5.3	Lee et al., 2001
		301 V	MF	bioassay	2.1	Reichl et al., 2002
		263 K	MF	W blot	≥ 3.5	Flan and Aubin, 2005
Fraction IV (IV$_1$/IV$_4$)	Albumin	263 K	BH	W blot	≥ 3.0	Foster et al., 2000
		263 K	BH	W blot	$\geq 4.2/\geq 4.1$	Lee et al., 2000
		263 K	BH	bioassay	3.7/4.6	Lee et al., 2001
		Sc237	BH/MF/CLD/PrP^{Sc}	CDI	3.2/3.4/3.2/2.2	Vey et al., 2002
		263 K	MF	W blot	≥ 4.3	Flan and Aubin, 2005
		263 K	MF, sonicated	W Blot	≥ 3.0	Yunoki et al., 2006

[a] Modified from Foster, 2006.

et al., 2000; 2004; Thyer et al., 2006a). Significant prion removal has been reported in the preparation of an immunoaffinity purified factor VIII concentrate, with infectivity being removed by 4.6 $\log_{10}$ and by 3.5 $\log_{10}$ by immunoaffinity and ion exchange chromatography respectively (Cervenakova et al., 2002). Less removal was observed with a heparin-affinity matrix when the product was eluted at high ionic strength and high pH (Foster et al., 2000). Prion infectivity can remain adsorbed to chromatography matrices following elution of product proteins, with the possibility that future product batches might be contaminated. Therefore, suitable cleaning procedures are necessary to ensure freedom from cross-contamination and there is evidence that treatment of chromatography media with sodium chloride and sodium hydroxide may be effective in this regard (Foster et al., 2004; Thyer et al., 2006b).

Removal of prions by nanofiltration

Filtration using membranes with a mean pore diameter of 35 nm and less has been shown to remove prion agents to a significant degree. However, prion infectivity has been detected in filtrates when bioassays were employed for determination (see Table 20.16). Nanofiltration is normally located near the end of manufacturing processes, following completion of protein purification. Any prion agent remaining at this point is likely to be soluble and well dispersed. Silveira et al. (2005) have examined the size distribution of prion particles and have observed that particles with the highest specific infectivity were 17–27 nm in diameter. Rohwer and Sato detected infectivity after nanofiltration through a 15 nm membrane where the prion 'spike' had been treated with detergent and by sonication in order to solubilize and disperse the infectivity (see Table 20.16), suggesting that nanofiltration

may not be fully effective in removing prion agents if infectivity is present in such a soluble, dispersed state.

Equipment cleaning

Effective cleaning of equipment and materials that come in contact with the product is necessary to avoid potential cross-contamination between product batches. Procedures recommended include heating at 134–138 °C for 18 minutes in a porous-load autoclave, treatment with 1 M sodium hydroxide for one hour at 20 °C, and treatment with 2% sodium hypochlorite for one hour at 20 °C (Taylor, 2003). However, these recommendations were based on the inactivation of relatively large quantities of infected brain tissue. In studies more relevant to plasma fractionation, treatment with 0.1 M sodium hydroxide for 15 minutes reduced abnormal prion protein by 3.5 and 4.0 $\log_{10}$ at 4 °C and 18 °C, respectively, with ≥ 4.5 $\log_{10}$ reduction after a 60-minute incubation with 0.1 M sodium hydroxide in which the detergent Sarkosyl was included (Bauman et al., 2006). In a similar study, Unal et al. (2007) obtained a 3.9 $\log_{10}$ reduction in scrapie ME7 infectivity by treatment with 0.1 M sodium hydroxide at 60 °C for two minutes or with 0.25 M sodium hydroxide at 30 °C for one hour.

Issues still to be resolved

Infective dose

The quantity of infectivity needed to transmit the agent of vCJD and to cause disease in humans in clinically relevant circumstances is not known. Nor is it known if there is a threshold of exposure below which infectivity is not transmitted. However, one study in mice found that repeated injection of sub-infectious

Table 20.15 Removal of prion agents by depth filtration in the preparation of immunoglobulin and albumin[a].

Solution filtered	Resultant product	Prion agent	Prion spike	Prion assay	Depth filter	Prion reduction factor ($\log_{10}$)	Reference
Supernatant III	IgG	301 V	MF	bioassay	Seitz KS80P	≥3.1	Reichl et al., 2002
		301 V	MF	bioassay	Millipore AP20	2.4	Reichl et al., 2002
		263 K	BH	W blot	Cuno Zetaplus	≥3.3	Van Holten and Autenrieth, 2003
Fraction II solution	IgG	263 K	MF	W blot	Seitz K200	≥2.8	Foster et al., 2000
		263 K	BH	bioassay	Cuno	≥4.9	Trejo et al., 2003
IGIV	IGIV	263 K	MF	W blot	Cuno Zetaplus 30LA	≥3.1	Yunoki et al., 2006
IGIV	IGIV	263 K	MF, sonicated	W blot	Cuno Zetaplus 30LA	≥2.4	Yunoki et al., 2006
Supernatant IV	Albumin	Sc237	BH/MF/CLD/PrP^{Sc}	CDI	Seitz Supra P80	≥0.9/≥1.1/≥0.9/≥2.4[b]	Vey et al., 2002
Fraction V solution	Albumin	263 K	MF	W blot	Seitz KS80P	≥4.9	Foster et al., 2000
	Albumin	263 K	MF	W blot	Cuno delipid-1	2.3	Foster et al., 2000
	Albumin	263 K	MF	W blot	Seitz AKS5	≥2.9	Flan and Aubin, 2005
	Albumin	263 K	MF	W blot	Cuno Zetaplus 90LA	≥3.1	Yunoki et al., 2006
	Albumin	263 K	MF, sonicated	W blot	Cuno Zetaplus 90LA	≥3.6	Yunoki et al., 2006

[a] Modified from Foster, 2006.

[b] Prion spike added prior to cold-ethanol precipitation and the resultant supernatant clarified by depth filtration.

Table 20.16 Removal of prion agents by nanofiltration of protein solutions[a].

Solution filtered	Prion agent	Prion spike	Prion assay	Nanofilter	Mean pore diameter, nm	Prion reduction factor (log$_{10}$)	Prion in filtrate	Reference
IgG	263 K	BH[b]	W blot	Millipore, Viresolve 180	30	≥3.0	no	Van Holten et al., 2002
Albumin	263 K	BH	W blot	Millipore, Viresolve 180	30	≥5.0	no	Gilligan et al., 2002
Albumin			Bioassay	Millipore, Viresolve 180	30	5.0	yes	Gilligan et al., 2002
Albumin	CJD	BH	Bioassay	Millipore, Viresolve 180	30	≥5.9	no	Tateishi et al., 1993
Albumin	ME7	BH	Bioassay	Asahi, Planova 35 N	35	4.9	yes	Tateishi et al., 2001
		BH[c]		Asahi, Planova 35 N	35	1.6	yes	Tateishi et al., 2001
IgG	263 K	MF[b]	W blot	Asahi, Planova 20 N	20	2.0/2.5	yes	Yunoki et al., 2006
Albumin	ME7	BH	Bioassay	Asahi, Planova 15 N	15	≥5.9	no	Tateishi et al., 2001
		BH[c]		Asahi, Planova 15 N	15	≥4.2	no	Tateishi et al., 2001
Protein	263 K	BH[d]	Bioassay	Asahi, Planova 15 N	15		yes	Sato and Rohwer, unpublished results

[a] Modified from Foster, 2006.
[b] BH clarified by sonication and filtration to 0.1 μM before spiking.
[c] Anionic detergent (0.5% Sarkosyl) added to BH to disaggregate prion protein.
[d] BH treated with detergent and ultrasonication prior to spiking.

doses of scrapie were cumulative and eventually caused infection (Jacquemot *et al.*, 2005).

State of the prion agent

For process investigational studies to be meaningful, the prion agent must be presented in a state in which it would be expected to exist naturally at the relevant stage of a manufacturing process. The agent responsible for vCJD has not been detected directly in human blood, nor in human plasma, nor in any intermediate fraction, nor in any plasma product. Its biochemical and biophysical state in these materials has not been determined. Therefore, the extent to which prion agents derived from brain or other tissue can represent prion agents that would be present naturally in a plasma fractionation process is not known. In order to resolve this issue it may be necessary to directly compare the behaviour of exogenous infectivity with that of endogenous infectivity, for each separation technology of interest.

Prion determination

The limit of detection of prion assays will determine the extent to which product safety can be established. Currently, the sensitivity of available assays, combined with dilution of the spike material and with limits on the quantity of sample that can be injected into rodents, means that even bioassays are insufficiently sensitive to determine if all infectivity has been removed. Advances in analytical technology are required to demonstrate that low levels of infectivity can be removed.

Impact of multiple steps

Most prion removal studies have examined process steps individually. The extent to which data from a series of individual steps can be combined is not clear. A progressive reduction in the concentration of prion agent has been observed over successive precipitation steps (Brown *et al.*, 1998; 1999; Cai *et al.*, 2002; Thyer *et al.*, 2006a), but when depth filtration was combined with precipitation (Reichl *et al.*, 2002) and when two different filtration procedures were combined (Reichl *et al.*, 2002; Trejo *et al.*, 2003) the degree of TSE removal over the combined steps was greater than that achieved with the first step alone, but less than that obtained by adding together individual $\log_{10}$ reductions. These observations suggest that results from individual steps may not necessarily be additive unless this has been shown to be the case experimentally.

Conclusion

Microbiological pathogens naturally present in the human population have been a major challenge to the preparation of pooled plasma products for many years. Scientific and technical advances during the 1980s have essentially removed the risks of transmission of HIV, HBV and HCV that were associated with coagulation factor concentrates. Rigorous regulatory requirements, introduced since, ensure a high degree of safety. Despite these advances, potential risks remain from small, non-enveloped viruses. Although the quantity of infective prions in large-volume pools of plasma is expected to be low compared

with viruses, such as HIV and HCV, and there is a body of data to indicate that prion agents should be removed to a high degree by existing manufacturing processes, current limits to knowledge of prion diseases mean that there is still uncertainty over the safety of plasma products in this regard.

Acknowledgements

We would like to acknowledge helpful contributions by our SNBTS colleagues, especially Jacqueline Barry, Bruce Cuthbertson, Tony Jones, Druscilla Rodger, Ronald McIntosh, Emma Waite and Anne Welch.

REFERENCES

Adcock, W. L., MacGregor, A., Davies, J. R., *et al.* (1998a) Chromatographic removal and heat inactivation of hepatitis A virus during the manufacture of human albumin. *Biotechnol Appl Biochem*, **28**, 85–94.

Adcock, W. L., MacGregor, A., Davies, J. R., *et al.* (1998b) Chromatographic removal and heat inactivation of hepatitis B virus during the manufacture of human albumin. *Biotechnol Appl Biochem*, **28**, 169–78.

Addiego, J. E., Gomperts, E., Liu, S. L., *et al.* (1992) Treatment of haemophilia A with highly purified factor VIII concentrate prepared by anti-FVIIIC immunoaffinity chromatography. *Thromb Haemost*, **67**, 19–27.

Aiuti, F., Carbonari, M., Scano, G., *et al.* (1986) Screening for antibodies to LAV/HTLV-III in recipients of immunoglobulin preparations. *Lancet*, **i**, 1091.

Allain, J.-P. (1984) Non-factor VIII related constituents in concentrates. *Scand J Haematol*, **33** (Suppl. 41), 173–80.

Allen, J. G., Enerson, D. M., Barron, E. S. G., *et al.* (1954) Pooled plasma with little or no risk of homologous serum jaundice. *JAMA*, **154**, 103–7.

Alter, H. J. (2000) You'll wonder where the yellow went: a 30 year perspective on the near-eradication of post-transfusion hepatitis. *Nat Med*, **6**, 1082–4.

Alving, B., Tankersley, D. L., Mason, B. L., *et al.* (1980) Contact-activated factors: contaminants of immunoglobulin preparations with coagulant and vasoactive activities. *J Lab Clin Med*, **96**, 334–6.

Anderson, H. D. and Gibson, S. T. (1957) Evaluation of the risk of transmitting hepatitis by the administration of dried fibrinogen (human) (a preliminary report). In *Hepatitis Frontiers*, eds F. W. Hartman, G. LoGrippo, J. G. Mateer and J. Barron, pp. 287–295. London, J. and A. Churchill Ltd.

Anderson, H. D., McCall, K. B., Sgouris, J. T., *et al.* (1966) The clinical use of dried fibrinogen (human) and the risk of transmitting hepatitis by its administration. *Transfusion*, **6**, 234–6.

Andrewes, C. H. and Horstmann, D. M. (1949) The susceptibility of viruses to ethyl ether. *J Gen Microbiol*, **3**, 292–7.

Aronson, D. L. (1990) The development of the technology and capacity for the production of factor VIII for the treatment of hemophilia A. *Transfusion*, **30**, 748–58.

Australian Senate (2004) Hepatitis C and the blood supply in Australia. *Report of the Community Affairs Reference Committee of the Australian Senate, June 2004*. Canberra, The Senate.

Atrah, H. I., Crawford, R. J., Dow, B. C., *et al.* (1985) Safety of intravenous immunoglobulin treatment. *J Clin Pathol*, **38**, 1192–3.

Aygoren-Pursen, E. and Scharrer, I. (1997) A multicenter pharmacosurveillance study for the evaluation of the efficacy and safety of recombinant factor VIII in the treatment of patients with hemophilia A. German Kogenate Study Group. *Thromb Haemost*, **78**, 1352–6.

Aymard, J. P., Janot, C., Chermann, J. C., *et al.* (1985) Prevalence of antibodies to lymphadenopathy-AIDS virus in French haemophiliacs. *Vox Sang*, **49**, 161–3.

Azimi, P. H., Roberto, R. R., Guralnik, J., *et al.* (1986) Transfusion-acquired hepatitis A in a premature infant with secondary nosocomial spread in an intensive care nursery. *Am J Dis Child*, **140**, 23–7.

Azzi, A., Ciappi, S., Zakvrzewska, K., *et al.* (1992) Human parvovirus B19 infection in hemophiliacs first infused with two high-purity, virally attenuated factor VIII concentrates. *Am J Hematol*, **39**, 228–30.

Azzi, A., De Santis, R., Morfini, M., *et al.* (2001) TT virus contaminates first-generation recombinant factor VIII concentrates. *Blood*, **98**, 2571–3.

Barbara, J., Howell, D., Briggs, M., *et al.* (1982) Post-transfusion hepatitis A. *Lancet*, **i**, 738.

Barker, L. F. and Murray, R. (1972) Relationship of virus dose to incubation time of clinical hepatitis and time of appearance of hepatitis-associated antigen. *Am J Med Sci*, **263**, 27–33.

Barré-Sinoussi, F., Chermann, J. C., Rey, F., *et al.* (1983) Isolation of a T-lymphotropic retrovirus from a patient at risk for acquired immune deficiency syndrome (AIDS). *Science*, **220**, 868–71.

Barrowcliffe T. W. (1993) Inhibitor development and activated factor VIII in concentrates. *Thromb Haemost*, **70**, 1065–6.

Bartolomi Corsi, O., Azzi, A., Morfini, M., *et al.* (1988) Human parvovirus infection in hemophiliacs first infused with treated clotting factor concentrates. *J Med Virol*, **25**, 165–70.

Barundun, S., Kistler, P., Jeunet, F., *et al.* (1962) Intravenous administration of human γ-globulin. *Vox Sang*, **7**, 157–74.

Bauman, P. A., Lawrence, L. A., Biesert, L., *et al.* (2006) Critical factors influencing prion inactivation by sodium hydroxide. *Vox Sang*, **91**, 34–40.

Becton, D., Manno, C., Green, D., *et al.* (1994) Viral safety of an affinity-purified coagulation factor IX concentrate (Alphanine SD). *Blood*, **84** (Suppl. 1), 198a.

Beeson, P. B. (1943) Jaundice occurring one to four months after transfusion of blood or plasma. Report of seven cases. *JAMA*, **121**, 1332–4.

Beeson, P. B., Chesney, G. and McFarlan, A. M. (1944) Hepatitis following injection of mumps convalescent plasma. *Lancet*, **i**, 814–15.

Bennett, B., Dawson, A. A., Gibson, B. S., *et al.* (1993) Study of viral safety of Scottish National Blood Transfusion Service factor VIII/IX concentrate. *Transfus Med*, **3**, 295–8.

Benveniste, R. E., Ochs, H. D., Fischer, S. H., *et al.* (1986) Screening for antibodies to LAV/HTLV-III in recipients of immunoglobulin preparations. *Lancet*, **i**, 1091–2.

Berg, R., Bjorling, H., Berntsen, K., *et al.* (1972) Recovery of Australia antigen from human plasma products separated by a modified Cohn fractionation. *Vox Sang*, **22**, 1–13.

Berg, W. van den, J. W., ten Cate, Breederveld, C., *et al.* (1986) Seroconversion to HTLV-III in haemophiliacs given heat treated factor VIII concentrate. *Lancet*, **I**, 803–4.

Berger, A., Doerr, H. W., Scharrer, I., *et al.* (1997) Follow-up of four HIV-infected individuals after administration of hepatitis C virus and GBV-C/hepatitis G virus contaminated intravenous immunoglobulin: evidence for HCV but not for GBV-C/HGV transmission. *J Med Virol*, **53**, 25–30.

Berntorp, E. (1996) Why prescribe highly purified factor VIII and IX concentrates. *Vox Sang*, **70**, 61–8.

Bidwell, E. (1955) The purification of bovine antihaemophilic globulin. *Br J Haematol*, **1**, 35–45.

Biesert, L. (1996) Virus validation studies of immunoglobulin preparations. *Clin Exp Rheumatol*, **14** (Suppl. 15), S47–S52.

Biesert, L. and Suhartono, H. (1998) Solvent/detergent treatment of human plasma – a very robust method for virus inactivation. Validated virus safety of OCTAPLAS. *Vox Sang*, **74** (Suppl. 1), 207–12.

Biesert, L., Lemon, S., Suhartono, H., *et al.* (1995) Virus validation experiments on the production process of OCTAVI SDPlus. *Blood Coagul Fibrinolysis*, **6** (Suppl. 2), S48–54.

Biggs, R. (1974) Supply of blood-clotting-factor VIII for treatment of haemophilia. *Lancet*, **i**, 1339.

Biggs, R. (1977) Haemophilia treatment in the United Kingdom from 1969 to 1974. *Br J Haematol*, **35**, 487–504.

Biggs, R. and MacFarlane, R. G. (1957) *Human Blood Coagulation and its Disorders*, 2nd edn. Oxford, Blackwell Scientific Publications.

Biggs, R., Douglas, A. S., MacFarlane, R. G., *et al.* (1952) Christmas disease. A condition previously mistaken for haemophilia. *BMJ*, **2**, 1378–82.

Biggs, R., Bidwell, E., Handley, D. A., *et al.* (1961) The preparation and assay of a Christmas factor (factor IX) concentrate and its use in the treatment of two patients. *Br J Haematol*, **7**, 349–64.

Bird, A. G., Codd, A. A. and Collins, A. (1985) Haemophilia and AIDS. *Lancet*, **i**, 162–3.

Biswas, R. M., Nedjar, S., Wilson, L. T., *et al.* (1994) The effect on the safety of intravenous immunoglobulin of testing plasma for antibody to hepatitis C. *Transfusion*, **34**, 100–4.

Björkander, J., Cunningham-Rundles, C., Lundin, P., *et al.* (1988) Intravenous immunoglobulin prophylax is causing liver damage in 16 of 77 patients with hypogammaglobulinemia or IgG subclass deficiency. *Am J Med*, **84**, 107–11.

Bjøro, K., Frøland, S. S., Yun, Z., *et al.* (1994) Hepatitis C infection in patients with primary hypogammaglobulinemia after treatment with contaminated immune globulin. *New Engl J Med*, **331**, 1607–11.

Blackburn, E. K. (1974) Treatment of haemophilia. *Lancet*, **ii**, 105.

Blanchard, M. C., Stokes, J., Hampil, B., *et al.* (1948) Methods of protection against homologous serum hepatitis II. The inactivation of hepatitis SH with ultraviolet rays. *J Am Med Assoc*, **138**, 341–3.

Blombäck, B. and Blombäck, M. (1956) Purification of human and bovine fibrinogen. *Arkiv Kemi*, **10**, 415–43.

Bloom, A. L., Forbes, C. D. and Rizza, C. R. (1985) HTLV-III, haemophilia and blood transfusion. *BMJ*, **290**, 1901.

Blumberg, B. S. (1964) Polymorphism of the serum proteins and the development of iso-precipitins in transfused patients. *Bull N Y Acad Med*, **40**, 377–86.

Blumberg, B. S., Gerstley, B. J. S., Hungerford, D. A., *et al.* (1967) A serum antigen (Australia antigen) in Down's syndrome, leukaemia and hepatitis. *Ann Intern Med*, **66**, 924–31.

Blümel, J., Schmidt, I, Wilkommen, H., *et al.* (2002) Inactivation of parvovirus B19 during pasteurization of human serum albumin. *Transfusion*, **42**, 1011–18.

Boklan, B. F. (1971) Factor IX concentrate and viral hepatitis. *Ann Intern Med*, **74**, 298.

Bos, O. J., Sunye, D. G., Nieuweboer, C. E., *et al.* (1998) Virus validation of pH 4-treated immunoglobulin products produced by the Cohn fractionation process. *Biologicals*, **26**, 267–76.

Boschetti, N., Niederhauser, I., Kempf, C., *et al.* (2004) Different susceptibility of B19 virus and mice minute virus to low pH treatment. *Transfusion*, **44**, 1079–86.

Boychyn, M., Yim, S. S., Bulmer, M., *et al.* (2004) Performance prediction of industrial centrifuges using scale-down models. *Bioprocess Biosyst Eng*, **26**, 385–91.

Boyer, P. D., Lum, F. G., Ballou, G. A., *et al.* (1946) The combination of fatty acids and related compounds with serum albumin. I. Stabilization against heat denaturation. *J Biol Chem*, **162**, 181–98.

Brackmann, H. H. and Egli, H. (1988) Acute hepatitis B infection after treatment with heat inactivated factor VIII concentrate. *Lancet*, **ii**, 967.

Bradley, D. W. and Maynard, J. E. (1983) Non-A, non-B hepatitis: research progress and current perspectives. *Developments in Biological Standardization*, 54, pp. 463–73. In *Viral Hepatitis: Standardization in Immunoprophylaxis of Infections by Hepatitis Viruses*, eds G. Papaevangelan and W. Hennessen. Basel, Karger.

Bradley, W. H., Loutit, J. F. and Maunsell, K. (1944) An episode of 'homologous serum jaundice'. *BMJ*, **2**, 268–9.

Breen, F. A. and Tullis, J. L. (1969) Prothrombin concentrates in treatment of Christmas disease and allied disorders. *J Am Med Assoc*, **208**, 1848–52.

Bremard-Ourcy, C., Courouce, A. M., Badillet, M., *et al.* (1986) Screening for antibodies to LAV/HTLV-III in recipients of immunoglobulin preparations. *Lancet*, **i**, 1090–1.

Bresee, J. S., Mast, S. E., Coleman, P. J., *et al.* (1996) Hepatitis C virus infection associated with administration of intravenous immune globulin: a cohort study. *J Am Med Assoc*, **276**, 1563–7.

Brettler, D. B., Alter, H. J., Dienstag, J. L., *et al.* (1990) Prevalence of hepatitis C virus antibody in a cohort of hemophilia patients. *Blood*, **76**, 254–6.

Brightman, I. J. and Korns, R. F. (1947) Homologous serum jaundice in recipients of pooled plasma. *J Am Med Assoc*, **135**, 268–72.

Brinkhous, K. M., Shanbrom, E., Roberts, H. R., *et al.* (1968) A new high-potency glycine-precipitated antihemophilic factor (AHF) concentrate. Treatment of classical hemophilia and hemophilia with inhibitors. *J Am Med Assoc*, **205**, 613–17.

British Pharmacopoeia (2005) Normal immunoglobulin. In *British Pharmacopoeia*, vol. III, pp. 2895–6. London, The Stationery Office.

Brown, P., Cervenakova, L. and McShane, L. M., *et al.* (1999) Further studies of blood infectivity in an experimental model of transmissible spongiform encephalopathy, with an explanation of why blood components do not transmit Creutzfeldt-Jacob disease in humans. *Transfusion*, **39**, 1169–78.

Brown, P., Rohwer, R. G., Dunstan, B. C., *et al.*, (1998) The distribution of infectivity in blood components and plasma derivatives in experimental models of transmissible spongiform encephalopathy. *Transfusion*, **38**, 810–16.

Burnouf, T. (1993) Chromatographic removal of viruses from plasma derivatives. *Developments in Biological Standardization*, **81**, 199–209.

Burnouf, T. and Radosevich, M. (2003) Nanofiltration of plasma-derived biopharmaceutical products. *Haemophilia*, **9**, 24–37.

Burnouf, T., Burnouf-Radosevich, M., Huart, J. J., *et al.* (1991) A highly purified factor VIII: C concentrate prepared from cryoprecipitate by ion exchange chromatography. *Vox Sang*, **60**, 8–15.

Burnouf, T., Michalski, C., Goudemand, M., *et al.* (1989) Properties of a highly purified human plasma factor IX: therapeutic concentrate prepared by conventional chromatography. *Vox Sang*, **57**, 225–32.

Burnouf-Radosevich, M., Appourchaux, P., Huart, J. J., *et al.* (1994) Nanofiltration, a new specific virus elimination method applied to high-purity factor IX and factor IX concentrates. *Vox Sang*, **67**, 132–8.

Burrell, C. J., Black, S. H. and Ramsay, D. M. (1978) Antibody to hepatitis B surface antigen in haemophiliacs on long-term therapy with Scottish factor VIII. *J Clin Pathol*, **31**, 309–12.

Butt, A. A. (2006) Hepatitis C virus infection: the new global epidemic. *Exp Rev Anti-Infect Ther*, **3**, 241–9.

Cabrera Chaves, T., Simon Marco, M. A., Gomollon Garcia, F., *et al.* (1996) Hepatitis C following administration of intravenous immunoglobulin. *Gastroenterologia y Hepatologia*, **19**, 305–8.

Cai, K., Gierman, T. M., Hotta, J. A., *et al.* (2005) Ensuring the biologic safety of plasma-derived therapeutic proteins. *Biodrugs*, **19**, 79–96.

Cai, K., Miller, J. L. C., Stenland, C. J., *et al.* (2002) Solvent-dependent precipitation of prion protein. *Biochim Biophys Acta*, **1597**, 28–35.

Callet-Fauquet, P., Giambattista, M., Draps, M. L., *et al.* (2004) An assay for parvovirus B19 neutralizing antibodies based on human hepatocarcinoma cell lines. *Transfusion*, **44**, 1340–3.

Cash, J. D., Dalton, R. G., Middleton, S., *et al.* (1975) Studies on the thrombogenicity of Scottish factor IX concentrates in dogs. *Thromb Diath Haemorrh*, **33**, 632–9.

Centers for Disease Control (1974) Viral hepatitis-B associated with transfusion of plasma protein fraction. *Morbidity and Mortality Weekly Report*, **23** (11), 98.

Centers for Disease Control (1981a) Pneumocystis pneumonia – Los Angeles. *Morbidity and Mortality Weekly Report*, **30**, 250–2.

Centers for Disease Control (1981b) Kaposi's sarcoma and Pneumocystis pneumonia among homosexual men – New York City and California. *Morbidity and Mortality Weekly Report*, **30**, 305–8.

Centers for Disease Control (1982a) Pneumocystis carinii among persons with hemophilia A. *Morbidity and Mortality Weekly Report*, **31**, 365–7.

Centers for Disease Control (1982b) Update on acquired immune deficiency syndrome (AIDS) among patients with hemophilia A. *Morbidity and Mortality Weekly Report*, **31**, 644–6, 652.

Centers for Disease Control (1982c) Possible transfusion-associated acquired immune deficiency syndrome (AIDS) – California. *Morbidity and Mortality Weekly Report*, **31**, 652–4.

Centers for Disease Control (1983) Prevention of acquired immune deficiency syndrome (AIDS): report of inter-agency recommendations. *Morbidity and Mortality Weekly Report*, **32**, 101–3.

Centers for Disease Control (1984) Update: acquired immunodeficiency syndrome (AIDS) in persons with hemophilia. *Morbidity and Mortality Weekly Report*, **33**, 589–91.

Centers for Disease Control (1986) Safety of therapeutic immune globulin preparations with respect to transmission of human T-lymphotropic virus type III/lymphadenopathy-associated virus infection. *Morbidity and Mortality Weekly Report*, **35**, 231–3.

Centers for Disease Control (1994) Outbreak of hepatitis C associated with intravenous immunoglobulin administration – United States, October 1993–June 1994. *Morbidity and Mortality Weekly Report*, **43**, 505–9.

Centers for Disease Control (1996) Hepatitis A among persons with hemophilia who received clotting factor concentrates – United States, September–December 1995. *Morbidity and Mortality Weekly Report*, **55**, 841–4.

Centers for Disease Control (2006) The global HIV/AIDS pandemic, 2006. *Morbidity and Mortality Weekly Report*, **55**, 841–4.

Cervenakova, L., Brown, P., Hammond, D. J., *et al.* (2002) Factor VIII and transmissible spongiform encephalopathy: the case for safety. *Haemophilia*, **8**, 63–75.

Chandra, S. and Brummelhuis, H. G. J. (1981) Prothrombin complex concentrates for clinical use. *Vox Sang*, **41**, 257–73.

Chandra, S., Groener, A. and Feldman, F. (2002) Effectiveness of alternative treatments for reducing potential viral contaminants from plasma-derived products. *Throm Res*, **105**, 391–400.

Charm, S. E. and Wong, B. L. (1974) An immunoadsorbent process for removing hepatitis antigen from blood and plasma. *Biotechnol Bioeng*, **16**, 593–607.

Cheinsong-Popov, R., Weiss, R. A., Dalgleish, A., *et al.* (1984) Prevalence of antibody to human T-lymphotropic virus type III in AIDS and AIDS-risk patients in Britain. *Lancet*, **ii**, 477–80.

Chen, B. P., Rumi, M. G., Colombo, M., *et al.* (1999) TT virus is present in a high frequency of Italian hemophilic patients transfused with plasma-derived clotting factor concentrates. *Blood*, **94**, 4333–6.

Cho, Y. K., Foley, B. T., Sung, H., *et al.* (2007) Molecular epidemiologic study of human immunodeficiency virus 1 outbreak in haemophiliacs B infected through clotting factor 9 after 1990. *Vox Sang*, **92**, 113–20.

Choo, Q.-L., Kuo, G., Weiner, A. J., *et al.* (1989) Isolation of a cDNA clone derived from a blood-borne non-A, non-B viral hepatitis genome. *Science*, **244**, 559–61.

Christie, J. M., Healey, C. J., Watson, J., *et al.* (1997) Clinical outcome of hypogammaglobulinaemic patients following outbreak of acute hepatitis C: 2-year follow up. *Clin Exp Immunol*, **110**, 4–8.

Chudy, M., Budek, I., Keller-Stanislawski, B., *et al.* (1999) A new cluster of hepatitis A infection in hemophiliacs traced to a contaminated plasma pool. *J Med Virol*, **57**, 91–9.

Coates, J. B. and McFetridge, E. M. (1964) The bovine and human albumin programmes. In *Blood Programmes in World War II*, eds. J. B. Coates and E. M. McFetridge, pp. 325–57. Washington, Office of the Surgeon General.

Cockburn, W. C., Harrington, J. A., Zeitlin, R. A., *et al.* (1951) Homologous serum hepatitis and measles prophylaxis. A report to the Medical Research Council. *BMJ*, **2**, 6–12.

Cohen, B. (1995) Parvovirus B19: an expanding spectrum of disease. *BMJ*, **311**, 1549–52.

Cohn, E. J. (1948) The history of plasma fractionation. In *Science in World War II. Advances in Military Medicine Made by American Investigators Working Under the Sponsorship of the Committee on Medical Research, Volume 1*, eds. E. C. Andrus, C. S. Keefer, D. W. Bronke, *et al.*, pp. 364–443. Boston, Little, Brown & Co.

Cohn, E. J., Gurd, F. R. N., Surgenor, D. M., *et al.* (1950) A system for the separation of the components of human blood: quantitative procedures for the separation of the protein components of human plasma. *J Am Chem Soc*, **72**, 465–74.

Cohn, R. J., Schwyzer, R. Field, S. P., *et al.* (1994) Acute hepatitis A in haemophiliacs. *Thromb Haemost*, **75**, 785–6.

Cohn, E. J., Strong, C. E., Hughes, W. L., *et al.* (1946) Preparation and properties of serum and plasma proteins IV: a system for the separation into fractions of the protein and lipoprotein components of biological tissues and fluids. *J Am Chem Soc*, **68**, 459–75.

Colombo, M., Carnelli, V., Gazengel, C., *et al.* (1985) Transmission of non-A, non-B hepatitis by heat treated factor VIII concentrate. *Lancet*, **ii**, 1–4.

Colvin, B. T. (1990) Prevention of hepatitis C infection in haemophiliacs. *Lancet*, **335**, 1474.

Colvin, B. T., Rizza, C. R., Hill, F. G. H., *et al.* (1988) Effect of dry-heating of coagulation factor concentrates at 80 °C for 72 hours on transmission of non-A, non-B hepatitis. *Lancet*, **ii**, 814–16.

Committee for Medicinal Products for Human Use (2004a) *Guideline on Assessing the Risk for Virus Transmission – New Chapter 6 of the Note for Guidance on Plasma-Derived Medicinal Products (CPMP/BWP/269/95)*. CPMP/BWP/5180/03. London, European Medicines Agency.

Committee for Medicinal Products for Human Use (2004b) *Position Statement on Creutzfeldt-Jakob Disease and Plasma-Derived and Urine-Derived Medicinal Products*. CPMP/BWP/2879/02/rev 1. London, European Medicines Agency.

Committee for Medicinal Products for Human Use (2004c) *Guideline on the Investigation of Manufacturing Processes for Plasma-Derived Medicinal Products with Regard to vCJD Risk*. CPMP/BWP/CPMP/5136/03. London, European Medicines Agency.

Committee for Medicinal Products for Human Use (2006) *Guideline on the Clinical Investigation of Human Anti-D Immunoglobulin for Intravenous and/or Intramuscular Administration*. CPMP/BPWG/575/99 rev.1. London, European Medicines Agency.

Committee for Proprietary Medicinal Products (1991) Validation of virus removal and inactivation procedures. *Biologicals*, **19**, 247–51.

Committee for Proprietary Medicinal Products (1992) Guidelines for medicinal products derived from human blood and plasma. *Biologicals*, **20**, 159–64.

Committee for Proprietary Medicinal Products (1995a) *Note for Guidance on Validation of Analytical Methods: Definitions and Terminology*. CPMP/ICH/381/95. London, European Agency for the Evaluation of Medicinal Products.

Committee for Proprietary Medicinal Products (1995b) *Intramuscular Immunoglobulins: Nucleic Acid Amplification Tests for HCV RNA Detection*. CPMP/117/95, annex 4. London, European Agency for the Evaluation of Medicinal Products.

Committee for Proprietary Medicinal Products (1996a) *Note for Guidance on Virus Validation Studies: the Design, Contribution and Interpretation of Studies Validating the Inactivation and Removal of Viruses*. CPMP/BWP/268/95 revised. London, European Agency for the Evaluation of Medicinal Products.

Committee for Proprietary Medicinal Products (1996b) *Note for Guidance on Plasma-Derived Medicinal Products*. CPMP/BWP/269/95. London, European Agency for the Evaluation of Medicinal Products.

Committee for Proprietary Medicinal Products (1997) *Note for Guidance on Quality of Biotechnological Products: Viral Safety Evaluation of Biotechnology Products Derived from Cell Lines of Human or Animal Origin*. CPMP/ICH/295/95. London, European Agency for the Evaluation of Medicinal Products.

Committee for Proprietary Medicinal Products (1998) *The Introduction of Nucleic Acid Amplification Technology (NAT) for the Detection of Hepatitis C Virus RNA in Plasma Pools*. CPMP/BWP/390/97. London, European Agency for the Evaluation of Medicinal Products.

Committee for Proprietary Medicinal Products (2001) *Note for Guidance on Plasma-Derived Medicinal Products*. CPMP/BWP/269/95 rev. 3. London, European Agency for the Evaluation of Medicinal Products.

Cossart, Y. E., Field, A. M., Cant, B., *et al.* (1975) Parvovirus-like particles in human sera. *Lancet*, **i**, 72–3.

Counts, R. B. (1977) Serum transaminase and HBsAb antibody in hemophiliacs treated exclusively with cryoprecipitate. In *Unsolved Therapeutic Problems in Hemophilia*, eds. J. C. Fratantoni and D. L. Aronson, pp. 71–3. Washington, US, Department of Health, Education, and Welfare, DHEW publication no. (NIH) 77–1089.

Craske, J., Dilling, N. and Stern, D. (1975) An outbreak of hepatitis associated with intravenous injection of factor-VIII concentrate. *Lancet*, **ii**, 221–3.

Craske, J., Kirk, P., Cohen, B., *et al.* (1978) Commercial factor VIII associated hepatitis, 1974–75, in the United Kingdom: a retrospective survey. *J Hyg (Lond)*, **80**, 327–36.

Crewdson, J. (2002) *Science Fictions*. Boston, Little, Brown and Company.

Cronberg, S., Belfrage, S. and Nilsson, I. M. (1963) Fibrinogen-transmitted hepatitis. *Lancet*, **i**, 967–9.

Crovari, P., De Flora, S. and Castagna, M. (1975) Distribution of hepatitis B surface antigen in plasma fractions extracted by the Cohn method. *Giornale di Igiene e Medicina Preventiva*, **16**, 3–12.

Cumming, R. A., Davies, S. H., Ellis, D., *et al.* (1965) Red cell banking and the production of a factor VIII concentrate. *Vox Sang*, **10**, 687–99.

Cunningham, C. J. (1980) Production of human immunoglobulin anti-D (RhO) for intravenous administration for a national Rh prophylaxis programme. *Biochem Soc Trans*, **8**, 178–9.

Cuthbert, R. J., Ludlam, C. A., Brookes, E., *et al.* (1988) Efficacy of heat treatment of factor VIII concentrate. *Vox Sang*, **54**, 199–200.

Cuthbertson, B., Perry, R. J., Foster, P. R., *et al.* (1987a) The viral safety of intravenous immunoglobulin. *J Infect*, **15**, 125–33.

Cuthbertson, B., Rennie, J. G., Aw, D., *et al.* (1987b) Safety of albumin preparations manufactured from plasma not tested for HIV antibody. *Lancet*, **ii**, 41.

Cutter Biological (1978) *Koate Antihemophilic Factor (Human) for Haemophilia A. Product Insert, October 1978*. Berkeley, California, Cutter Laboratories Inc.

Dane, D. S., Cameron, C. H. and Briggs, M. (1970) Virus-like particles in serum of patients with Australia-antigen-associated hepatitis. *Lancet*, **i**, 695–8.

Darnell, M. E. and Taylor, D. R. (2006) Evaluation of inactivation methods for severe acute respiratory syndrome coronavirus in noncellular blood products. *Transfusion*, **46**, 1770–7.

De Filippi, F., Castelli, R., Cicardi, M., *et al.* (1998) Transmission of hepatitis G virus in patients with angioedema treated with steam-heated plasma concentrates of C1 inhibitor. *Transfusion*, **38**, 302–11.

Del Duca, V. and Eppes, R. B. (1966) Hepatitis transmitted by anti-hemophilic globulin. *N Eng Med*, **275**, 965–6.

Department of Health (1998) *Committee on Safety of Medicines Completes Review of Blood Products*, press release no. 98/102. London, Department of Health.

Department of Health (1999) *The Good Laboratory Practice Regulations 1999*. UK Department of Health, Statutory Instruments 1999 No. 3106. London, The Stationery Office Limited.

Department of Health (2002) *Department of Health Secures Guaranteed Long-Term Supplies of Plasma for NHS Patients*, press release no. 2002/0524. London, Department of Health.

Dichtelmuller, H., Rudnick, D., Breuer, B., *et al.* (1993) Validation of virus inactivation and removal for the manufacturing procedure of two immunoglobulins and a 5% serum protein solution treated with beta-propiolactone. *Biologicals*, **21**, 259–68.

Dichtelmuller, H., Rudnick, D., Rinscheid, V., *et al.* (1998) Removal of viruses by Asahi 35nm nanofiltration of IVIG. In *Proceedings of Planova® Workshop, Oslo, 27 June 1998*, pp. 27–37. Tokyo, Asahi Chemical Industry Co. Ltd.

Didisheim, P., Loeb, J., Blatrix, C., *et al.* (1959) Preparation of a human plasma fraction rich in prothrombin, proconvertin, Stuart factor, and PCT and a study of its activity and toxicity in rabbits and man. *J Lab Clin Med*, **53**, 322–30.

Dietrich, S. L., Mosley, J. W., Lusher, J. M., *et al.* (1990) Transmission of human immunodeficiency virus type 1 by dry-heated clotting factor concentrates. *Vox Sang*, **59**, 129–35.

Dike, G. W. R., Bidwell, E. and Rizza, C. R. (1972) The preparation and clinical use of a new concentrate containing factor IX, prothrombin and factor X and of a separate concentrate containing factor VII. *Br J Haematol*, **22**, 469–90.

DiLeo, A. J. and Allegrezza, A. E. (1991) Validatable virus removal from protein solutions. *Nature*, **351**, 420–21.

Dittmann, S., Roggendorf, M., Dürkop, J., *et al.* (1991) Long-term persistence of hepatitis C virus antibodies in a single source outbreak. *J Hepatol*, **13**, 323–7.

Dormandy, K. M. (1974) Blood fractions for haemophilia. *Lancet*, **ii**, 155.

Drake, M. E., Hampil, B., Pennell, R. B., *et al.* (1952) Effect of nitrogen mustard on virus of serum hepatitis in whole blood. *Proceedings of the Society of Experimental Biology and Medicine*, **80**, 310–13.

Echevarria, J. M., Leon, P., Domingo, C. J., *et al.* (1996) Laboratory diagnosis and molecular epidemiology of an outbreak of hepatitis C virus infection among recipients of human intravenous immunoglobulin in Spain. *Transfusion*, **36**, 725–30.

Editorial (1947) Homologous serum hepatitis. *Lancet*, **ii**, 691–2.

Edsall, J. T. (1984) Stabilization of serum albumin to heat, and inactivation of the hepatitis virus. *Vox Sang*, **46**, 338–40.

Edwards, C. A., Piet, M. P., Chin, S., *et al.* (1987) Tri-n-butyl phosphate/detergent treatment of licensed therapeutic and experimental blood derivatives. *Vox Sang*, **52**, 53–9.

Eibl, J., Barret, N., Hämmerle, T., *et al.* (1996) Nanofiltration of immunoglobulin with 35-nm filters fails to remove substantial amounts of HCV. *Biologicals*, **24**, 285–7.

Einarsson, M., Kaplan, L., Nordenfelt, E., *et al.* (1981) Removal of hepatitis B virus from a concentrate of coagulation factors II, VII, IX and X by hydrophobic interaction chromatography. *J Virol Methods*, **3**, 213–28.

Einarsson, M., Prince, A. M. and Brotman, B. (1985) Removal of non-A, non-B hepatitis virus from a concentrate of the coagulation factors II, VII, IX and X by hydrophobic interaction chromatography. *Scand J Infect Dis*, **17**, 141–6.

Emile-Weil, P. (1906) Etude du sang chez les hémophiles. *Bulletins et Mémoires de la Société Médicale des Hôpitaux de Paris*, **23**, 1001–18.

Enders, J. F. (1944) Chemical, clinical, and immunological studies on the products of human plasma fractionation. X. The concentrations of certain antibodies in globulin fractions derived from human blood plasma. *J Clin Invest*, **23**, 510–30.

Enoki, C., Higashi, S., Oohata, M., *et al.* (2002) A case of acute erythroblastic anemia due to infection with human parvovirus B19 after coronary bypass grafting. *Kyobu Geka*, **55**, 116–9.

Esteban, J. I., Esteban, R., Viladomui, L., *et al.* (1989) Hepatitis C virus antibodies among risk groups in Spain. *Lancet*, **ii**, 294–7.

Ettingshausen, C. E. and Kreuz, W. (2006) Recombinant vs. plasma-derived products, especially those with intact VWF, regarding inhibitor development. *Haemophilia*, **12** (Suppl. 6), 102–6.

European Pharmacopoeia (2004) Validation of nucleic acid amplification techniques (NAT) for the detection of hepatitis C virus (HCV) RNA in plasma pools: guidelines. In *European Pharmacopoeia*, 5th edn, vol. 1, pp. 176–177. Strasburg, Council of Europe.

Evatt, B. L. (2006) The tragic history of AIDS in the hemophilia population 1982–1984. *J Thromb Haemost*, **4**, 2295–301.

Evatt, B. L., Gomperts, E. D., McDougal, J. S., *et al.* (1985) Coincidental appearance of LAV/HTLV-III antibodies in hemophiliacs and the onset of the AIDS epidemic. *N Eng J Med*, **312**, 483–6.

Evensen, S. A., Rollag, H. and Glomstein, A. (1995) Hepatitis C virus seroconversion in a haemophiliac treated exclusively with solvent/detergent-treated clotting factor concentrate. *Eur J Clin Microbiol Infect Dis*, **14**, 631–2.

Fanning, L. J. (2002) The Irish paradigm on the natural progression of hepatitis C virus infection: an investigation in a homogeneous patient population infected with HCV 1b (review). *Int J Mol Med*, **9**, 179–84.

Farshid, M., Mitchell, F., Biswas, R., *et al.* (1997) Prevalence of hepatitis G virus in hepatitis C virus (HCV)-infected patients and in HCV-contaminated intravenous immunoglobulin products. *J Vir Hepat*, **4**, 415–19.

Feinstone, S. M., Kapikian, A. Z. and Purcell, R. H. (1973) Hepatitis A: detection by immune electron microscopy of a virus-like antigen associated with acute illness. *Science*, **182**, 1026–8.

Feinstone, S. M., Kapikian, A. Z., Purcell, *et al.* (1975) Transfusion-associated hepatitis not due to viral hepatitis type A or B. *N Eng J Med*, **292**, 767–70.

Feinstone, S. M., Mihalik, K. B., Kamimura, T., *et al.* (1983) Inactivation of hepatitis B virus and non-A, non-B hepatitis by chloroform. *Infect Immun*, **41**, 816–21.

Feissley, R. (1924) Recherches sur la pathogénie at la thérapeutique des états hémophiliques. *Schweizerische Medizinische Wochenschrift*, **55**, 81–4.

Felding, P., Nilsson, I. M., Hansson, B. G., *et al.* (1985) Absence of antibodies to LAV/HTLV-III in haemophiliacs treated with heat-treated factor VIII concentrate of American origin. *Lancet*, **ii**, 832–3.

Feldman, F., Klekamp, M. S., Hrinda, M. E., *et al.* (1989) *Stabilization of Biologicals and Pharmaceutical Products during Thermal Inactivation of Viral and Bacterial Contaminants*. US Patent, no. 4876241.

Feldman, P. and Roberts, P. (1998) Virus-filtration of factor IX – an approach to process validation. In *Proceedings of Planova® Workshop, Oslo, 27 June 1998*, pp. 47–55. Tokyo, Asahi Chemical Industry Co. Ltd.

Fernandes, P. M. (1997) *Deposition in JKB vs. Armour Pharmaceutical Corporation, et al., 25 January 1997*. Vallejo, California, Doucette Legal Services.

Fernandes, P. M. and Lundblad, J. L. (1984) *Pasteurised Therapeutically Active Protein Compositions*. US Patent, no. 440679.

Findlay, G. M., MacCallum, F. O. and Murgatroyd, F. (1939) Observations bearing on aetiology of infective hepatitis (so-called catarrhal jaundice). *Trans R Soc Trop Med Hyg*, **32**, 575–86.

Finlay, T. A. (1997) *Report of the Tribunal of Inquiry into the Blood Transfusion Service Board*. Dublin, Government Publications.

Finlayson, J. S. and Tankersley, D. L. (1990) Anti-HCV screening and plasma fractionation: the case against. *Lancet*, **335**, 1274–5.

Fiore, J. W., Olson, W. P. and Holst, S. L. (1980) Depth filtration. In *Methods of Plasma Protein Fractionation*, ed. J. M. Curling, London, Academic Press. pp. 239–68.

Fitzpatrick, J. and Kennedy, C. C. (1969) Serum hepatitis in a haemophiliac. *BMJ*, **4** (5678), 299.

Flan, B. and Aubin, J. T. (2005) Evaluation de l'efficacité des procédés de purification des protéines plasmatique à éliminer les agents transmissible non-conventionnels. *Virologie*, **9**, 545–56.

Forbes, C. D. and Prentice, C. R. M. (1977) Mortality in haemophilia – a United Kingdom survey. In *Unsolved Therapeutic Problems in Hemophilia*, eds. J. C. Fratantoni and D. L. Aronson, pp. 15–22. Washington US Department of Health, Education, and Welfare, DHEW publication no. (NIH) 77–1089.

Foster, P. R. (1994) Protein precipitation. In *Engineering Processes for Bioseparation*, ed. L. R. Weatherley. Oxford, Butterworth-Heinemann, pp. 73–109.

Foster, P. R. (1999) Assessment of the potential of plasma fractionation processes to remove causative agents of transmissible spongiform encephalopathy. *Transfus Med*, **9**, 3–14.

Foster, P. R. (2000) Prions and blood products. *Annals of Medicine*, **32**, 501–13.

Foster, P. R. (2005) Fractionation, plasma. In *The Kirk-Othmer Encyclopedia of Chemical Technology*. 5th edn, volume 12, ed. A. Seidel. New York, John Wiley & Sons, Inc. pp. 128–59.

Foster, P. R. (2006) Plasma products. In *Creutzfeldt-Jakob Disease: Managing the Risk of Transmission by Blood, Plasma, and Tissues*, ed. M. L. Turner. Bethesda, Maryland, AABB Press. pp. 187–213.

Foster, P. R., Cuthbertson, B., McIntosh, R. V., *et al.* (1997a) Safer clotting factor concentrates. In *Hemophilia*, eds C. D. Forbes, L. Aledort and R. Madhok, pp. 307–32. London, Chapman & Hall Medical.

Foster, P. R., Cuthbertson, B., Perry, R. J., *et al.* (1988b) Coagulation factor VIII concentrates and the marketplace. *Lancet*, **ii**, 43.

Foster, P. R., Dickson, I. H., Macleod, A. J., *et al.* (1983a) Zinc fractionation of cryoprecipitate. *Thromb Haemost*, **50**, 117.

Foster, P. R., Dickson, I. H., McQuillan, T. A., *et al.* (1983b) Factor VIII stability during the manufacture of a clinical concentrate. *Thromb Haemost*, **50**, 117.

Foster, P. R., Dickson, I. H., McQuillan, T. A., *et al.* (1988a) Studies on the stability of VIII:C during the manufacture of a factor VIII concentrate for clinical use. *Vox Sang*, **55**, 81–9.

Foster, P. R., Griffin, B. D., Bienek, C., *et al.* (2004) Distribution of a bovine spongiform encephalopathy-derived agent over ion exchange chromatography in the preparation of concentrates of fibrinogen and factor VIII. *Vox Sang*, **86**, 92–9.

Foster, P. R., McIntosh, R. V. and Welch, A. G. (1995) Hepatitis C infection from anti-D immunoglobulin. *Lancet*, **346**, 372.

Foster, P. R., Patterson, M. R., Dickson, A. J., *et al.* (1980b) Intermediate purity factor VIII concentrate: changes in antigen and coagulant activity during production. *Br J Haematol*, **46**, 334.

Foster, P. R., Patterson, M. R., Johnson, A. J., *et al.* (1980a) Thrombogenicity of factor IX concentrates and polyethylene glycol processing. *Thrombosis Research*, **17**, 273–9.

Foster, P. R., Welch, A. G., Cuthbertson, B., *et al.* (1997b) Immunoglobulin for intravenous use. *Transfus Med*, **7**, 67–9.

Foster, P. R., Welch, A. G., McLean, C., *et al.* (2000) Studies on the removal of abnormal prion protein by processes used in the manufacture of human plasma products. *Vox Sang*, **78**, 86–95.

Fox, J. P., Manso, C., Penna, H. A., *et al.* (1942) Observations on the occurrence of icterus in Brazil following vaccination against yellow fever. *Am J Hyg*, **36**, 68–116.

Funk, M., Ebener, U. and Kreuz, W. (1993) Immune status of HIV and HCV negative haemophiliacs treated with intermediate-purity factor VIII concentrates. *Lancet*, **342**, 933–4.

Gaboulaud, V., Parquet, A., Tahiri, C., *et al.* (2002) Prevalence of IgG antibodies to human parvovirus B19 in haemophilia children treated with recombinant factor (F) VIII only or with at least one plasma-derived FVIII or FIX concentrate: results from the French haemophilia cohort. *Br J Haematol*, **116**, 383–9.

Gallo, R. C., Popovic, M. and Sarngadharan, M. G. (1985) Serological detection of antibodies to HTLV-III in sera of patients with AIDS and pre-AIDS conditions. US Patent no. 4 520 113.

Gallo, R. C., Salahuddin, S. Z., Popovic, M., *et al.* (1984) Frequent detection and isolation of cytopathic retroviruses (HTLV-III) from patients with AIDS or at risk from AIDS. *Science*, **224**, 500–3.

Galpin, S. A., Karayiannis, P., Middleton, S. M., *et al.* (1984) The removal of hepatitis B virus from factor VIII concentrates by fractionation on ethylene maleic anhydride polyelectrolyte. *J Med Virol*, **14**, 229–33.

Garcia, T., Lopez, A., Quintana, M., *et al.* (1996) HGV in coagulation factor concentrates. *Lancet*, **348**, 1032.

Gazengel, C., Torcher, M. F., Boneu, B., *et al.* (1988) Viral safety of solvent/detergent treated factor VIII concentrate. Results of a French multicenter study. In *Proceedings of 18th International Congress of World Federation of Hemophilia*, eds G. Papaevangelon and W. Hennessen, p. 59. Madrid, World Federation of Hemophilia.

Gedye, R. (1993) German AIDS scandal infects Europe. *BMJ*, **307**, 1229.

Gellis, S. S., Neefe, J. R., Stokes, J., *et al.* (1948) Chemical, clinical and immunological studies on the products of human plasma fractionation. XXXVI. Inactivation of the virus of homologous serum hepatitis in solutions of normal human serum albumin by means of heat. *J Clin Invest*, **27**, 239–44.

Gerety, R. J. (1985) Safety aspects. Discussion. In *Plasma Fractionation and Blood Transfusion*, eds. C. Th. Smit Sibinga and P. C. Das, p. 181. Boston, Kluwer Academic Publishers.

Gerety, R. J. and Aronson, D. L. (1982) Plasma derivatives and viral hepatitis. *Transfusion*, **22**, 347–51.

Gerolami, V., Halfon, P., Chambost, H., *et al.* (1997) Prevalence of hepatitis G virus RNA in a population of French haemophiliacs. *Br J Haematol*, **99**, 209–14.

Gerolami, V., Halfon, P., Chambost, H., *et al.* (1998) Transfusion transmitted virus. *Lancet*, **352**, 1309.

Gerritzen, A., Schneweis, K. E., Brackmann, H. H., *et al.* (1992b) Acute hepatitis A in haemophiliacs. *Lancet*, **340**, 1231–2.

Gerritzen, A., Scholt, B., Kaiser, R., *et al.* (1992a) Acute hepatitis C in haemophiliacs due to 'virus inactivated' clotting factor concentrates. *Thromb Haemost*, **68**, 781.

Gilligan, K. J., Pizzi, V. F., Stenland, C., *et al.* (2002) The use of size exclusion composite membrane to remove TSE infectious particles from a model protein solution filtration. *Poster PS 1020EN00*. Bedford, MA, Millipore Publications.

Glied, S. (1999) The circulation of the blood. AIDS, blood, and the economics of information. In *Blood Feuds. AIDS, Blood, and the Politics of Medical Disaster*, eds. E. A. Feldman and R. Bayer, pp. 322–347. New York, Oxford University Press.

Gocke, D. J., Raska, K., Pollack, W., *et al.* (1986) HTLV-III antibody in commercial immunoglobulin. *Lancet*, **i**, 37–8.

Gomperts, E. D. (1994) HCV and Gammagard in France. *Lancet*, **344**, 201.

Gomperts, E. D. (1996) Gammagard and reported hepatitis C virus episodes. *Clin Therap*, **18** (Suppl. B), 3–8.

Gonzaga, A. L. and Bonecker, C. (1990) Follow-up of hemophiliacs using solvent/detergent treated FVIII and FIX concentrates. In *Proceedings of 19th International Congress of the World Federation of Hemophilia*, eds. F. Brown and A. S. Lubiniecki, p. 25. Washington, World Federation of Hemophilia.

Goudemand, J., Laurian, Y. and Calvez, T. (2006b) Risk of inhibitors in haemophilia and the type of factor replacement. *Curr Opin Hematol*, **13**, 316–22.

Goudemand, J., Rothschild, C., Demiguel, V., *et al.* (2006a) Influence of the type of factor VIII concentrate on the incidence of factor VIII inhibitors in previously untreated patients with severe hemophilia A. *Blood*, **107**, 46–51.

Gregori, L., Maring, J. A., MacAuley, C., *et al.* (2004) Partitioning of TSE infectivity during ethanol fractionation of human plasma. *Biologicals*, **32**, 1–10.

Griffin, M. (1991) Ultrapure plasma factor VIII produced by anti-FVIIIC immunoaffinity chromatography and solvent/detergent viral inactivation. Characterisation of the Method M process and Hemofil M antihemophilic factor (human). *Ann Hematol*, **63**, 131–7.

Grosse-Bley, A., Eis-Hubinger, A. M., Kaiser, R., *et al.* (1994) Serological and virological markers of human parvovirus B19 infection in sera of haemophiliacs. *Thromb Haemost*, **72**, 503–7.

Grossman, C. M. and Saward, E. W. (1946) Homologous serum jaundice following the administration of commercial pooled plasma. A report of eight cases including one fatality. *N Eng J Med*, **234**, 181–3.

Guérois, C. Rothschild, C., Laurian, Y., *et al.* (1993) Incidence of inhibitors specific for factor VIII. Inhibitor development in severe haemophilia patients treated with only one brand of highly purified plasma-derived concentrate. *Thromb and Haemost*, **73**, 215–8.

Gunson, H. H. and Rawlinson, V. I. (1991) Screening of blood donations for HIV-1 antibody: 1985–1991. *Communicable Disease Report Review*, **1** (no. 13), R144–6.

Hamalainen, E., Suomela, H. and Ukkonen, P. (1992) Virus inactivation during intravenous immunoglobulin production. *Vox Sang*, **63**, 6–11.

Hamamoto, Y., Harada, S., Kobayashi, K., *et al.* (1989) A novel method for removal of human immunodeficiency virus: filtration with porous polymeric membranes. *Vox Sang*, **56**, 230–6.

Hanley, J. P., Jarvis, L. M., Hayes, P. C., *et al.* (1998) Patterns of hepatitis G viraemia and liver disease in haemophiliacs previously exposed to non-virus inactivated coagulation factor concentrates. *Thromb Haemost*, **79**, 291–5.

Harasawa, R. and Sasaki, T. (1995) Sequence analysis of the 5' untranslated region of pestivirus RNA demonstrated in interferons for human use. *Biologicals*, **23**, 263–9.

Harris, R. B., Johnson, A. J., Semar, M., *et al.* (1979) Freedom from transmission of hepatitis-B of gamma-globulin and heat-inactivated plasma protein fraction prepared from contaminated human plasma by fractionation with solid-phase polyelectrolytes. *Vox Sang*, **36**, 129–36.

Hart, H., Hart, W. G., Crossley, J., *et al.* (1994b) Effect of terminal (dry) heat treatment on non-enveloped viruses in coagulation factor concentrates. *Vox Sang*, **67**, 345–50.

Hart, H., Hart, W. G. and Foster, P. R. (1995) Virus inactivation in intravenous immunoglobulin: a comparison with SD treatment of factor VIII. *Transfus Med*, **5** (Suppl. 1), 41.

Hart, H., Jones, A., Cubie, H., *et al.* (1994a) Distribution of hepatitis A antibody over a process for the preparation of a high-purity factor VIII concentrate. *Vox Sang*, **67** (Suppl. 1), 51–5.

Hart, H., McIntosh, R. V. and Foster, P. R. (1996) Safety of coagulation factor concentrates: reducing the infectious bioburden. *Haemophilia*, **2** (Suppl. 1), 23.

Hartman, W. H., Kelly, A. R. and LoGrippo, G. A. (1955) Four-year study concerning the inactivation of viruses in blood and plasma. *Gastroenterology*, **28**, 244–56.

Hartman, F. W., LoGrippo, G. A. and Kelly, A. R. (1956) Procedure for sterilisation of plasma using combinations of ultra violet irradiating and beta-propiolactone. *Federation Proceedings*, **15**, 518.

Hayakawa, F., Imada, K., Towatari, M., *et al.* (2002) Life-threatening human parvovirus B19 infection transmitted by intravenous immune globulin. *Br J Haematol*, **118**, 1187–9.

Healey, C. J., Sabharwal., McOmish, F., *et al.* (1996) Outbreak of acute hepatitis C following the use of anti-HCV screened intravenous immunoglobulin therapy. *Gastroenterology*, **110**, 1120–6.

Hedlund, K. (1973) Hepatitis B antigen: removal from protein solutions in a recognizable form by an insoluble lipophilic matrix of silicic acid. *Life Sci*, **13**, 1491–7.

Heimburger, N., Schwinn, H., Gratz, P., *et al.* (1981a) A factor VIII concentrate highly purified and heated in solution. *Haemostasis*, **10** (Suppl. 1), 204.

Heimburger, N., Schwinn, H., Gratz, P., *et al.* (1981b) Factor VIII concentrate highly purified and heated in solution. *Arzneimittel-Forschung*, **31**, 619–22.

Heimburger, N., Schwinn, H. and Mauler, R. (1980) Factor VIII concentrate – now free from hepatitis risk: progress in the treatment of haemophilia. *Die gelben Hefte*, **4**, 165–74.

Heimburger, N., Wormsbacher, W. and Kumpe, G. (1986) Process for the Production of a Pasteurized Isoagglutinin-free Factor VIII Preparation from a Cryoprecipitate. European Patent no. EP0173242.

Heldebrandt, C. M., Gomperts, E. D. Kasper, C. K., *et al.* (1985) Evaluation of two viral inactivation methods for the preparation of safer factor VIII and factor IX concentrates, *Transfusion*, **25**, 510–5.

Hellerstein, L. J. and Deykin, D. (1971) Hepatitis after Konyne administration. *N Eng J Med*, **284**, 1039–40.

Henin, Y., Maréchal, V., Barré-Sinoussi, F., *et al.* (1988) Inactivation and partition of human immunodeficiency virus during Kistler and Nitschmann fractionation of human blood plasma. *Vox Sang*, **54**, 78–83.

Herring, S. W., Abildgaard, C., Shitanishi, K. T., *et al.* (1993) Human coagulation factor IX: assessment of thrombogenicity in animal models and viral safety. *J Lab Clin Med*, **121**, 394–405.

Hershgold, E. J., Pool, J. G. and Pappenhagen, A. R. (1966) The potent antihemophilic globulin concentrate derived from a cold insoluble fraction of human plasma: characterization and further data on preparation and clinical trial. *J Lab Clin Med*, **67**, 23–32.

Heystek, J., Brummelhuis, H. G. J. and Krijnen, H. W. (1973) Contributions to the optimal use of human blood. II. The large-scale preparation of prothrombin complex. A comparison between two methods using the anion exchangers DEAE-cellulose DE52 and DEAE-Sephadex A-50. *Vox Sang*, **25**, 113–23.

Hile, J. P. (1978) Fibrinogen (human) revocation of licenses. *Federal Register*, **43**, 1131–2.

Hilfenhaus, J. and Nowak, T. (1994) Inactivation of hepatitis A virus by pasteurization and elimination of picornaviruses during manufacture of factor VIII concentrate. *Vox Sang*, **67** (Suppl. 1), 62–6.

Hilfenhaus, J., Geiger, H., Lemp, J., *et al.* (1987) A strategy for testing established human plasma protein manufacturing procedures for their ability to inactivate or eliminate human immunodeficiency virus. *J Biol Stand*, **15**, 251–63.

Hilfenhaus, J. W., Gregersen, J. P., Mehdi, S., *et al.* (1990) Inactivation of HIV-1 and HIV-2 by various manufacturing procedures for human plasma proteins. *Cancer Detec Preven*, **14**, 369–75.

Hilfenhaus, J., Herrmann, A., Mauler, R., *et al.* (1986) Inactivation of the AIDS-causing retrovirus and other human viruses in antihemophilic plasma protein preparations by pasteurisation. *Vox Sang*, **50**, 208–11.

Hino, M., Ishiko, O., Honda, K. I., *et al.* (2000) Transmission of symptomatic parvovirus B19 infection by fibrin sealant used during surgery. *Br J Haematol*, **108**, 194–5.

Hino, M., Yamamura, R., Nishiki, S., *et al.* (1999) Human parvovirus B19-induced aplastic crisis in a patient treated with fibrin sealant. *Japanese J Clin Hematol*, **40**, 145–9.

Hoag, M. S., Johnson, F. F., Robinson, J. A., *et al.* (1969) Treatment of hemophilla B with a new clotting-factor concentrate. *N Eng J Med*, **280**, 581–6.

Hollinger, F. B., Doland, G., Thomas, W., *et al.* (1984) Reduction in risk of hepatitis transmission by heat-treatment of a human factor VIII concentrate. *J Infect Dis*, **150**, 250–62.

Hollinger, F. B., Khan, N. C., Oefinger, P. E., *et al.* (1983) Post-transfusion hepatitis type A. *J Am Med Assoc*, **250**, 2313–17.

Hoofnagle, J. H. and Barker, L. F. (1976) Hepatitis B virus and albumin products. In *Proceedings of the Workshop on Albumin*, eds. J. T. Sgouris and A. René, pp. 305–14. Washington, Department of Health, Education, and Welfare, DHEW Publication No. (NIH) 76–925.

Hoofnagle, J. H. and Waggoner, J. G. (1980) Hepatitis A and B virus markers in immune serum globulin. *Gastroenterology*, **78**, 259–63.

Hoofnagle, J. H., Aronson, D. and Roberts, H. (1975) Serological evidence for hepatitis B virus infection in patients with hemophilia B. *Thrombosis et Diathesis Haemorrhagica*, **33**, 606–9.

Hoofnagle, J. H., Gerety, R. J., Thiel, J., *et al.* (1976) The prevalence of hepatitis B surface antigen in commercially prepared plasma products. *J Lab Clin Med*, **88**, 102–13.

Hooper, J. A. (1997) Production and properties of intravenous immunoglobulins. In *Intravenous Immunoglobulins in Clinical Practice*, eds M. L. Lee and V. Strand, pp. 37–55. New York, Marcel Dekker Inc.

Hooper, J. A., Alpern, M. and Mankarious, S. (1988) Immunoglobulin manufacturing procedures. In *Immunoglobulins*, eds H. W. Krijnen, P. F. W. Strengers and W. G. van Aken, pp. 361–80. Amsterdam, Central Laboratory of the Netherlands Red Cross.

Hoppe, H. H., Krebs, H. J., Mester, T., *et al.* (1967) Production of anti-Rh gamma globulin for preventive immunisation. *Munchener Medizinische Wochenschrift*, **109**, 1749–52.

Hoppe, H. H., Mester, T., Hennig, W., *et al.* (1973) Prevention of Rh-immunization. Modified production of IgG anti-Rh for intravenous application by ion exchange chromatography (IEC). *Vox Sang*, **25**, 308–16.

Horowitz, B. (1989) Investigations into the application of tri-n-butyl phosphate/detergent mixtures to blood derivatives. In *Virus Inactivation in Plasma Products*, ed. J. J. Morgenthaler, pp. 83–96. Basel, Karger.

Horowitz, B. (1991) Potential accumulation of tri-n-butyl phosphate in solvent-detergent virus-inactivated plasma products (reply). *Transfusion*, **31**, 871.

Horowitz, B. and Ben-Hur, E. (2000) Efforts in minimizing risk of viral transmission through viral inactivation. *Ann Med*, **32**, 475–84.

Horowitz, B., Lazo, A., Grossberg, H., *et al.* (1998) Virus inactivation by solvent/detergent treatment and the manufacture of SD-plasma. *Vox Sang*, **74** (Suppl. 1), 203–6.

Horowitz, B., Wiebe, M. E., Lippin, A., *et al.* (1985) Inactivation of viruses in labile blood derivatives. I. Disruption of lipid-enveloped viruses by tri-n-butyl phosphate detergent combinations. *Transfusion*, **25**, 516–22.

Horowitz, M. S., Rooks, C., Horowitz, B., *et al.* (1988) Virus safety of solvent/detergent-treated antihemophilic factor concentrate in previously untreated patients. *Lancet*, **ii**, 186.

Horzinek, M. C. (1981) *Non-Arthropod-Borne Togaviruses*. London, Academic Press.

Hrindra, M. E., Feldman, F. and Schrieber, A. B. (1990) Preclinical characterisation of a new pasteurised monoclonal antibody purified factor VIIIC. *Semin Hematol*, **27** (2, Suppl. 2), 19–24.

Hrindra, M. E., Huang, C., Tarr, G. C., *et al.* (1991) Preclinical studies of a monoclonal antibody-purified factor IX, Mononine™. *Semin Hematol*, **28** (3, Suppl. 6), 6–14.

Hsia, D.Y.-Y., Kennell, J. H. and Gellis, S. S. (1953) Homologous serum-hepatitis following the use of Fraction IV prepared from postpartum plasma. A report of four cases. *Am J Med Sci*, **226**, 261–4.

Hubbard, A. R., Weller, L. J. and Bevan, S. A. (2002) A survey of one-stage and chromogenic potencies in therapeutic factor VIII. *Br J Haematol*, **117**, 247–8.

Hyland (1975) *Hemofil AHF Products, Product Insert. December 1975*. Costa Mesa, California, Hyland Division Travenol Laboratories Inc.

Ikeda, Y., Hirano, T. and Murakami, H. (1986) Screening for antibodies to LAV/HTLV-III in recipients of immunoglobulin preparations. *Lancet*, **i**, 1092.

Imbach, P., Perret, B. A., Babington, R., *et al.* (1991) Safety of intravenous immunoglobulin preparations: a prospective multicenter study to exclude the risk of non-A, non-B hepatitis. *Vox Sang*, **61**, 240–3.

Ingram, G. I. C. (1974) Blood fractions for treatment of haemophilia. *Lancet*, **ii**, 56–7.

Ireland, T., Lutz, H., Siwak, M., et al. (2004) Viral filtration of plasma-derived human IgG: a case study using Viresolve NFP. *BioPharm International*, **17** (11), 38–44.

Iwarson, S., Einarsson, M., Smallwood, L., et al. (1987) Chromatographic removal of hepatitis B virus from a factor IX concentrate. Experimental studies in chimpanzees. *Transfusion*, **27**, 171–3.

Jacobson, I. M., Dienstag, J. L., Werner, B. G., et al. (1985) Epidemiology and clinical impact of hepatitis D virus (delta) infection. *Hepatology*, **5**, 188–91.

Jacquemot, C., Cuche, C., Dormont, D., et al. (2005) High incidence of scrapie induced by repeated injection of sub-infectious prion doses. *J Virol*, **79**, 8904–8.

Jakubik, J. J., Vicik, S. M., Tannatt, M. M., et al. (2004) West Nile virus inactivation by the solvent/detergent steps of the second and third generation manufacturing processes from B-domain deleted recombinant factor VIII. *Haemophilia*, **10**, 69–74.

Janeway, C. A. (1948) Clinical use of blood derivatives. *J Am Med Assoc*, **138**, 859–65.

Jantsch-Plunger, V., Beck, G. and Maurer, W. (1995) PCR detection of a low viral load in a prothrombin complex concentrate that transmitted hepatitis B virus. *Vox Sang*, **69**, 352–4.

Jason, J., McDougal, J. S., Holman, R. C., et al. (1985) Human T-lymphotropic retrovirus type III/lymphadenopathy-associated virus antibody. Association with hemophiliacs' immune status and blood component usage. *J Am Med Assoc*, **253**, 3409–15.

Jason, J. M. (1984) HTLV-I/II and HTLV-III seroprevalence in blood product recipients. Presentation at The Ninth Annual Symposium on Blood Transfusion, Gronigen, The Netherlands, 2 November 1984.

John, T. J., Ninan, G. T., Rajagopalan, M. S., et al. (1979) Epidemic hepatitis B caused by commercial immunoglobulin. *Lancet*, **i**, 1074.

Johnson, A. J., MacDonald, V. E., Semar, M., et al. (1978) Preparation of the major plasma fractions by solid-phase polyelectrolytes. *J L Clin Med*, **92**, 194–210.

Johnson, A. J., Newman, J., Howell, M. B., et al. (1967) Purification of antihemophilic factor (AHF) for clinical and experimental use. *Thrombosis Diathesis Haemorrhagica*, **26** (Suppl.), 377–81.

Johnson, A. J., Semar, M., Newman, J., et al. (1976) Removal of hepatitis B surface antigen (HBsAg) from plasma fractions. *J Lab Clin Med*, **88**, 91–101.

Johnson, Z., Thomson, L., Tobin, A. et al. (1995) An outbreak of hepatitis A among Irish haemophiliacs. *International Journal of Epidemiology*, **24**, 821–8.

Johnston, A., MacGregor, A., Borovec, S., et al. (2000) Inactivation and clearance of viruses during the manufacture of high purity factor IX. *Biologicals*, **28**, 129–6.

Jones, P. (1974) Blood fractions for haemophilia. *Lancet*, **ii**, 155.

Jordan, R. T. and Kempe, L. L. (1957) Virus inactivation with gamma radiation from cobalt[60]. In *Hepatitis Frontiers*, eds F. W. Hartman, G. A. LoGrippo, J. G. Mateer and J. Barron, pp. 343–54. London, J. & A. Churchill Ltd.

Josic, D., Hoffer, L., Buchacher, A., et al. (2000) Manufacturing of a prothrombin complex concentrate aiming at low thrombogenicity. *Thromb Res*, **100**, 433–41.

Kappeler, A., Lutz-Wallace, C., Sapp, T., et al. (1996) Detection of bovine polyomavirus contamination in fetal bovine sera and modified live viral vaccines using using polymerase chain reaction. *Biologicals*, **24**, 131–5.

Karcher, H. (1991) German haemophilic patients infected with HIV. *BMJ*, **303**, 1352–3.

Kasermann, F., Kempf, C. and Boschetti, N. (2004) Strengths and limitations of the model virus concept. *PDA J Pharm Sci Technol*, **58**, 244–9.

Kasper, C. K. and Kipnis, S. A. (1972) Hepatitis and clotting-factor concentrates. *J Am Med Assoc*, **221**, 510.

Kasper, C. K., Lusher, J. M., Silberstein, C. E., et al. (1993) Recent evolution of clotting factor concentrates for hemophilia A and B. *Transfusion*, **33**, 422–34.

Kawamura, M., Sawafuji, M., Watanabe, M., et al. (2002) Frequency of transmission of human parvovirus B19 infection by fibrin sealant used during thoracic surgery. *Ann Thorac Surg*, **73**, 1098–1100.

Kekwick, R. A. and MacKay, M. E. (1954) *The Separation of Protein Fractions from Human Plasma with Ether*. Medical Research Council Special Report Series No. 286. London, Her Majesty's Stationery Office.

Kekwick, R. A. and Wolf, P. (1957) A concentrate of antihemophilic factor; its use in six cases of haemophilia. *Lancet*, **i**, 647–50.

Kempf, C., Jentsch, P., Barré-Sinoussi, F., et al. (1991) Inactivation of human immunodeficiency virus (HIV) by low pH and pepsin. *J Acquir Immune Defic Syndr*, **4**, 828–30.

Kenny-Walsh, E. (1999) Clinical outcomes after hepatitis C infection from contaminated anti-D immune globulin. Irish hepatology research group. *N Eng J Med*, **340**, 1228–33.

Kernoff, P. B. A., Miller, E. J., Savidge, G. F., et al. (1987) Reduced risk of non-A, non-B hepatitis after a first exposure to 'wet heated' factor VIII concentrate. *Br J Haematol*, **67**, 207–11.

Kingdon, H. S. (1970) Hepatitis after Konyne. *Ann Intern Med*, **73**, 656–7.

Kirchebner, Ch., Sölder, E. and Schönitzer, D. (1994) Prevention of rhesus incompatibility and viral safety. *Infusionsther Transfusionsmed*, **21**, 281–3.

Kistler, P. and Nitschmann, H. (1962) Large-scale production of human plasma fractions. Eight years' experience with the alcohol fractionation procedure of Nitschmann, Kistler and Lergier. *Vox Sang*, **7**, 414–24.

Kleim, J. P., Bailly, E., Schneweis, K. E., et al. (1990) Acute HIV-1 infection in patients with haemophilia B treated with β-propiolactone-UV-inactivated clotting factor. *Thromb Haemost*, **64**, 336–7.

Kreil, T. R. (2004) West Nile virus: recent experience with the model virus approach. *Dev Biol (Basel)*, **118**, 101–5.

Kreil, T. R., Berting, A., Kistner, O., et al. (2003) West Nile virus and the safety of plasma derivatives: verification of high safety margins, and the validity of predictions based on model virus data. *Transfusion*, **43**, 1023–28.

Kreil, T. R., Wieser, A., Berting, A., et al. (2006) Removal of small nonenveloped viruses by antibody-enhanced nanofiltration during the manufacture of plasma derivatives. *Transfusion*, **46**, 1143–51.

Kreuz, W., Auerswald, G., Brachmann, C., et al. (1992) Prevention of hepatitis C virus infection in children with haemophilia A and B von Willebrand's disease. *Thromb Haemost*, **67**, 184.

Kumar, J., Shaver, M. J. and Abul-Ezz, S. (2005) Long-term remission of recurrent parvovirus-B associated anemia in a renal transplant recipient induced by treatment with immunoglobulin and positive seroconversion. *Transpl Infect Dis*, **7**, 30–33.

Kupfer, B., Oldenburg, J., Brackmann, H. H., et al. (1995) Beta-propiolactone UV inactivated clotting factor concentrate is the source of HIV-infection of 8 hemophilia B patients: confirmed. *Thromb Haemost*, **74**, 1386–7.

Kuo, G., Choo, Q. L., Alter, H. J., et al. (1989) An assay for circulating antibodies to a major etiologic virus of human non-A, non-B hepatitis. *Science*, **244**, 362–4.

Lane, R. S. (1983) Non-A, non-B hepatitis from intravenous immunoglobulin. *Lancet*, **ii**, 974–5.

Lane, S. (1840) Successful transfusion of blood. *Lancet*, **i**, 185–8.

Laub, R., Giambattista, M. D., Fondu, P., et al. (1997) Restricted epitope specificity for factor VIII inhibitors which appeared in previously treated haemophiliacs after infusion with OCTAVI SD plus. *Thromb Haemost*, **77** (Suppl.), 590.

Laurian, Y., Dussaix, E., Parquet, A., et al. (1994) Transmission of human parvovirus B19 by plasma derived factor VIII concentrates. *Nouvelle Revue Française Hématologie*, **36**, 449–53.

Leary, T. P., Muerhoff, A. S., Simmonds, J. N., et al. (1996) Sequence and genomic organization of GBV-C a novel member of the Flaviviridae associated with human non-A-E hepatitis. *J Med Virol*, **48**, 60–2.

Lederman, M. M., Ratnoff, O. D., Evatt, B. L., et al. (1985) Acquisition of antibody to lymphadenopathy-associated virus in patients with classical hemophilia (factor VIII deficiency). *Ann Intern Med*, **102**, 753–7.

Lee, C. A. (1995) Hepatitis C virus and haemophilia: the natural history of HCV in haemophilia patients. *Haemophilia*, **1** (Suppl. 4), 8–12.

Lee, C. A., Kernoff, P. B., Karayiannis, P., et al. (1985) Interaction between hepatotropic viruses in patients with haemophilia. *J Hepatol*, **1**, 379–84.

Lee, D. C., Stenland, C. J., Hartwell, R. C., et al. (2000) Monitoring plasma processing steps with a sensitive Western blot assay for the detection of the prion protein. *J Virol Methods*, **84**, 77–89.

Lee, D. C., Stenland, C. J., Miller, J. L. C., *et al.* (2001) A direct relationship between partitioning of the pathogenic prion protein and transmissible spongiform encephalopathy infectivity during purification of plasma proteins. *Transfusion*, **41**, 49–55.

Lee, M. L., Kingdon, H. S., Hooper, J., *et al.* (1987) Safety of an intravenous immunoglobulin preparation: lack of seroconversion for human immunodeficiency virus. *Clin Thera*, **9**, 300–3.

Leen, C. L. S., Yap, P. L., Neil, G., *et al.* (1986) Serum ALT levels in patients with primary hypogammaglobulinaemia receiving replacement therapy with intravenous immunoglobulin or fresh frozen plasma. *Vox Sang*, **50**, 26–32.

Lefrere, J. J., Loiseau, P., Martinot-Peignoux, M., *et al.* (1996) Infection by hepatitis C virus through contaminated intravenous immune globulin: results of a prospective national inquiry in France. *Transfusion*, **36**, 394–7.

Lehane, D., Kwantes, C. M. S., Upward, M. G. and Thomson, D. R. (1949) Homologous serum jaundice. *BMJ*, **2**, 572–4.

Lesses, M. F. and Hamolsky, M. W. (1951) Epidemic of homologous serum hepatitis apparently caused by human thrombin. *J Am Med Assoc*, **147**, 727–30.

Levene, C. and Blumberg, B. S. (1969) Additional specificities of Australia antigen and the possible identification of hepatitis carriers. *Nature*, **221**, 195–6.

Lever, A. M. L., Webster, A. D. B., Brown, D., *et al.* (1984) Non-A, non-B hepatitis occurring in agammaglobulinaemic patients after intravenous immunoglobulin. *Lancet*, **ii**, 1062–4.

Levy, J. A., Mitra, G. A., Wong, M. F., *et al.* (1985) Inactivation by wet and dry heat of AIDS-associated retroviruses during factor VIII purification from plasma. *Lancet*, **i**, 1456–7.

Lewis, J. H. (1970) Hemophilia, hepatitis and HAA. *Vox Sanguinis*, **19**, 406–9.

Lewis, J. H., Maxwell, N. G. and Brandon, J. M. (1974) Jaundice and hepatitis B antigen/antibody in hemophilia. *Transfusion*, **14**, 203–11.

Lindsay, A. (2002) *Report of the Tribunal of Inquiry into the Infection with HIV and Hepatitis C of Persons with Haemophilia and Related Matters*. Dublin, Government of Ireland Publications.

Linnen, L., Wages, J., Zhangekeck, Z. Y., *et al.* (1996) Molecular cloning and disease association of hepatitis G virus. A transfusion transmissible agent. *Science*, **271**, 505–8.

Littlewood, J. D., Dawes, J., Smith, J. K., *et al.* (1987) Studies on the effect of heat treatment on the thrombogenicity of factor IX concentrates in dogs. *Br J Haematol*, **65**, 463–8.

Llewelyn, C. A., Hewitt, P. E., Knight, R. S. G., *et al.* (2004) Possible transmission of variant Creutzfeldt-Jakob disease by blood transfusion. *Lancet*, **363**, 417–21.

LoGrippo, G. A. and Rupe, C. E. (1957) Chemical sterilization of whole blood and plasma with beta-propiolactone. In *Hepatitis Frontiers*, eds. F. W. Hartman, G. A. LoGrippo, J. G. Mateer and J. Barron, pp. 371–85. London, J. & A. Churchill Ltd.

Louie, R. E., Galloway, C. J., Dumas, M. L., *et al.* (1994) Inactivation of hepatitis C virus in low pH intravenous immunoglobulin. *Biologicals*, **22**, 13–9.

Lubetsky, A., Hoffman, R., Zimlichman, R., *et al.* (2004) Efficacy and safety of a prothrombin complex concentrate (Octaplex®) for rapid reversal of oral anticoagulation. *Thromb Res*, **113**, 371–8.

Ludlam, C. A. (1997) New-variant Creutzfeldt-Jakob disease and treatment of haemophilia. *Lancet*, **350**, 1704.

Ludlam, C. A., Chapman, D., Cohen, B., *et al.* (1989) Antibodies to hepatitis C virus in haemophilia. *Lancet*, **ii**, 560–1.

Ludlam, C. A., Tucker, J., Steel, C. M., *et al.* (1985) Human T-lymphotropic virus type III (HTLV-III) infection in seronegative haemophiliacs after transfusion of factor VIII. *Lancet*, **ii**, 233–6.

Lürman, A. (1885) Eine icterusepidemic. *Berliner Klinischhe Wochenschrift*, **22**, 20–3.

Lynch, T., Weinstein, M. J., Tankersley, D. L., *et al.* (1996) Considerations of pool size in the manufacture of plasma derivatives. *Transfusion*, **36**, 770–5.

Machin, S. J., McVerry, B. A., Cheinsong-Popov, R., *et al.* (1985) Seroconversion for HTLV-III since 1980 in British haemophiliacs. *Lancet*, **i**, 336.

MacLeod, A. J., Cuthbertson, B. and Foster, P. R. (1984) Pasteurisation of factor VIII and factor IX concentrates. In *Abstracts of 18th Congress of the International Society of Blood Transfusion*, p. 34. Basel, Karger.

MacNalty, A. S. (1938) Acute infective jaundice and administration of measles serum. In *On the State of the Public Health. Annual Report of the Chief Medical Officer of the Ministry of Health for the Year 1937*, pp. 38–9. London, His Majesty's Stationery Office.

Madhok, R., Melbye, M., Lowe, G. D., *et al.* (1985) HTLV-III antibody in sequential plasma samples: from haemophiliacs 1974–84. *Lancet*, **i**, 524–5.

Mainwaring, R. L. and Brueckner, G. G. (1966) Fibrinogen-transmitted hepatitis. A controlled study. *J Am Med Assoc*, **195**, 437–41.

Mannucci, P. M. (1974) Blood fractions for haemophilia. *Lancet*, **ii**, 584.

Mannucci, P. M. (1992) Outbreak of hepatitis A among Italian patients with haemophilia. *Lancet*, **339**, 819.

Mannucci, P. M. (1993) Clinical evaluation of viral safety of coagulation factor VIII and IX concentrates. *Vox Sang*, **64**, 197–203.

Mannucci, P. M. (2003) AIDS, hepatitis and hemophilia in the 1980s: memoirs from an insider. *J Thromb Haemost*, **1**, 2065–69.

Mannucci, P. M. and Colombo, M. (1988) Virucidal treatment of clotting factor concentrates. *Lancet*, **ii**, 782–5.

Mannucci, P. M. and Colombo, M. (1989) Revision of the protocol recommended for studies of safety from hepatitis of clotting factor concentrates. *Thromb Haemost*, **61**, 532–4.

Mannucci, P. M., Capitanio, A., Del Ninno, E., *et al.* (1975) Asymptomatic liver disease in haemophiliacs. *J Clin Pathol*, **28**, 620–4.

Mannucci, P. M., Gdovin, S., Gringeri, A., *et al.* (1994) Transmission of hepatitis A to patients with haemophilia by factor VIII concentrates treated with organic solvent and detergent to inactivate viruses. *Ann Intern Med*, **120**, 1–7.

Mannucci, P. M., Schimpf, K., Brettler, D. B., *et al.* (1990) Low-risk for hepatitis in hemophiliacs given a high-purity, pasteurized factor VIII concentrate. *Ann Intern Med*, **113**, 24–32.

Mariani, G., Dipaolantonio, T., Baklaya, R., *et al.* (1991) Prospective hepatitis C safety evaluation of a high purity solvent detergent treated FVIII concentrate. *Blood*, **78** (Suppl. 1), 55a.

Mariani, G., Dipaolantonio, T., Baklaya, R., *et al.* (1993) Prospective study of the evaluation of hepatitis C virus infectivity in a high-purity, solvent/detergent-treated factor VIII concentrate: parallel evaluation of other markers for lipid-enveloped and non-lipid-enveloped virus. *Transfusion*, **33**, 814–8.

Matsui, H., Sugimoto, M., Tsuji, S., *et al.* (1999) Transient hypoplastic anemia caused by a primary human parvovirus B19 infection in a previously untreated patient with hemophilia transfused with a plasma-derived, monoclonal antibody-purified factor VIII concentrate. *J Pediatr Hematol Oncol*, **21**, 74–6.

Mauser, E., Marjolen, D., Zaaijer, H., *et al.* (1998) Hepatitis G virus RNA and E2 antibodies in Dutch haemophiliac patients. *Blood*, **92**, 2164–6.

Mauser-Bunschoten, E. P., Varon, D., Savidge, G. F., *et al.* (1993) Effects of chronic use of monoclate, pasterized in patients with haemophilia A previously unexposed to factor VIII concentrate or other blood products. *Blood*, **82** (Suppl. 7), 153.

Maycock, W. d'A. (1964) Transmission of hepatitis by blood and blood products. *Proceedings of Royal Society of Medicine*, **57**, 1077–80.

Maycock, W. d'A., Evans, S., Vallet, L., *et al.* (1963) Further experience with a concentrate containing human antihaemophilic factor. *Br J Haemato*, **9**, 215–35.

McCall, K. B., Gordon, F. H., Bloom, F. C., *et al.* (1957) Methods for the preparation and ultraviolet irradiation of human fibrinogen for intravenous use. *J Am Pharma Assoc*, **46**, 295–8.

McDougal, J. S., Martin, L. S., Court, S. P., *et al.* (1985) Thermal inactivation of the acquired immunodeficiency syndrome virus T-cell lymphotropic virus-III/lymphadenopathy-associated virus, with special reference to antihemophilic factor. *J Clin Invest*, **76**, 875–7.

McGrath, K. M., Thomas, K. B., Herrington, R. W., *et al.* (1985) Use of heat-treated clotting-factor concentrates in patients with haemophilia and a high exposure to HTLV-III. *Med J Aust*, **143**, 11–3.

McIntosh, R. V., Dickson, A. J., Smith, D., *et al.* (1990) Freezing and thawing plasma. In *Cryopreservation and Low Temperature Biology in Blood Transfusion*, eds C. Th. Smit Sibinga, P. C. Das and H. T. Meryman, pp. 11–24. Norwell, MA, Kluwer Academic Publishers.

McIntosh, R. V., Docherty, N., Fleming, D., *et al.* (1987) A high yield factor VIII concentrate suitable for advanced heat treatment. *Thromb Haemost*, **58**, 306.

McIntosh, R. V., Rogers, P., Latto, D., *et al.* (1996) Safety of coagulation factor concentrates: validation of equipment for virus inactivation. *Haemophilia*, **2** (Suppl. 1), 23.

McGhee, S. A., Kaska, B., Liebhaber, M., *et al.* (2005) Persistent parvovirus-associated chronic fatigue treated with high dose intravenous immunoglobulin. *Pediatr Infect Dis J*, **24**, 272–4.

McMillan, C. W., Diamond, C. L., and Surgenor, D. M. (1961) Treatment of classic hemophilia: the use of fibrinogen rich in factor VIII for hemorrhage and for surgery. *N Eng J Med*, **265**, 224–30.

Meer, J. van der, Daenen, S., van Imhoff, G. W., *et al.* (1986) Absence of seroconversion for HTLV-III in haemophiliacs intensively treated with heat treated factor VIII concentrates. *British Medical Journal (Clinical Research Edition)*, **292**, 1049.

Meisel, H., Reip, A., Faltus, B., *et al.* (1995) Transmission of hepatitis C virus to children and husbands by women infected with contaminated anti-D immunoglobulin. *Lancet*, **345**, 1209–11.

Melbye, M., Biggar, R. J., Chermann, J. C., *et al.* (1984) High prevalence of lymphadenopathy virus (LAV) in European haemophiliacs. *Lancet*, **ii**, 40–1.

Michalski, C., Bal, F., Burnouf, T., *et al.* (1988) Large-scale production and properties of a solvent-detergent-treated factor IX concentrate from human plasma. *Vox Sang*, **55**, 202–10.

Middleton, S. M., Bennett, I. H. and Smith, J. K. (1973) A therapeutic concentrate of coagulation factors II, IX and X from citrated, factor VIII-depleted plasma. *Vox Sang*, **24**, 441–56.

Ministry of Health (1943) Homologous serum jaundice. Memorandum prepared by Medical Officers of the Ministry of Health. *Lancet*, **i**, 83–8.

Minot, G. R. and Taylor, F. H. L. (1947) Hemophilia: the clinical use of antihemophilic globulin. *Ann Intern Med*, **26**, 363–7.

Minot, G. R., Davidson, C. S., Lewis J. H., *et al.* (1945) The coagulation defect in hemophilia: the effect, in hemophilia, of the parenteral administration of a fraction of the plasma globulins rich in fibrinogen. *J Clin Invest*, **24**, 704–7.

Mitra, G., Dobkin, M. B., Wong, M. F., *et al.* (1989) Virus inactivation/elimination in therapeutic protein concentrates. In *Virus Inactivation in Plasma Products*, ed. J.-J. Morgenthaler, pp. 34–43. Basel, Karger.

Mitra, G., Wong, M. F., Mozen M. M., *et al.* (1986) Elimination of infectious retroviruses during preparation of immunoglobulins. *Transfusion*, **26**, 394–7.

Miyagawa, E., Yoshida, T., Takahashi, H., *et al.* (1999) Infection of the erythroid cell line, KU812Ep6 with human parvovirus B19 and its application to titration of B19 infectivity. *J Virol Methods*, **83**, 45–54.

Mondorf, A. W., Stephan, W., Uthemann, H., *et al.* (1981) A clinical study of the tolerance and safety of a beta-propiolactone-treated immunoglobulin. *Arzneimittel-Forschung*, **31**, 1928–30.

Montagnier, L., Chermann, J. C., Barré-Sinoussi, F., *et al.* (1983) Diagnosis of Lymphadenopathy and Acquired Immune Deficiency Syndrome. US Patent application, No. 558 109.

More, J. E. and Harvey, M. J. (1991) Purification technologies for human plasma albumin. In *Blood Separation and Plasma Fractionation*, ed. J. R. Harris, pp. 261–306. New York, John Wiley & Sons, Inc.

Morfini, M., Mannucci, P. M., Ciaverella, N., *et al.* (1994) Prevalence of infection with the hepatitis C virus among Italian hemophiliacs before and after the introduction of virally inactivated clotting factor concentrates: a retrospective evaluation. *Vox Sang*, **67**, 178–82.

Morgado, A. F. and da Fonte, J. G. (1979) An outbreak of hepatitis attributable to inoculation with contaminated gamma globulin. *Bull Pan Am Health Organ*, **13**, 177–86.

Morgan, H. V. and Williamson, D. A. J. (1943) Jaundice following administration of human blood products. *BMJ*, **1**, 750–53.

Morgenthaler, J. J., Maring, J. A. and Rentsch, M. (2002) Method for the Removal of Causative Agent(s) of Transmissible Spongiform Encephalopathies from Protein Solutions. USA Patent, No. 6 407 212.

Mortimer, P. P., Jesson, W. J., Vandervelde, E. M., *et al.* (1985) Prevalence of antibody to human lymphotropic virus type III by risk group and area, United Kingdom 1978–1984. *BMJ (Clinical Research Edition)*, **290**, 1176–8.

Mortimer, P. P., Luban, N. L. C., Kelleher, J. F., *et al.* (1983) Transmission of parvovirus-like virus by clotting factor concentrates. *Lancet*, **ii**, 482–4.

Mösseler, J., Schimpf, K., Auerswald, G., *et al.* (1985) Inability of pasteurised factor VIII preparations to induce antibodies to HTLV-III after long-term treatment. *Lancet*, **i**, 111.

Murphy, W. P. and Workman, W. G. (1953) Serum hepatitis from pooled irradiated dried plasma. *Journal of the American Medical Association*, **152**, 1421–3.

Murray, R. (1955) Viral hepatitis. *Bull N Y Acad Med*, **31**, 341–58.

Murray, R. and Diefenbach, W. C. L. (1953) Effect of heat on the agent of homologous serum hepatitis. *Proceedings of the Society of Experimental Biology and Medicine*, **84**, 230–1.

Murray, R. and Ratner, F. (1953) Safety of immune serum globulin with respect to homologous serum hepatitis. *Proceedings of the Society of Experimental Biology and Medicine*, **83**, 554–5.

Murray, R., Diefenbach, W. C., Geller, H., *et al.* (1955a) The problem of reducing the danger of serum hepatitis from blood and blood products. *N Y State J Med*, **55**, 1145–60.

Murray, R., Oliphant, J. W., Tripp, J. T., *et al.* (1955b) Effect of ultraviolet radiation on the infectivity of icterogenic plasma. *J Am Med Assoc*, **157**, 8–14.

Murray, R., Ratner, F., Diefenbach, W. C. L., *et al.* (1954) Effect of storage at room temperature on infectivity of icterogenic plasma. *J Am Med Assoc*, **155**, 13–5.

Mussgay. M. (1964) Studies on the structure of a hemagglutinating component of a group A arbovirus (Sindbis). *Virology*, **23**, 573–81.

Neurath, A. R., Vernon, S. K., Dobkin, M. B., *et al.* (1972) Characterization of subviral components resulting from treatment of rabies virus with tri-n-butyl phosphate. *J Gen Virol*, **14**, 33–48.

Newman, J., Johnson, A. J., Karpatkin, M. H., *et al.* (1971) Methods for the production of clinically effective intermediate and high purity factor VIII concentrates. *Br J Haematol*, **21**, 1–20.

Ng, P. K. and Dobkin, M. B. (1985) Pasteurisation of antihemophilic factor and model virus inactivation studies. *Thromb Res*, **39**, 439–47.

Nilsson, I. M., Blömback, M. and Ramgren, O. (1962) Haemophilia in Sweden. VI. Treatment of haemophilia with the human antihaemophilia factor preparation (fraction I-0). *Acta Medica Scandinavia*, **379** (Suppl.), 61–110.

Nishizawa, T., Okamoto, H., Konishi, K., *et al.* (1997) A novel DNA virus (TTV) associated with elevated transaminase levels in post-transfusion hepatitis of unknown etiology. *Biochem Biophys Res Commun*, **241**, 92–7.

Noble, R. C., Kane, M. A., Reeves, S. A., *et al.* (1984) Post-transfusion hepatitis A in a neonatal intensive care unit. *J Am Med Assoc*, **252**, 2716–21.

Noel, L., Guerois, C., Maisonneuve, P., *et al.* (1989) Antibodies to hepatitis C virus in hemophilia. *Lancet*, **ii**, 560.

Nowak. T., Gregersen, J. P., Klockmann, U., *et al.* (1992) Virus safety of human immunoglobulins: efficient inactivation of hepatitis C and other human pathogenic viruses by the manufacturing procedure. *J Med Virol*, **36**, 209–16.

Nowak, T., Niedrig, M., Bernhardt, D., *et al.* (1993) Inactivation of HIV, HBV, HCV related viruses and other viruses in human plasma derivatives by pasteurisation. *Dev Biol (Basel)*, **81**, 169–76.

Nubling, C., Chudy, M. and Lower, J. (1999) Validation of HCV-NAT assays and experience with NAT application for blood screening in Germany. *Biologicals*, **27**, 291–4.

Nubling, C., Groner, A. and Lower, J. (1998) GB virus C/hepatitis G virus and intravenous immunoglobulin. *Vox Sang*, **75**, 189–92.

Nubling, C., Willkommen, H. and Lower, J. (1995) Hepatitis C transmission associated with intravenous immunoglobulins. *Lancet*, **345**, 1174.

Ochs, H. D., Fischer, S. H., Virant, F. S., *et al.* (1985) Non-A, non-B hepatitis and intravenous immunoglobulin. *Lancet*, **i**, 404–5.

Ochs, H. D., Fischer, S. H., Virant, F. S., *et al.* (1986) Non-A, non-B hepatitis after intravenous immunoglobulin. *Lancet*, **i**, 322–3.

Offergeld, R., Faensen, D., Ritter, S., *et al.* (2005) Human immunodeficiency virus, hepatitis C and hepatitis B infections among blood donors in Germany 2000–2002: risk of virus transmission and impact of nucleic acid amplification testing. *Euro Surveill*, **10**, 8–11.

Office of Biologics Research and Review (1987) *Points to Consider in the Manufacture and Testing of Monoclonal Antibody Products for Human Use*. Bethesda, MD, Food and Drug Administration.

Oliphant, J. W. and Hollaender, A. (1946) Homologous serum jaundice: experimental inactivation of etiological agent in serum by ultraviolet irradiation. *Public Health Rep*, **61**, 598–602.

Omar, A. and Kempf, C. (2002) Removal of neutralized model parvoviruses and enteroviruses in human IgG solutions by nanofiltration. *Transfusion*, **42**, 1005–10.

Omar, A., Kempf, C., Immelmann, A., *et al.* (1996) Virus inactivation by pepsin treatment at pH 4 of IgG solutions: factors affecting the rate of virus inactivation. *Transfusion*, **36**, 866–72.

Oncley, J. L., Melin, M., Richert, D. A., *et al.* (1949) The separation of the antibodies, isoagglutinins, prothrombin, plasminogen and β_1-lipoprotein into subfractions of human plasma. *J Am Chem Soc*, **71**, 541–50.

Onions, D. (2004) Animal virus contaminants of biotechnology products. *Dev Biol*, **118**, 155–63.

Over, J. (1998) Nanofiltration, the EPFA experience. In *Proceedings of Planova® Workshop, Oslo, 27 June 1998*, pp. 5–15. Tokyo, Asahi Chemical Industry Co. Ltd.

Paine, R. S. and Janeway, C. A. (1952) Human albumin infusions and homologous serum jaundice. *J Am Med Assoc*, **150**, 199–202.

Palmer, J. W. (1976) The evolution of large-scale human plasma fractionation in the United States. In *Proceedings of the Workshop on Albumin*, eds J. T. Sgouris and A. René, pp. 255–269. Washington, Department of Health, Education, and Welfare, DHEW Publication No. (NIH) 76–925.

Pasi, K. J., Evans, J. A., Skidmore, S. J., *et al.* (1990) Prevention of hepatitis C infection in haemophiliacs. *Lancet*, **335**, 1473–4.

Patek, A. J. and Taylor, F. H. L. (1937) Hemophilia II. Some properties of a substance obtained from normal plasma effective in accelerating the coagulation of hemophilic blood. *J Clin Invest*, **16**, 113–24.

Pattison, C. P., Klein, C. A., Leger, R. T., *et al.* (1976) An outbreak of type B hepatitis associated with transfusion of plasma protein fraction. *Am J Epidemiol*, **103**, 399–407.

Paul-Ehrlich-Institut (1994) Reducing the risk of transmission of haematologenous viruses in medicinal products derived from human plasma by fractionation. *Bundesanzeiger*, **101**, 9243–4.

Payne, W. W. and Steen, R. E. (1929) Haemostatic therapy in haemophilia. *BMJ*, **1**, 1150–2.

Peden, A. H., Head, M. W., Ritchie, D. L., *et al.* (2004) Preclinical vCJD after blood transfusion in a PRNP codon 129 heterozygous patient. *Lancet*, **364**, 529–31.

Peerlinck, K. and Vermylen, J. (1993) Acute hepatitis A in patients with haemophilia. *Lancet*, **341**, 189.

Peerlinck, K., Arnout, J., Giambattista, M. D., *et al.* (1997) Factor VIII inhibitors in previously treated haemophilia A patients with a double virus-inactivated plasma derived factor VIII concentrate. *Thromb Haemost*, **77**, 80–6.

Peerlinck, K., Arnout, J., Gilles, J. G., *et al.* (1993) A higher than expected incidence of factor VIII inhibitors in multi-transfused haemophilia A patients treated with an intermediate purity pasteurised factor VIII concentrate. *Thromb Haemost*, **69**, 115–8.

Peerlinck, K., Goubau, P., Coppens, G., *et al.* (1994) Is the apparent outbreak of hepatitis A in Belgian haemophiliacs due to a loss of previous passive immunity? *Vox Sang*, **67** (Suppl. 1), 14–7.

Pennell, R. B. (1957) The distribution of certain viruses in the fractionation of plasma. In *Hepatitis Frontiers*, eds F. W. Hartman, G. A. LoGrippo, J. G. Mateer and J. Barron, pp. 297–309. London, J. & A. Churchill Ltd.

Petrilli, F. L., Crovari, P. and De Flora, S. (1977) Hepatitis B in subjects treated with a drug containing immunoglobulins. *J Infect Dis*, **135**, 252–8.

Phillips, L. L. (1965) Homologous serum jaundice following fibrinogen administration. *Surg Gynecol and Obstet*, **121**, 551–6.

Piszkiewicz, D., Andrews, J., Holst, S., *et al.* (1986a) Safety of immunoglobulin preparations containing antibody to LAV/HTLV-III. In *Progress in Immunodeficiency Research and Therapy II*, eds J. Vossen and C. Griscelli, pp. 197–200. Amsterdam, Elsevier.

Piszkiewicz, D., Mankarious, S., Holst, S., *et al.* (1986b) HIV antibodies in commercial immune globulins. *Lancet*, **i**, 1327.

Piszkiewicz, D., Sun, C. S. and Tondreau, S. C. (1989) Inactivation and removal of human immunodeficiency virus in monoclonal purified antihemophilic factor (human) (Hemofil M). *Thromb Res*, **55**, 627–34.

Pocchiari, M. (1991) Methodological aspects of the validation of purification procedures of human/animal-derived products to remove unconventional slow viruses. *Dev Biol (Basel)*, **75**, 87–95.

Pollmann, H. and Richter, H. (1994) Prevalence of hepatitis and HIV in a group of haemophiliacs. In *Proceedings of the 21st International Congress of the World Federation of Hemophilia*, p. 309. Mexico City, World Federation of Hemophilia.

Pool, J. G. and Robinson, J. (1959) Observations on plasma banking and transfusion procedures for haemophilic patients using a quantitative assay for antihaemophilic globulin (AHG). *Br J Haematol*, **5**, 24–30.

Pool, J. G. and Shannon, A. E. (1965) Production of high-potency concentrates of antihemophilic globulin in a closed-bag system. Assay in vitro and in vivo. *N Engl J Med*, **273**, 1443–7.

Pool, J. G., Hershgold, E. J. and Pappenhagen, A. R. (1964) High-potency antihaemophilic factor concentrate prepared from cryoglobulin precipitate. *Nature*, **203**, 312.

Porter, J. E., Shapiro, M., Maltby, G. L. *et al.* (1953) Human thrombin as a vehicle of infection in homologous serum hepatitis. *J Am Med Assoc*, **153**, 17–9.

Porter, R. R. (1960) γ-Globulins and antibodies. In *The Plasma Proteins, volume 1. Isolation, Characterization, and Function*, ed. F. W. Putnam, pp. 241–77. New York, Academic Press.

Powell, J. S., Bush, M., Harrison, J., *et al.* (2000) Safety and efficacy of solvent/detergent-treated antihaemophilic factor with an added 80°C terminal dry heat treatment in patients with haemophilia A. *Haemophilia*, **6**, 140–9.

Power, J. P., Lawlor, E., Davidson, F., *et al.* (1994) Hepatitis C viraemia in recipients of Irish intravenous anti-D immunoglobulin. *Lancet*, **344**, 1166–7.

Preece, M. A. (1986) Creutzfeldt-Jakob disease: implications for growth hormone-deficient children. *Neuropathol Appl Neurobiol*, **12**, 509–15.

Prescott, L. E. and Simmonds, P. (1998) Global distribution of transfusion-transmitted virus. *N Engl J Med*, **339**, 776–7.

Preston, F. E., Hay, C. R. M., Dewar, M. S., *et al.* (1985) Non-A, non-B hepatitis and heat-treated factor VIII concentrates. *Lancet*, **ii**, 213.

Prikhod'ko, G. G. (2005) Dry-heat sensitivity of human B19 and porcine parvoviruses. *Transfusion*, **45**, 1692–3.

Prince, A. M., Brotman, B., Grady, G. F., *et al.* (1974) Long-incubation post-transfusion hepatitis without serological evidence of exposure to hepatitis-B virus. *Lancet*, **ii**, 241–6.

Prince, A. M., Horowitz, B. and Brotman, B. (1986) Sterilization of hepatitis and HTLV-III viruses by exposure to tri-n-butyl phosphate and sodium cholate. *Lancet*, **i**, 706–10.

Prince, A. M., Horowitz, B., Brotman, B., *et al.* (1984) Inactivation of hepatitis B and Hutchinson strain non-A, non-B hepatitis viruses by exposure to Tween 80 and ether. *Vox Sang*, **46**, 36–43.

Prince, A. M., Horowitz, B., Dichtelmueller, H., *et al.* (1985) Quantitative assays for evaluation of HTLV-III inactivation procedures: tri-n-butyl phosphate: sodium cholate and beta-propiolactone. *Cancer Res*, **45** (Suppl.), 4592S.

Propert, S. A. (1938) Hepatitis after prophylactic serum. *BMJ*, **2**, 677–8.

Prothero, J. L. (1974) Blood fractions for haemophilia. *Lancet*, **ii**, 300–1.

Prowse, C. V., Griffin, B., Pepper, D. S., *et al.* (1981) Changes in factor VIII complex activities during the production of a clinical intermediate-purity factor VIII concentrate. *Thromb Haemost*, **46**, 597–601.

Purcell, R. H., Gerin, J. L., Popper, H., *et al.* (1985) Hepatitis B virus, hepatitis non-A, non-B virus and hepatitis delta virus in lyophilized antihemophilia factor: relative sensitivity to heat. *Hepatology*, **5**, 1091–9.

Rabenau, H., Ohlinger, V., Anderson, J., *et al.* (1993) Contamination of genetically engineered CHO-cells by epizootic haemorrhagic disease virus (EHDV). *Biologicals*, **21**, 207–14.

Ramsay, R. B., Palmer, E. L., McDougal, J. S., *et al.* (1984) Antibody to lymphadenopathy-associated virus in haemophiliacs with and without AIDS. *Lancet*, **ii**, 397–8.

Raut, S., Di Giambattista, M., Bevan, S. A., *et al.* (1998) Modification of factor VIII in therapeutic concentrates after virus inactivation by solvent-detergent and pasteurisation. *Thromb Haemost*, **80**, 624–31.

Redeker, A. G., Hopkins, C. E., Jackson, B., *et al.* (1968) A controlled study of the safety of pooled plasma stored in the liquid state at 30–32 °C for six months. *Transfusion*, **8**, 60–64.

Reichl, H. E., Foster, P. R., Li, Q., *et al.* (2002) Studies on the removal of a bovine spongiform encephalopathy-derived agent by processes used in the manufacture of human immunoglobulin. *Vox Sang*, **83**, 137–45.

Reid, K. G., Cuthbertson, B., Jones A. D. L., *et al.* (1988) Potential contribution of mild pepsin treatment at pH4 to the viral safety of human immunoglobulin products. *Vox Sang*, **55**, 75–80.

Remington, K. M., Trejo, S. R., Buczynski, G., *et al.* (2004) Inactivation of West Nile virus, vaccinia virus and viral surrogates for relevant and emergent viral pathogens in plasma-derived products. *Vox Sang*, **87**, 10–8.

Remis, R. S., O'Shaughnessy, M., Tsoukas, C., *et al.* (1990) HIV transmission to patients with hemophilia by heat-treated donor screened factor concentrate. *Can Med Assoc J*, **142**, 1247–54.

Ristol, P., Gensana, M., Fernandez, J., *et al.* (1996) Evaluation of viral safety of a high-purity human factor VIII concentrate submitted to two specific virus inactivation treatments (FANDHI). *Sangre (Barcelona)*, **41**, 131–6.

Rizza, C. R., Fletcher, M. L. and Kernoff, P. B. A. (1993) Confirmation of viral safety of dry heated factor VIII concentrate (8Y) prepared by Bio Products Laboratory (BPL): a report on behalf of UK haemophilia centre directors. *Br J Haematol*, **84**, 269–72.

Rizza, C. R., Spooner, R. J. D. and Giangrande, P. L. F. (2001) Treatment of haemophilia in the United Kingdom 1981–1996. *Haemophilia*, **7**, 349–59.

Rizzetto, M., Canese, M. G., Arico, S., *et al.* (1977) Immunofluorescence detection of a new antigen-antibody system (δ/anti-δ) associated to hepatitis B virus in liver and in serum of HBsAg carriers. *Gut*, **18**, 997–1003.

Rizzetto, M., Hoyer, B., Canese, M. G., *et al.* (1980) δ agent: association of δ antigen with hepatitis B surface antigen and RNA in serum of δ-infected chimpanzees. *Proceedings of the National Academy of Sciences USA*, **77**, 6124–8.

Rizzetto, M., Morello, C., Mannucci, P. M., *et al.* (1982) Delta infection and liver disease in hemophilic carriers of hepatitis B surface antigen. *J Infect Dis*, **145**, 18–22.

Roberts, P. (2000) Resistance of vaccinia virus to inactivation by solvent/detergent treatment of blood products. *Biologicals*, **28**, 29–32.

Roberts, P. L. and Hart, H. (2000) Comparison of the inactivation of canine and bovine parvoviruses by freeze-drying and dry-heat treatment in two high-purity factor VIII concentrates. *Biologicals*, **28**, 185–8.

Roberts, P. L., El Hana, C. and Saldana, J. (2006) Inactivation of parvovirus B19 and model viruses in factor VIII by dry heat treatment at 80 °C. *Transfusion*, **46**, 1648–50.

Roggendorf, M., Deinhardt, F., Rasshofer, R., *et al.* (1989) Antibodies to hepatitis C virus. *Lancet*, **ii**, 324–5.

Rosenberg, G. Y., Kiselev, A. E., Barinsky, I. F., *et al.* (1971) On the thermoinactivation of Botkin's hepatitis virus in dry fibrinogen and albumin preparations. In *Proceedings of the 12th Congress of the International Society of Blood Transfusion, Moscow 1969, Bibliotheca Haematalogica, No. 38, part II*, pp. 474–8. Basel, Karger.

Rosendaal, F. R., Niewenhuis, H. K., van den Berg, H. M., *et al.* (1993) A sudden increase in factor VIII inhibitor development in multitransfused haemophilia A patients in the Netherlands. *Blood*, **81**, 2180–6.

Rosenthal, N., Bassen, F. A. and Michael, S. R. (1950) Probable transmission of viral hepatitis by ultraviolet-irradiated plasma: report of three cases. *J Am Med Assoc*, **144**, 224–6.

Rosina, F., Saracco, G. and Rizzetto, M. (1985) Risk of post-transfusion infection with the hepatitis delta virus. A multicenter study. *N Eng J Med*, **312**, 1488–91.

Rossi, G., Tucci, A., Cariani, E., *et al.* (1997) Outbreak of hepatitis C virus infection in patients with haematological disorders treated with intravenous immunoglobulin: different prognosis according to immune status. *Blood*, **90**, 1309–14.

Rotblat, F., O'Brien, D. P., O'Brien, F. J., *et al.* (1985) Purification of human factor VIII: C and its characterization by Western blotting using monoclonal antibodies. *Biochemistry*, **24**, 4294–300.

Roussell, R. H. and McCue, J. P. (1991) Antibody purification from plasma. In *Blood Separation and Plasma Fractionation*, ed. J. R. Harris, pp. 307–40. New York, John Wiley & Sons, Inc.

Rouzioux, C., Brun-Vezinet, F., Courouce, A. M., *et al.* (1985) Immunoglobulin G antibodies to lymphadenopathy-associated virus in differently treated French and Belgian hemophiliacs. *Ann Intern Med*, **102**, 476–9.

Rubinstein, A. (1984) Heat Treatment of Lyophilized Blood Clotting Factor VIII Concentrate. US Patent, No. 4456590.

Rubinstein, A. and Dodds, W. J. (1982) Heat treated lyophilised factor VIII concentrate and factor IX concentrate studies in hemophilia A and B dogs. In *Proceedings of the 19th Congress of the International Society of Haematology and the 17th Congress of the International Society of Blood Transfusion, Budapest, 1–7 August 1982*, p. 360. Budapest, Akadémiai Nyomda.

Rumi, M. G., Colombo, M., Gringeri, A., *et al.* (1989) High prevalence of antibody to hepatitis C virus in multitransfused hemophiliacs with normal transaminase levels. *Ann Intern Med*, **112**, 379–80.

Saldanha, J. and Minor, P. (1996) Detection of human parvovirus B19 DNA in plasma pools and blood products derived from these pools: implications for the efficiency and consistency of removal of B19 DNA during manufacture. *Br J Haematol*, **93**, 714–9.

Sarngadharan, M. G., Popovic, M., Bruch, L., *et al.* (1984) Antibodies reactive with human T-lymphotropic retroviruses (HTLV-III) in the serum of patients with AIDS. *Science*, **224**, 506–8.

Savage, M. and Hinskens, W. (1997) Use of Structured Depth Filters for Virus Removal. European Patent Application, No. EP0 798 003.

Savage, M., Torres, J., Franks, L., *et al.* (1998) Determination of adequate moisture content for efficient dry-heat viral inactivation in lyophilized factor VIII by loss on drying and near infrared spectroscopy. *Biologicals*, **26**, 119–24.

Sawyer, W. A., Meyer, K. F., Eaton, M. D., *et al.* (1944) Jaundice in army personnel in the Western region of the United States and its relation to vaccination against yellow fever (parts II, III and IV). *Am J Hyg*, **39**, 35–107.

Scatchard, G., Strong, L. E., Hughes, W. L., *et al.* (1945) Chemical clinical and immunological studies on the products of human plasma fractionation. XXVI. The properties of solutions of serum albumin of low salt content. *J Clin Invest*, **24**, 671–9.

Scheidler, A., Rokos, K., Reuter, T., *et al.* (1998) Inactivation of viruses by beta-propiolactone in human cryo poor plasma and IgG concentrates. *Biologicals*, **26**, 135–44.

Scheinberg, I. H., Kinney, T. D. and Janeway, C. A. (1947) Homologous serum jaundice. *J Am Med Assoc*, **134**, 841–8.

Schimpf, K., Brachmann, H. H., Kreuz, W., *et al.* (1989) Absence of anti-human immunodeficiency virus types 1 and 2 seroconversion after treatment of hemophilia A and B or von Willebrand's disease with pasteurized factor VIII concentrate. *N Eng J Med*, **321**, 1148–52.

Schimpf, K., Mannucci, P. M., Kreuz, W., *et al.* (1987) Absence of hepatitis after treatment with a pasteurized factor VIII. *N Eng J Med*, **316**, 918–22.

Schmidt, I., Blümel, H., Seitz, H., *et al.* (2001) Parvovirus B19 DNA in plasma pools and plasma derivatives. *Vox Sang*, **81**, 228–35.

Schneider, B., Becker, M., Brackmann, H. H., *et al.* (2004) Contamination of coagulation factor concentrates with human parvovirus B19 genotype 1 and 2. *Thromb Haemost*, **92**, 838–845.

Schreiber, A. B., Hrindra, M. E., Newman, J., *et al.* (1989) Removal of viral contaminants by monoclonal antibody purification of plasma proteins. In *Virus Inactivation in Plasma Products*, ed. J.J Morgenthaler, pp. 146–153. Basel, Karger.

Schroeder, D. B. and Mozen, M. M. (1970) Australia antigen distribution during Cohn ethanol fractionation. *Science*, **168**, 1462–4.

Schulman, S., Lindgren, A. C., Petrini, P., *et al.* (1992) Transmission of hepatitis C with pasteurised factor VIII. *Lancet*, **340**, 305–6.

Schuurman, R., van Steenis, B., van Strien, A., *et al.* (1991) Frequent detection of bovine polyomavirus in commercial batches of calf serum by using the polymerase chain reaction. *J Gen Virol*, **72**, 2739–45.

Schwarz, T. F., Roggendorf, M., Hottenräger, B., *et al.* (1991) Removal of parvovirus B19 from contaminated factor VIII during fractionation. *J Med Virol*, **35**, 28–31.

Schwinn, H. (1996) *Deposition in Corson vs. Gulf Coast Regional Blood Center, et al., 2 August 1996*. New York, Doyle Reporting, Inc.

Schwinn, H., Heimburger, N., Kumpe, G., *et al.* (1981) Blood Coagulation Factors and Process for their Manufacture. US patent, no. 4297344.

Seeberg, S., Brandberg, A, Hermodsson, S., *et al.* (1981) Hospital outbreak of hepatitis A secondary to blood exchange in a baby. *Lancet*, **i**, 1155–6.

Seremetis, V. S., Aledort, L. M., Bergman, G. E., *et al.* (1993) Three-year randomised study of high-purity or intermediate-purity factor VIII concentrates in symptom-free HIV-seropositive haemophiliacs: effects on immune status. *Lancet*, **342**, 700–3.

Sergiev, P. G., Tareev, E. M., Gontaeva, A. A., *et al.* (1940) Virusnaya sheltukha: Epidemicheski gepatit v sviasi s immunizatchiei tchelovetscheskoi syvorotkoi. *Terapevticheski Archiv*, **18**, 595–611.

Sexton, D. J., Rollin, P. E., Breitschwerdt, E. B., *et al.* (1997) Life-threatening Cache Valley virus infection. *N Eng J Med*, **336**, 547–9.

Shepard, C. W., Simard, E. P., Finelli, L., *et al.* (2006) Hepatitis B virus infection: epidemiology and vaccination. *Epidemiologic Rev*, **28**, 112–25.

Sherertz, R. J., Russell, B. A. and Reuman, P. D. (1984) Transmission of hepatitis A by transfusion of blood products. *Arch Intern Med*, **144**, 1579–80.

Shikata, T., Karasawa, T., Abe, K., *et al.* (1978) Incomplete inactivation of hepatitis B virus after heat treatment at 60 °C for 10 hours. *J Infect Dis*, **138**, 242–4.

Shimizu, Y. K., Feinstone, S. M., Purcell, R. H., *et al.* (1979) Non-A, non-B hepatitis: ultrastructural evidence for two agents in experimentally infected chimpanzees. *Science*, **205**, 197–200.

Shopnick, R. I., Bolivar, E. and Brettler, D. B., *et al.* (1996) Hepatitis C seropositivity in HIV-negative children with severe haemophilia. *Haemophilia*, **2**, 100–3.

Silva, L. C., Sette, H., Antonacio, F., *et al.* (1977) Commercial gammaglobulin (CGG) as a possible vehicle of transmission of HBsAg in familial clustering. *Revista do Instituto de Medicina Tropical de São Paulo*, **19**, 352–4.

Silveira, J. A., Raymond, G. J., Hughson, A. G., *et al.* (2005) The most infectious prion protein particles. *Nature*, **437**, 257–61.

Simmonds, P., Davidson, F., Lycett, C., *et al.* (1998) Detection of a novel DNA virus (TTV) in blood donors and blood products. *Lancet*, **352**, 191–5.

Skidmore, S., Boxall, E. and Ala, F. (1982) A case report of post-transfusion hepatitis A. *J Med Virol*, **10**, 223.

Skinner, J. S. (1957) Serum hepatitis: occurrence following the use of human fibrinogen. *Mo Med*, **54**, 740–4.

Smith, D. B., Lawlor, E., Power, J., *et al.* (1999) A second outbreak of hepatitis C virus infection from anti-D immunoglobulin in Ireland. *Vox Sang*, **76**, 175–8.

Smith, M. P., Rice, K. M. and Savidge, G. F. (1997) Successful clinical use of a plasma-derived, dual virus inactivated factor VIII concentrate incorporating solvent-detergent and dry heat treatment. *Thromb Haemost*, **77**, 406–7.

Snape, T. J. (1987) Quality control in the development of coagulation factor concentrates. *Devel Biol* (*Basel*), **67**, 141–67. In *Viral Hepatitis: Standardization immunoprophylaxis of Infections by Hepatitis Viruses*, eds P. Schiff and W. Hennessen. Basel, Karger.

Soper, F. L. and Smith, H. H. (1938) Yellow fever vaccination with cultivated virus and immune and hyperimmune serum. *Am J Trop Med*, **18**, 111–34.

Soucie, J. M., Richardson, L. C., Evatt, B. L., *et al.* (2001) Risk factors for infection with HBV and HCV in a large cohort of haemophiliac males. *Transfusion*, **41**, 338–43.

Soulier, J. P., Blatix, C., Courouce, A. M., *et al.* (1972) Prevention of virus B hepatitis (SH hepatitis). *Am J Dis Child*, **123**, 429–34.

Spire, B., Dormont, D., Barré-Sinoussi, F., *et al.* (1985) Inactivation of lymphadenopathy-associated virus by heat, gamma rays, and ultraviolet light. *Lancet*, **i**, 188–9.

Spurling, N., Shone J. and Vaughan, J. (1946) The incidence, incubation period, and symptomatology of homologous serum jaundice. *BMJ*, **2**, 409–12.

Stephan, W. (1975) Undegraded human immunoglobulin for intravenous use. *Vox Sang*, **28**, 422–37.

Stephan, W. (1989) Inactivation of hepatitis viruses and HIV in plasma and plasma derivatives by treatment with β-propiolactone/UV irradiation. In *Virus Inactivation in Plasma Products*, ed. J. J. Morgenthaler, pp. 275–36. Basel, Karger.

Stirling, M. L., Murray, J. A., Mckay, P., *et al.* (1983) Incidence of infection with hepatitis B virus in 56 patients with haemophilia A 1971–1979. *J C Pathol*, **36**, 577–80.

Stokes, J., Blanchard, M., Neefe, J. R., *et al.* (1948) Methods of protection against homologous serum hepatitis SH virus; studies on protective value of gamma-globulin. *J Am Med Assoc*, **138**, 336–41.

Strong, L. E. (1948) Blood fractionation. In *Encyclopedia of Chemical Technology*, volume 2, eds R. E. Kirk and D. F. Othmer, pp. 1–29. New York, The Interscience Encyclopedia, Inc.

Stucki, M., Moudry, R., Kempf, C., *et al.* (1997) Characterisation of a chromatographically produced anti-D immunoglobulin product. *J Chromatogr*, **700**, 241–8.

Sumazaki, R., Yamada-Osaki, M., Kajiwara, Y., *et al.* (1998) Transfusion transmitted virus. *Lancet*, **352**, 1308–9.

Surgenor, D. M. (2002) *Edwin J. Cohn and the Development of Protein Chemistry*, p. 221. Boston, Centre for Blood Research, Inc.

Tabor, E. (1999) The epidemiology of virus transmission by plasma derivatives: clinical studies verifying the lack of transmission of hepatitis B and C viruses and HIV type 1. *Transfusion*, **39**, 1160–8.

Tabor, E. and Gerety, R. J. (1979) Transmission of hepatitis B by immune serum globulin. *Lancet*, **ii**, 1293.

Takahashi, M., Koike, T., Moriyami, Y., *et al.* (1991) Neutralizing activity of immunoglobulin preparation against erythropoietic suppression of human parvovirus. *J Hematol*, **37**, 68.

Tateishi, J., Kimoto, T., Ishikawa, G., *et al.* (1993) Removal of causative agent of Creutzfeldt-Jakob disease (CJD) through membrane filtration method. *Membrane*, **18**, 357–62.

Tateishi, J., Kimoto, T., Mohri, S., *et al.* (2001) Scrapie removal using Planova virus removal filters. *Biologicals*, **29**, 17–25.

Taylor, D. M. (2003) Inactivation of TSE agents: safety of blood and blood derived products. *Transfusion Clinique et Biologique*, **10**, 23–5.

Taylor, F. H. L., Davidson, C. S., Tagnon, H. J., *et al.* (1945) Studies in blood coagulation: the coagulation properties of certain globulin fractions of normal human plasma in vitro. *J Clin Invest*, **24**, 698–703.

Tedder, R. S., Uttley, A. and Cheinsong-Popov, R. (1985) Safety of immunoglobulin preparation containing anti-HTLV-III. *Lancet*, **i**, 815.

Temperley, I. J., Coter, K. P. Walsh, T. J., *et al.* (1992) Clotting factors and hepatitis A. *Lancet*, **340**, 1466.

Terpstra, F. G., Parkinen, J., Tola, H., *et al.* (2006) Viral safety of Nanogam, a new nm-filtered liquid immunoglobulin product. *Vox Sang*, **90**, 21–32.

Theiler, M. (1957) Action of sodium desoxycholate on arthropod-borne viruses. *The Proceedings of the Society of Experimental Biology and Medicine*, **96**, 380–2.

Thyer, J., Unal, A., Hartel, G., *et al.* (2006b) Investigation of prion removal/inactivation from chromatographic gel. *Vox Sang*, **91**, 301–8.

Thyer, J., Unal, A., Thomas, P., *et al.* (2006a) Prion-removal capacity of chromatographic and ethanol precipitation steps used in the production of albumin and immunoglobulin. *Vox Sang*, **91**, 292–300.

Torchin, N. G. (1987) Patent Interference No. 101 574 17 September 1987. Washington, US Department of Commerce, Patent and Trade Mark Office.

Trejo, S. R., Hotta, J. A., Lebing, W., *et al.* (2003) Evaluation of virus and prion reduction in a new intravenous immunoglobulin manufacturing process. *Vox Sang*, **84**, 176–87.

Trepo, C., Hantz, O., Jacquier, M. F., *et al.* (1978) Different fates of hepatitis B virus markers during plasma fractionation. A clue to infectivity of blood derivatives. *Vox Sang*, **35**, 143–8.

Troccoli, N. M., McIver, J., Losikoff, A., *et al.* (1998) Removal of viruses from human intravenous immunoglobulin by 35 nm nanofiltration. *Biologicals*, **26**, 321–9.

Trump, J. G. and Wright, K. A. (1957) Inactivation of the hepatitis virus by high energy electrons. In *Hepatitis Frontiers*, eds. F. W. Hartman, G. A. LoGrippo, J. G. Mateer and J. Barron, pp. 333–41. London, J. & A. Churchill Ltd.

Uemura, Y., Yang, Y. H. L., Heldebrant, C. M., *et al.* (1994) Inactivation and elimination of viruses during preparation of human intravenous immunoglobulin. *Vox Sang*, **67**, 246–54.

UK Regional Haemophilia Centre Directors (1992) Recommendations on choice of therapeutic products for the treatment of patients with haemophilia A, haemophilia B and von Willebrand's disease. *Blood Coagul Fibrinolysis*, **3**, 205–14.

Unal, A., Thyer, J., Uren, E., *et al.* (2007) Investigation by bioassay of the efficacy of sodium hydroxide treatment on the inactivation of mouse-adapted scrapie. *Biologicals*, **35**, 161–4.

Van Holten, R. W. and Autenrieth, S. M. (2003) Evaluation of depth filtration to remove prion challenge from immune globulin preparation, *Vox Sang*, **85**, 20–4.

Van Holten, R. W., Ciavarella, D., Oulundsen, G., *et al.* (2002) Incorporation of an additional viral-clearance step into a human immunoglobulin manufacturing process. *Vox Sang*, **83**, 227–33.

Vey, M., Baron, H., Weimer, T., *et al.* (2002) Purity of spiking agents affects partitioning of prions in plasma protein purification. *Biologicals*, **30**, 187–96.

Wagner, R. H. (1967) Report of the sub-committee on human factor VIII (AHF) preparations. *Thrombosis Diathesis Haemorrhagica*, **26** (Suppl.), 371–5.

Wagner, R. H., Roberts, H. R., Webster, W. P., *et al.* (1968) Glycine-precipitated antihemophilic factor concentrates and their clinical uses. *Thromb Diath Haemorrh*, **35** (Suppl.), 41–8.

Wain-Hobson, S., Vartanian, J. P., Henry, M., *et al.* (1991) LAV revisited: origins of early HIV-1 isolates from Institute Pasteur. *Science*, **252**, 961–5.

Wang, J., Horner, G. W. and O'Keefe, J. S. (2004) Detection and molecular characterisation of bovine polyomavirus in bovine sera in New Zealand. *N Z Vet J*, **53**, 26–30.

Watanabe, K. K., Busch, M. P., Schreiber, G. B., *et al.* (2000) Evaluation of the safety of Rh immunoglobulin by monitoring viral markers among Rh-negative female blood donors. *Vox Sang*, **78**, 1–6.

Watson, H. G. and Ludlam, C. A. (1992) Immunological abnormalities in haemophiliacs. *Blood Rev*, **6**, 26–33.

Webster, A. D. B., Dalgleish, A. G., Malkovsky, M., *et al.* (1986) Isolation of retroviruses from two patients with 'common variable' hypogammaglobulinaemia. *Lancet*, **i**, 581–3.

Webster, W. P., Roberts, H. R., Thelin, G. M., *et al.* (1965) Clinical use of a new glycine-precipitated antihemophilic fraction. *Am J Med Sci*, **250**, 643–51.

Weiland, O., Mattsson, L. and Glaumann, H. (1986) Non-A, non-B hepatitis after intravenous gamma globulin. *Lancet*, **i**, 976–7.

Weisser, J. (1988) Transmission of human immunodeficiency virus by a dry heat treated factor VIII concentrate. *Klinische Pediatrie*, **200**, 307–9.

Welch, A. G., Cuthbertson, B., McIntosh, R. V., *et al.* (1983b) Non-A, non-B hepatitis from intravenous immunoglobulin. *Lancet*, **ii**, 1198–9.

Welch, A. G., McIntosh, R. V. and Foster, P. R. (1983a) Human immunoglobulin for clinical use. *Lancet*, **i**, 358.

Welch, J., Bienek, C., Gomperts, E., *et al.* (2006) Resistance of porcine circovirus and chicken anemia virus to virus inactivation procedures used for blood products. *Transfusion*, **46**, 1951–8.

Wells, M. A., Wittek, A. E., Epstein, J. S., *et al.* (1986) Inactivation and partitioning of human T-cell lymphotropic virus, type III, during ethanol fractionation of plasma. *Transfusion*, **26**, 210–3.

White, G. C., Matthews, T. J., Weinhold, K. J., *et al.* (1986) HTLV-III seroconversion associated with heat-treated factor VIII concentrate. *Lancet*, **i**, 611–2.

Whittaker, J. A. and Brown, M. J. (1969) Serum hepatitis in a haemophiliac. *BMJ*, **3**, 597.

Widell, A., Zhang, Y. Y., Andersson-Gare, B., *et al.* (1997) At least three hepatitis C virus strains implicated in Swedish and Danish patients with intravenous immunoglobulin-associated hepatitis C. *Transfusion*, **37**, 313–20.

Wiese, M., Grüngreiff, K., Güthoff, W., *et al.* (2005) Outcome in a hepatitis C (genotype 1b) single source outbreak in Germany – a 25-year multicenter study. *Journal of Hepatology*, **43**, 590–8.

Will, R. G., Ironside, J. W., Zeilder, M., *et al.* (1996) A new variant of Creutzfeldt-Jakob disease in the UK. *Lancet*, **347**, 921–5.

Williams, M. D., Cohen, B. J., Beddal, A. C., *et al.* (1990b) Transmission of human parvovirus B19 by coagulation factor concentrates. *Vox Sang*, **58**, 177–81.

Williams, M. D., Skidmore, S. J. and Hill, F. G. H. (1990a) HIV seroconversion in haemophilic boys receiving heat treated factor VIII concentrate. *Vox Sang*, **58**, 135–6.

Williams, P. E., Yap, P. L., Gillon, J., *et al.* (1989) Transmission of non-A, non-B hepatitis by pH4-treated intravenous immunoglobulin. *Vox Sang*, **57**, 15–8.

Winkelman, L. (1988) Purification of Blood Coagulation Factor VIII by Precipitation with Sulfated Polysaccharides. US Patent, No. 4 789 733.

Winkelman, L., Owen, N. E., Evans, D. R., *et al.* (1989) Severely heated therapeutic factor VIII concentrate of high specific activity. *Vox Sang*, **57**, 97–103.

Winkelman, L., Owen, N. E., Haddon, M. E., *et al.* (1985) Treatment of a new, high, specific activity, factor VIII concentrate to inactivate viruses. *Thromb Haemost*. **54**, 19.

Wolf, A. M., Mason, J., Fitzpatrick, W. J., *et al.* (1947) Ultraviolet irradiation of human plasma to control homologous serum jaundice. *J Am Med Assoc*, **135**, 476–7.

Wolfs, T. F., Breederveld, C., Krone, W. J., *et al.* (1988) HIV-antibody seroconversions in Dutch haemophiliacs using heat-treated and non-heat-treated coagulation factor concentrates. *Thromb Haemost*, **59**, 396–9.

Wong-Staal, F., Ratner, L., Shaw, G., *et al.* (1985) Molecular biology of human T-lymphotropic retroviruses. *Cancer Research*, **45** (9 Suppl.), 4539–44S.

World Health Organization (1966) The use of human immunoglobulin. Report of a WHO Expert Committee. *World Health Organization Technical Report Series*, No. 327. Geneva, World Health Organization.

World Health Organization (1971) Prevention of Rh sensitisation. Report of a WHO scientific group. *World Health Organization Technical Report Series*, No. 468. Geneva, World Health Organization.

World Health Organization (2005) WHO recommendations on the production, control and regulation of human plasma for fractionation. *56th Meeting of the WHO Expert Committee on Biological Standardization*. Geneva, World Health Organization.

Wroe, S. J., Pal, S., Siddique, D., *et al.* (2006) Clinical presentation and pre-mortem diagnosis of variant Creutzfeldt-Jakob disease associated with blood transfusion: a case report. *Lancet*, **368**, 2061–7.

Wu, C. G., Mason, B., Jong, J., *et al.* (2005) Parvovirus transmission by a high-purity factor VIII concentrate. *Transfusion*, **45**, 1003–10.

Yamada-Osaki, M., Sumazaki, R. and Kajiwara, Y. (1998) Natural course of HGV in haemophiliacs. *Br J Haematol*, **102**, 616–21.

Yap, P. L. (1996) The viral safety of intravenous immunoglobulin. *Clin Expl Immunol*, **104** (Suppl. 1), 35–42.

Yei, S., Yu, M. W. and Tankersley, D. L. (1992) Partitioning of hepatitis C virus during Cohn-Oncley fractionation of plasma. *Transfusion*, **32**, 824–8.

Yokoyama, T., Murai, K., Wakisaka, A., *et al.* (2004) Removal of small non-enveloped viruses by nanofiltration. *Vox Sang*, **86**, 225–9.

Yu, M. W., Mason, B. L., Guo, Z. P., *et al.* (1995) Hepatitis C transmission associated with intravenous immunoglobulins. *Lancet*, **345**, 1173–4.

Yu, M. Y. (1996) Follow-up studies of hepatitis C association with an intravenous immunoglobulin. In *Developments in Biological Standardization*, **88**, pp. 215–6. Basel, Karger.

Yu, M. Y., Bartosch, B., Zhang, P., *et al.* (2004) Neutralizing antibodies to hepatitis C virus (HCV) in immune globulins derived from anti-HCV-positive plasma. *Proceedings of the National Academy of Sciences*, **101**, 7705–10.

Yu, M. Y., Mason, B. L. and Tankersley, D. L. (1994) Detection and characterization of hepatitis C virus RNA in immune globulins. *Transfusion*, **34**, 596–602.

Yunoki, M., Urayama, T. and Kuta, K. (2006) Possible removal of prion agents from blood products during the manufacturing process. *Future Virology*, **1**, 659–74.

Yunoki, M., Urayama, T., Yamamoto, I., *et al.* (2004) Heat sensitivity of a SARS-associated coronavirus introduced into plasma products. *Vox Sang*, **87**, 302–3.

Zanetti, A. R., Ferroni, P., Colombo, M., *et al.* (1985) Anti-LAV/HTLV-III antibodies in groups of individuals at high risk of infection in Italy. *La Ricera in Clinica e in Laboratorio*, **15**, 357–64.

Zuckerman, A. J. (1975) *Human Viral Hepatitis*, 2nd edn. Amsterdam, North-Holland Publishing Company.

SECTION 3: SURVEILLANCE, RISK AND REGULATION

21 SERIOUS HAZARDS OF TRANSFUSION (SHOT); HAEMOVIGILANCE

Elizabeth M. Love

The Serious Hazards of Transfusion scheme (SHOT), is the UK's approach to the surveillance of complications associated with the transfusion of blood and blood components. It was established as part of the UK's response to a European Commission (EC) resolution in 1995 on 'Blood safety and self-sufficiency in the Community' (Council Resolution, 1995). This identified that one of the main activities needed to improve public confidence in the safety of the blood supply was the development of a haemovigilance system 'based on the existing networks for the collection of data related to the blood transfusion safety chain'. Certain aspects of haemovigilance are now a requirement in Europe, as specified in the EU Directive 'Setting standards of quality and safety for the collection, testing, processing, storage and distribution of human blood and blood components' (EU Directive, 2002). These requirements are now adopted in UK law (The Blood Safety and Quality Regulations, 2005).

What is haemovigilance?

Haemovigilance is a broad term which is defined in Council of Europe Guidelines as comprising the detection, gathering and analysis of untoward and unexpected effects of blood transfusion (Council of Europe, 2005). These may contribute to the safety of blood transfusion by:

(1) Providing the medical community with a reliable source of information about untoward effects of blood transfusion.
(2) Indicating corrective measures required to prevent the recurrence of some accidents or dysfunctions in the transfusion process.
(3) Warning hospitals and blood transfusion services about adverse events that could involve more individuals than a single recipient.

Its scope may cover the entire transfusion process, from collection of the donation to transfusion of the recipient and follow-up of the transfusion.

The overall goal is to make clinical care safer for patients requiring transfusion and to demonstrate to the public, patients and professionals the safety of existing transfusion systems (McClelland et al. 1998). It can be approached in a number of different ways, as illustrated by the variety of systems which have been developed in different countries in recent years (Andreu et al., 2002; Linden et al., 2000; Noel et al., 1998; Williamson and Love, 1998). Issues which must be considered when devising a scheme of national haemovigilance or surveillance include the following:

- Its scope: should it be very comprehensive or more restricted with respect to the data it sets out to collect? For example,

severe versus all complications; microbial only versus all; patient data only or the inclusion of donor data.
- Voluntary versus compulsory reporting.
- Confidentiality and anonymity.
- The types of information to be collected.
- 'Ownership' of the scheme: professionals, regulators or government?
- Sources and level of funding.

The choice for an individual country will be influenced by a number of factors, which are governed by the overall organization of blood services within that country. Such factors include, for example, the regulatory and legal environment, the modus operandi for other reporting systems covering complications of medical interventions, priorities in health care development and the level of financial resources available.

Two of the earliest haemovigilance schemes to be set up, those in the UK and France, clearly demonstrate fundamentally different approaches on which several other countries have based their own schemes. The French Haemovigilance scheme is an example of a very comprehensive national system created by law and comprising a complex network of local and regional personnel entrusted with the responsibility of collecting reports and relaying them to the central blood agency. There is a legal obligation on all health care personnel to report any unexpected or undesirable effect of transfusion (Noel et al., 1998). This generates a large body of data which not only comprises serious adverse outcomes of transfusion but also encompasses minor events and those which eventually turn out to be completely unassociated with the transfusion.

The French system contrasts with the much more restricted, confidential and anonymized SHOT scheme in the UK. Both have their advantages and disadvantages and both suffer to a greater or lesser extent from the limitation of lack of denominator data concerning recipients and blood usage (Noel et al., 1998). Many other countries have now established haemovigilance systems based on one or other of the above models. These include the Republic of Ireland, the Netherlands, Denmark, Greece, Canada, Japan and South Africa (Faber, 2004). Other schemes, such as that for New York State (Linden et al., 2000), have been in existence for a number of years, and in Germany surveillance of adverse events of transfusion falls within the remit of pharmacovigilance which is the responsibility of the Paul-Ehrlich-Institut, the regulatory authority in Germany. The requirements of the European Directive, referred to earlier, mean that it will be mandatory for European countries to implement haemovigilance systems.

Transfusion Microbiology, eds John A. J. Barbara, Fiona A. M. Regan and Marcela C. Contreras. Published by Cambridge University Press. © Cambridge University Press 2008.

The transfusion process and the organization of transfusion services in the UK

Ensuring that the right blood is transfused to the right patient at the right time is a complex, multi-step process which crosses several managerial and professional boundaries and may involve many individuals (McClelland *et al.*, 1996; Williamson *et al.*, 1998).

In many countries, responsibility for the transfusion process is divested in a number of different organizations or authorities. These tend to fall into three main categories: first, the blood agency or service (local, regional or national) with responsibility for selection of donors and processing, testing, storage and issue of donations; second, the hospital blood bank, which is responsible for component storage, selection and compatibility testing; third, hospital staff such as nurses, doctors, phlebotomists and porters who are responsible for taking patient samples, prescribing treatment, collecting blood from its storage site, administering the transfusion and monitoring the patient. Mistakes may arise at any point in this process and are often multiple, as SHOT data illustrate, later in this chapter.

In the UK, regulation and training in these three areas fall under a variety of organizations comprising health services and other agencies which set policies and standards, licensing and accreditation bodies, professional organizations which draw up guidelines and recommendations and hazard reporting systems such as SHOT (2000). All contribute to various aspects of blood safety, but as yet there is no national organization with overall responsibility for coordinating blood safety, although this is beginning to be addressed.

The SHOT reporting system: organization and practice

The SHOT scheme was launched in November 1996 following two years of intensive development by a small working group comprising hospital and blood service consultant haematologists, a blood bank scientist and a clinical transfusion nurse specialist. In devising the scheme the working group examined the practice of other confidential enquiry systems in the UK and also the French Haemovigilance scheme. Following discussions with the Department of Health, the Royal College of Pathologists and relevant professional societies it was concluded and agreed that a voluntary, confidential and anonymized reporting scheme, focusing on serious hazards only, would be a pragmatic solution for the UK. Since then, as SHOT has provided increasingly authoritative analysis of serious hazards of transfusion, instructions to hospitals to participate in SHOT have been issued in two directives from the UK Departments of Health (Better Blood Transfusion, 1998; 2002). Therefore, strictly speaking, participation in SHOT is no longer voluntary and with the adoption of the EU Directive, certain aspects of haemovigilance have become a legal requirement.

Ownership of the scheme resides with a multidisciplinary steering group, comprising representatives from all the medical and nursing Royal Colleges and other professional bodies, including

health service management. It is chaired by a hospital-based consultant haematologist and provides the SHOT scheme with strategic direction. Affiliation to the Royal College of Pathologists, gained one year after implementation, strengthens the professional standing of the scheme.

A standing working group, accountable to the steering group through a national medical coordinator, is responsible for the operational working of the scheme. Day-to-day activities are organized in two ways. Non-infectious hazard reports are handled by a small secretariat working under the direction of the national medical coordinator. The latter is currently a part-time role of a consultant haematologist. Reports of infectious complications are collated and analysed by a second national coordinator who has a shared appointment between the National Blood Service (NBS), England and the Health Protection Agency (HPA). Funding is provided by the four UK blood services (England, Scotland, Wales and Northern Ireland).

Services Hazards of Transfusion (SHOT) invites reports of major adverse events surrounding the transfusion of single or small pool blood components supplied by blood centres (red cells, platelets, fresh frozen plasma (FFP), methylene blue FFP and cryoprecipitate). It does not cover complications of fractionated plasma products (coagulation factors, albumin, immunoglobulin) which are licensed medicinal products and covered under a different scheme. However, for purposes of comparison, complications of treatment with solvent/detergent treated FFP should also be reported to SHOT. Hospitals report events under the following categories:

- Incorrect blood component transfused regardless of whether or not harm results (IBCT).
- Acute transfusion reaction (within 24 hours) (ATR).
- Delayed transfusion reaction (beyond 24 hours) (DTR).
- Transfusion-associated graft versus host disease (TA-GVHD).
- Transfusion-related acute lung injury (TRALI).
- Post-transfusion purpura (PTP).
- Transfusion-transmitted infection including bacterial contamination (TTI).
- Autologous pre-deposit incidents.
- 'Near miss' events.

At hospital level, hazards are reported to the local haematologist. Suspected transfusion-transmitted infections must be reported to the supplying blood centre to ensure prompt withdrawal of other implicated components and appropriate follow-up of donors and other possible recipients. (Please refer to Chapter 22.) Blood centre personnel are then responsible for onward reporting to HPA. Non-infectious hazards may be reported directly to the SHOT office using a simple 'initial report' form. This is followed up using a detailed questionnaire specific to the reported event. Once complete, anonymized data is entered using a unique identification number and the paper records are then shredded to prevent traceback to individual cases. Each year an annual report and summary are published and distributed widely to hospitals. This is made freely available on the SHOT website (http//www.shot-uk.org) together with presentations from SHOT, annual update meetings and other information about the SHOT scheme. SHOT has no authority to implement its recommendations for improvement

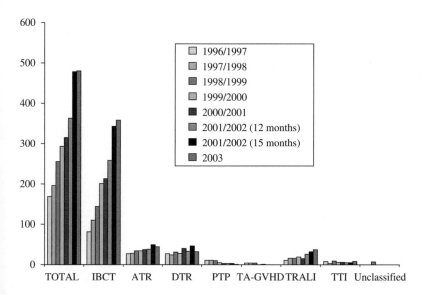

Figure 21.1 Comparison of initial reports of incidents since reporting began in 1996. IBCT: incorrect blood component transfused; ATR: acute transfusion reaction; DTR: delayed transfusion reaction; PTP: post-transfusion purpura; TRALI: transfusion-related acute lung injury; TA-GVHD: transfusion-associated graft versus host disease; TTI: transfusion-transmitted infection.

but relies on education, professional influence and persuasion to achieve its aims.

In an anonymized and confidential scheme such as SHOT, denominator data, in which to place transfusion hazards in the overall context of blood transfusion, is hard to obtain. However, to assess the number of hospitals participating annually in the scheme and their workload in terms of units of red cells handled, hospitals have been invited each year to submit a 'nil events' card. By this means in 2003, 85% of hospitals indicated that they participated, but only 47% of hospitals submitted actual reports, suggesting that, in fact, the completeness of reporting by hospitals is quite variable (SHOT, 2004). In 2003, the use of a confidential code number linked to levels of blood issues to hospitals has allowed more accurate information to be obtained about the context of transfusion errors. A survey about hospital laboratory activity (workload and timing) has also provided useful information and further work is planned to obtain additional benchmarking data (Stainsby, 2004).

Serious Hazards of Transfusion Scheme key findings October 1996–December 2003: cumulative data from seven years of reporting

From 1996–2003 the SHOT scheme collected a powerful body of data on serious transfusion complications in the UK from which to make firm recommendations for improvements in transfusion safety (SHOT, 2004). The four UK blood services issue about 3.5 million blood components each year, although issues of red cells by the NBS have been falling since 2001 as a result of reducing demand by hospitals, linked to more appropriate blood use. Reports to the scheme have risen year on year over seven years of reporting and those in the category 'incorrect blood component transfused' (IBCT) are the main contributors to the increase (see Figure 21.1). Despite these increases, there is now a downward trend in reports of ABO incompatible transfusions (see Figure 21.2), suggesting that improvements in transfusion practice may be starting to take effect.

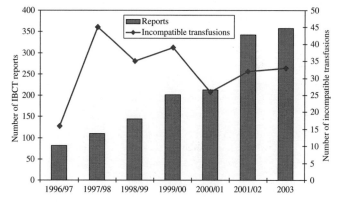

Figure 21.2 ABO incompatible transfusions since 1996.

Of 2087 fully analysed reports, 1393 (66.7%) were 'wrong blood' incidents. Of these, 226 were ABO incompatible transfusions leading to 12 deaths and 49 cases of major morbidity (see Figure 21.3 and Table 21.1). Multiple errors characterized about 48% of cases. Approximately 48% of errors involved mis-identification at the point of collection from the hospital storage site and/or bedside administration, whilst laboratories and prescription/sampling/request errors contributed 29% and 20% respectively.

The single most important cause resulting in mis-transfusion was failure of some aspect of the bedside checking procedure immediately prior to administering the transfusion. Contributory factors included confusion over patients with the same or similar names, checking remotely from the patient's bedside, interruption between completion of the checking procedure and administration of the transfusion and failure to note discrepancies between compatibility and donation labels where a preceding laboratory labelling error had occurred. Unusual circumstances contributed to a small proportion of these incidents but in the majority, no clear explanation for the failures was apparent. Missing wristbands or other formal means of patient identification also contributed to bedside errors in some instances. Withdrawal of the wrong component from its storage location in the hospital preceded a bedside

Table 21.1 Overall mortality/morbidity figures 1996/97–2003 (n = 2087).

		Total	IBCT	ATR	DTR	PTP	TA-GVHD	TRALI	TTI
Deaths definitely attributed to transfusion		43	5	2	6	1	13	8	8
Probably attributed		9	2	2	1	0	0	4	0
Possibly attributed		38	9	6	1	1	0	21	0
	Sub total 1	**90**	**16**	**10**	**8**	**2**	**13**	**33**	**8**
Major morbidity		249	85	5	23	13	0	89	34
Minor or no morbidity		1580	1191	194	158	26	0	9	2
	Sub total 2	**1829**	**1276**	**199**	**181**	**39**	**0**	**98**	**36**
Death unrelated to transfusion		146	90	21	23	3	0	8	1
Outcome unknown		15	11	3	1	0	0	0	0
	TOTAL[a]	**2080**	**1393**	**233**	**213**	**44**	**13**	**139**	**45**

[a] Excludes seven cases from 1998–1999 which were not classified.

IBCT – Incorrect blood component transfused; ATR – Acute transfusion reaction; DTR – Delayed transfusion reaction; PTP – Post-transfusion purpura; TRALI – Transfusion-related acute lung injury; TA-GVHD – Transfusion-associated graft versus host disease; TTI – Transfusion-transmitted infection.

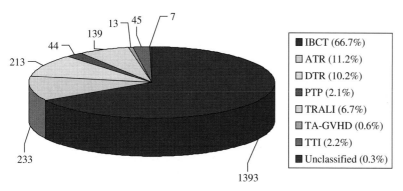

13 — 45 — 7
139
44
213
233
1393

- ■ IBCT (66.7%)
- ☐ ATR (11.2%)
- ☐ DTR (10.2%)
- ■ PTP (2.1%)
- ☐ TRALI (6.7%)
- ■ TA-GVHD (0.6%)
- ■ TTI (2.2%)
- ■ Unclassified (0.3%)

Figure 21.3 Questionnaires by incident 1996–2003 (n = 2087). IBCT: incorrect blood component transfused; ATR: acute transfusion reaction; DTR: delayed transfusion reaction; PTP: post-transfusion purpura; TRALI: transfusion-related acute lung injury; TA-GVHD: transfusion-associated graft versus host disease; TTI: transfusion-transmitted infection. (See colour plate section).

administration error in a significant proportion of cases. The laboratory environment within blood centres and hospital transfusion laboratories is subject to robust quality assurance systems, including strict process control and operation in accordance with good manufacturing practice and good laboratory practice, whereas the stages of the transfusion process which lie outside the laboratory environment are less readily amenable to implementation of equivalent systems.

Immune complications comprised about 31% of reports. There were 139 cases of possible TRALI over seven years, resulting in a fatal outcome in 23% (see Table 20.1). Leucodepletion of all blood components was implemented in the UK in 1999 and since then, reports of PTP and TA-GVD have reduced, although overall numbers of case reports are small.

Transfusion-transmitted infection (TTI) comprised only 2.2% of reports (see Figure 21.3) and of 45 confirmed TTIs, 29 were due to bacterial contamination, 25 of these being associated with platelet transfusions. In this group there were seven deaths, six of which occurred in recipients of contaminated platelets, the majority of which were three or more days old. The source of contamination was confirmed as the donor's skin in 40% of cases, and suspected in many others. In less than 10%

of cases was the donor's blood (i.e. endogenous bacteria) believed to be the source of contamination. There were ten cases where donations transmitted hepatitis B, nine of which were due to donations collected in the acute phase (window period) from donors testing negative for hepatitis B surface antigen using a sensitive test (personal communication). (Please refer to Chapters 1 and 11.)

'Near miss' data collection commenced in 1997 and was originally limited to small pilot studies but has since been extended to all hospitals. Reports are entered under five error categories: sample request, laboratory sampling/handling, laboratory component selection, handling/storage and component issues, and transport and patient identification. Analysis of 2427 reports received up to December 2003 showed that sample errors comprised 57% of the total. The 2003 SHOT report (SHOT, 2004) notes that only 41% of eligible hospitals actually submitted reports in 2003, probably reflecting the difficulty in sustaining external reporting of large numbers of events. However, despite this limitation, the distribution of errors each year has been consistent, highlighting that, as with 'wrong blood' incidents, mistakes involving bedside identification head the list of transfusion errors.

Contribution of haemovigilance data to decision making in blood safety

Developed originally as a response to highly publicized and damaging outbreaks of transfusion-transmitted infections, such as human immunodeficiency virus and hepatitis C, the growth of haemovigilance systems has raised the profile of other complications of transfusion which previously received scant attention. As SHOT data demonstrates, the risk of contracting a transfusion-transmitted viral infection is now very small in comparison with other adverse events such as 'wrong blood to patient', transfusion-related acute lung injury and bacterial contamination incidents.

Although transfusion in the developed world is now probably safer than at any other time, there is continuing pressure to further reduce the already very low risk of infection transmission, by using genomic detection assays, viral inactivation processes and the extension of mandatory testing. (Please refer to Chapter 26.) In addition, the UK has had to face the possibility that vCJD may be transmissible in the blood supply, leading to highly expensive precautionary measures, including leucodepletion of all blood components, outsourcing of plasma for fractionation from non-UK suppliers and the deferral of donors who have themselves received blood component transfusions since 1 January 1980. (Please refer to Chapter 9.) With ever increasing pressures on health care resources, data which helps to establish the relative risks of transfusion can be used to set priorities for further initiatives to improve transfusion safety, a process which requires clear decision-making pathways (Williamson, 2002).

A further benefit of transparent systems of adverse event reporting such as SHOT is their contribution to public confidence, by demonstrating the safety of existing systems, whilst also showing that, where problems exist, these are recognized and effectively tackled in a culture of 'no blame'. This is in keeping with a recent Department of Health (England) development of a system for reporting and analysing all adverse health care events (*An Organization with a Memory*, 2000).

In the UK, SHOT's increasingly authoritative analysis of serious transfusion hazards has provided an evidence base for several blood safety initiatives, policies and guidelines (SHOT, 2004). Attention has been drawn to three main areas for improvement:

(1) Errors in the transfusion process, particularly those resulting in ABO incompatibility.
(2) Transfusion-related acute lung injury (TRALI).
(3) Bacterial contamination of platelet concentrates.

(Please refer back to Chapter 7.) As a result, a number of new safety initiatives have been implemented to reduce the risk of TRALI and bacterial contamination events. The SHOT Annual Report 2003 (SHOT, 2004) made 46 recommendations, targeted at specific groups and organizations to maximize effectiveness. However, it concluded that the most important contribution that could now be made to the safety of the blood transfusion process would be to improve the pre-transfusion bedside checking procedure. This is likely to involve investment in evaluating suitable computerized systems as well as further education and audit (Cohen, 2004).

A further contribution to transfusion safety has been the growth in hospital transfusion teams, as a result of the Chief Medical Officers' (UK) 'Better Blood Transfusion' initiative (Better Blood Transfusion, 2002). These specialists in transfusion practice help to raise awareness of SHOT as well as leading on education, audit and the development of hospital transfusion practice policies and guidelines.

Comparison of SHOT with other haemovigilance schemes

In recent years, a number of national haemovigilance schemes have been established and have reported their data (Faber, 2004). In general, these schemes have been based either on SHOT or the French Haemovigilance scheme, incorporating those aspects considered most appropriate for the individual country, for example, Ireland and Canada follow the French model (Andreu *et al.*, 2002; National Haemovigilance Office Annual Report, 2003; Robillard *et al.*, 2004). Precise comparisons are difficult because of differences in a number of factors, including the range and type of data collected, lack of common definitions and different national requirements. For example, the UK collects information on TRALI but does not do so for transfusion-associated circulatory overload (TACO), whereas in France, until 2003, data was collected on TACO but not TRALI (Andreu *et al.*, 2002 and Rebibo *et al.*, 2004). In France, TRALI reports are now included and in Ireland both complications are reported (National Haemovigilance Office Annual Report, 2003).

Further limitations of haemovigilance include:

- Lack of denominator data to set transfusion hazards in the overall context of transfusion practice.
- The potential for under-reporting, even in mandatory schemes.
- Delayed complications, such as post-transfusion viral infections, are not easily captured as they may escape recognition. (Please refer to Chapters 1 and 4.)

Nevertheless, despite these difficulties, similar key findings have been reported, pointing to common problems and priorities for action, namely:

- Transfusion errors leading to ABO incompatibility.
- TRALI.
- Bacterial contamination of platelets.

In addition, TACO has been highlighted in some schemes as an important cause of transfusion-related morbidity and mortality (Andreu *et al.*, 2002; Rebibo *et al.*, 2004).

Conclusion

Despite a high level of blood safety in the developed world, haemovigilance data has identified a number of areas where further improvements could be made. However, investing in costly measures to reduce already very low residual risk of transfusion-transmitted viral infections, for example, may be inappropriate in the setting of finite resources and more pressing health care needs. It is therefore essential that clear decision-making pathways be established for using haemovigilance data to influence blood safety policy and to prioritize the allocation of resources (Cohen, 2004).

Since its inception, the SHOT scheme has collected a powerful body of data about serious transfusion complications in the UK and has made many recommendations for improvements in transfusion safety. However, in common with other haemovigilance schemes, three main areas for improvement (errors, TRALI and bacterial contamination of platelets) have been highlighted. These findings have contributed to a number of new safety initiatives, policies and guidelines and there are encouraging signs that improvements in transfusion safety are beginning to take effect. However, the single most important cause resulting in mis-transfusion was failure of some aspect of the bedside checking procedure immediately prior to administering the transfusion. These 'wrong blood' incidents are avoidable errors. Efforts should be directed at developing computerized bedside identification systems to reduce human error. These can be linked to secure systems to reduce errors at the point of collection from storage and are also applicable in the drugs administration setting.

Acknowledgements

The author would like to thank the following, without whose significant contributions to SHOT this chapter could not have been written: Hannah Cohen, Dorothy Stainsby, Lorna Williamson, Hilary Jones, Katy Davison, Kate Soldan, Aysha Boncinelli, past and present members of the annual report writing group, standing working group and steering group and all participating hospitals.

REFERENCES

Andreu, G., Morel, P., Forestier, F. *et al.*, (2002) Hemovigilance in France: organisation and analysis of immediate transfusion incident reports from 1994–1998. *Transfusion*, **42**, 1356–64.

An Organization with a Memory. Report of an Expert Group on Learning from Adverse Events in the NHS, Chaired by the Chief Medical Officer. (2000) HMSO, London, The Stationery Office.

Better Blood Transfusion (2002) *Appropriate use of Blood*. Circular no. HSC 2002/009. London, Department of Health.

Better Blood Transfusion (1998) Circular no. HSC 1998/1224. London, Department of Health.

Cohen, H. (2004) *Highlights from the 7th SHOT Report – Taking SHOT Recommendations Forward. Presentations from SHOT meeting 2004.* (available at: http//www.shot-uk.org/presentationsindex.htm).

Council of Europe (2005) *Guide to the Preparation, Use and Quality Assurance of Blood Components.* 11th edn. Council of Europe Publishing.

Council of Europe (1995) Council Resolution of 2 June 1995 on blood safety and self-sufficiency in the Community (95/c 164/01) OJ No. C164, 30.6.95, p1.

European Parliament (2002) EU Directive 2002/98/EC of the European Parliament L33/30 8.2.2003.

Faber, J.-C. (2004) Worldwide overview of existing haemovigilance systems. *Transfusion and Apheresis Science*, **31**, 99–110.

Linden, J. V., Wagner, K., Voytovich A. E., *et al.* (2000) Transfusion errors in New York State: an analysis of 10 years' experience. *Transfusion*, **40**, 1207–13.

McClelland, B., Love, E., Lowe, S., *et al.* (1998) Haemovigilance: concept, Europe and UK Initiatives. *Vox Sang*, **74** (Suppl. 2), 431–9.

McClelland, D. B. L., McMenamin, J. J., Moores, H. M., *et al.* (1996) Reducing risks in blood transfusion: process and outcome. *Transfus Med*, **6**, 1–10.

National Haemovigilance Office Annual Report 2003 (available at: www.ibts.ie).

Noel, L., Debeir, J. and Cosson, A. (1998) The French Hemovigilance System. *Vox Sang*, **74** (Suppl. 2), 441–5.

Rebibo, D., Hauser L., Slimani A., *et al.* (2004) The French Hemovigilance System: organisation and results for 2003. *Transfusion and Apheresis Science*, **31**, 145–53.

Robillard, P., Nawej, K. I. and Jochem, K. (2004) The Quebec Hemovigilance System: description and results from the first two years. *Transfusion and Apheresis Science*, **31**, 111–22.

Serious Hazards of Transfusion, SHOT Annual Report 2003 (2004) ISBN 0 9532 789 6 4. Manchester, UK, SHOT Publishers.

Serious Hazards of Transfusion, SHOT 3rd Annual Report 1998–1999 (2000), ISBN 0 9532 789 2 1. Manchester, UK, SHOT Publishers.

Stainsby, D. (2004) Benchmarking SHOT data. Presentations from SHOT meeting 2004 (available at: http//www.shot-uk.org/presentationsindex.htm). Manchester, UK, SHOT Publishers.

The Blood Safety and Quality Regulations (2005) (available at: www.hmso.gov/uk/si2005/2005.2005.htm).

Williamson, L. M. and Love, E. M. (1998) Reporting serious hazards of transfusion: the SHOT program. *Transfus Med Rev*, **12**, 28–35.

Williamson, L. M., Lowe, S., Love, E. *et al.* (1998) Serious Hazards of Transfusion Annual Report 1996–1997. ISBN 09532 789 05 18.

Williamson, L. M. (2002) Transfusion hazard reporting: powerful data but do we know how best to use it? *Transfusion*, **42**, 1249–52.

Patricia E. Hewitt and Chris Moore

This chapter is primarily concerned with the investigation of reports of infection in transfusion recipients, in order to determine whether the infection was transmitted to the patient by transfusion. In addition, the question of 'look-back' is briefly considered. We describe our experience in the National Blood Service (NBS), England.

Introduction

The NBS provides a service to England and North Wales from 12 centres sited throughout the country. All staff involved in the investigation of post-transfusion infection work to national policies and procedures which have been developed as a result of experience over the last 25 years.

The NBS is part of the National Health Service and therefore has strong links and good communication with hospital clinicians, hospital transfusion laboratories and general practitioners. Since the late 1990s there have been NBS hospital liaison staff whose role is to work closely with the hospital transfusion laboratories and hospital transfusion committees. This initiative has strengthened the flow of information and communication between the NBS and the hospitals it serves.

Reports of possible infection associated with blood transfusion may arise from a number of sources, but within the NBS all reports reach one central office which has close links with the Serious Hazards of Transfusion scheme (SHOT). (Please refer to Chapter 21.) Although the investigation of possible transfusion-transmitted infection involves liaison locally with hospitals and donors, the process is managed centrally within the transfusion microbiology clinical function of the NBS and each case is reviewed at the close of the investigation.

It should be noted that up to 100 investigations are carried out by the NBS each year, but on average only one case of transfusion-transmitted infection is confirmed. Furthermore, in all other cases it is usual to demonstrate definitely that transfusion is not the source. (SHOT reports can be viewed at: www.shotuk.org.)

The investigation

The reasons for carrying out a post-transfusion infection investigation are several. Any or all may apply in an individual case:

- To identify an infectious donor, who can then be removed from the donor panel and referred for clinical care. Systems are in place to ensure that if such a donor does by any chance donate in the future, these donations cannot be issued for clinical use. This is particularly important in the rare cases where infection in the donor has not been detected by routine donation screening.

- To satisfy the need of the recipient, or recipient's family, for information about the source of the infection. In rare cases where transfusion-transmission is confirmed, this may lead to a claim for compensation, or legal action. On occasions, the NBS first learns about a possible case of transfusion-transmitted infection through legal action, indicating a potential claim. Investigation will be necessary in order to defend the claim.

- To satisfy the clinicians that blood transfusion was not the source of infection, so that other hospital-based sources of infection may be explored.

The chapter is divided into investigations of non-bacterial (including parasites) and bacterial transmissions. Reference should be made to Chapters 6, 7 and 8 for more detail about specific infectious agents.

Non-bacterial agents

In the UK, all blood donations are currently screened for evidence of infection with the microbial agents listed:

- Hepatitis B virus (HBV)
- Hepatitis C virus (HCV)
- Human immunodeficiency viruses (HIV 1 and 2)
- Human lymphotropic virus types I and II (HTLV-I/II)
- *Treponema pallidum*.

In addition, selected donations are screened for evidence of infection with:

- Cytomegalovirus (CMV)
- Malaria
- *Trypanosoma cruzi*.

Non-bacterial post-transfusion infection investigations are usually restricted to cases involving donations which have been screened for the organism in question. Very rarely, the investigation concerns an organism for which the blood has not been screened.

The basis of investigation of a post-transfusion infection in a recipient is to show:

- That the recipient was not infected prior to transfusion but had markers of infection thereafter.

- Whether any of the donors whose blood components the recipient received could have been infectious for the agent in question at the time of donation.

It is often not possible to show conclusively that the recipient was free of infection prior to transfusion. The identification of an infectious agent in the recipient may be made years after the

Transfusion Microbiology, John A. J. Barbara, Fiona A. M. Regan and Marcela C. Contreras. Published by Cambridge University Press. © Cambridge University Press 2008.

transfusion event, perhaps only when the recipient shows symptoms of disease (e.g. in the case of HIV and HCV infection). In most cases the patient will not have been tested for evidence of the infection prior to transfusion. A pre-transfusion blood sample is almost always unavailable. It is important, therefore, to make an assessment of the facts of the case before embarking on an investigation. The assessment should take into account the clinical details, the likely timing of the infection, any other possible sources of infection, and the test results. As a very minimum, a copy of the patient's test results should be obtained, together with relevant clinical details. The likelihood of transfusion being the cause of the infection will depend in part on the residual risk of infection, and this will vary from place to place, depending upon the donor population and the routine tests which are performed on donated blood. For example, in the UK in 2005–2006 the estimated residual risk for HIV infection was 1 in 4 to 5 million and for HCV 1 in 45 million donations (see position statement: www.transfusionguidelines). It follows that transfusion will usually not be the source of HIV or HCV infection. Nevertheless, many investigations are carried out, even when the likelihood of transfusion-transmission is remote (Regan *et al.*, 1999), to satisfy patients and clinicians, and almost without exception the blood donors are eliminated as the source of infection.

Before commencing the investigation, a complete list of the blood components received by the patient and their dates of issue or transfusion is required. Wherever possible, a printed list, preferably generated electronically from laboratory computer records, is produced.

The following information is sought from the hospital:

(1) Patient details
  (a) full name
  (b) address
  (c) date of birth
  (d) sex
  (e) ethnic origin.
(2) Clinical details
  (a) consultant, with speciality
  (b) reason for transfusion
  (c) underlying diagnosis
  (d) current condition
  (e) clinical evidence of post-transfusion infection.
(3) Laboratory results
  (a) copies of laboratory reports for infectious markers
  (b) any test results on samples prior to transfusion
  (c) liver function test results (hepatitis cases).
(4) Transfusion details
  (a) computer printout of transfusion history.

Once a decision has been made to start an investigation, and the list of components has been received, the donors of those blood components are identified. This is a relatively easy task when computerized records are available, but searches involving paper records are often very time consuming. When tracing records, care is taken to ensure that all the available information, such as blood group, date of donation and issue, expiry date and fate (i.e. hospital receiving the component) is consistent.

The donor records are then reviewed, together with the results of routine testing of any donations given subsequent to the one which the infected recipient received (the 'index donation'). An assessment of what (if any) further investigation is required can then be performed.

The following action is then taken:

- Collect recipient information.
- Identify donations.
- Examine relevant donor records.
- Assess test results of index and subsequent donations from each donor.
- Determine need for additional testing (and additional samples).
- Review results.
- Report conclusion to clinician, hospital laboratory, etc.

Investigation of possible human immunodeficiency virus, hepatitis C virus and human-T cell virus transmission

Routine serological testing of blood donations for transfusion-transmissible agents other than HBV depends upon the presence of antibody as a marker of past exposure. Lack of antibody in the transfused blood component will usually reflect absence of infection (Hewitt, 1994). A false-negative antibody test could occur in two situations: where the donor is in the early acute phase of infection ('window period') before detectable antibodies have developed, or where there is an error in testing. Both these possibilities can be excluded if the donor has given a further donation, which is also negative in routine antibody screening tests. The existence of infection in the absence of detectable antibody on two different samples is theoretically possible, but extremely unlikely (Durand & Beauplet 2000). In addition, all samples associated with the donations will have been pooled and subjected to genomic testing for HCV (and possibly HIV), making the existence of infection in donations tested by two methodologies remote in the extreme.

As most blood recipients have other possible sources of infection (e.g. hospital admission, invasive medical procedures, infected sexual partner, or vertical transmission) and have not been proven free of infection before the transfusion, an exhaustive search for a rare 'antibody negative but infectious' blood donor is virtually never justified.

In the NBS, archive samples are kept from all donations, stored at minus 30 °C for a minimum of three years. The volume of sample is in the order of 150 ul, so it is important to undertake only those investigations which will provide the necessary information. Where archive samples or subsequent donations from a donor are not available, the donor(s) will have to be approached and asked to provide blood samples for further testing. A request for fresh blood samples can be made using a standard letter sent to all donors for whom a subsequent sample is not available. The letter should contain an explanation of why a sample is required and the donor should be told which infection is being investigated. Although this information may be alarming, donors should not be asked for samples without being told the reason. The likelihood that the donor is the source of infection is remote, and therefore the letter can be reassuring; placing emphasis on the need to eliminate the donors as a source of infection, rather than the expectation of identifying one as such. It is important to give detailed information about how the blood sample can be obtained, how long the results are likely to take, how the donor will be given these results and a contact telephone number for donors who are anxious or who have questions. Once a donor has been eliminated from the inquiry he/she should be informed, preferably in writing.

Investigation of cases of possible hepatitis B virus transmission

Please refer back to Chapter 1.

In the UK, routine screening for HBV is by hepatitis B surface antigen (HBsAg) alone. In other countries routine screening for antibody to hepatitis B core (anti-HBc) is also performed. Anti-HBc appears early during the course of HBV infection and is detectable for probably the rest of the lives of individuals who have had HBV infection. However, it does not appear before HBsAg and therefore its presence in the blood, in the absence of HBsAg, is indicative of past rather than current infection.

Transmission of HBV to a recipient can theoretically occur because of failure of routine screening, either through laboratory errors, or because levels of HBsAg (or anti-HBc) in the donated blood are below the sensitivity of the assays in use. These very low levels of HBsAg can occur at the start of an acute HBV infection, in which case no other markers of HBV infection will be detectable, or after lifelong carriage of HBV when viral levels have dropped. In this case, anti-HBc will be detectable (Allain *et al.*, 1999) .

It is entirely possible for a blood donor to have an inapparent acute HBV infection with full recovery, including elimination of HBsAg and possibly development of anti-HBs, in the time interval between two blood donations. We have recently identified a routine blood donor who has had an inapparent acute HBV infection and whose test results changed from HBsAg only, with no other markers, to HBsAg negative, with low levels of anti-HBs, within the space of six weeks. Therefore, a negative HBsAg result on an index and a subsequent donation is not sufficient to eliminate any donor from an inquiry.

To do so, it is necessary to demonstrate:

- That the donor was not infected with HBV at the time of giving the index donation, and ideally
- That the donor has never had HBV infection.

In the UK, where only HBsAg testing is routinely performed, additional testing is required to give absolute assurance that a donor has not transmitted HBV to a recipient. It is logical to test any archive samples from the index donation for the presence of HBV DNA, to exclude an infection undetectable by HBsAg screening, and to look for anti-HBc in a subsequent donation or sample from the donor, in order to demonstrate absence of past or present HBV infection. The absence of anti-HBc in a follow-up sample and a negative test for HBV DNA on the index archive sample is sufficient evidence to eliminate a donor from the inquiry.

Investigations involving other viruses

On rare occasions reports are received of possible transfusion-transmission of other viral infections (e.g. hepatitis A, cytomegalovirus, human herpes virus 8). In these cases the principles described above are followed, but in addition it is usually necessary to seek expert virological advice about the most suitable tests to perform. This applies especially when archive samples have to be used, so that small volume samples are not wasted. In other situations specialist laboratory investigations may be required and the conditions under which blood samples are obtained from the implicated donors and transported for specialist testing need to be specified.

Parasitic infections

All transfusion-transmissable parasitic infections are rare in the UK, but there were five cases of malaria transmission between 1985 and 2005 by blood transfusion (Kitchen *et al.*, 2005). In contrast, there have been no reports of possible transfusion-transmitted *Trypanosoma cruzi*, and in over 15 years of selective screening of blood donations, only one donor has been confirmed to possess antibodies to this parasite. The increased popularity of travel to 'exotic' locations, many of which are endemic for malaria, and the increase in immigration to the UK of individuals from malarious areas of the world has resulted in the UK having the highest number of reported cases of malaria of any non-endemic country. Figures from the Health Protection Agency report an average of 2000 confirmed cases of malaria each year in the UK, in travellers returning from abroad.

The investigation of a possible case of transfusion-transmitted malaria is triggered by a report of malaria in a transfused patient. The donors of the implicated components are identified as in any post-transfusion investigation, but we have found it helpful, before performing any tests, to speak to the donors and confirm their travel history. Donors who have never visited, or lived in, areas endemic for malaria can be eliminated from the inquiry immediately. The guidelines for selection of donors in the UK provide specific instructions about risks associated with travel and history of malaria or feverish illness (see: www. transfusionguidelines.org.uk), and some donors identified as being part of an investigation may have been tested for malaria antibodies at the time of donating the component which the infected patient received. We review these results and may repeat the tests. The archive samples from the remaining components which the patient received are also tested, with the exception of those from the donors already eliminated by travel history. In each of two cases in recent years, a donor with strongly positive antibodies to malaria parasites has been identified following testing as part of an investigation, and reported as the probable source of the patient's infection. The donors were selected correctly according to the guidelines at the time, which did not require antibody testing prior to the use of these donations. The implication of these donors in transmission of infection resulted in changes to the guidelines (Caffrey *et al.*, 1998).

Bacterial infections

Please refer back to Chapter 7.

In England, approximately 70–80 cases of possible bacterial contamination of blood components are referred for investigation each year, but a proportion relate to component investigations (components rejected for abnormal appearance) and only about 30 relate to transfusion reactions in recipients. In the vast majority of these reactions, no bacterial contamination of the component can be demonstrated.

The investigation of severe transfusion reactions in recipients will usually follow a report from the hospital transfusion laboratory. At this point, the cause of the reaction may be unknown and exclusion of bacterial contamination may be part of a larger investigation. On the other hand, the first indication of a severe reaction due to bacterial transmission may be given only when the hospital has partially investigated a transfusion reaction and identified bacteria either within the pack or in a patient's blood cultures.

In all cases, it should be borne in mind that the investigation may have been initiated and partly performed by the hospital. The pack may already have been sampled, not only for bacterial culture, but also to obtain samples for checking of ABO groups and compatibility testing. The method by which the pack has been sampled may influence further investigation for bacterial contamination.

A record of the original notification, clinical details and any investigations carried out by the hospital is made by the blood centre. All available information is assessed, any additional information obtained as necessary and the consultant in charge reviews all clinical information and decides the degree of investigation required, including whether recall of other components from the same donation is necessary. The component under suspicion is sent for bacterial investigation, either at the blood centre or to a designated laboratory. The hospital may have taken blood cultures from the patient and will probably have taken cultures from the pack. If the patient has died without blood samples being obtained after transfusion, it may be necessary to arrange for a post-mortem blood sample to be collected.

The appearance of the component (e.g. colour change, etc.) is recorded and a note taken of any important documentary evidence which might be available from the pack, for example attached labels, signatures, etc. The storage conditions of the pack since the incident occurred is also recorded. The contents of the primary pack and of any constituent sealed off parts are subjected to Gram stain and culture. If the cultures on the pack are negative, no further investigation of the donation or donor is necessary.

Where there is a high index of suspicion of bacterial contamination, other components from the same donation(s) are isolated or recalled, without awaiting results of the initial investigations, and are also sent for bacterial investigation. If other components have been transfused, the outcome and fate of the recipients is recorded.

If bacterial contamination of the blood component is established, the possible source will need to be investigated. (Please refer back to Chapter 7.) The commonest source of bacterial contamination is from the donor's arm (Jacobs et al., 2001) and therefore the investigation centres around obtaining swabs from the venepuncture site for bacterial investigation. An explanation of the reason for requesting these swabs is given to the donor. It is possible to provide this explanation without giving details of the potential seriousness of the incident, especially in the rare cases resulting in recipient fatality. The donor should not be left with a burden of guilt. It is made clear that this is a routine investigation and that even if organisms are detected, this is quite normal since all skin carries bacteria. At the same time, it is helpful to establish whether there has been any recent illness which could have sparked a bacteraemic episode (McDonald et al., 1996). When taking the swabs, the extent of any scarring or the presence of any skin lesions at the venepuncture site is noted. It is usual to take swabs both before and after the standard skin cleansing procedure, used prior to donation, has been carried out.

Investigation of flora identified on the donor's arm may include molecular typing for comparison with the contaminant in the blood component; samples may therefore need referral to a specialist bacteriology laboratory (McDonald et al., 1998).

Once investigations are complete, the donors are advised about future donation. Only rarely is it necessary to exclude a donor, for example when an organism has been isolated from the donor's arm which cannot be removed by the standard skin cleansing procedure, probably because of gross scarring from multiple venepunctures. A full explanation is always given when a donor has to be excluded.

Occasionally, it is necessary to carry out further investigation of the environment in which the component was processed and stored, both at the blood centre and the hospital. This type of investigation will usually come under the auspices of the hospital or blood centre's quality management systems, and is outside the scope of this chapter. The incident should also be reported to the Serious Hazards of Transfusion or other relevant haemovigilance scheme. (Please refer to Chapter 21.)

The following action is required:

- Collect recipient information, including blood culture results.
- Identify implicated donations and arrange for bacteriological testing.
- Assess results (if donations are negative on culture, transfusion is not implicated).
- Determine whether any further investigation of the donor(s) is required.
- Review results.
- Report conclusions to clinicians.

Look-back investigations

The term 'look-back' is often used synonymously with 'post-transfusion infection investigation', which is incorrect. Whereas post-transfusion infection investigations are triggered by the detection of an infected recipient, look-back investigations commence at the other end of the transfusion process, with a newly identified infected donor. Once an infected donor has been identified, a look-back is conducted on previous donations which might have presented a risk to recipients. The rationale is that, once a potential risk to the recipient is identified, the recipient should have the information and should be offered the possibility of testing. In rare situations, notification of the recipient may be considered inadvisable, but these cases are the exception.

There are two particular situations in which look-back investigations are used. The first is following the introduction of a new screening test applied to all blood donations. The new test will identify a cohort of donors whose previous donations have been transfused to recipients, but which are now recognized to present an infectious risk. All previous and therefore untested donations will be of similar risk, and all previous recipients could have been infected. A look-back will identify the donations through to their ultimate fate, which will usually be transfusion to a recipient. In the UK, look-back exercises have been carried out following the introduction of screening for HIV (Hewitt et al., 1988 HCV (NBS Look-back Collaborators, 2002) and most recently, HTLV.

The second look-back situation is where a previously tested donor has been newly identified as infected, that is, the donor has seroconverted. The previous donation, although tested, could have been donated in the 'window period' and could therefore have presented a risk to the recipient. In this situation, an assessment of the likelihood of a window-period donation can be made by reviewing the information obtained from the donor about likely source and timing of infection, and by subjecting the archived sample of the last 'negative' donation to genomic testing. This information, taken together, can inform the assessment of risk from the donation. Our practice is to provide the assessment to the clinician caring for the recipient so that appropriate decisions can be made about the advisability of notifying the recipient and offering testing. In the case of a seroconverting donor, there is no justification in pursuing look-back beyond the last donation found negative by the most sensitive assays.

Conclusion

Currently, the vast majority of reports of possible post-transfusion infection in developed countries, such as the UK, lead to a conclusion, further to appropriate investigations, that blood transfusion was not the source of the infection. This conclusion must be reported, as soon as possible, to the clinicians caring for the patient so that the patient is aware of the outcome of the investigation. Furthermore, there may be other possible sources of infection which need investigating. As blood transfusions are usually carried out in the hospital setting, there may be a need to conduct a hospital-based investigation. In many cases, it is likely that the recipient was already infected before the hospital admission and blood transfusion. This is not surprising, since the incidence of these infections in the blood donor population is significantly lower than in the general (and even more so, the hospital patient) population.

Investigation of post-transfusion infection and transfusion look-back share a common need for a designated individual, usually a medical consultant, who carries ultimate responsibility for these procedures. Good documentation systems are vital for all cases. It is recommended that an investigation file is made for each infection investigation, which contains all the associated documents, such as the initial report/request, laboratory reports, records of transfused units, clinical information, instructions and actions taken throughout the investigation. Information from hospitals demonstrating the fate of components should form a clear audit trail. As the investigation file may be considered as part of the recipient's 'medical record', it is advisable not to keep any personal donor information in such files, but to use a cross-reference system.

It is becoming more common for infection in transfusion recipients to be the trigger to a claim for compensation. It is not unusual for such a claim to appear years after the initial investigation. In some cases, notification of a potential claim is the first indication that an infection has been attributed to blood transfusion, and investigation is started years after the transfusion in question. In other cases, notification and investigation have been carried out promptly, but a claim is much delayed. In this climate, it is wise to consider that all investigation files may be subject to scrutiny by lawyers and medical experts at some point in the future. Careful attention to documentation and recording of all aspects of the investigation at the time can save much work and worry in the future. See also Chapter 9.

REFERENCES

Allain, J.-P., Hewitt, P. E., Tedder, R. S., et al. (1999) Evidence that anti-HBc and HBV DNA testing of blood donations would not overlap in preventing HBV transmission by transfusion. Br J Haematol, 107(1), 186–95.
Caffrey, E. A., Hewitt, P. E. and Boralessa, H. (1998) Improved blood safety following a fatal transmission of malaria. Abstract: Transfus Med 8 (Suppl. 1), 18.
Durand, F. and Beauplet, A. (2000) Evidence of hepatitis C viraemia without detectable antibody to hepatitis C virus in a blood donor. Ann Intern Med, 133 (1), 74–5.
Hewitt, P. E. (1994) Investigation of post-transfusion HIV infection. Abstract: Transfus Med, 4 (Suppl. 1), 4.
Hewitt, P. E., Moore, M. C. and Barbara, J. (1988) Look-back experience of a UK blood transfusion centre. Abstract: IV International Conference on AIDS, Stockholm, June 1988. Book 2, Abstract 7714, p. 353.
Jacobs, M. R., Palavecino, E. and Yomtovian, R. (2001) Don't bug me: the problem of bacterial contamination of blood components – challenges and solutions. Transfusion, 41, 1331–4.
Kitchen, A. D., Barbara, J. A. J. and Hewitt, P. E. (2005) Documented cases of post-transfusion malaria occurring in England: a review in relation to current and proposed donor-selection guidelines. Vox Sang, 89, 77–80.
McDonald, C. P., Barbara, J. A. J., Hewitt, P. E., et al. (1996) Yersinia enterocolitica transmission from a red cell unit 34 days old. Transfus Med, 6, 61–3.
McDonald, C. P., Hartley, S., Orchard, K., et al. (1998) Fatal Clostridium perfringens sepsis from a pooled platelet transfusion. Transfus Med, 8, 19–22.
Regan, F. A. M., Hewitt, P. E., Barbara, J. A. J., et al. (1999) Prospective investigation of transfusion-transmitted infection in the recipients of over 20 000 units of blood. BMJ, 320, 403–6.
The English National Blood Service HCV Look-back Collaborators (2002) Probability of receiving testing in a national look-back program: the English HCV experience. Transfusion, 42, 1140–5.

Patricia E. Hewitt and Chris Moore

This chapter describes the notification of confirmed positive, indeterminate and false-positive microbiological test results to donors and the circumstances and objectives of the subsequent discussion. We have based our chapters on extensive experience and describe examples of arrangements in England.

Introduction

The procedures described in this chapter have been developed over many years. Historically, notification of donors with significant test results began within the National Blood Service (NBS) in the early 1970s with the introduction of routine screening for hepatitis B virus (HBV).

The introduction of screening tests for antibody to human immunodeficiency virus (HIV) throughout the UK in October 1985 initiated a more formal approach to 'donor counselling', and the NBS, which covers England and North Wales, now has national formal standard procedures for donor notification. The role and value of HIV counselling consultation meetings, which began in 1985, and which have now been widened to include discussion of issues relating to other microbiological markers, has also been recognized (Miller et al., 1989).

In addition, as part of the National Health Service, the NBS has excellent links with hospital clinicians and general practitioners, which facilitates donor referral to specialist services. Within England there are 12 blood centres which deal in an average year with 200–300 confirmed infections out of approximately 2 to 2.25 million blood donations (see Table 23.1).

The majority of these infections will be detected in first-time blood donors. We are aware that most individuals will not expect to hear that they have positive test results, and some will be extremely anxious and distressed to learn this information. On the other hand, a small minority of individuals appear to 'ignore' the information and need active management to ensure that they seek appropriate medical advice. Donor notification can therefore be a challenging activity which demands special skills from the staff involved, who should always be prepared to meet new challenges and help donors come to terms with their newly discovered status.

We have a small team of specialist clinical staff, working within transfusion microbiology as part of their post, and split across the 12 sites covering England and North Wales. This ensures, as far as possible, that each donor is treated as an individual. Staffing levels at each centre are reviewed annually to ensure that numbers are appropriate: too few donors per clinician and staff lose their expertise, too many and donors may receive less individual care. Clinical staff with responsibility for transfusion microbiology work within their local area but form part of a national clinical team, the National Transfusion Microbiology Clinical Group. They attend regular meetings, both to review and implement changes to ensure best practice and to provide training, including up-dates on clinical practice from specialists.

In other countries the logistics of donor notification will be affected by donor numbers and geographical area, but the same principles of purpose, confidentiality, standard approach and staff training can be applied.

Confirmed positive microbiological test results

Please refer to Chapter 12.

In accordance with the principle of duty of care it is usual practice to inform donors who are confirmed positive for any microbiological marker. The blood service should therefore ensure that appropriate arrangements are in place to enable this to happen efficiently and professionally (Miller et al., 1998).

The management of donors with confirmed positive microbiological markers is a clinical task and it is preferable for a senior member of the medical staff, usually a consultant, to take ultimate responsibility for this function, ensuring that all the necessary facilities are in place and that suitably trained staff are available, when required. In order to maintain staff experience and expertise, the number of staff should be kept at the minimum level necessary to provide the service.

Donors will often be seen in person, but in some circumstances (e.g. long distance from a blood centre) it may be more appropriate for the discussion to be held over the telephone. In these cases staff should ensure that the correct individual is on the telephone, and that circumstances are convenient to the donor, particularly with regard to confidentiality. It is our practice always to see HIV positive donors in person, since we would not be confident of being able to offer immediate appropriate support by telephone to a very distressed donor. It is not recommended that donors are seen in their own homes.

Whenever possible, before taking any action to refer the donor for further care, a second blood sample should be taken to confirm that the results are consistent and relate to that individual. The donor should be notified of the test results of this second sample. The method chosen will depend upon the individual circumstances.

Consent, which should normally be in writing, is required before information about donors' test results, medical or risk history is disclosed to any third party. When consent is obtained,

Table 23.1 Number of donors per year with confirmed infections

	2004	2005	2006
hepatitis B virus	94	91	68
hepatitis C virus	102	66	68
HIV	18	30	25
Human T-lymphotropic virus (HTLV)	16	15	9
Treponemal infection	85	76	82

whether written or verbal, this should be documented. It may be necessary, on rare occasions, to consider disclosure without consent. Such a decision should be taken only after appropriate consultation.

The objectives of the notification discussion

- To explain the meaning of the test results and why further donation is not possible.
- To repeat the tests on a further blood sample.
- To explore the consequences for the donor's future health and circumstances.
- To arrange appropriate medical referral.
- To reduce the risk of onward transmission.
- To obtain information about the source of infection.
- To maintain confidentiality.

In addition, valuable information can be obtained which will inform donor selection criteria (MacLennan et al., 1994).

Planning for donor contact

It is advisable to make a file for each case, including copies of the donor's microbiological test results (both screening and confirmatory), details of the donor's record, and any documentation completed by or about the donor at the time of blood donation. Consent to refer the donor for medical assessment and/or care will be required in most cases and a standard form may be used. It is advisable to have an information sheet for the donor to take away, a list of relevant specialist referral sites and standard forms for gathering demographic information and information about possible sources of the infection.

Before notification, the test results and donor details should be reviewed and contingency plans made for any particular issues which may be relevant, for example health care workers who may need specific occupational advice.

For HIV positive donors, options for direct specialist referral should be explored before seeing the donor.

The accommodation for the discussion of the test results should be provisionally booked and should provide the following:
- Confidentiality
- Pleasant surroundings
- A waiting area for those who may accompany the donor

- Suitable facilities for taking blood samples (this may be a donor clinic in the vicinity)
- Reasonable access to a telephone.

Ideally, it should be possible to provide refreshments for the donor, and the staff member should be able to alert other staff or have access to a 'panic' button in case of need, for example, an anxious donor may faint.

Notification of donors

It is our standard practice to use letters as the primary means of contact for all donors, except in cases of clinical urgency (e.g. probable acute hepatitis B infection), when the telephone may be used. Except in the case of HIV and syphilis, we name in the letter the microbiological marker which is positive and send the donor an information leaflet about the infection. Letters bear the name of the senior member of the medical staff who is taking responsibility, and are posted to arrive at a time when there is a clinician available to speak to the donor, should he/she have concerns on receipt of the letter. Copies of all correspondence are kept in the donor's file.

Secretarial/clerical staff are available to receive a reply from the donor and to make the necessary arrangements for the donor either to be seen, or to discuss the test results with clinical staff by telephone.

An out-of-hours message service is helpful for donors who ring out of office hours.

Action if no response received to initial letter

If no response is received, we send a further letter. Timing will depend on the availability of staff to discuss the results with donors subsequently, but the following are suggested intervals for sending further letters:
- One week for results meriting an early interview, as these donors present a risk to sexual contacts, or may benefit from early intervention: HIV, acute HBV, acute syphilis, HBV e antigen positive individuals and HCV seroconversion.
- Two to four weeks for results not considered clinically urgent: HBV e antibody positive, HCV positive, HTLV positive and non-acute syphilis infections.
- We recommend using a delivery method which allows tracking and confirmation of delivery of the letter.

If no response is received to subsequent letters we will often telephone the donor to check whether our letter has been received. In some cases we may send a letter to the donor's general practitioner whose identity can be traced from central NHS records. In exceptional circumstances, in the best interests of the donor and for public health reasons, it may be necessary to breach confidentiality by informing the general practitioner or other clinician of the donor's test results. In these circumstances the case will have been discussed with colleagues, and in particular with the clinician in charge, and these discussions and reasons for breaking confidentiality are documented.

The discussion with donors

We find that many donors can be managed by a telephone discussion with a clinician who has wide experience of this type of interaction, but face-to-face discussions are, in our view, necessary for HIV positive donors and for those where communication is difficult, for example extreme anxiety or language difficulties (Hewitt and Moore, 1989).

For face-to-face interviews, the appointment should be arranged to allow about an hour for the session. The donor must be given the opportunity to be seen alone and, initially at least, the presence of others should be discouraged. This is essential when the infectious agent has not been disclosed in the letter. When donors are aware of what is for discussion, however, they may choose to include others and should be able to do so. Individuals from outside agencies should not be included at this stage, since this would be a breach of confidentiality.

Immediately after the introductions have been made and the donor is seated and attentive, the test results and their implications are fully explained to the donor in clear terms that are easy to understand. The donor's response is observed and he/she is given time to absorb the information and to ask questions. It is often necessary to repeat the information several times and staff need to be satisfied that the donor has understood.

The discussion should help the donor to identify and express particular concerns. These may include some or all of the following:

- Implications for future health
- Medical referral/investigations/treatment
- Transmission to others
- Lifestyle changes
- Sexual practices
- Pregnancy
- Implications for employment, finances and insurance
- Confidentiality
- Whom to tell/concerns about telling partners
- Concerns about early death/care for dependants
- What the donor will do immediately after leaving the session
- A plan for future action.

The donor's mental state and reaction to the information is assessed. This may include, on occasion, an assessment of suicide risk.

The importance of a further blood sample is explained, and permission sought to take it. The donor is told that the test result on the original sample has been confirmed, that a different result is not expected, but that it is important to show the same results on a second sample to exclude any possibility of error. The means by which the donor will be given the second test result is agreed, and recorded in the file.

Specialist referral is recommended for all donors, except for known, treated cases of syphilis or yaws where discretion is used. Informed consent to contact the donor's general practitioner and/or for a direct referral is obtained, normally in writing, and the donor is given clear information about when the general practitioner/specialist is likely to be informed. In the UK, the donor is offered a copy of the letter sent to the general practitioner or referral centre, as is normal practice with letters written about patients. In some cases, the donor may not want to read a letter detailing information about him/herself and how the infection was caught, and if this is the case it is noted in the file.

At the end of the session:

- The donor's main concerns should have been addressed.
- A course of action, whether it be another appointment, direct referral to a specialist or advice about seeing the donor's general practitioner, should have been agreed.
- The donor should be offered an information leaflet, if he/she has not already received one.

Documentation

All contacts with the donor, including telephone conversations, and a summary of the content are recorded in the file. Copies of all letters to the donor and clinicians are kept in the donor file, and all documentation associated with the discussion session is completed and kept in the file.

For medico-legal reasons, advice given to the donor, such as the importance of medical referral, is noted, as should be a donor's agreement to take part in research, if applicable. Similarly, it is important to record when a donor, whose sexual partner is also a donor, has been advised to inform his/her partner that they may not be eligible to donate blood.

All donor files are held securely and placed in locked filing cabinets when not under direct supervision. The security of the cabinets is the responsibility of nominated individuals. If recording information on computerized records, these details are confidentially coded and cross-referenced with the files held in the locked filing cabinets.

Staff

All staff involved with the handling of information relating to donors should be reminded of their obligation to preserve donor confidentiality and any legal provisions such as data protection legislation. Within the NBS, only clinical staff who have been trained and assessed will carry out notification discussions with donors. We have found it helpful, particularly in difficult cases, for two staff to be present, but staffing levels are not always sufficient.

Staff training, monitoring and assessment are essential to ensure a high quality service. Recommendations with regard to training include regular local and national meetings, and assessment and review of individual skills at local level. These meetings help to identify what has been going well, any difficulties, new issues and interesting cases for discussion. All staff should benefit from the opportunity for regular discussion. Links with clinicians should be fostered to facilitate referral and two-way information flow.

Training may include:
- A theoretical and ethical overview
- Observing experienced staff

- Discussion session with donors in the presence of experienced staff
- A system of review.

Confirmation and referral

Unless the general practitioner has already been involved, the results of repeat testing are usually available before the donor's general practitioner is informed and/or specialist referral made. Results are sent by letter to donors' general practitioners, or directly to the specialist unit, whether or not there has been any telephone contact. Letters to general practitioners usually recommend referral to a specialist, and a list of geographically appropriate specialists is often included. A request for follow-up information from the specialist may be required in some cases, in particular those where 'look-back' may be indicated and timing and source of infection is unclear.

Letters are copied to the donor, depending on the donor's wishes.

Non-living donors

On occasion, non-living donors (e.g. deceased tissue donors) are shown to have confirmed positive microbiological test results, and then decisions need to be made about the notification of family members and/or sexual partners of the deceased. These decisions are based on the need to inform only those known, or thought to be, at risk of infection. On occasion, further questioning of the next of kin may reveal hitherto unknown family members who will need to be traced and informed.

Each case is assessed on an individual basis and discussed with colleagues.

Falsely reactive and indeterminate test results

Please refer to Chapter 12.

Before consideration can be given to notifying donors about falsely reactive or indeterminate test results a decision has to be made about the likely significance of the test result to the donor's health. We have a policy document which is applicable to all staff who have contact with these donors.

Falsely reactive test results are of no significance to the health of the donor, but for quality assurance reasons donations giving false reactions cannot be used. It is considered unethical to continue taking donations from these donors, and they should be informed of the problem. We inform donors about false reactions and explain what will happen next.

It is appropriate to inform the donor by letter and to provide a telephone number in case of concerns or questions. The letter refers to 'reactive' rather than 'positive' results and emphasizes that the result is of no significance to the donor's health. It does not mention the infectious agent for which the screening test has given a reactive result. This information will need to be given if the donor makes contact and asks a direct question, but is best avoided if possible, since once the infectious agent is mentioned the donor is likely to ask questions about the infection and come

to believe that he/she is infected. A leaflet explaining the general principles of false reactions, their relative frequency in comparison with confirmed infection and the routine nature of management is sent with the letter. The letter also explains what the donor should expect with regard to future donations, for example whether donation may be possible after providing a further blood sample, how and when such a sample will be obtained, and how results will be given to the donor. In all cases the routine nature of the procedure helps to reassure the donor, and any staff answering questions about false reactions are sufficiently knowledgeable about the interpretation of the test results to be confident about the advice they give to the donor. In most cases, false reactions are transitory in nature and following a repeat test, after a statutory interval, the donor can continue to donate.

Indeterminate test results apply almost exclusively to hepatitis C antibody tests. These results require interpretation to determine whether the result should be regarded as a false reaction, or whether it may relate to infection. Those regarded as false reactions are managed as above, and in some cases it is possible for the donor to return to donation. Indeterminate test results that may be of clinical significance will usually require a notification discussion and resampling of the donor. This notification discussion is arranged in a similar way to the discussion for confirmed positive results, with the following considerations:

- Enclosing an information leaflet about the infection with the notification letter is probably not appropriate since infection has not been confirmed.
- A second blood sample is required to assist clarification of the meaning of the results, but it may be most appropriate to conduct the discussion on the telephone and arrange for a sample to be taken locally.
- The possible explanations for the indeterminate result are explained to the donor and explored with the donor as part of the discussion. These include, early infection too soon for full development of antibody, a 'scar' or reflection of infection long ago, or false reactivity.
- Possible exposures to infection, both recent and in the past are discussed.
- A conclusion that infection is, or has been, present leads to referral for a medical assessment in the same way as for donors with confirmed positive results.

Future tests

The above protocols have been developed over a number of years and provide a standard approach for the management of donors with 'not negative' microbiological test results. The introduction into the NBS of any new microbiological screening test for donations also involves consideration of the arrangements for donor notification. These considerations include predicted workload (projected prevalence of the infection within the donor population), staffing numbers and distribution, training issues, specific notification considerations, and specialist referral. All these issues must be addressed before the introduction of a new test. In this way, we aim to provide a high quality service to those who come forward to donate their blood, and facilitate prompt management of those donors found to have infections which may have consequences for their future health.

REFERENCES

Hewitt, P. and Moore, C. (1989) HIV counselling in the National Blood Transfusion Service. *Couns Psychol Q*, **2** (1), 59–64.

MacLennan, S., Moore, M. C., Hewitt, P. E., *et al.* (1994) A study of anti-hepatitis C positive blood donors: the first year of screening. *Transfus Med*, **4**, 125–33.

Miller, R., Hewitt, P., Moore, C., *et al.* (1989) The role and value of HIV counselling consultation meetings at the North London Blood Transfusion Centre (1986–1989). Abstract. V International Conference on AIDS, Montreal, June 1989 (abstract MBP155).

Miller, R., Hewitt, P. E., Warwick, R., *et al.* (1998) Review of counselling in a transfusion service: the London (UK) experience. *Vox Sang*, **74**, 133–9.

24

RESEARCHING THE NATURAL HISTORY OF TRANSFUSION-TRANSMITTED INFECTIONS: THE UK HEPATITIS C (HCV) NATIONAL REGISTER

Helen Harris

Introduction

On the rare occasions when infections are acquired following transfusion, a unique opportunity can arise to study the natural history of the infectious agent in question. These studies are particularly useful when little is known about the outcome of the infection, for example when the agent is newly discovered or if it is rare. When recipients of potentially infected blood are traced during a look-back exercise, large groups of patients who may have acquired the infection are identified (HCV Look-back Collation Collaborators, 2002). Patients who are traced in this way can be invited to participate in natural history studies because the precise dates when they acquired their infections are usually known. Information about transfusion recipients who test negative for the agent in question can be equally useful as they can sometimes provide control data for comparison. Because the date of acquisition of infection is usually known, it is possible to study the natural history of infections that have a relatively benign early course from the precise date of acquisition. Under normal circumstances such infections may not be detected until much later, when patients present with symptoms. If no symptoms develop then the infections may never be detected.

The recruitment and subsequent collection of regional or national data into a central database, or register, is a prerequisite for undertaking such natural history studies. An example of such a database is the UK hepatitis C (HCV) national register.

Hepatitis C virus and the UK HCV national register

The hepatitis C virus (HCV) was cloned in 1989 (Choo *et al.*, 1989) and has subsequently been found to be responsible for practically all of the post-transfusion hepatitis that could not be attributed to either hepatitis A or hepatitis B. Since HCV has been identified only relatively recently, there is still much to learn about its natural history and the disease it can cause. Hepatitis C virus is now known to be one of the most common causes of liver disease, (Seeff, 1998) and is a major health problem worldwide (WHO, 1999). Since both the acute and chronic phases of HCV infection are predominantly asymptomatic, and because the chronic illness runs a course measured in decades rather than months, it has been difficult to define the frequency and rate at which infection progresses to symptomatic or end-stage liver disease.

Much of the current information about the natural history of HCV infection has been accrued from studies of patients with established chronic liver disease (Tong *et al.*, 1995). Unfortunately, such studies exclude individuals with clinically inapparent infection and those who have clinically apparent liver disease but have not been tested for HCV. This approach inevitably biases the data in favour of more severe disease outcomes. For these reasons it is important to undertake other natural history studies that follow individuals from the date that they were first exposed, regardless of whether they have developed any HCV-related disease or not. This then allows a more complete description of the spectrum of HCV-related disease. Opportunities for prospective studies of HCV-related disease are rare and the best known include cohorts of women exposed to contaminated immunoglobulin (Dittmann *et al.*, 1991; Kenny-Walsh, 1999). These studies suggest that HCV-related liver disease is relatively mild, but they involve women who were young at the time of acquisition. As both female sex and young age are independently associated with a favourable outcome, (Poynard *et al.*, 1997) such studies may in turn underestimate the impact of HCV-related liver disease in the wider population.

When anti-HCV testing of donated blood was introduced in the UK in 1991, some of the anti-HCV positive donors identified had donated blood before the introduction of testing. In early 1995, the UK Health Departments announced that a look-back at recipients of blood or blood components derived from these donations would be undertaken (Chief Medical Officer, 1995). Recipients were identified from local hospital records, and those who were not known to have died were contacted and offered counselling, serological testing, and treatment for HCV infection, where appropriate. Cases of transfusion-acquired HCV infection are unusual in having a known date of acquisition, an identifiable source, and often, in having been identified relatively early in the course of infection by a process largely unrelated to any HCV disease progression. As a consequence of the exclusion of HCV infected donors from the donor panel, the incidence of transfusion-acquired HCV in the UK has fallen to the extent that such infections are now extremely rare. Thus, the patients who were traced during the HCV look-back formed a rare cohort of individuals who offered an unrepeatable opportunity to study the natural history of HCV infection in the UK. In order to do this, the UK HCV national register was set up (Harris *et al.*, 2000).

Recruitment and enrolment

Individuals who satisfied the following case definition were eligible for inclusion in the register: 'A transfusion recipient traced during the UK HCV look-back exercise who tested either positive or indeterminate for antibodies to HCV.'

The UK blood services invited clinicians, by letter, to register their eligible patients. The clinicians were asked to provide

Transfusion Microbiology, eds John A. J. Barbara, Fiona A. M. Regan and Marcela C. Contreras. Published by Cambridge University Press. © Cambridge University Press 2008.

PATIENT DETAILS	ANTIVIRAL DRUG TREATMENT
Age Sex Ethnic group Country of birth Clinician Risk factors for HCV infection Other infections/medical conditions	Treatment dates Drug details Drug dosages Drug schedules Response to therapy Drug trials
TEST RESULTS	**CURRENT CLINICAL STATUS**
Hepatitis B status Hepatitis C status Hepatitis C genotype Liver function Liver biopsy	Deceased? Signs and symptoms of liver disease
	CURRENT MANAGEMENT
	Admissions (dates/type) Alcohol consumption

Figure 24.1 Information collected by the UK HCV national registry.

anonymized information on the patients' background, clinical status, test results, treatment and management using a standard form (see Figure 24.1) (Harris *et al.*, 2000). Any available clinical data for patients who had died were also collected. Registered patients were 'flagged' in the UK National Health Service central registers (Botting *et al.*, 1995) for notification of death, cancer and movement within or between health authorities. Each registered patient was given a unique case reference number under which his or her anonymized data were stored. All clinical data were then linked to infection data that were collected during the HCV look-back programme and to death data that were reported from the UK National Health Service central registers. By the end of 2002, more than 1000 patients had been enrolled throughout the UK (see Figure 24.2).

Comparative data sources

One of the limitations of transfusion recipients as a group for natural history studies is that their morbidity and mortality are likely to differ from that observed in the general population. This means that study results might not be applicable to the general population. This could lead researchers to overestimate the burden of disease that is attributable to the infectious agent in question. For this reason, data from patients who were traced during the HCV look-back but who tested negative for HCV were also collected. These data could then be compared with data from the HCV positive patients, thus controlling for any excess mortality that might be observed in a transfused population. With HCV, it is unethical and not feasible to follow any control group as intensively as registered cases (Harris *et al.*, 2000; Seeff, 1997), and therefore mortality was the most reliable outcome for comparison between the infected and non-infected cohorts of patients. All patients in the HCV register had been flagged in the UK National Health Service central registers for notification of cause of death, as had a group of HCV negative transfusion recipients who were ascertained by the same mechanism (Harris *et al.*, 2000). In this way, deaths from all causes as well as those from specific liver diseases could be compared between infected

and non-infected individuals. This information was also supplemented with routinely collected death data from the general population.

Long-term follow-up

With diseases like HCV, that can run their course over several decades, it is often necessary to follow patients prospectively for many years. In practice this is difficult to achieve because resources are always finite and long-term commitment to research projects is difficult to obtain. At the UK HCV national registry, cases are followed up every two years. Standard forms, identifying the patients by their unique case reference numbers and the clinicians' own identifiers, are sent directly to the relevant clinicians. These clinicians provide data on the patients' current clinical status, test results, treatment and management (Harris *et al.*, 2000). Placing a 'flag' in the UK National Health Service Central Registers against those patients who are enrolled in the register also ensures that cases do not become lost to follow-up. For diseases like HCV, with a long natural history, it is essential that contact with relevant individuals is not lost as this will result in biases that can invalidate study results.

Hepatitis C virus-related morbidity and mortality in the first decade of infection

Thus far, data from the UK HCV national register have been used to investigate HCV-related morbidity and mortality in the first decade of infection (Harris *et al.*, 2002). These analyses have shown that HCV infection does not have a great impact on all-cause mortality in the first decade of infection. Mortality from all causes during the first decade of infection among transfusion recipients who tested anti-HCV positive or indeterminate was 1.4 times greater than that observed in a similarly traced group of HCV negative transfusion recipients (see Figure 24.3). However, this excess mortality was not statistically significant. The risk of dying directly from liver disease was almost six-fold higher amongst HCV infected individuals

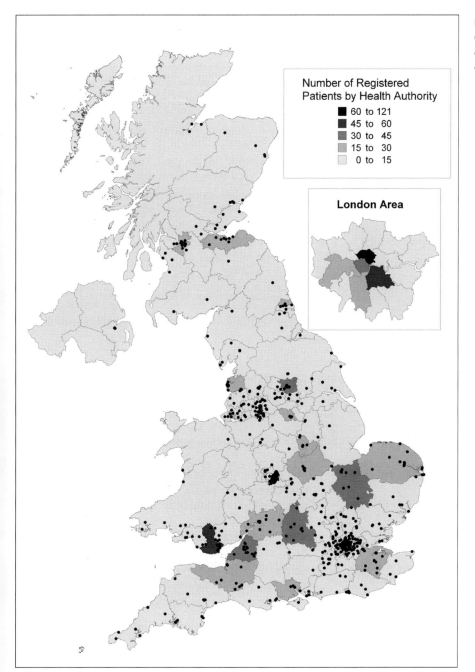

Figure 24.2 Geographical distribution of patients enrolled in the UK HCV national register (transfusion-acquired infections with known dates of acquisition).

than negative controls, but again this difference was not formally significant. Excessive alcohol consumption was implicated in at least one-third of the deaths from liver disease amongst HCV infected cases (Harris *et al.*, 2002). It is likely that the baseline prevalence of risk factors, like alcohol consumption, will explain the differential rates of progression that have also been observed in other cohorts of patients. For example, an excess of deaths from liver disease was only seen in two of the five cohorts studied by Seeff *et al.* (1992) and these were the only two cohorts not to have excluded individuals with alcoholic liver disease.

The vast majority of patients in the UK HCV national register had no signs or symptoms of liver disease, but nearly 40% had abnormal liver function tests and 90% of those biopsied had abnormal liver histology (see Figure 24.4). Patients who had developed physical signs or symptoms of liver disease were significantly more likely to have been infected for longer, to be positive for HCV ribonucleic acid, and to have acquired their infections at an older age. Those with clinical features of severe liver disease were also more likely to be male.

Long-term hepatitis C virus-related morbidity and mortality

The natural history of HCV after the first decade of infection remains controversial and will only be established as the results

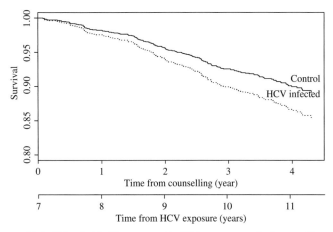

Note: This cohort had been exposed to HCV seven years prior to counselling.

Figure 24.3 Survival of HCV positive cases and HCV negative controls in the UK HCV national register: Cox's proportional hazards model (*British Medical Journal* 2002, **324**, 451. Reproduced with permission from the BMJ Publishing Group).

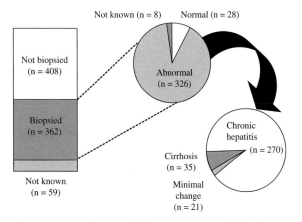

Figure 24.4 Liver biopsy results from 826 cases enrolled in the UK HCV national register.

of long-term cohort studies become available. In the USA, Seeff *et al.* followed-up a cohort of transfusion recipients with non-A, non-B hepatitis who had been identified in the early 1970s, and compared their mortality with a control group of matched transfused patients without hepatitis from the same studies (Seeff *et al.*, 1992). This study is now able to inform the natural history of HCV-related liver disease after 25 years of infection, and shows that all-cause mortality, although high, was not significantly different between test cases and controls (Seeff *et al.*, 2001). However, the relatively low level of liver-related mortality (<3%) was found to be significantly higher among test cases (4.1%) than controls (1.3%; P = 0.05).

At the present time, few cohort studies have exceeded 25 years of follow-up and therefore critical information has not been available beyond this time point. This is a problem because the only alternative to these data are those that are obtained from retrospective studies of individuals who have presented with chronic

symptomatic disease. These studies tend to overestimate HCV-related disease because they exclude individuals with mild or sub-clinical disease as well as those who have not been tested for HCV or who have resolved their infections. Forty-five-year follow-up has been achieved by one retrospective cohort study that used archived serum collected in the 1940s and 1950s to test for group A streptococcal infection and acute rheumatic fever (Seeff *et al.*, 2000). Although the results of this study may have been limited by the quality of the specimens following prolonged storage and the representativeness of the sample (predominantly male US military recruits), HCV positive individuals in this study had low liver-related morbidity and mortality rates. Like those studies of women who were exposed to HCV contaminated immunoglobulin (Dittmann *et al.*, 1991; Kenny-Walsh, 1999), this study suggests that otherwise healthy HCV positive persons might be at less risk of progressive liver disease than was previously thought.

The UK hepatitis C virus register as a national resource

Data from the UK HCV national register can be used to help make predictions about the future burden of HCV related disease and to help identify those groups of patients who are at greatest risk of developing liver disease and/or cancer. Such ongoing analyses are important as they allow health care resources to be targeted to those groups that need them most. These analyses can help identify:

(1) Those patients who respond best to therapy
(2) Those to whom preventive efforts might best be targeted
(3) Those groups that should be screened for the virus.

Because the UK HCV national register is one of the largest cohorts of patients with known dates of acquisition of infection, it is uniquely placed to help achieve these aims. National or regional registries can also support other external research projects by supplying large, reliable, statistically powerful, anonymous data sets that would otherwise be costly or impossible to access at local level.

Conclusion

Consideration should always be given to setting up national or regional disease registers when studying the natural history of newly discovered or rare transfusion-transmitted infections. Opportunities to establish such registries often arise following the introduction of a new screening test, for example the tests that have been introduced in the UK to detect antibodies to the hepatitis C virus or the human T-lymphotropic virus in the UK blood supply. The look-back programmes that are subsequently initiated to trace any recipients of potentially infected blood offer a unique opportunity to study the natural history of the infectious agent in question.

REFERENCES

Botting, B., Reilly, H. and Harris, D. (1995) Use of Office of Population Censuses and Surveys records in medical research and clinical audit. *Health Trends*, **27**, 4–7.

Chief Medical Officer (1995) *Hepatitis C and Blood Transfusion Look-back.* London, HMSO.

Choo, Q. L., Kuo, G., Weiner, A. J., *et al.* (1989) Isolation of a cDNA clone derived from a blood-borne non-A, non-B viral hepatitis genome. *Science*, **244**, 359–62.

Dittmann, S., Roggendorf, M., Durkop, J., *et al.* (1991) Long-term persistence of hepatitis C virus antibodies in a single source outbreak. *J Hepatol*, **13**, 323–7.

Harris, H. E., Ramsay, M. E. Andrews, N., *et al.* (2002) Clinical course of hepatitis C virus during the first decade of infection: cohort study. *B Med J*, **324**, 450–53.

Harris, H. E., Ramsay, M. E., Heptonstall, J., *et al.* (2000) The HCV National Register: towards informing the natural history of hepatitis C infection in the UK. *J Viral Hep*, **7**, 420–7.

HCV Look-back Collation Collaborators (2002) Transfusion transmission of HCV infection before anti-HCV testing of blood donations in England: results of the national HCV look-back programme. *Transfusion*, **42**, 1146–53.

Kenny-Walsh, E. (1999) Clinical outcomes after hepatitis C infection from contaminated anti-D immune globulin. Irish Hepatology Research Group. *N Eng J Med*, **340**, 1228–33.

Poynard, T., Bedossa, P. and Opolon, P. (1997) Natural history of liver fibrosis progression in patients with chronic hepatitis C. The OBSVIRC, METAVIR, CLINIVIR and DOSVIRC groups. *Lancet*, **349**, 825–32.

Seeff, L. B. (1997) Natural history of hepatitis C. *Hepatology*, **26** (Suppl. 1), 21–28S.

Seeff, L. B. (1998) The natural history of hepatitis C. A quandary. *Hepatology*, **28**, 1710–2.

Seeff, L. B., Blaine Hollinger, F., Alter, H. J., *et al.* (2001) Long-term mortality and morbidity of transfusion-associated non-A, non-B, and type C hepatitis: a National Heart, Lung, and Blood Institute Collaborative Study. *Hepatology*, **33**, 455–63.

Seeff, L. B., Buskell-Bales, Z., Wright, E. C., *et al.* (1992) Long-term mortality after transfusion-associated non-A, non-B hepatitis. The National Heart, Lung and Blood Institute Study Group. *N Eng J Med*, **327**, 1906–11.

Seeff, L. B., Miller, R. N., Rabkin, C. S., *et al.* (2000) Forty-five-year follow-up of hepatitis C virus infection in healthy young adults. *Ann Intern Med*, **132**, 105–11.

Tong, M. J., El-Farra, N. S., Reikes, A. R., *et al.* (1995) Clinical outcomes after transfusion-associated hepatitis C. *N Eng J Med*, **332**, 1463–6.

World Health Organization (1999) Hepatitis C global prevalence (update). *Wkly Epidemiol Rec*, **74**, 425–7.

25

HOW TO ASSESS RISK: PROSPECTIVE STUDIES AND CALCULATIONS

Kate Soldan and Katy Davison

Introduction

Assessing, or quantifying, the risk of transfusion-transmission of infection can be attempted by several approaches, each having different costs, advantages and limitations. Surveillance systems, as described in Chapter 21, can monitor diagnosed transfusion-transmitted infections. However, several factors common to transfusion-transmitted infections, and to transfusion recipients, are likely to contribute to a lack of clinically apparent symptoms and therefore to under-diagnosis of infections. For example, other therapies may negate or modify symptoms. Many transfusion recipients are receiving antibiotic drugs and are therefore less likely to suffer observable consequences from bacterial infections. Transfusion recipients may be sick or injured, are often elderly, and have high mortality from other causes. Furthermore, the recipients who receive relatively large numbers of transfusions, and are therefore at the highest risk of transfusion-transmitted infections, have the highest comorbidity and mortality rates. Long pre-symptomatic periods are common for persistent blood-borne virus infections and occurrence of disease may be far removed in time from the transfusion-exposure. This period may be shortened by a relatively large dose of the infectious agent, and in recipients who are older, already ill or immunocompromised. Such characteristics are common amongst transfusion recipients, but even so, transfusion may be overlooked as a possible route of infection due to some delay in diagnosis. For some infections (for example hepatitis A and parvovirus B19), naturally acquired immunity may be quite high – especially in older age groups – meaning that transmission of infection may be considerably less frequent than the number of infectious units of blood transfused. Also, asymptomatic infection is more common amongst the younger age groups who have lower levels of naturally acquired immunity; so transmission may not result in any disease. For many reasons, therefore, recognized and reported cases of transfusion-transmitted infections are likely to be biased towards those with more apparent, and more severe, clinical consequences, and will not necessarily be representative of actual transmissions either in absolute frequency of occurrence, or in nature and outcome. There are therefore considerable ascertainment biases and limitations in an assessment of risk based on reports of diagnosed transfusion-transmitted infections alone, although these cases provide crucial information on clinical outcomes of the risk of transmission. Other useful methods for assessing risk include prospective observational studies and calculation of expected risk.

Prospective studies

General description and usage

Prospective studies that actively follow-up transfused recipients and observe and/or test them for evidence of transfusion-transmitted infections can overcome many of the limitations of haemovigilance and case reports mentioned above. A more complete picture of transmissions can be seen by this approach, as sub-clinical and undiagnosed infections can be detected. There may still be 'blind-spots' due to mortality of recipients prior to follow-up measures. There may also be complications to deal with, concerning the effects of naturally acquired immunity and of infections acquired from other routes during the post-transfusion follow-up.

Limitations

In many countries (particularly countries with highly developed donor selection and donation testing systems) transfusion-transmission of infection with observed clinical consequences is rare – both in absolute terms and relative to incidents of infection acquired by other routes. The number of recipients that need to be followed up in order to obtain a precise estimate of transmission rates is therefore very large and such studies have thus become prohibitively expensive and unwieldy. Table 25.1 shows some examples, using the rule of three to estimate binomial confidence intervals (Armitage and Colton, 1998) of the number of subjects needed in a prospective cohort study to produce a 95% CI that excludes a given transmission rate in studies that observe no cases, that is, the minimum sample size needed to demonstrate that the true transmission rate is lower than the given rate (in left column). These simple power calculations assume no loss to follow-up and no error in recipient tracing, and therefore are optimistic estimates of the power that can be obtained by real studies.

A study of over 22 000 units issued in the UK (London and the south-east) in the late 1990s found no transfusion-transmitted HIV, HBV, HCV or HTLV I and II infections (Regan et al., 2000). Although an impressive size in terms of requisite effort, the results of this study could not exclude with 95% confidence a frequency of transfusion-transmission of 1 in 10 000 units transfused.

Designs that, for example, over-sample recipients of multiple transfusions, or recipients with relatively long life expectancy address these limitations to some extent, and may be able to do better in the future. However, these design factors usually come at

Transfusion Microbiology, eds John A. J. Barbara, Fiona A. M. Regan and Marcela C. Contreras. Published by Cambridge University Press. © Cambridge University Press 2008.

Table 25.1 Sample size calculations for prospective transmission studies.

Transmission rate (per number of units transfused)	Number needed in cohort for 95% CI on transmission rate of zero (i.e. when no transmissions observed) to exclude given rate
1 in 10 000	30 000
1 in 100 000	300 000
1 in 3 million	9 million
1 in 10 million	30 million

a cost of some additional selection biases that may limit the interpretation or extrapolation of findings.

Studies in settings with higher rates of transfusion-transmitted infections are not necessarily easier to conduct and interpret. Where transmission of infection by transfusion is relatively common, so usually is transmission of infection by other mechanisms. Distinguishing transfusion-transmitted infections from infections from other sources is therefore more demanding and prone to introduce greater uncertainties and errors.

Another problem with prospective studies is that the results are out of date as soon as either the epidemiology of the infections considered, or transfusion service practices, change. This is a particular concern as these studies usually take a long time to conduct, meaning that the value of the final results can be difficult to predict at the outset.

Prospective studies often involve complicated and costly procedures for requesting the necessary consent from patients prior to their participation, particularly if the study aims to store biological samples as a resource for further testing (see below). In some countries, those conducting such studies may face severe restrictions due to ethical and/or legal concerns.

Advantages/rewards

The prime value of prospective studies, when they can be designed to overcome the problems above, is that they are based on direct observation of actual events. They can therefore give an evidence base to theoretical expectations of risk, and uncover, or at least suggest, modifying factors that were not expected by theory, nor evident from cases of transmission picked up by surveillance. An important aspect of this observation of 'reality' is the provision of information about the consequences of transfusion-transmitted infections in patients. One other feature of these studies that has very high potential value for understanding the risk of transfusions, is the repository of biological specimens used for the baseline and follow-up testing of the recipients. This value is greatly enhanced if specimens from the transfusions given to the recipients are also stored, and these specimens can be matched (donor and recipient) and used to investigate the presence and transmission of other infections that raise concerns for transfusion safety in the years following the study. In this way, these studies can contribute to vigilance for, and relatively rapid assessment of, new risks.

Another beneficial spin-off can be the identification of infections with a known date of infection. For blood-borne infections with long asymptomatic periods it is often impossible to accurately determine the time of infection retrospectively, once the clinical diagnosis is made years later. Individuals with transfusion-transmitted infections can aid in the study of the natural history of such infections, and prospective studies discover these individuals in a relatively unbiased way.

Summary

Prospective studies have some very desirable theoretical advantages for the measurement of the risk of infection transmission by transfusion. However, they are severely limited in practice by the high costs and difficult logistics involved in conducting definitive studies.

Calculations

General description and usage

Another approach to assessing risk is to calculate estimates of the number (or frequency) of infectious donations that current donation testing is *not* expected to remove from the donations collected. This approach requires first, identifying the circumstances that could allow an infectious donation to be issued into the blood supply, and second, assessing the likelihood, or frequency, of each and any of those circumstances occurring. To do this, information is needed about:

(1) The frequency of infections in the population donating blood
(2) The development and persistence of the markers that are tested for
(3) The tests and testing systems used.

Even in the presence of good testing for an infection, several circumstances can lead to infectious donations entering the blood supply:

(1) Collection of donations during the infectious period of sero-negativity (the infectious 'window period') prior to detectable levels of antibody or antigen, following infection.
(2) Donations testing falsely negative due to test sensitivities less than 100% (including insensitivity to certain existing or new subtypes or variants). See Chapter 11.
(3) Donations erroneously issued as negative due to an error in sample collection and labelling, retrieval of the sample for testing or conduct of the test, or due to an error in recording test results, or identifying and removing positive donations. Please refer to Chapter 17. Even in the presence of stringent controls on every part of the testing and information-management process, experience shows that systems are rarely infallible and can be evaded by unforeseen circumstances.
(4) Collection of donations from individuals who are seronegative and infectious during post-acute stages of infection, either temporarily due to fluctuating or waning levels of serological markers, or permanently due to atypical or absent serological markers, for example at the end of HBsAg carriage in some cases (please refer back to Chapter 1).

Table 25.2 Key information for estimating the risk of donations infectious for known pathogens entering the blood supply despite donation testing.

	Information needed and source of that information	
Component of risk	Derived from donation testing	Other sources
(1) Risk of seronegative infectious donation being collected during early infection (2) Risk of seropositive donation entering the blood supply through test failure or process error (3) Risk of seronegative infectious donation being collected from donors with established (not early) infection	• Incidence of infection in donors • Prevalence of marker used to indicate infectivity in donations	• Length of the infectious seronegative window period following infection • Sensitivity of tests for the marker • Rate of errors that could lead to failure to identify or withdraw a positive donation • Frequency of seronegative, infectious individuals (other than those in the window period following infection) amongst blood donors

The probability of a donation being collected during the infectious window-period of negativity, when the tests used cannot detect evidence of infection, depends upon the incidence (i.e. the rate of occurrence of new infections) of the infection and the length of the window-period (see later in chapter for methods). The probability of symptoms that may prevent donation occurring during this period may be an important modifier for some infections and may also need to be considered. Incidence rates are usually calculated using observations of seroconversions in repeat donors, or observations of signs (either clinical or serological) of acute infections in donors.

The probability of a positive donation being released into the blood supply due to a false-negative test, and due to a failure, or error, in the testing system, depends upon the sensitivity of the test and the probability of a failure or error, respectively, and upon the prevalence of the infectious marker in the donations undergoing testing. The risk of a seropositive donation not being identified by testing is the probability of a false-negative (FN) test result. This can be estimated using the sensitivity of the test and the prevalence of the marker.

$$\text{FN risk} = \frac{(\text{prevalence})}{\text{sensitivity}} \times (1 - \text{sensitivity})$$

Process error can be defined as error in the testing, recording, or discarding of infectious donations. This error rate was estimated to be 0.5%, based on data from USA (Linden, 1994; Linden and Kaplan, 1994). The risk of a process error (PE) (i.e. any technical or human error) involving an infectious donation can be estimated using the estimated frequency of process errors and the prevalence of the marker.

$$\text{PE risk} = \text{prevalence} \times \text{process error frequency}$$

The fourth circumstance, that of true seronegativity in infectious individuals (during post-acute infection), can occur, for example, in immunosuppressed individuals (usually thought to be negligible amongst healthy adults selected for donation), and in the end stages of some infections (e.g. at end of HBsAg carriage).

The total risk is the sum of the frequencies of each risk component, minus the product of any mutually exclusive risks. For donor panels with relatively high prevalence of some infections, or high correlation of different infections amongst donors, it may also be appropriate to adjust for the probability that an undetected infectious donation is discarded due to detected infectivity for another infection.

Table 25.2 summarizes these key items of information required to calculate theoretical estimates of the risk of a donation infectious for a given organism entering the blood supply due to these three circumstances. The range of values in which each of the variables in Table 25.2 might lie depends on the sample used to estimate the variable, the biological variability involved, and the assumptions made in obtaining the working value. As the influence of each parameter varies with the others, it is often worthwhile to include a sensitivity analysis in risk estimation studies to determine which parameters are the most important. This can suggest which parameters to concentrate on measuring more accurately in order to improve the estimates, and also which parameters affect the risk to patients the most, and therefore may be the most fruitful focus for risk reduction strategies. Many studies have explored changes to the parameters concerning testing in order to predict benefits of new tests. Some have explored changes to the prevalence and incidence that may result from different donor recruitment strategies (e.g. lower age groups) and different donor selection criteria (e.g. deselection of men who have sex with men (Germain *et al.*, 2003; Soldan and Sinka, 2003a)).

The provision of good incidence and prevalence data is a prerequisite for these calculations. These measures are usually obtained from surveillance of infections in donors and the following section considers the methods for securing these data from testing and surveillance systems.

Surveillance of infections in donors

The key parameters needed from the surveillance of infections in donors are the prevalence and the incidence of the infections being assessed. For accurate measurements of prevalence, surveillance of donation testing needs to provide the number of donations tested and the number of donations with confirmed markers of infection. To assess risk for sub-groups of donors, these data must be available for each sub-group. Ideally, data would be available for the whole donor panel, but where this is not possible, or efficient, data should be obtained from a representative sample of donors.

Incidence is a harder parameter to measure as it requires observation of discrete events (new infections) over time. Incidence rates in repeat donors can be derived from the observation of seroconversion between donations. Repeat donors who have seroconverted for infections under risk assessment can be routinely identified from surveillance systems, or by a retrospective survey of blood centre records. The results of screening and confirmatory tests performed on the last negative, and the first positive, donation may need to be reviewed for some infections in order to check that an apparent change of infection status is most likely to be due to a new infection, rather than to introduction of a new test or even slight differences in performance in different batches from the same kit manufacturer to testing, or any other reason. A seroconverter can be defined as a donor who has made a seropositive donation during the study period and had made a seronegative donation within a defined period prior to the positive donation – the length of this period can result in different estimates of incidence. The shorter this look-back period, the fewer seroconverters will be defined. However, as the interval between donations for the 'excluded' seroconverters is very long, the contribution these make to the risk of a window-period donation is likely to be small, and may be negligible in many studies. Incidence rates in repeat donors can then be calculated as the number of seroconverting donors divided by the total number of person years at risk. The number of person years at risk can be observed directly (summed from date intervals between donations by all donors in the study period). This is normally easy for the seroconverting donors, but may not be feasible for all donations, so can be estimated by multiplying the number of donations made by repeat donors by the best available estimate of the average interval (in years) between donations from repeat donors.

In circumstances where complete information needed to define seroconverters (or prevalent infections) is not available (e.g. if confirmatory testing is not always performed), an estimate may be made by multiplying the identified numbers of seroconverters (or prevalent infections) amongst a sample by 1/the proportion of all possible cases that were sampled.

Hepatitis B surface antigen is generally transient in individuals infected with HBV as adults, and therefore in newly infected donors the HBsAg test can revert to negative before the time of their next donation. Hepatitis B surface antigen testing alone is therefore expected to identify all persistent carriers and only some of the donors who experience acute, resolving infection and have a transient period of antigenaemia. Estimates of HBV incidence need to take this transient antigenaemia into account by calculating the weighted probability that donation testing would detect seroconversion. For example, Korelitz et al. (1997) assumed that 70% of infected donors would have transient antigenaemia lasting an average of 63 days (the mid-point of two published estimates (Hoofnagle and Schaffer, 1986; Mimms et al., 1993), that 25% of infected donors would have no antigenaemia and that 5% would have persistent antigenaemia,

making the adjustment for HBV incidence = (63/IDI in days × 0.7) + (0 × 0.25) + (1 × 0.05). Other studies have somewhat varied the proportions reaching each outcome, but basically used a similar approach to calculating true HBV incidence from HBsAg seroconversions.

Another approach to estimating the incidence of HBV – at least in theory – can be based on direct assessment of the presence of anti-HBc IgM in blood donors and assumptions about the validity and duration of anti-HBc IgM as a marker of acute infection. The advantage of this method is that it can be done using single samples, and so may be used to estimate incidence in new donors.

The incidence of infections such as HIV and HCV in new donors cannot be measured directly from current routine test results. However, an estimate of the extent to which the incidence of infection differs in new donors can sometimes be derived, and applied to incidence measured in repeat donors to estimate incidence in new donors. Methods to estimate this new donor incidence adjustment depend on the infection and the available data. Some examples are:

(1) The ratio of the frequency of acute HBV in donations from new donors to the frequency of acute HBV in donations from repeat donors.

(2) A method used in a study by Lackritz et al. (1995) that is based on the understanding that at the start of testing, when no repeat donors have been excluded because of a positive test result, the seroprevalence of a persistent marker of infection is equivalent to the cumulative incidence of the infection. The ratio of the seroprevalence in new donors and repeat donors during the first period of testing (weighted for different time at risk if appropriate, e.g. if exposure to infection starts in adolescence and new donors are younger) provides an estimate of the new donor incidence multiplier.

(3) A method used by Cumming et al. (1989) was to use the time at risk to convert prevalence rates (the results of cumulative incidence) to annual incidence rates.

An alternative approach to measuring incidence is available for some infections if there are non-routine tests that can directly identify recent infections. For example, specialized tests such as anti-HCV avidity testing, and more recently 'de-tuned' anti-HIV testing have been used to detect recent infections and to derive incidence (Janssen et al., 1998; McFarland et al., 1999). De-tuned tests work by applying a sensitive and a less-sensitive (de-tuned) assay to samples and classifying samples that are positive in the sensitive assay and negative in the less-sensitive assay as early infections. This approach to measuring incidence is based on an expectation, that has been shown to hold true by the testing of samples from well characterized infections, that antibody levels during early infection are below the detection levels of less-sensitive assays (Kothe et al., 2003).

For most calculations, donations must be sub-classified into donations from new donors and donations from repeat donors. The exact working definition of a new and repeat donor for the purposes of this data collection may differ between blood services and should be described in each case, but normally new donors should be new to the test for the infection under risk assessment, and repeat donors should have been previously tested. Information systems should be able to identify positive donations from donors classified as 'repeat donors' who have not in fact been previously found negative for the test in question, for example if they attended but did not donate due to a failed haemoglobin test, or last attended before the test in question was introduced, or were previously found to be positive and asked not to donate again, but have done so this time.

A look at the frequency of infections detected in donations from new donors compared to repeat donors typically shows much higher frequencies amongst new donors. This is to be expected, as repeat donors have been tested before and asked not to donate again if found to be positive. This means, however, that, for non-perfect testing systems, donations from new donors should be expected to bear a higher risk of being 'false-negatives' missed by testing. It is also often the case that not only the prevalence of infection, but the ongoing risk of infection is higher in individuals who are new donors than in individuals who are repeat donors. This higher incidence of infection can be measured by the three methods mentioned above. In the UK, the mean of the results of these methods suggests new donors have an approximately four-fold risk of acquiring HBV, a six-fold risk of acquiring HCV and a two-fold risk of acquiring HIV, compared to repeat donors. Comparison of the frequency of HCV-NAT positive anti-HCV negative donations from new and repeat donors in the US (Schreiber et al., 2002) has suggested that new donors have an approximately 2.4-fold risk of acquiring HCV. Higher incidence amongst individuals who are new donors is probably due to higher frequency of behaviours involving possible exposure to infection. This hypothesis is supported by the association of younger age with higher incidence in other population groups, and the generally younger age of new donors compared to repeat donors in many countries at least. This higher incidence means that donations from new donors should also be expected to bear a higher risk of being window-period donations. Taking these factors into account in the UK, the estimated risks of HBV, HCV and HIV infections amongst donations supplied from new donors are four-fold, thirteen-fold and three-fold the risks amongst donations from repeat donors (Soldan et al., 2005).

Different methods of risk estimation

Estimates of the risks of transfusion-transmitted viral infections have now been published for a number of different blood services and different periods of time. The results have varied: the methods and scope of the estimates have also varied. Table 25.3 shows some results, and some characteristics, of studies from the UK and other countries.

Differences in the estimated risk of HIV infectious donations in Europe and North America between the early days of HIV testing and more recent years have been due largely to reductions in the window period of HIV tests. In the USA, studies in the late 1980s estimated the risk of HIV infectious units issued at 0.46 to 2.6 per 100 000 donations issued (Brookmeyer and Gail, 1994; Cumming et al., 1989; Ward, 1988); studies in the early 1990s produced estimates of around 0.2 per 100,000 donations issued

(Lackritz et al., 1995; Schreiber et al., 1996). This fall was largely due to a reduction in the length of the window period used in the risk calculations, from 56 days to 22 days. Differences between populations with high HIV infection prevalence and incidence and countries of low infection prevalence and incidence show clearly in the risk estimates produced for different countries. Calculations in Thailand estimated the risk of HIV infectious donations in the early 1990s at 200 per million donations issued (Kitayaporn et al., 1996), which is markedly higher than estimates in Europe and North America, largely as a result of the higher incidence of HIV infection in Thailand than in Europe and North America (and also partly due to a longer window period of 45 days for the test in use in Thailand).

Such large differences in risk are usually evident when risk estimates are compared. However, some variations in the methods used to calculate risk estimates can mean that estimates produced by countries using similar testing systems and with similar epidemiology are not directly comparable and any differences should be interpreted carefully, with cognisance of the effects of methodological differences in both the testing and surveillance systems generating the data that are used, and in the calculations performed on these data.

Studies have varied in the possible components, or contributions, to risk that they have considered. Most studies include estimation of the risk of window-period donations, based on the window period of tests and the incidence of infection. Only some studies (see Table 25.3) have also included estimation of the risk of false-negative results and errors; these risks are dependent on the prevalence of infections amongst donors, rather than the incidence.

Studies have also varied in whether they have estimated the risk from all donations, or just from donations from repeat donors. New (i.e. first-time) donors differ from repeat donors in ways that can affect the risk of an infectious donation entering the blood supply. Probably most important is that new donors have not previously undergone testing for infectious disease by the blood service. As this testing leads to diagnosis and exclusion of donors with prevalent infections, new donors have a higher prevalence of infections. Incidence may also be higher due to common risk factors for prevalence and incidence of blood-borne infections, and to higher age-specific incidence, as new donors tend to be younger and young adults tend to be at higher risk of certain infections.

Most studies have used a method of calculating the window-period risk that has been called the 'incidence' method. The probability of a seronegative donation being made during the window period is calculated as equal to the incidence of infection in donors, multiplied by the length of the infectious window period during acute infection.

$$\text{WP risk} = \text{incidence} \times \text{infectious window period}$$

As the period immediately after infection, before much replication of the organism in its new host, is unlikely to be infectious, the infectious window period is usually taken to be several days shorter than the total window period from infection to positive detection of evidence of the infection in the blood.

Table 25.3 Results from selected published studies of estimated risks of transfusion-transmissible infections, UK and worldwide.

Year of data/estimates (reference)	Estimated risk of infectious donations per million donations (range[a])	Length of infectious window period used in days (range)	False-negative (FN) and error risk estimated	Test sensitivity (S) and error rate (ER) used	Estimate for new donor donation included
UK					
1986–1987 (Hickman and Mortimer, 1988)	HIV: 1986 3.2	56	Yes	S: 98%	Partially WP = no FN = yes
	HIV: 1987 1.1		No	—	
1993–2001 (Soldan et al., 2003b)	HIV: 0.15 (0.07–0.29)	HIV: 22(6–38)	Yes	S-HIV: 99.9%	Yes
	HCV: 1.66 (1.52–2.89)	HCV: 66(38–94)		S-HCV: 99.0%	
	HBV: 3.88 (1.76–7.80)	HBV: 59(37–87)		S-HBV: 100% ER: 0.5%	
1996–2003 (Soldan et al., 2005)	HIV: 0.14	HIV: 8–15	Yes	S-HIV: 99.9%	Yes
	HCV: 0.80	HCV: 4–59		S-HCV: 99.0%	
	HBV: 1.66	HBV: 80.5		S-HBV: 100% ER: 0.1%	
Rest of Europe					
France, 1992–1994 (Courouce and Pillonel, 1996)	HIV: 1.75 (0.3–4.6)	22 (6–38)	No	—	No
	HTLV: 0.17 (0.0–1.6)	56 (24–128)	No	—	
	HCV: 4.48 (1.7–10.0)	66 (38–94)			
	HBsAg: 3.13 (0.9–11.2)	51 (36–72)			
	HBV: 8.45 (2.8–25.2)				
France, 1998–2000 (Pillonel et al., 2002)	HIV: 0.73 (0.12–2.06)	22 (6–38)	No	—	No
	HCV: 1.16 (0.33–2.25)	66 (38–94)			
	HBV: 2.13 (0.59–6.56)	56 (25–109)			
France, 2001–2003 (Pillonel and Laperche, 2005)	HIV: 0.32 (0.0–1.1)	12–22	No	—	No
	HCV: 0.10 (0.0–0.8)	10–66			
	HBV: 1.57 (0.5–4.7)	56			
Italy, 1996–2000 (Velati et al., 2002)	HIV: 2.5 (0.9–4.1)	22	No	—	No
	HCV: 7.9 (5.7–10.0)	70			
Spain, 1997–1999 (Alvarez et al., 2002)	HIV: 1.95 (0.37–4.71)	22 (6–38)	No	—	No
	HCV: 6.69 (2.74–13.06)	66 (38–94)			
	HBV: 13.51 (5.31–30.08)	59 (37–87)			
Germany and Austria, 1993 (Schwartz et al., 1995)	HIV (Austria): 1.9 (0.7–4.8)	22	Yes	S: 99% ER: 0.1%	Yes
	HIV (Germany): 1.1 (0.4–2.6)		Yes		
Austria and Germany, 1994–2005 (Riggert et al., 1996)	HCV (Austria): 111 (61–161)	74	Yes	S: 98% ER: 0.1%	Yes
	HCV (Germany): 208 (25–756)		Yes		
Germany, 1990–1995 (Koerner et al., 1998)	HCV: 1995 5(0.7–10) repeat	74	Yes	S: 98% ER: 0.1%	Yes
	HCV: 1995 50(36–67) new		Yes		
Germany, 1996 (Gluck et al., 1998)	HIV: 0.53 (0.21–1.39)	22	No	—	No
	HCV: 8.8 (3.3–31)	82	No	—	
	HBV: 4.3 (1.6–7.5)	56			

Study (reference)	Residual risk	Window period (days)			
Germany, 2001–2002 (Offergeld et al., 2005)	HIV: 0.18 HCV: 0.23 HBV: 1.62	11 10 45	No	—	No
Switzerland, 2001–2003 (Niederhauser et al., 2005)	HIV: 0.53 HCV: 0.45 HBV: 8.70	22 66 59	No	—	No
EPFA countries[b], 1997 (Muller-Breitkreutz, 2000)	HIV: 0.43 (0.05–1.41) HCV: 1.61 (0.43–4.97) HBV: 2.51 (0.92–6.44)	HIV: 22 (6–38) HCV: 66 (38–94) HBV: 59 (37–87)	No No	— —	No
Rest of world					
USA, 1986–1987 (Ward et al., 1988)	HIV: 26	56 (28–98)	Yes No	S: 99% —	Partially WP = No FN = Yes
USA, 1987 (Cumming et al., 1989)	HIV: 6.5 (3.33–11.33)	56	No Yes	— ER: 0.1%	Yes
USA, 1987 (Brookmeyer and Gail, 1994)	HIV 4.64	56	No	—	Yes
USA, 1991–1993 (Schreiber et al., 1996)	HIV: 2.03 (0.36–4.95) HTLV: 1.56 (0.50–3.90) HCV: 9.70 (3.47–36.11) HBV: 15.83 (6.82–31.97)	22 (6–38) 51 (36–72) 82 (54–192) 59 (37–87)	No No No	— —	No
USA, 1992–1993 (Lackritz et al., 1995)	HIV: 1.52–2.22	Average of 25	No Yes	— ER: 0.5%	Yes
USA, 1999–2001 (Dodd et al., 2002)	HIV: 0.47 HCV: 0.52 HBV: 4.88	11 10 59	No	—	No
Australia, 1985–1990 (Dax et al., 1992)	HIV: 1.08	28–42	Yes No	S: 99.69%	Yes
Australia, 1994–95 (Whyte and Savoia, 1997)	HIV: 0.79 (0.22–1.37) HCV: 4.27 (2.82–10.01) HBV: 6.45 (4.05–9.52)	22 (6–38) 82 (54–192) 59 (37–87)	No No	— —	No
South Africa (Sitas et al., 1994)	HIV: 22(11–39)	34–98	Yes Yes	S: 99.9% ER: 0.1%	Yes
Thailand, 1990–1993 (Kitayaporn et al., 1996)	HIV: 1990 380 (210–650) HIV: 1991 190 (100–340) HIV: 1992 200 (110–360) HIV: 1993 190 (50–670)	45	No No	— —	No

[a] Various methods.

[b] Not-for-profit blood services in Denmark, England, France, Finland, Germany, Scotland, Switzerland (NB data and estimates for Australia and American Red Cross are also included in paper).

An alternative approach to estimating the risk of a window period does not work from incidence, but sums the probability that previous donations from donors showing seroconversion (SC) were made during the window period.

$$\text{WP risk} = \frac{\text{number of SC} \times (\text{WP/median pre-SC donation interval})}{\text{number of repeat donor donations}}$$

This method, used by Gluck et al., 1998 and Muller-Breitkreutz, 2000, has the advantage of directly accommodating the effect of different inter-donation intervals found in donors who seroconvert compared with other donors.

The amount of difference between the results of these two methods depends on the difference in donation frequency between the minority of donors who acquire new infections (i.e. who seroconvert) and the majority of donors who do not. If donors who seroconvert have shorter or longer inter-donation intervals between their pre-seroconversion donation and their seroconversion donation than the majority of donors, the probability of a window-period donation may actually be greater or less than the average probability that is calculated by the 'incidence' method. For example, if infected donors had inter-donation intervals three times the length of ordinary inter-donation intervals, the chance of the final day of their inter-donation interval occurring during a window period of X days that falls randomly during their inter-donation interval would be one-third the chance of the final day of a non-seroconverting donor's inter-donation interval occurring during a random X days' period. The basic calculation of the frequency of window-period donations by the 'incidence' method can be multiplied by an adjustment factor to accommodate for this effect.

$$P\ WP = \text{incidence} \times WP \times S$$

where

$$S = \frac{\text{inter-donation interval for non-seroconverting donors}}{\text{inter-donation interval for seroconverting donors}}$$

There has been no standard approach to the calculation of ranges around point estimates. Some studies have repeated the calculations using the 'best' and 'worst' values of some or all variables (e.g. window-period length) to give a range from best-case to worst-case estimates. Some studies have generated a range by repeating the calculations using the 95% confidence intervals around observed rates to allow for sampling variability in the data used. The next step is to combine these variabilities, and add others, and use computer simulations to generate distributions of results from which ranges can be read, for example the range within which 95% of the results fall.

Ideally, the same methods would be used to compare risks at different times and places. This was done to produce comparable estimates for Germany and Austria (Riggert et al., 1996; Schwartz et al., 1995). Another initiative has produced combined estimates using comparable data from a larger collection of blood services – those blood services collaborating in the European Plasma Fractionation Association's viral marker surveillance (Muller-Breitkreutz, 2000) (see Table 25.3 for results). A collection of papers from the USA and Europe published in 2002 used similar methods for window-period risk amongst repeat donors (and varying methods to include other risks and new donors) to estimate the risks in these countries at the end of the 1990s (Alvarez et al., 2002; Dodd et al., 2002; Glynn et al., 2002; Pillonel et al., 2002; Velati et al., 2002), and a collection of studies focusing on the impact of nucleic acid testing in Europe was published in 2005 (Alvarez et al., 2005; Niederhauser et al., 2005; Offergeld et al., 2005; Pillonel and Laperche, 2005; Soldan et al., 2005; Velati et al., 2005) (see Table 25.3).

During the tail-end of HBV carriage, HBsAg may fall below detectable levels for a considerable period of time before HBV infectivity is lost (Hoofnagle and Schaffer, 1986). Transmission of infection from such donors has been observed (Soldan et al., 1999) and this risk may need to be considered in estimates of total risk for blood services that use HBsAg alone as a marker of HBV infective donations. One way to estimate the contribution this risk makes to the total risk of transfusion-transmitted HBV is to look at the contribution it makes amongst observed and investigated post-transfusion HBV cases. If half of post-transfusion HBV cases are shown to be due to donors with late-stage HBV infections, then approximately half the estimated total risk of transfusion-transmitted HBV should be contributed by this cause, and the ratio in observed cases may be used to scale up the estimated risk accordingly.

Limitations

Studies frequently state that the risk of a donation being collected during the window period is the largest remaining risk of infection transmission (for those infections that donations are tested for). Although this may often be the case, in certain circumstances it may not be true. The relative importance of each possible component of the risk of issuing infectious donations varies between blood services, depending on the specifications of donation testing, the proportion of donations collected from new donors and the rates of incidence and prevalence in the donating population. Figure 25.1 shows how the percentage of the total risk estimate due to the window period of early infection can vary with different prevalences and incidences. The greater the prevalence of infection, the more important the risk of false-negative tests and errors in the exclusion of seropositive donations.

The estimates of risk associated with window-period donations are highly dependent on accurate and complete identification of seroconversion in blood donors. The identification of true seroconversions in repeat donors can, for some infections, require detailed information about the first seropositive donation and the last seronegative donation. Not all donor testing systems and surveillance systems provide enough detail for accurate determination of seroconversion. The assumptions used to estimate incidence in new donors often result in considerable uncertainty around the estimates of the risks of window-period donations from new donors.

The risk from donors who donate during an infectious window period, but do not re-attend to give a post-seroconversion seropositive donation is not included. There are plausible reasons why donors may be more likely to donate only, or for the last time,

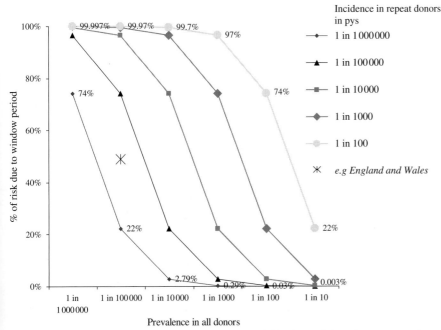

Incidence in repeat donors in pys

—◆— 1 in 1 000 000

—▲— 1 in 100 000

—■— 1 in 10 000

—◆— 1 in 1000

—●— 1 in 100

✻ e.g England and Wales

Figure 25.1 Variation in components of risk with varying prevalence and incidence (in person years at risk, pys).

For an infection with a 22 day window period, using tests with 99.5% sensitivity and an error rate of 0.5%, e.g. HIV, and 11% donations from new donors.

during an infectious window period. Despite alternative testing options and donor education, people who have a self-perceived exposure risk may attend donation sessions in order to be tested for infectious markers, and these donation attendances may occur in the seronegative window period. Also, in the course of a donation attendance a donor may become aware that he/she is not eligible to donate due to a recent exposure risk, and never return.

Many studies omit separate calculations for donations from new donors. However, as mentioned above, donations from new donors consistently have higher prevalence and there are good reasons to expect they will also have higher incidence. The greater the proportion of donations collected from new donors, the larger their contribution to the true overall risk. A study conducted in Thailand (Kitayaporn *et al.*, 1996) reported that 76% of all donations were collected from new donors. However, the risk calculated was based on incidence in repeat donors. According to calculations for England (Soldan *et al.*, 2003b) for 1993–2001, the component of risk due to the window period accounted for 66%, 47% and 89% of the total estimated risk of issuing an HIV, HBV and HCV infectious donation respectively.

In most risk estimation studies, estimates of incidence based on seroconversions have been a key element, and have not been adjusted for differing inter-donation intervals amongst donors who acquire infections, as mentioned above (in different methods). The basic estimate of incidence from seroconversions (incidence = seroconversions/person years observed) assumes that donors are not more likely to self-defer, either temporarily or permanently, after they have seroconverted and that the probability of an individual donating blood does not vary over the course of antibody development after infection. There are some observations, such as longer than average inter-donation intervals in donors who have seroconverted for antibodies to HCV

(Soldan *et al.*, 1998), and fewer than expected HIV p24 antigen positive, HIV antibody negative donations in the USA (Schreiber *et al.*, 2002), that suggest that donors are more likely to self-defer during the window phase. This may be due to a perception of recent risk, symptomatic primary infection, or perhaps just a disrupted life less conducive to donation around the time of exposure to infection. An inter-donation interval that is simply longer can be adjusted for (as above); however, the behavioural factors that may affect the timing of donation in relation to infection are far more difficult to understand and incorporate in the estimation process.

Several other scenarios that could lead to infectious donations entering the blood supply are seldom considered in risk estimates. The sensitivity of assays is typically estimated using a panel of samples considered representative of the population positive for the marker concerned. The potential of newly recognized subtypes and variants of viral infections (e.g. sub-types of HIV other than sub-type B for which tests have usually been tailored (Gurtler, 1998) or mutant HBV infections, not detected by HBsAg tests (Jongerius *et al.*, 1998) to escape detection by routine screening assays is not addressed by most risk estimation studies that tend to focus on the more predictable components of risk and use sensitivity on a limited range of samples.

Besides these internal limitations in the data and assumptions used, there are also external, and more basic limitations to this approach for assessing risk. Only those components of risk that are known about can be estimated, meaning this approach does not contribute to vigilance for new risks. This is not a problem with the estimates themselves, but could be a problem if they are used inappropriately to focus attention and resources on these measured risks and thereby detract efforts from the control of greater threats to blood safety.

Data that could verify or refute the results of risk estimation studies are rare. The introduction of nucleic acid testing (NAT) of donations is now detecting infectious donations missed by current serological tests and is therefore providing some data to compare with the estimates. However, if the estimates from Europe and the USA are close to, or higher than, the true risk, many years of data collection from NAT will be needed to test the accuracy of the estimates for risk in the presence of serological testing only.

The comparability of these estimates to other risks of morbidity is not straightforward. Infectious donations entering the blood supply do not directly translate to infected recipients and the actual risk of disease depends upon many other factors, including the viability of the infectious agent during processing and storage, the transmission rate, the susceptibility of the recipient and the natural history of transfusion-transmitted infections in recipients.

Also, the communication and use of these risk estimates is often difficult, and misunderstanding of these estimates, or ignorance of their limitations or wide probable ranges, can lead to a false sense of confidence or a false sense of alarm in the microbial safety of transfusion.

As risks become lower, the estimates become more fragile and vulnerable to errors in assumptions and to errors in generalizations. As for prospective studies, it can also be true that these calculations lack the precision to accurately detect true risks – at least not with accuracy good enough to, for example, evaluate the relative expected benefit from two alternative approaches to improving blood safety.

Advantages/bonuses

The advantages of estimating transmission risk using routinely available data and evidence-based assumptions include the speed and low cost, and the ease of revision in the light of new data or changing circumstances.

Calculations of risk are relatively quick and economical, and therefore can be done to assess the risk for a range of different situations, especially when the level of risk is extremely low (as in many developed countries currently). The additional safety that may be gained by strategic policy changes such as more stringent donor selection, donation testing or by performing viral inactivation procedures on tested components may be estimated by appropriate alteration to the data and assumptions used in the calculations described. This can be useful both for providing information and choices to health providers and patients, and for comparing different risk-reduction strategies. When comparing the results of these estimations, limitations in knowledge of the common parameters that are therefore a constant error for all risks being compared, become less important.

Although comparability of different studies has been described here as an area deserving some caution, this approach has the potential to produce comparable results from a wide range of circumstances and countries. Calculations can be applied in a standardized manner in countries with different languages, cultures, health care systems, ethical restrictions and resources in a way that observational studies (e.g. prospective studies) cannot.

Conclusion

Calculations of the risk of issuing infectious donations for transfusion can be of great value, and a very efficient way to assess risk on an ongoing and standardized basis. The quality of the results depends upon how correctly the contributions to total real risk are represented in the calculations, and on the accuracy of the parameters used in these calculations. Good surveillance of infections in blood donors (preferably on a national scale) is usually a prerequisite to provision of the necessary data.

Studies that omit some components of risk or only consider donations from repeat/established donors are likely (to an extent dependent on their epidemiology and selection and testing practices) to underestimate the risk of issuing an infected donation. A commonly used method for estimating the window-period risk does not allow for the effect of infected donors leaving longer, or shorter, than average intervals between donations; this may also result in overestimation, or underestimation of the risk respectively.

These estimates are, by their nature, ignorant and uninformative about new, as yet unidentified, risks. Risk estimates may even detract from blood safety if they give the misleading impression that the true and total infectious risks of transfusion are known.

There are three main approaches to assessing and monitoring the risk of the transmission of blood-borne infections by blood transfusion.

Surveillance of clinically identified adverse events following transfusion are discussed in Chapter 21.

Prospective examination of transfusion recipients.

Calculations of estimated infectious donations issued for transfusion, based on data from surveillance of infections in donors, and other sources.

Prospective studies can give the truest picture, with fewest assumptions; however, only if done well and on large numbers and even then only for one point in time. As time moves on, the applicability of their results starts to involve more and more assumptions, and the advantage over calculations therefore lessens. These approaches complement each other quite well. Calculations can enable realistic design and appropriate sample size to be determined for prospective studies, and prospective studies can validate or suggest corrections to the calculations, and can provide data for further calculations, such as prevalence of and transmission rates of new infections, as well as providing information about the end result of the events under study, that is, morbidity and mortality in infected recipients.

The ideal strategy for the assessment of the risk of transfusion-transmitted infections is one that utilizes all three approaches, with the design and priorities of each being determined by information obtained from the others.

REFERENCES

Alvarez, M., González, R., Hernández, J. M., *et al.* (2005) Residual risk of transfusion-transmitted viral infections in Spain, 1997–2002, and impact of nucleic acid testing. *Euro Surveill*, **10**(2), 20–2.

Alvarez, M., Oyonarte, S., Rodriguez, P. M., *et al.* (2002) Estimated risk of transfusion-transmitted viral infections in Spain. *Transfusion*, **42**, 994–8.

Armitage, P. and Colton, T. (editors-in-chief) (1998) Binomial confidence intervals when no events are observed. *Encyclopedia of Biostatistics*, **1**, 358.

Atrah, H. I., Ala, F. A., Ahmed, M. M., *et al.* (1996) Unexplained hepatitis C virus antibody seroconversion in established blood donors. *Transfusion*, **36**, 339–43.

Barrera, J. M., Francis, B., Ercilla, G., *et al.* (1995) Improved detection of anti-HCV in post-transfusion hepatitis by a third-generation ELISA. *Vox Sang*, **68**, 15–18 (and personal communication with authors).

Brennan, M. T., Hewitt, P. E., Moore, C., *et al.* (1995) Confidential unit exclusion: the North London Blood Centre's experience. *Transfus Med*, **5**, 51–6.

Brookmeyer, R. and Gail, M. H. (1994) *Epidemiology: a Quantitative Approach.* Buckingham, Open University Press. Oxford, UK.

Busch, M. P., Lee, L. L., Satten, G. A., *et al.* (1995) Time course of detection of viral and serological markers preceding human immunodeficiency virus type 1 seroconversion: implications for screening of blood and tissue donors. *Transfusion*, **35**, 91–7.

Courouce, A. M. and Pillonel, J. (1996) Estimation du risque de transmission des virus des hepatitis B et C, et des retrovirus par transfusion de derives sanguins labiles. *Bulletin Epidemiologique Hebdomadaire*, **11**, 54–5.

Crawford, R. J., Mitchell, R., Burnett, A. K., *et al.* (1987) Who may give blood? *BMJ*, **294**, 572.

Cumming, P. D., Wallace, E. L., Schorr, J. B., *et al.* (1989) Exposure of patients to HIV through the transfusion of blood components that test antibody negative. *N Eng J Med*, **321**, 941–6.

Dax, E. M., Healey, D. S. and Crofts, N. (1992) Low risk of HIV-1 infection from blood donation: a test-based estimate (letter). *Med J Aust*, **157**, 69.

Dodd, R. Y., Notari, E. P. and Stramer, S. L. (2002) Current prevalence and incidence of infectious disease markers and estimated window-period risk in the American Red Cross blood donor population. *Transfusion*, **42**, 975–9.

Durand, F. and Baeuplet, A. (2000) Evidence of hepatitis C virus viraemia without detectable antibody to hepatitis C virus in a blood donor (letter). *Ann Intern Med*, **133**(1), 74.

Germain, M., Remis, R. S. and Delage, G. (2003) The risks and benefits of accepting men who have had sex with men as blood donors. *Transfusion*, **43**, 25–33.

Gluck, D., Kubanek, B., Maurer, C., *et al.* (1998) Seroconversion of HIV, HCV, and HBV in blood donors in 1996 – risk of virus transmission by blood products in Germany. *Infusion Therapy and Transfusion Medicine*, **25**, 82–4.

Glynn, S. A., Kleinman, S. H., Wright, D. J., *et al.* (2002) International application of the incidence rate/window period model. *Transfusion*, **42**, 966–72.

Gurtler, L. (1998) The impact of HIV subtypes and variants on the stability of HIV screening assays. *Infusion Therapy and Transfusion Medicine*, **25**(2), 9.

Hewitt, P. E., Kendall, B. and Barbara, J. A. J. (1997) Hepatitis A transmitted by red cell transfusion. *Transfus Med*, **7**(Suppl. 1), 48 (abstract).

Hickman, M. and Mortimer, J. Y. (1988) Donor screening for HIV: how many false negatives? (letter). *Lancet*, **28**, 1221.

Hoofnagle, J. H. and Schaffer, D. F. (1986) Serological markers of hepatitis B virus infection (review). *Seminars in Liver Disease*, **6**(1), 1–10.

Hoofnagle, J. H., Seeff, L. B., Buskell-Bales, Z., *et al.* (1978) Serological responses in HB. In *Viral Hepatitis: a Contemporary Assessment of Aetiology, Epidemiology, Pathogenesis and Prevention*, eds. G. N. Vyas, S. N. Cohen and R. Schmid, pp. 219–42. Philadelphia, Franklin Institute Press.

Janssen, R. S., Satten, G. A., Stramer, S. L., *et al.* (1998) New testing strategy to detect early HIV-1 infection for use in incidence estimates and for clinical and prevention purposes. *JAMA*, **280**(1), 42–8.

Jongerius, J. M., Wester, M., Cuypers, H. T. M., *et al.* (1998) New hepatitis B virus mutant form in a blood donor that is undetectable in several hepatitis B surface antigen screening assays. *Transfusion*, **38**, 56.

Kitayaporn, D., Kaewkungwal, J., Bejrachandra, S., *et al.* (1996) Estimated rate of HIV-1 infectious but seronegative blood donations in Bangkok, Thailand. *AIDS*, **10**, 1157–62.

Koerner, K., Cardoso, M., Dengler, T., *et al.* (1998) Estimated risk of transmission of hepatitis C virus by blood transfusion. *Vox Sang.* **74**(4), 213–6.

Korelitz, J. J., Busch, M. P., Kleinman, S. H., *et al.* (1997) A method for estimating hepatitis B virus incidence rates in volunteer blood donors. *Transfusion*, **37**, 634–40.

Kothe, D., Byers, R. H., Caudill, S. P., *et al.* (2003) Performance characteristics of a new less sensitive HIV-1 enzyme immunoassay for use in estimating HIV seroincidence. *J Acquir Immune Defic Syndr*, **33**(5), 15 Aug 625–34.

Lackritz, E. M., Satten, G. A., Aberle-Grasse, J., *et al.* (1995) Estimated risk of transmission of the human immunodeficiency virus by screened blood in the United States. *N Eng J Med*, **333**, 1721–5.

Linden, J. V. (1994) Error contributes to the risk of transmissible disease. *Transfusion*, **34**, 1016.

Linden, J. V. and Kaplan, H. S. (1994) Transfusion errors: causes and effects. *Transfus Med Rev*, **8**, 169–83.

Martlew, V. J., Carey, P., William C. Y., *et al.* (2000) Post-transfusion HIV infection despite donor screening: a report of three cases. *J Hosp Infect*, **44**(2), 93–7.

McFarland, W., Busch, M. P., Kellogg, T. A., *et al.* (1999) Detection of early HIV infection and estimation of incidence using a sensitive/less-sensitive enzyme immunoassay testing strategy at anonymous counselling and testing sites in San Francisco. *J Acquir Immune Defic Syndr*, **22**(5), 484–9.

Mimms, L. T., Mosley, J. W., Hollinger, F. B., *et al.* (1993) Effect of concurrent acute infection with hepatitis C on acute hepatitis B virus infection. *BMJ*, **307**, 1095–7.

Muller-Breitkreutz, K. (2000) Results of viral marker screening of unpaid blood donations in 1997 and probability of window period donations. *Vox Sang*, **78**, 149–57.

Medical Devices Agency Report (1995). PHLS Kit Evaluation Group, Hepatitis and Retrovirus Laboratory, Medical Devices Agency.

Niederhauser, C., Schneider, P., Fopp, M., *et al.* (2005) Incidence of viral markers and evaluation of the estimated risk in the Swiss blood donor population from 1996 to 2003. *Euro Surveill*, **10**(2), 14–6.

Offergeld, R., Faensen, D., Ritter, S., *et al.* (2005) Human immunodeficiency virus, hepatitis C and hepatitis B infections among blood donors in Germany 2000–2002: risk of virus transmission and the impact of nucleic acid amplification testing. *Euro Surveill*, **10**(2), 8–11.

Pillonel, J. and Laperche, S. (2005) Trends in risk of transfusion-transmitted viral infections (HIV, HCV, HBV) in France between 1992 and 2003 and impact of nucleic acid testing (NAT). *Euro Surveill*, **10**(2), 5–8.

Pillonel, J., Laperche, S., Saura, C., *et al.* (2002) Trends in residual risk of transfusion-transmitted viral infections in France between 1992 and 2000. *Transfusion*, **42**, 980–8.

Regan, F. A. M., Hewitt, P. E., Barbara, J. A. J., *et al.* (2000) Prospective investigation of transfusion-transmitted infection in recipients of over 20 000 units of blood. *BMJ*, **320**, 403–6.

Look-back Coordinators, Transfusion transmission of HCV infection prior to anti-HCV testing of blood donations in England: results of the national HCV lookback programme. *Transfusion*, 2001 (in press).

Riggert, J., Schwartz, D. W., Uy, A., *et al.* (1996) Risk of hepatitis C virus (HCV) transmission by anti-HCV-negative blood components in Austria and Germany. *Ann Hematol*, **72**(1), 35–9.

Schreiber, G. B., Busch, M. P. and Kleinman, S. H. (1996) The risk of transfusion-transmitted viral infections. *New England Journal Medicine*, **334**, 1685–90.

Schreiber, G. B., Glynn, S. A., Satten, G. A., *et al.* (2002) HIV seroconverting donors delay their return: screening test implications. *Transfusion*, **42**(4), 414–21.

Sitas, F., Fleming, A. F. and Morris, J. (1994) Residual risk of transmission of HIV through blood transfusion in South Africa. *S Afr Med J*, **84**(3), 142–4.

Soldan, K. and Sinka, K. (2003a) Evaluation of the de-selection of men who have had sex with men from blood donation in England. *Vox Sang.* **84**(4), 265–73.

Soldan, K., Barbara, J. A. J., Ramsay, M., *et al.* (2003b) Estimation of the risk of hepatitis B virus, hepatitis C virus and human immunodeficiency virus infectious donations entering the blood supply in England, 1993–2001. *Vox Sang*, **84**(4), 274–86.

Soldan, K., Barbara, J. A. J. and Heptonstall, J. (1998) Incidence of seroconversion to positivity for hepatitis C antibody in repeat blood donors in England, 1993–1995. *BMJ*, **316**, 1413–7.

Soldan, K., Davison, K. and Dow, B. (2005) Estimates of the frequency of HBV, HCV and HIV infectious donations entering the blood supply in the United Kingdom, 1996 to 2003. *Euro Surveill*, **10**(2), 17–9.

Soldan, K. Ramsay, M. and Collins, M. (1999) Acute hepatitis B infection associated with blood transfusion in England and Wales, 1991–1997: review of database. *BMJ*, **318**, 95.

Schwartz, D. W., Simson, G., Baumgarten, K., *et al.* (1995) Risk of human immunodeficiency virus (HIV) transmission by anti-HIV-negative blood components in Germany and Austria. *Ann Hematol*, **70**(4), 209–13.

Velati, C., Fomiatti, L., Baruffi, L., *et al.* (2005) Gruppo Italiano per lo Studio delle Malattie Trasmissibili con la Trasfusione. Impact of nucleic acid amplification technology (NAT) in Italy in the three years following implementation (2001–2003). *Euro Surveill*, **10**(2), 12–4.

Velati, C., Romano, L., Baruffi, L., *et al.* (2002) Residual risk of transfusion-transmitted HCV and HIV infections by antibody-screened blood in Italy. *Transfusion*, **42**, 989–93.

Ward, J. W., Holmberg, S. D., Allen, J. R., *et al.* (1988) Transmission of HIV by blood transfusions screened as negative for HIV antibody. *N Eng J Med*, **318**, 473–8.

Whyte, G. S. and Savoia, H. F. (1997) The risk of transmitting HCV, HBV or HIV by blood transfusion in Victoria. *Med J Australia*, **166**, 584–6.

26 RISK MANAGEMENT

Arturo Pereira

Introduction

In the fight against transfusion-transmitted infections (TTI), transfusion medicine has traditionally focused on assessing risk and deploying preventive measures, and less attention has been paid to other elements of risk management, such as implementing good risk communication practices or establishing a fair and balanced decision-making framework. The tragedy of transfusion-transmitted AIDS, with its aftermath of judicial, political and social effects, shaped the way transfusion medicine has faced the risk of TTI over the past two decades. Times have changed, however, and current challenges are quite different from those of the early 1980s. The risk for major TTI (HIV, HCV and HBV) has decreased to negligible levels, but public concern seems unabated, so the challenge now is finding how to communicate effectively with the public rather than how to further reduce risk. Nevertheless, resources continue to be detracted from areas of the health care system where they are urgently needed, to be allocated to preventive measures that may themselves be riskier than the risks of TTI they intend to prevent. While early risk reduction measures were unanimously accepted by all involved in transfusion safety, recent proposals have been more controversial, and some, such as universal leucoreduction, have produced a deep division among specialists. There is an increasing perception that risk assessment is biased toward product quality focusing on TTI at the expense of process safety, that regulations issued by governmental agencies are excessively self-protective, that some risk reduction measures are driven by the industry, and that a paradoxical reduction of transfusion safety may have resulted from all this (Dzik *et al.*, 2000). If the latter statement proves to be the case, the challenge would be how to reframe a fair and balanced risk management process.

On the other hand, concern is rising about the risk that emerging infectious agents could gain entry into the blood supply. Dealing with this concern poses the challenge of how to manage risks, the mere existence of which is unknown, since over-reaction against an unconfirmed hazard would be as detrimental to transfusion safety as an inadequate response against a real one might be.

All of this emphasizes the need for checking whether the current process of risk management in transfusion medicine, which is the result of incidents that happened two decades ago, continues to be the most appropriate approach for the challenges we face at present or may face in the future. This chapter tries to convey an overview of risk management and how it applies to TTI. The first two sections deal with the concept of risk, how it is assessed, and what risk management means. Then, the distinctive features of TTI and specific preventive measures are reviewed from the perspective of risk management. The prominent aspects of risk perception and risk communication are addressed next, and the final sections are devoted to cost-effectiveness analysis.

The nature of risk and how it is assessed

Risk is a word used in many different ways by different disciplines. In medicine and public health the term usually means the chance for a hazard or health loss either as a consequence of the physical world, disease or human action. Risk implies uncertainty about what the future holds. Interest in future events arises from the recognition that their advent and the consequences they may have upon our lives are often the result of decisions we make at present.

Future events do not arise from nothing, they are the result of a system – a mechanism or a particular sequence of events – that may be explicit or stand totally or partially hidden from our knowledge. Uncertainty arises from the natural variability in the system or from our imperfect knowledge of how the system works. According to our level of knowledge of the underlying mechanism, there are two conceptually different categories of risk. First, a risk of harm really exists because it has been observed and measured (e.g. the risk of being hit by lightning), but a given person has no way of knowing whether he/she will be hit or not. Second, the very existence of risk is unknown because the harm has not been observed in the past, but it does not mean that it cannot happen in the future. Real and hypothetical risks require assessment methods that are quite different from one another.

Mortality tables predict that about 3% of 49-year-old Western Europeans will die before their fiftieth birthday, but nobody can say for certain who exactly will die. On the other hand, nobody knows whether or not an epidemic of transfusion-transmitted vCJD will unfold anytime in the future because our knowledge of the mechanisms behind such a terrible outcome is as yet quite imperfect.

Observation and statistical analysis allow us to deal with known risks and to gain control over future events. We know that the probability of dying among 49-year-olds is higher, for instance, among smokers, car drivers, or those who suffer from cardiac disease. Risk increases when there is a history of heavy cigarette smoking, previous car crashes or recent myocardial infarction. Driven by our knowledge of the mechanisms causing mortality in middle-aged people we may continue subdividing the population of 49-year-old Europeans into different risk groups until we get quite an accurate profile of every person's risk of death. We cannot reach absolute certainty for a given person, but we can get quite a good approximation. Insurance companies make use

Transfusion Microbiology, eds John A. J. Barbara, Fiona A. M. Regan and Marcela C. Contreras. Published by Cambridge University Press. © Cambridge University Press 2008.

of these statistical models every day. In addition, knowledge about the causes of mortality allows us to undertake the appropriate preventive measures to reduce the risk outcome, and to forecast by how much the risk will be reduced. Natural variability will continue to impose a limit to our level of certainty, but we will have gained a substantial degree of control over the future risk outcome.

A quite different approach must be applied to the example of vCJD and transfusion because data are not available for us to apply to our statistical armamentarium. Since we cannot observe the whole system, we have to make guesses about how the system works to predict the risk outcome. Investigators of the psychology of prediction have shown that human ability to make accurate evaluations of risk is severely limited by systematic biases (Kahneman *et al.*, 1982), so we need a more reliable method than a mere 'gut feeling'. The rational method that science has developed to appraise this kind of uncertainty is the risk simulation model. The tools we have at hand for building such a model include research aimed at increasing our knowledge of the system, logical thinking, and comparison of the predictions made by the model with emerging observations. A risk model is much like a scientific theory. It is useful as long as data generated by the model allow us to predict accurately the risk outcome. It must be modified, or even discarded, when new observations do not match model predictions.

Any risk assessment requires a model of the underlying system, even such a simple one as 'the near future will be much like the recent past'. When an appreciable level of knowledge about the system driving the risk outcome has been accrued, we can apply statistical methods to our data in order to assess system variability. Conversely, if the risk is new or merely hypothetical, we need to construct de novo a simulation model. The nuclear power industry and the space exploration agencies have refined the methods to conduct risk assessment analyses of systems that have never existed before (Wilson and Crouch 2001). First, a complex system is split into smaller and simpler pieces. All the imaginable outcomes and the sequence of events that bring these outcomes are listed and evaluated for causal relationship. Thereafter, a tree model of chance nodes and associated outcomes conveying all the causal relationships is built, and each node is given a range of probabilities. The risk associated with every possible outcome is then calculated using the rules of conditional probability. Decision nodes may be included into the tree in order to test the effect of preventive interventions.

Since the future is intrinsically unknown, a risk model is necessarily based on assumptions. The only condition that model assumptions must fulfil is consistency with the current scientific knowledge and with the rules of logic. Assumptions and the assigned probabilities should be tested in sensitivity analyses. Critical components in the model are changed by a meaningful amount or varied from worst case to best case, and final risk is recalculated. The resulting difference provides some indication of how sensitive the risk estimate is to model assumptions. When sensitivity is high, conclusions are not robust, and there is a strong case for conducting more empirical research aimed at reducing uncertainty.

The most difficult and critical step in model building is probability assignment, since all the required data are rarely available to the analyst. When empirical data are insufficient to derive a probability estimate, the analyst has to rely on expert opinions. There are refined techniques (e.g. the Delphi method) to elicit reliable quantitative estimates from experts (Ayyub, 2001). This may sound rather strange to physicians and practitioners well versed in evidence-based medicine, but sceptics must acknowledge that much valuable information on how a system works is qualitative and is held in the mind of experts. Risk models based on subjective probabilities, analyst assumptions and expert opinions are not easily accepted in medicine because they are regarded as a form of non-scientific 'data cooking'. However, such kinds of model are commonplace in other technological and scientific disciplines, and will become more familiar to transfusion medicine specialists as they are increasingly involved in decision making about emerging, never previously encountered risks. The power of models based on expert opinions to get accurate quantitative risk estimates is illustrated in the following anecdote, updated from a quote in the book by Ayyub (2001).

At the beginning of the space shuttle project, NASA sponsored a study to assess the risk of catastrophic outcome. In this study, Bayesian analysis utilizing prior experience with solid rocket motor failures, engineering knowledge, system analysis and subjective probabilities get an estimate of 1 in 35 launches. The estimate was disregarded by NASA, and managers and administrators dictated a 1 in 100 000 number. The catastrophic Challenger explosion occurred on the 25th launch of the space shuttle, and Columbia disintegrated during reentry on the 107th mission. At the bottom line, one catastrophic outcome every 53 missions, on average.

There are some examples of very influential risk models in the field of TTI. The famous incidence window-period model, developed by REDS (Retrovirus Epidemiology Donor Study) investigators to appraise the risk for major TTI, is an archetype of statistical models (Schreiber *et al.*, 1996). It will be discussed in detail later on. On the other hand, the model on the risk of transfusion-transmitted vCJD built by Det Norske Veritas, a Norwegian risk assessment firm, for the British Health Service in the late 1990s, and which triggered the introduction of universal leucoreduction in most of Western Europe, gathers all the characteristics of a risk simulation (Kleinman, 1999). More recently, the model built by Centers for Disease Control (CDC) investigators on West Nile virus transmission through transfusion can be regarded as a mixed one, since statistical analysis of known data were combined with simulation to infer a risk that was unknown at that time (Biggerstaff and Petersen 2002).

What does risk management mean?

Risk management is a systematic approach to the discovery and treatment of risk. The goal is to help to state objectively, document and rank risk, and to prepare a plan for implementation of risk reduction measures and effective risk communication. The scope of risk management is, therefore, broader than merely assessing risk and deploying preventive measures.

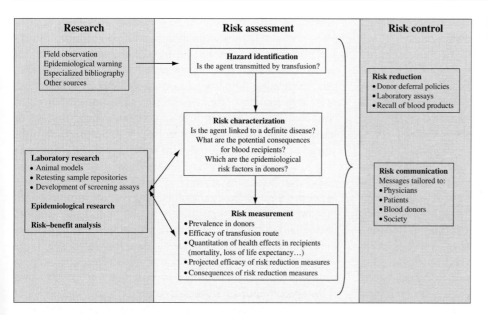

Figure 26.1 Elements of comprehensive risk management.

Disciplines related to technology assessment, engineering, environmental sciences and public health have developed comprehensive methods for risk management. Figure 26.1 shows a scheme applicable to TTI that is inspired by one of the milestones in the field of risk management: the 'red book' published by the US National Academy of Sciences in 1983 (NAS, 1983). The fundamental principles of comprehensive risk management are outlined next. Further details can be found in the specialized bibliography (Morgan, 1993; NAS, 1994; Stern and Fineberg, 1996; Wilson and Crouch, 2001).

Experts in risk management agree on the necessity for activities of risk assessment, risk reduction and risk communication to be clearly separated from one another, so that the former cannot be influenced by the prejudices of managers on how risk is to be reduced or communicated to the public. In 1983, concern about the consequences of implementing blood donor deferral policies based on the epidemiological risk factors for AIDS led to downplaying the risk that the disease was transmitted through transfusion. In the early 1990s, the risk that BSE could pass to humans through the food chain was trivialized through fear of public overreaction.

Pre-established protocols or procedural guidelines on how to conduct the risk management process are very important. They safeguard against the neglects of improvization, help save time and increase efficacy and objectivity. Guidelines make it difficult for managers to move the focus from the main issue under the pressure of the media or interested parties.

Scientific research aimed at decreasing uncertainty should be encouraged and financed at the early stages of risk management. This is particularly urgent when uncertainty is high, the hypothetical harm may be severe or the preventive measures are costly, of doubtful efficacy or potentially harmful themselves. It is amazing that several years after universal leucoreduction was implemented to prevent the risk of prion transmission through the transfusion, efficacy of this measure has not yet been tested in the laboratory, despite the availability of suitable animal models

which have been used extensively for other purposes, and research could have been done at a fraction of the annual cost of leucoreduction.

Interventions aimed at reducing risk should be evaluated for effectiveness, safety and efficiency. Risk–benefit and cost-effectiveness analyses should be conducted using the same measurement units that were employed in assessing risk. Usage of a common yardstick prevents managers from implementing risk reduction measures that may result in more risk from them than from the initial threat.

While assessment of risk must be done by those who have the requisite expertise, all interested parties should be informed on time, listened to by the managers, and invited to participate in the process of risk management. Nevertheless, whatever the number and eminence of participants, rules of democracy demand that ultimate decisions must be taken by elected representatives or public officers who are politically accountable. In democratic societies, the whole process of decision making must be accessible to the public. In this respect, it is noteworthy that both the Blood Product Advisory Committee of the FDA and the Advisory Committee on Blood Safety and Availability of the USA Department of Health and Human Services publish the complete transcripts of meetings on the Internet.

Good risk communication should be exercised from the very beginning of the risk management process. The objective is to provide people with the basis for making informed decisions. Poor communication practices have repeatedly proved a failure, since they result in social amplification of risk, public distrust of managers, and high-order social and economic effects.

Risk identification and characterization

A thorough search for post-transfusion clinical case reports is the most basic method of establishing that a disease is transmitted by transfusion. The first evidence that AIDS was transfusion-transmitted emerged from the report of recipients of blood products who had no other known risk factors (CDC, 1982), and this triggered more extensive investigations. However, a causal relationship to the previous transfusion is difficult to substantiate on the basis of isolated case reports, as the recipient may have acquired the infection from other sources. On occasion, molecular characterization of the infectious agent in the blood recipient and the involved donor helps confirm (Muder *et al.*, 1992) or refute the thesis (Engstrand *et al.*, 1995) that transfusion was the source of infection. Clinical case reporting is subject to the biases of under-diagnosis and under-reporting, mainly when physicians and patients are not aware of the new TTI, or the clinical manifestations of disease are ill defined or very delayed.

Look-back studies consist of investigating whether an infection has appeared in recipients when the blood bank becomes aware that the implicated donor has developed an infection that is potentially transmissible by blood transfusion, and is another method for detecting that an infectious agent is transmitted by transfusion (Please refer to Chapter 24). Look-back studies have been used to investigate the occurrence of rare or hypothetical TTI, such as classical CJD (Heye *et al.*, 1994). Close surveillance of patients who have received blood from donors who later developed vCJD is being conducted in the UK in order to establish whether or not the disease is transmitted by transfusion (please refer to Chapters 22 and 23). Here again, the existence of potential sources of infection other than transfusion may preclude scientists from establishing a causal relationship on the basis of scattered positive look-back cases. Poor traceability from donor to recipient and the short survival of many transfused patients (due to underlying diseases) decrease the effectiveness of look-back studies, as many of the recipients of potentially infectious blood units cannot be reached and transmission cannot be confirmed.

Close surveillance of patients on chronic transfusion support is another way of gaining insight into TTI. Patients with congenital coagulation factor deficiency, who are regularly transfused with factor concentrates derived from large pools of donor plasma, and patients with constitutional anaemia, such as sickle-cell disease or thalassaemia, who receive frequent red cell transfusions, have historically played this role of 'mine canary' or sentinel for the benefit of all transfusion recipients. The first three patients reported with transfusion-transmitted AIDS were haemophiliacs (CDC, 1982), and HIV was first successfully isolated from the blood of a French patient with haemophilia and AIDS (Montagnier, 2002). More recently, evidence against CJD transmission by blood products was obtained from post-mortem neuropathological analyses of haemophilic patients who had died from AIDS or other CJD-unrelated causes (Evatt *et al.*, 1998; Lee *et al.*, 1998). Lack of reference to haemophilia, sickle-cell disease or thalassaemia as an associated disorder in death certificates of patients who died from classical CJD was regarded as further evidence that the disease is not transmitted by transfusion (Holman *et al.*, 1996).

Case-control studies, population-based investigation and other kinds of epidemiological studies can be useful in suggesting that infectious agents may be transmitted by blood transfusion. The rationale is that should the agent be transfusion-transmitted, the resulting disease would be more frequent in people who have received transfusions than in un-transfused controls.

Alternatively, if transfusion is a significant source of infection, history of blood transfusion should be more common among patients having the disease than in controls. The first irrefutable evidence that hepatitis was significantly transmitted by transfusion was provided by the large and detailed epidemiological studies conducted by Allen in the 1950s (Allen and Sayman, 1962). Case-control studies conducted in the late 1990s did not find that a history of transfusion was more frequent in patients with classical CJD than in healthy controls (Van Duijn *et al.*, 1998; Wientjens *et al.*, 1996). Epidemiological studies have several drawbacks. They need to be large enough to detect minor differences, are expensive and difficult to conduct, and do not permit a causal relationship between transfusion and disease to be established, since transfusion may be merely a confounding variable. In addition, results of prospective epidemiological studies are usually too delayed to be useful in the presence of an emerging TTI.

Recently, the first empirical evidence that West Nile virus was transmitted through transfusion emerged from investigation of blood or solid organ recipients who developed the disease shortly thereafter, and in whom transfused blood or transplanted organs could be traced back to donors who were retrospectively found to be viraemic at the time of blood donation or organ harvest (Iwamoto *et al.*, 2003; Pealer *et al.*, 2003). This quick and successful epidemiological achievement was possible, at least in part, because physicians were already aware of the possibility that West Nile virus was transmissible by transfusion. A theoretical model based on the biology and epidemiology of West Nile virus had alerted the medical community that the agent might be transmitted by blood or blood components, even though no post-transfusion case had been documented in other international epidemics of West Nile virus (Biggerstaff and Petersen, 2002).

As emerging infectious agents will continue to pose real or hypothetical threats to the safety of the blood supply, proactive surveillance for such agents is of paramount importance. Kitchen and Barbara (2000) have summarized the attributes that a biological agent has to possess to be transmissible by transfusion, which may help decide which agents are candidates for close surveillance.

Attributes of transfusion-transmissible agents

First, the agent must be present in the bloodstream, either free in plasma (e.g. HCV or HBV), within the leucocytes (e.g. HTLV or CMV) or within the red cells (e.g. plasmodia or babesia). It may be in a form that is directly infectious or in a latent form that needs to be activated in the recipient, as in the case of CMV.

Second, the agent must be infectious when transmitted through the parenteral route. Hepatitis B and C virus and HIV are very effectively transmitted by blood, even at low concentrations. The respiratory viruses are poorly transmitted, although they might be present in the bloodstream. In some cases, transmission is a matter of dose. For instance, the hepatitis A virus may be transmitted if the donor is highly viraemic at the time of donation, though the usual route of transmission is faeco-oral.

Third, clinical disease should be preceded by an asymptomatic incubation period, as the carrier would not come to donate blood if he/she were too ill, nor would the blood service accept the donation. The longer the incubation period, the higher the risk that the infectious donor is not deferred and also the longer the delay until disease develops in blood recipients and is recognized as transfusion-transmitted. Viruses of African haemorrhagic fevers, such as the Ebola virus, are present in the bloodstream and are very effectively transmitted by the parenteral route, but they seem to have a very short incubation period to pose a transfusion risk, even though they can 'escape' from their current geographical niches.

Finally, the agent needs to be stable upon storage. Before they are transfused into the recipient, red cells are stored at 4 °C for up to 42 days in some countries, platelets are stored at 22 °C for up to 5–7 days, and plasma is frozen at −30 °C or less for several months. *Treponema pallidum* is the most conspicuous example of a potential blood-borne agent that has nearly disappeared from the records of TTI because it does not survive for more than three days at 4 °C (and also because many recipients of blood are treated with antibiotics).

In addition to the above attributes, an agent that is transmissible through blood transfusion needs to fulfil some additional conditions in order to pose a threat to public health. One condition is that the agent reaches an epidemic level among blood donors, which requires an effective way of transmission from person to person other than blood transfusion. In addition, the epidemiological risk factors for the infectious agent must be different from those that already constitute the basis for donor deferral, or carriers would be indirectly excluded from blood donation. West Nile virus is a good example of the above two characteristics, as it is transmitted by mosquito bite and reached epidemic levels in some areas of the USA during mosquito seasons. Finally, but no less important, the agent must cause a definite illness in blood recipients, or at least in some groups of susceptible recipients, such as immunocompromised patients. GB virus C (so called 'hepatitis G virus') is transmitted by blood transfusion, but to date it has not been linked to any definite disease.

Direct measurement of risk

Because of under-diagnosis, under-reporting and lack of follow-up of blood recipients, clinical case reporting and look-back studies are severely biased and cannot provide accurate risk estimates. In addition, as the population size from which the reported cases are extracted is usually unknown, lack of denominators may make it impossible for epidemiologists to get any risk estimate. Active haemovigilance programmes, such as those established in Great Britain, France and other European countries, decrease under-reporting and yield more precise denominators, but cannot eliminate the problem of under-diagnosis. (Please refer to Chapter 21). Haemovigilance programmes are appropriate for detection of known, acute transfusion complications, but are probably less effective in detecting TTI with a long incubation period or new infections of which physicians are unaware.

A prospective controlled study of transfusion recipients is the most accurate method of directly establishing the risk of TTI.

Patients undergoing cardiac surgery have been the ideal candidates for this kind of study, since they are usually transfused only at the time of surgery and long post-transfusion follow-up is feasible. The recipients are monitored for clinical disease, and blood specimens are collected prior to transfusion and at periodic intervals during follow-up for laboratory evidence of TTI. Ideally, serum samples from patients and donors are stored frozen in a repository, so they may be re-tested when more sensitive assays become available or a new TTI is suspected. Since the mid-1970s the National Heart, Lung and Blood Institute in the USA has funded several large-scale, prospective studies on the risk of transfusion-transmitted hepatitis virus and retrovirus infections. Study design and results have recently been summarized by Kleinman and Busch (2000).

An alternative approach to direct estimation of risk involves holding large repositories of donor specimens, testing for TTI agents in these specimens, and follow-up of selected recipients. Two studies based on this design were conducted in the late 1980s to measure the rate of HIV and HTLV I/II infection in blood donors, the level of transmission to recipients, and the clinical outcomes of infection (Kleinman and Busch, 2000). From 1991 to 1995, the REDS group has built up a large repository of over 600 000 donor samples from five areas in the USA, which represented about 8% of all allogeneic blood collected in the USA during the period under study (Zuck et al., 1995). The repository and the large database of blood donors proved to be very useful in monitoring the risk of TTI (Glynn et al., 2000), and in gaining further understanding of donor characteristics associated with increased risk of TTI.

From the early 1990s onwards, the frequency of the major TTI (HIV, HBV and HCV) in screened blood donors has become so low that direct measurement of transmission rates is no longer feasible. Prospectively followed-up cohorts had to be so large that study became impractical or very expensive. However, large repositories of donor and patient specimens will continue to render several benefits in the study of new TTI. Although any prevalence figure for the new agent derived from these repositories would be outdated, rapid testing of a large number of samples will provide information on whether the agent is new or newly detected, and valuable data on the level of transmission and the clinical outcomes in the recipient (Kleinman and Busch, 2000).

Risk modelling

Modelling the mechanism behind a TTI is the only available way of getting an estimate of risk when the infection is very rare or the risk is hypothetical (please refer to Chapter 25).

In the mid-1990s, REDS investigators developed a mathematical model to quantify the residual risk of transmission through blood screened for the major TTIs (Kleinman et al., 1997; Schreiber et al., 1996). Potential mechanisms behind residual risk include blood collected during the early stage of infection, when the donor is infectious but has negative results at the laboratory screening (window period); blood given by asymptomatic carriers with chronic immunosilent infection; and the existence of viral variants that pass undetected by laboratory

Table 26.1 Example of incidence rate calculation[a].

Donor	Previous donation		Last donation		Incident case	Time-interval (months)	Persons-month at risk
	Date	Result	Date	Result			
(1)	January 1998	Negative	April 2000	Negative	No	15	15
(2)	March 1998	Negative	March 2000	Negative	No	24	24
(3)	April 1998	Negative	November 1999	Positive	Yes	19	9.5[b]
(4)	May 1998	Negative	March 1999	Positive	Yes	10	5[b]

There are two incident cases observed during $15 + 24 + 9.5 + 5 = 53.5$ person-months at risk. Incidence = 2 seroconverters/53.5 person-months = 0.0373 seroconverters per person-month = 0.448 seroconverters per person-year at risk.

[a] According to Kleinman *et al.* (1997).

[b] Seroconversion is assumed to happen at the midpoint between the last seronegative and the first seropositive donation, so that the person-months at risk of seroconverting is half (the first half of) the observed period.

screening of donated blood. Laboratory errors (especially if process control is inadequate) are another contributor to risk. Based on available data, REDS investigators assumed that window-period donation was the main reason for the residual risk of HIV, HCV and HBV transmission in developed countries (Kleinman and Busch, 2000).

The incidence window-period model provides an estimate of risk by calculating the probability of collecting a unit of blood within the seronegative window period. Two parameters are needed for such calculation: the length of the window period for a particular laboratory assay and the incidence of infection in the population of donors over a specific time interval. The incidence is obtained from repeat donors who seroconvert for the infectious agent, and is measured as the number of newly infected donors (seroconverters) divided by the observed person-year at risk. Table 26.1 shows a simple example of how incidence is calculated. Length of window period is estimated from serial samples taken from people who have recently been exposed to the infectious agent. Such samples would need to be collected at closely spaced intervals, from a large number of infected individuals, with a known date of infection, to accurately establish the mean and range of the window period.

There are two kinds of sample sets that fit these criteria. One source is samples from transfusion recipients that were prospectively enrolled in TTI studies, and which can be retrospectively tested when a new assay becomes available (please refer to Chapter 24). Since the date of transfusion is known, these samples provide an accurate estimate of the window-period duration. A second sample source is panels of seroconverters selected from paid plasmapheresis donors. These have the advantage of very closely spaced donations and a large volume of sample, as many paid plasma donors donate up to twice a week for long periods and entire units of plasma are often available. However, as the exact date of infection is usually unknown, this kind of repository is more suitable for determining by how much a new test closes an already established analytical window than for establishing the duration of an unknown window period (see Figure 11.8). The above kinds of sample sets have provided a direct measurement of window period duration for HCV and HBV, but not HIV.

For the latter, the infectious window period was estimated from transfusion recipients known to have received a unit of blood from a donor who later seroconverted for HIV (Petersen *et al.*, 1994). As closely spaced samples were not available from these blood recipients, the window-period estimate required some mathematical modelling. Subsequent studies used samples from high-risk cohorts (i.e. intravenous drug users or men who have sex with men) to determine the window-period reduction yielded by new HIV assays (Busch *et al.*, 1995b). Table 26.2 shows window-period estimates for the major TTI, according to source of data and kind of assay.

Once the incidence and window-period duration are known, the risk for an incident case of donation during the window period is calculated by multiplying both parameters. (See Table 26.3.)

The incidence window-period model has several weaknesses. First, there is some uncertainty in the way that the window period was measured for major TTI. As previously stated, the duration of the window period for HIV is the result of mathematical modelling rather than direct measurement. For HCV and HBV, length of the window period has been determined on a relatively small number of seroconverting cases, so it may not be representative of what occurs in the whole population of donors. In addition, window-period duration has been calculated in people who became infected by transfusion of several hundred millilitres of blood. It is possible that exposure by other routes or to smaller inocula might give rise to longer window periods (Kleinman *et al.*, 1997). In the case of HIV, the real infectious period might be shorter than the time elapsed from exposure to seroconversion. Data from a chimpanzee model indicate that there would be an 'eclipse period' ranging from days to weeks after exposure, during which HIV is replicating in regional lymph nodes before being released to peripheral blood (Murthy *et al.*, 1999).

The second weakness involves the calculation of incidence. Incidence in first-time donors is not observable by monitoring seroconversion, so that the model assumes that it is equivalent to that measured in repeat donors. However, there are data indicating that incidence of HIV infection may be increased in first-time donors. On the one hand, history of high-risk behaviour undisclosed at the time of donation is more frequent in first-time

Table 26.2 Data source and method for estimates of window-period (WP) length.

Virus	Assays	Population	Method	WP days; mean (range)	Source
HCV	EIA-1/EIA-2	9 transfusion recipients	Direct measurement of length	EIA-1: 82 (54–192); EIA-2: 65 (20–130)	Lelie *et al.* (1992)
HCV	EIA-2/EIA-3	21 transfusion recipients	Direct measurement of length		Barrera *et al.* (1995b)
HCV	EIA-2/EIA-3	71 seroconversion panels	WP length as compared with HCV NAT	EIA-2: 63 (24–>180) EIA-3: 46 (0–135)	Tobler *et al.* (2003)
HBV	HBsAg	12 transfusion recipients	Direct measurement of length	59 (37–87)	Mimms *et al.* (1993)
HIV	Anti-HIV 1	Look-back study of 179 seroconverting donors and 36 blood recipients.	Mathematical modelling	45	Petersen *et al.* (1994)
HIV	10 anti-HIV EIAs p24 antigen RNA PCR	81 seroconverting persons from high-risk groups	WP reduction as compared with the above estimate Mathematical modelling	EIA HIV 1 + 2: 22 (12–38) p24: 16 (8–24) RNA PCR: 10 (0–20)	Busch *et al.* (1995b)

Table 26.3 Example of risk calculation using the incidence window-period model.

Hypothetical data of number of seroconverters (SC) and window-period length

Incidence rate:	2 SC per 100 000 persons-year (or 0.00002 per person-year).
Window period:	22 days (or 0.06 years).
Risk of window period donation:	2 SC × 0.06 years = 0.12 per 100 000 donations collected per year.

Expected risk reduction by introduction of new test

(Suppose the new test could detect infection 6 days (0.016 years) earlier than existing tests)

Expected yield:	0.016 years × 2 SC = 0.032 per 100 000 donations collected per year.
New risk of window period donation:	2 SC × (22 – 6 days = 0.044 years) = 0.09 per 100 000 donations per year.

Application to a geographical area where 10 million donations are collected per year

(1) Existing tests:

Number of window period donations:	0.12/100 000 donations × 10 million donations = 12 per year.
Number of infected recipients:	12 × 1.6 = 19 per year.

(Since, on average, 1.6 blood components are transfused from each donation.)

(2) New test:

Number of window period donations:	0.09/100 000 donations × 10 million donations = 9 per year.
Number of infected recipients:	9 × 1.6 = 14 per year.
Decrease in the number of infected recipients:	19 – 14 = 5 per year.

(This is like multiplying the yield of the new test × 10 million donations × 1.6 transfused components per donation.)

donors than in repeat donors (Chiavetta *et al.*, 2000; Williams *et al.*, 1997). On the other hand, application of a sensitive/less-sensitive dual HIV antibody assay to seroconverters has shown that incidence of HIV infection in first-time donors is two-fold higher that in repeat donors (Janssen *et al.*, 1998). Because epidemiological risk factors for HIV infection imply an increased risk for HBV and HCV infection, incidence for the latter virus might also be higher in first-time donors, though no direct measurement is available. Two recent studies add further support to the existence of increased risk among first-time donors. First, based on reasonable assumptions and using mathematical modelling, authors from the UK have estimated the risk of major TTI from donations from new donors to be approximately seven-fold

higher than the risk from donations from repeat donors (Soldan *et al.*, 2003). Second, a study conducted in the USA has shown that blood donation within the serological window period for HCV and HIV (antibody negative, NAT positive) was three to four times as frequent among first-time donors as among repeat donors (Stramer *et al.*, 2004).

The incidence window-period model assumes that infection in seroconverters occurs just in the middle of the period between the last negative and the first positive donation. If this were not the case because the donor came to donate early after infection, the probability of window-period collection would be greater than the model estimate. Early blood donation after infection may occur with test-seekers, that is, donors who make use of the blood bank as a means of becoming aware of their HIV serological status after a risky behaviour, such as casual high-risk sex. Studies conducted in the USA indicate that the contrary is true: that repeat donors recently infected with HIV delay their next donation (Schreiber *et al.*, 2002). Whether or not this finding can be extrapolated to other countries remains to be established. In the experience of the author of this chapter, test-seekers pose a significant threat to the safety of the blood supply.

An additional limitation of the incidence window-period model is the way HBV incidence is calculated. As seroconversion for HBsAg is transient, incidence estimates based on HBsAg will underestimate the number of new HBV infections in blood donors, some of whom may have acquired HBV infection and cleared HBsAg before the next blood donation. In order to cope with this problem, REDS investigators adjusted the HBV incidence by taking into account the interdonation interval for HBsAg seroconverters, which increased by 2.4-fold the observed incidence (Kleinman *et al.*, 1997).

Finally, as sensitive laboratory assays have decreased the risk of window-period donation to negligible levels, alternative mechanisms for the residual risk of major TTI, initially dismissed as irrelevant, must be given more consideration. Seronegative, chronic carriers have been described for HCV (Prat *et al.*, 2003) and HBV (Chemin *et al.*, 2001), and some genetic variants of TTI viruses are less effectively detected at laboratory screening (Bøgh *et al.*, 2001). If new tests, such as mini-pool NAT, fail to detect some of these variant cases, the risk reduction they actually provide would be less than projected by the incidence window-period model.

Another potential source of residual risk for TTI is laboratory error. However, automation of data management and testing systems, technological developments, such as colour change reagents, and stringent quality control requirements, have made testing errors extremely rare in the developed world. A study conducted in the early 1990s, when the degree of laboratory automation was below the current level, found a frequency of error of 1 in 2000 blood donations tested (Busch *et al.*, 2000). Since error would have to involve a seropositive blood donation before it could lead to transfusing an infectious unit, this number must be multiplied by the prevalence of seropositive donations. For instance, if prevalence of anti-HIV positive donors is 2 in 10 000, the risk of an HIV infectious unit passing undetected because of laboratory error would be $1/2000 \times 2/10\,000 = 1$ in 10 million.

In a large-scale prospective study to directly assess errors in HBsAg screening, results from parallel testing by haemagglutination and radioimmunoassay were compared between 1974 and 1984. In manual testing systems, one in 60 HBsAg positives might have been erroneously released. The causes of errors included failure to sample, incorrect tube sampled, incorrect reagent addition, misreading results and re-testing of the wrong initially reactive sample tube (Barbara and Howell, 1994).

Despite the above drawbacks, the incidence window-period model has gained widespread acceptance as a means of estimating the risk of transfusion-transmitted HIV, HBV and HCV infection because it has some notable advantages. The model provides an inexpensive estimate of the current risk that can be easily compared with actual data when new (more sensitive) screening procedures such as NAT or deferral criteria are introduced. Risk estimates can be compared across different geographical areas and, in fact, several countries have applied the model to produce their own estimates (see Table 26.4). Finally, and perhaps more importantly, the model can make predictions about the safety yield of new screening procedures, since only the shortening of the window period provided by the new test is needed to generate the new risk estimate. (Please refer to Chapter 17.)

As stated above, implementation of new laboratory tests provides the opportunity to validate empirically projections made by the incidence window-period model. Results, however, have been somewhat conflicting. Although the observed yield was within the range of predicted values for HIV and HCV NAT in the USA and Australia (Kleinman *et al.*, 2000; Seed *et al.*, 2002), it was below model predictions in some European countries (Eiras *et al.*, 2003; Roth *et al.*, 2002). The yield provided by the HIV p24 test in the USA was also below model predictions (Kleinman and Busch, 2000). Whether these incongruities can be ascribed to inaccuracies in the model or to a lower than expected sensitivity of the new assays when performed under daily working conditions has not been settled (Sanz and Pereira, 2003).

Risk per unit versus risk per patient

The current standard practice for expressing the risk of TTI is on a per blood donation or per transfused unit basis (e.g. 1 in 100 000; 0.00001 per unit; or 0.001%). Since one whole blood donation is divided into red cells, platelets and plasma (and occasionally cryoprecipitate) that are usually transfused into different patients, a single infectious whole blood donation can transmit the agent to more than one recipient. On the other hand, not all blood components produced from whole blood are eventually transfused. The shelf life of blood components may expire before they are transfused and many plasma units are used as source for manufactured derivatives (i.e. albumin and coagulation factor concentrates) that are rendered virus-free during the production process. On average, one whole blood donation gives rise to 1.5–1.8 transfused components, so this is the expected number of blood recipients that will get infected from a single infectious donation. This assumes that every blood component derived from an infectious donation can transmit the agent to the recipient. While this is true for HIV, HCV and HBV, it is not so for intracellular agents. Human T-cell lymphotropic virus and CMV, which are located within the leucocytes, are probably not transmitted by plasma or by leucodepleted cellular components. For intracellular agents the risk of transmission is also greater with fresher components. Intra-erythrocytic agents, like plasmodia or babesia, are only borne by red cell units, though they may also be transmitted by platelet units that are heavily contaminated by erythrocytes.

From the perspective of a blood recipient, the risk per unit transfused needs to be adjusted for the number of units of blood from different donors that he/she has received. The mathematically correct method to estimate the risk per patient is by

Table 26.4 Incidence rate and residual risk of window-period donation for selected countries.

Country (period; reference)	HIV			HCV			HBV		
	Incidence rate (per 100 000 persons-year)	Assay	Residual risk (per million donations)	Incidence rate (per 100 000 persons-year)	Assay	Residual risk (per million donations)	Incidence rate (per 100 000 persons-year)	Assay	Residual risk (per million donations)
USA-REDS (1991–1993; Schreiber et al. 1996)	3.37	Anti-HIV 1 + 2	2.03 (0.36–4.95)	4.32	EIA-2	9.70 (3.47–36.11)	9.8	HBsAg	15.83 (6.82–31.97)
USA American Red Cross (2000–2001; Dodd et al. 2002)	1.55	mp NAT	0.47	1.89	mp NAT	0.52	3.02	HBsAg	4.88
England (1993–1995; Soldan et al. 2003)	0.27	Anti-HIV 1 + 2	0.08 (0.02–0.21)	0.25	EIA-2	0.5 (0.32–1.72)	1.24	HBsAg	2.38 (1.22–4.15)
England (1999–2001; Soldan et al. 2003)	0.35	Anti-HIV 1 + 2	0.09 (0.02–0.22)	0.28	mp NAT	0.03 (0.01–0.07)	0.98	HBsAg	0.97 (0.4–1.9)
Canada (1999–2000; Chiavetta et al. 2003)	0.55	Anti-HIV 1 + 2 + p24	0.24 (0.03–0.62)	1.35	mp NAT	0.70 (0.08–3.13)	5.27	HBsAg	8.52 (4.44–15.11)
Italy, Northern and Central (1996–2000; Tosti 2002)	3.8	Anti-HIV 1 + 2	2.3 (1.7–3.0)	4.1	EIA-3	7.9 (5.7–10)	—	—	—
Italy, Lombardy (1994–1999; Velati et al. 2002)	4.06	Anti-HIV 1 + 2	2.45 (0.13–12.33)	2.41	EIA-3	4.35 (0.30–22.39)	9.77	HBsAg	15.78 (1.16–84.23)
France (1998–2000; Pillonel et al. 2002)	1.21	Anti-HIV 1 + 2	0.73(0.12–2.08)	0.64	EIA-3	1.16 (0.33–3.33)	1.39	HBsAg	2.13 (0.58–6.66)
Spain (1997–1999; Alvarez et al. 2002)	3.23	Anti-HIV 1 + 2	1.95 (0.37–4.71)	3.7	EIA-3	6.69 (2.74–13.06)	8.36	HBsAg	13.51(5.31–30.08)

Table 26.5 Annual risks associated with major TTI.

Probability per blood unit of infection undetected on screening assay[a]	
HIV (mini-pool NAT)	1 in 2 000 000
HCV (mini-pool NAT)	1 in 2 000 000
HBV (HBsAg EIA)	1 in 200 000
Lifelong probability of death from TTI (for infected recipients)	
HIV[b]	40%
HCV[c]	9.2%
HBV[d]	0.97%
Years of life lost to TTI (per infected recipient)	
HIV[b]	3.26
HCV[c]	0.754
HBV[d]	0.178
Risk of death from TTI (per 100 000 transfused persons)[e]	
HIV	0.06
HCV	0.0046
HBV	0.00049
Risk of death from TTI (per 100 000 persons in general population)[f]	
HIV	0.0012
HCV	0.00092
HBV	0.000097

[a] Obtained from Dodd et al. (2002).

[b] Data derived from Pereira (1999) and probably outdated, since expected survival of HIV infected patients on modern anti-retroviral treatment is significantly longer that in mid-1990s.

[c] According to Pereira and Sanz (2000).

[d] Derived from Pereira (2003).

[e] Calculated from the above data. Median age at transfusion was assumed to be 67 years; median post-transfusion survival was estimated at 4.2 years (Vamvakas, 2003); and median number of blood units for the average transfused patient was assumed to be three.

[f] The annual probability of being transfused for people in the general population was 0.0089, according to Vamvakas and Taswell (1994a).

subtracting the probability that at least one transfused unit was infectious from 1 (100% or certainty). If p represents the probability of infection per unit and n the number of transfused units, $1 - p$ is the probability that a unit is free of infection, and $(1-p)^n$ is the probability that all n units are infection free. Therefore, the probability that a recipient received at least one infectious unit is $1 - (1 - p)^n$. For risks that are very small (i.e. <1%) the result is similar to simply multiplying p × n.

Infection rates versus clinical outcomes

A distinction must be made between infection and disease. Since many major TTIs have a long asymptomatic or subclinical incubation period, acquiring such an infection through transfusion does not always imply that clinical disease will inevitably develop in the recipient. Several factors contribute to reduce the overall impact that a TTI has on the recipient's health.

On the one hand, about 95% of people acutely infected with HBV (Lee, 1997), and 20%–30% of patients with recent HCV infection (Barrera et al., 1995a), clear the virus within the first year of transfusion. Among patients with persistent viraemia, only in a minority will the infection progress to hepatic cirrhosis or liver cancer after 20–40 years from transfusion. For HBV there is a possibility for severe hepatic failure early after infection, but the risk is low, probably about 1%. In the case of HIV infection, the median time for the natural progression from transfusion to clinical AIDS is about five years (Ward, 1993).

On the other hand, follow-up of transfused patients and data from look-back studies have shown that 36% of blood recipients will die within the first year of transfusion and only 47% will survive more than five years (Vamvakas, 2003). In the UK, approximately 50% of blood is transfused to patients who die within one year (personal communication – Dr Barbara). This high mortality rate is not due to transfusion itself but to the advanced age of the majority of blood recipients and the severity of the underlying disease(s) that triggered transfusion. At the author's institution, the median age of patients who are transfused is 67 years, with first and third quartiles being 52 and 76 years, respectively. Similar figures have been communicated from other American and European centres (Tynell, 2001; Vamvakas, 1996; Zimmerman et al., 1997). In addition, since survival decreases with the number of transfused units (Vamvakas and Taswell, 1994b), because heavy transfusion is associated with more severe disease, the likelihood is about 50% that an infectious transfused unit will be given to a patient who will die within the following year. As older patients are increasingly being subjected to aggressive treatments, which, in the recent past were reserved for younger patients, it is conceivable that post-transfusion survival will continue to decrease over the coming years. In fact, by comparing survival between patients transfused in 1981 (Vamvakas and Taswell, 1994b) and a decade later (Vamvakas, 2003) it can be estimated that post-transfusion survival has been decreasing at a rate of about 1% per year.

Using mathematical models that include demographic and survival data of transfused patients and quantitative information on infection progression in blood recipients, it has been possible to get estimates of clinical outcomes for the major TTI (see Table 26.5). Clinical outcomes, particularly death rates and loss of life expectancy, allow risk to be compared across different sources of potential harm by means of a common yardstick. These estimates are very informative for risk managers, since they help put a particular risk into a broader perspective. For the sake of comparison, Tables 26.6 and 26.7 show risk estimates for a variety of non-medical and medical activities. By comparing data on these tables and Table 26.5 it can be inferred that, for an average person in the general population, the risk of death from a major TTI (HIV, HCV or HBV) is seven-fold lower than the risk of being killed by lightning. For the average blood recipient (i.e. transfused with three units of blood) the risk of acquiring HIV through transfusion is 96-fold smaller than the risk of having an acute haemolytic reaction, and 792-fold lower than the risk of dying from a preventable adverse event during a hospital admission.

However, no matter how impressive these comparisons might be, their usefulness is limited by the fact that perception of risk by

Table 26.6 Annual risk of death for selected exposures[a].

Source of risk	Deaths (per 100 000 exposed)
Daily life	
Accidental falls	49
Motor vehicle accident (total)	15
Home accidents (all ages)	11
Being run over while walking	2
Yearly coast to coast flight (USA)	1
Bicycling	0.3
Car accident while using cellular phone	0.15
Rail trespassing accident	0.15
Lightning	0.016
Being hit by falling aircraft	0.004
Recreational	
White water rafting	105
Water skiing	47
Children's toys (all ages)	37
Snow skiing	14
Playing football at college	1.4
Playing basketball	0.4
Occupational	
Fire fighters	61
Police officers killed in line of duty	47
Coal mining (accidents)	24
Construction (accidents)	14
Tractor fatalities	10
Airline pilots (accidents only)	10
Natural disasters	
Drought or heatwave	0.4
Floods	0.045
Lightning	0.016
Tornadoes	0.015
Tropical cyclones and hurricanes	0.009

[a] Extracted from Wilson and Crouch, (2001).

Table 26.7 Risk of death or severe complications in health care.

Risk of non-infectious, severe transfusion complications	
Acute haemolytic reaction[a]	1 in 13 000 transfused units.
Major allergic reaction[a]	1 in 23 000 transfused units.
Transfusion-related acute lung injury[b]	1 in 5000 plasma-containing transfusions.
Volume overload[a]	1 in 7000 transfused units.
Risk of death or severe complications during hospital stay	
Death due to preventable adverse events[c]	1 in 526 admissions.
Preventable death or permanent disability because of[c] operative complications	1 in 185 admissions.
Drug prescription, preparation or administration	1 in 585 admissions.
Accidental fall	1 in 10 256 admissions.
Medical error resulting in death[d]	1 in 10 000 admissions.
Death related to anesthesia[e]	1 in 15 000 interventions.
Death or permanent disability due to unexpected adverse events[f]	1 in 167 admissions.

[a] Kleinman et al., 2003
[b] Popovsky and Moore, 1985
[c] Thomas et al., 2000
[d] Hayward and Hofer, 2001
[e] Gabel, 2002
[f] Brennan et al., 1991

most laypersons depends less on sheer numbers than on qualitative, often intangible attributes of the potential harm, as discussed later. For experts and managers, objective parameters of harm, such as the number of preventable deaths, provide a common yardstick from which risk-comparison analyses can be conducted for preventive measures. For instance, if the risk of dying from a major TTI is about 1 in 1.5 million for the average blood recipient (see Table 26.5), any intervention aimed at further reducing this risk must prove that it does not carry a similar or higher risk, which may be a challenging task.

Risk reduction measures

In modern transfusion medicine, protection from TTI is built on a multi-layered structure (incremental interventions) with each layer planned to exclude infectious units that had 'leaked'

through the preceding barrier. The first line of defence comprises donor education and exclusion/deferral policies based on epidemiological data derived from high-risk populations. Such policies are put into practice in two ways: blanket exclusion based on donor location or donor group (e.g. inmates in prisons), and a pre-donation interview aimed at eliciting any detail of the donor's behaviour or medical history that may be associated with an increased risk of having contracted a TTI. Blood donated by 'qualified' donors is then tested for the major TTIs by sensitive laboratory assays. Because donor history and laboratory testing cannot eliminate all risk of TTI, viral inactivation methods are applied on those blood products for which this is technically feasible. Finally, limiting allogeneic transfusion to patients in whom the expected benefit clearly outweighs the associated hazards is a key step to reducing the overall risk of transfusion.

The effectiveness of this in-depth defence system has been dramatic, and HIV, HCV and HBV have almost been eliminated as TTIs (see Figure 26.2). This undeniable success has led physicians, policy-makers, and the public to believe that further emphasis on risk reduction measures will bring us closer to a zero-risk blood supply. However, as the risk of major TTI approaches zero, the risk of the blood safety measures themselves, once dismissed as trivial, becomes increasingly important,

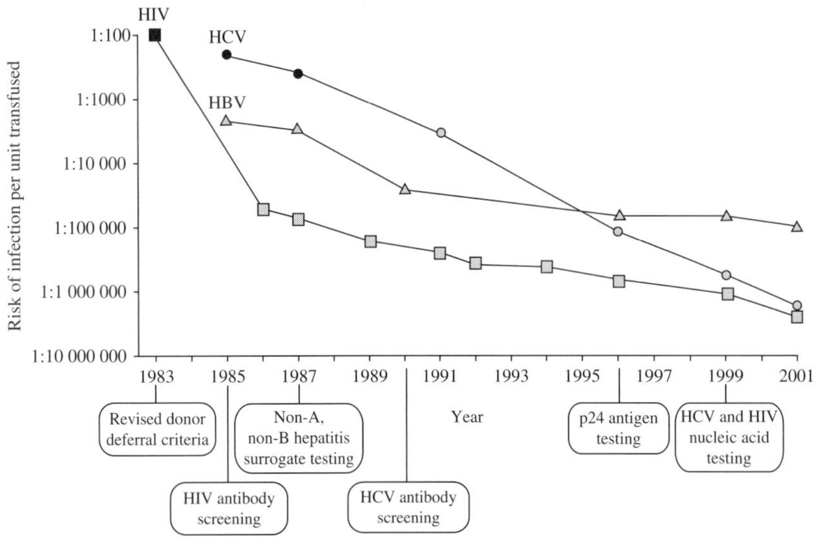

Figure 26.2 Decline in major TTI over the past two decades.

Reproduced courtesy of Busch *et al.* (2003) Current and emerging infectious risks of blood transfusion. *JAMA.*

since the negative consequences of some measures may outweigh the purported benefits (AuBuchon *et al.*, 1997).

Human actions take place in the physical world and cannot evade the laws of nature. The first law of thermodynamics states that energy can neither be created nor destroyed, it can only be transformed, and Newton's second law of motion states that for every action there is an equal and opposite reaction. Since the level of 'energy' or resources (time, personnel, capital, mental commitment, etc.) is fixed in the short run, every fraction of resource we allocate to reducing a particular risk will necessarily be detracted from other activities. Likewise, and to some extent as a consequence of the above 'law', every intervention aimed at reducing a given risk will give rise to a new risk or will increase an existing one elsewhere. That we were unable or unwilling to identify or quantify the resulting new risk neither negates its existence nor prevents its effects. Lack of recognition of these facts of life is the seed of many disagreements and misunderstandings about the worthiness of some recent measures aimed at further reducing the risk from TTI. This is becoming increasingly pertinent as the 'precautionary principle' becomes more commonly invoked. If there is concern about a possible or potential risk, even if it is yet unproven, then precautionary interventions are implemented. The efficacy of the interventions may only be theoretical, but if the 'dread factor' is high (such as for vCJD), there is great pressure for their implementation. On the one hand, there is the argument for not waiting until dire consequences are proven before measures are implemented. On the other hand, there may be new risks as a result of the implementation and a potential unnecessary diversion of resources. Currently, it is becoming increasingly difficult to know 'where to draw the line'. Although not proven to be effective, the introduction of leucodepletion of all blood components and the exclusion of donors who have received transfusions of blood, as measures that seem likely, among other measures, to reduce the risk of vCJD from transfusion, are examples of the precautionary principle.

Donor selection based on epidemiological criteria is the only available method for 'screening out' TTIs for which there are no routine laboratory tests. It is also important in providing protection against collecting blood during the window period of those TTIs for which donated blood is routinely tested. The method, however, has poor specificity and a large number of safe donors are likely to be deferred in order to prevent a single infectious unit from entering the blood supply. Stringent donor selection criteria undoubtedly increase the safety of donated blood, but they also increase the risk of an inadequate blood supply by shrinking the donor base. For instance, this may happen in the UK after exclusion of blood recipients as donors in order to prevent vCJD transmission by transfusion (Bird, 2004). In addition, when a new deferral criterion is publicized through the media a diffusion effect can occur, and eligible donors may erroneously feel themselves as potentially deferrable and refrain from going to donate. This is the reason why introduction of new deferral criteria may decrease the blood supply by a factor larger than previously expected, as has recently been the case in the USA, with deferral of donors who had stayed for some time in the UK or other European countries (as a precaution against vCJD transmission). Furthermore, emphasis on excluding donors at risk for a given TTI may lead to increased risk of another TTI. Blanket exclusion of donors older than 50 years has been proposed as a precautionary measure to avoid collecting blood from people with asymptomatic CJD disease. However, as older donors are the safest with respect to recent infection with the major transfusion-transmitted viruses, the measure would increase the risk for HIV, HBV, and HCV transmission by 10% to 20% (Busch *et al.*, 1997).

Exclusion based on laboratory tests is more specific, but also poses potential and real risks to the safety of the blood supply. Availability of new tests for infections (especially for HIV) may attract some high-risk persons to donate just to obtain such testing in a free, socially acceptable setting. Since test-seekers have an incentive to lie at the pre-donation interview, this magnet effect increases the risk of collecting blood during the window period for HIV, HBV and HCV infections (Korelitz *et al.*, 1996).

Inactivation of microbes in plasma and cellular blood components is a very appealing new technology since it may confer on labile components the same level of safety already achieved in manufactured blood products. In addition, pathogen inactivation is the only line of defence that may be effective against any new blood-borne agent before it is recognized as transfusion-transmitted after occurrence of cases and appropriate safety measures are deployed. At present there are methods to inactivate lipid-enveloped viruses in transfused plasma, and a wide range of viruses and bacteria in platelet concentrates. Research is continuing to make inactivation methods available for red cells. Inactivation of viruses in plasma by treatment with solvent/ detergent entails pooling several hundred units of plasma, with this step therefore increasing the risk of transmitting to many recipients any non-lipid enveloped virus present in a single donation. According to one analysis, a non-enveloped virus that causes an AIDS-like syndrome would have to be present in the population only at an undetectably low level (1 in 71 million donors) before all the benefits of avoiding lipid-enveloped viruses were entirely negated (AuBuchon and Birkmeyer, 1994). Virus inactivation in plasma by methylene blue and light is done in individual units and does not increase the risk of spreading agents that resist inactivation. However, methylene blue and light produces photo-oxidative damage of the fibrinogen molecule and other coagulation proteins, so that more plasma has to be transfused to attain the desired haemostatic effect, which increases the non-infectious risks of plasma transfusion (Atance et al., 2001). On occasion, the poor haemostatic quality of methylene blue treated plasma makes it necessary to resort to manufactured fibrinogen or prothrombin complex concentrates, which are derived from plasma pools of several thousand donors (Pereira, 2004). Although no formal risk comparison study has been conducted on this issue, it is quite possible that the drawbacks of using this kind of plasma outweigh the potential benefits. In addition to monitoring the quality of virus inactivated blood products, any chemical inactivation method must be scrutinized for the toxic potential of residual decontaminants. Psoralens, which are used for microbial inactivation in platelet concentrates and are under investigation for their applicability in red cells, are phototoxic, mutagenic in vitro (and thus have the potential to be genotoxic and carcinogenic), and may lead to the formation of neoantigens. Conventional toxicological studies conducted by the manufacturers have failed to show any significant toxicity for humans (Ciaravino et al., 2003), but a potential remains for delayed or very infrequent adverse effects.

Excessive emphasis on avoiding allogeneic transfusion can induce physicians and patients to select alternatives that may be more hazardous than the risk of acquiring a TTI. Blood donation by a healthy person is considered innocuous for the donor, but this may not be true for patients with overt or hidden coronary or cerebrovascular disease. Pre-operative autologous blood donation implies a risk of 1:17 000 for a reaction so serious that hospitalization is required (Popovsky et al., 1995). By using risk figures for the major TTIs that were nearly one order of magnitude larger than the current ones, one study conducted in the early 1990s concluded that a risk of death from a donation

reaction of only 1 in 101 000 would negate all the benefits of pre-operative autologous blood donation (Birkmeyer et al., 1994), and no study to date has been large enough to fully document that risk. By comparison, the current risk of dying from HIV, HBV or HCV infection transmitted through screened blood is estimated to lie below 1 in 4 million transfused units (see Table 26.5). Even the efforts to lower transfusion thresholds, once regarded as very desirable on the basis that a number of blood transfusions were unnecessary, must be carefully scrutinized, as the risks of not giving a transfusion when indicated are increasingly being recognized (Wu et al., 2001).

A fair risk management process requires that proof on the safety of preventive measures be in congruence with the expected health benefit. The smaller the latter is, the more conclusive the proof should be. This seems not to be happening in the field of TTI. There is a growing perception among transfusion medicine specialists that implementation of new blood safety measures is being driven more by political agendas and industrial interests than by a careful assessment of risks and benefits. Much energy has been allocated to reducing some risks at any cost, without questioning whether other risks were worthy of being addressed instead, or whether the new measures were actually riskier than the hazards they intended to prevent. Such a biased approach to risk reduction is also apparent in the asymmetric availability of information. While we have accurate estimates for the risk of major TTI, similar estimates for the risks inherent to some preventive measures are lacking, mainly because the necessary studies have not yet been conducted, which precludes any sound risk–benefit analysis. Even the precautionary principle is used asymmetrically, as it is frequently invoked in support of new safety interventions and rarely for safeguarding against the unknown safety of the intervention. This flaw in the risk assessment process has much to do with the way risk is perceived by society, how it is communicated to interested parties, and how stakeholders play their role in the process of risk management.

Perception of risk

Public concern about a danger is more linked to how the hazard is perceived than to any quantitative estimate of risk. Psychologists and sociologists have long studied the reasons why some risks are ignored or downplayed by society while others are responded to with anxiety, fear and anger, and why perception of a risk differs so much between experts and laypersons (Slovic, 2000). Some conclusions are consistent across studies. First, perceived risk is quantifiable and predictable, so that reaction by society when confronted with a new risk can be quite accurately foreseen. Second, expert judgements correlate highly with technical estimates of annual fatalities, whereas judgements made by laypersons are related more to qualitative hazard attributes than to potential impact on mortality. Third, society uses some kind of cost–benefit analysis in judging risks, as acceptability of risk from an activity is roughly proportional to the benefit from that activity. Finally, people tend to make qualitative rather than quantitative valuations, so that a risk is judged as acceptable or

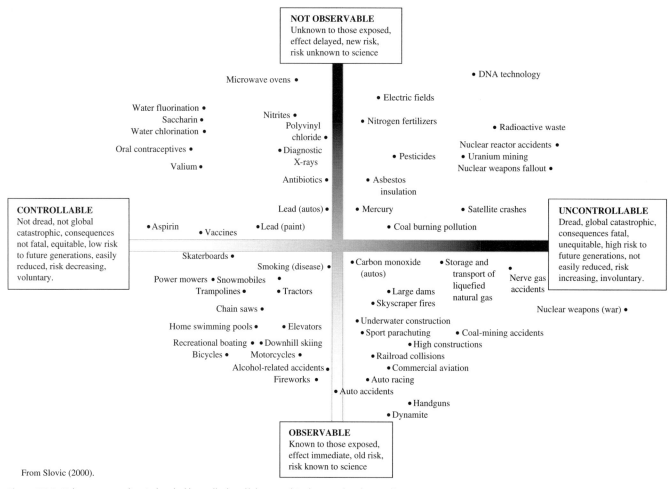

From Slovic (2000).

Figure 26.3 Risk space according to level of hazard's dreadfulness and to degree of understanding.

unacceptable, without any intermediate degree of acceptability. The perceived fairness and efficacy of government agencies, industry and others involved in risk management, as well as the possibility of assigning blame to one of the major participants in the risk-related decision making, have also been identified as major factors shaping public reaction to a risk (Lupton, 1999). In general, polls conducted in Western countries show that people believe that life is becoming more dangerous even though most objective measurements show the contrary to be true (Wilson and Crouch, 2001). This general sentiment decreases the acceptability of new risks and increases distrust of the ability of political officers to manage risky situations (Lupton, 1999).

Psychometric studies pioneered by Paul Slovic (reviewed in Slovic, 2000) have shown that the qualitative hazard attributes that influence the perception and acceptability of a risk can be summarized in a two-vector space (see Figure 26.3). On the horizontal axis, risk acceptability decreases with increased dread, perceived lack of control, catastrophic potential and inequitable distribution of risk and benefits. Nuclear power scores high on this scale. On the vertical axis, acceptability decreases for hazards judged to be unobservable, unknown, new and delayed in their manifestation of harm. Nucleic acid technologies attain a high score on this factor. Level of dreaded risk, as measured on the horizontal axis, is more influential on final acceptability than degree of knowledge and control, represented on the vertical axis.

A number of authors have recently applied the above psychometric paradigm to the study of how the risk of TTI is perceived by physicians and laypersons (Ferguson *et al.*, 2001; Finucane *et al.*, 2000; Lee *et al.*, 2003a;b; Lowe and Ferguson, 2003). Although laypersons agree with experts that blood transfusion conveys very important benefits, a substantial number of people (at least in the USA) still believe that blood transfusion is an unsafe and risky procedure, mainly because it invokes images of AIDS and HIV. The greatest risk from blood transfusion is perceived by the less educated people, who also manifest the greatest worry about many other hazards, from pesticides to nuclear power. According to Finucane *et al.* (2000), these people have relatively high perceptions of risk because they feel themselves as more vulnerable, have less control, and benefit less from new technologies. Tackling these feelings is beyond risk management and goes into the domain of social policies, but verification that blood transfusion is still believed to be unsafe because it could cause AIDS, at the present moment, when the risk of transfusion-transmitted HIV is below 1 in a million, denotes a spectacular failure of risk communication.

Table 26.8 Risk events with high potential signal value[a].

Event	Perceived message
Report that BSE has been identified in cattle.	A new and possibly catastrophic risk has emerged.
Scientists say that BSE is transmitted through carcasses used to feed cattle.	Unnatural practices are jeopardizing public health.
There is no scientific evidence of a risk for humans: do business as usual.	Managers are insensitive to public concerns.
Statement by regulators that the risk is very low as compared with everyday life risks.	Managers do not care about people who will be harmed.
Scientific dispute over the validity of an epidemiological study.	Experts do not understand the risk.
Resignation of regulators or corporate officials 'in conscience'.	Top managers are trying to conceal the risk: they cannot be trusted.

[a]Adapted from Slovic (2000, p. 244).

Risk communication

On occasion, relatively minor risks, as assessed by experts, result in strong public reaction, disproportionate cost in the form of stricter regulation or public opposition, and even an increased physical risk from the measures aimed at controlling the starting hazard (Slovic, 2000). This phenomenon of social amplification of risk is one of the most challenging tasks confronted by risk managers, and has much to do with the way messages on risk are delivered to society.

As many people have no direct experience with dramatic accidents or risks, individuals learn about a hazard from their network of social contacts and the media. The latter are particularly important in transmitting the qualitative attributes of risk that determine how it will be perceived by individuals. Communications science provides some clues on how social amplification of minor risks may occur (Slovic, 2000). Beside factual information, messages may contain inferential, value-related and symbolic meanings that are relevant to the receiver within a sociocultural context. These non-factual attributes of a message may give rise to a 'signal event', that is, an apparently trivial event that triggers high-order social and economic impacts because it is interpreted to mean that the risk is not well understood, not controllable, or not competently managed, thus implying that further, and possibly worse mishaps are likely (see Table 26.8). Technical experts tend to over-emphasize the factual content of risk communication, and to forget that cultural symbols embedded in the message are key factors in triggering the attention of receivers and in shaping their decoding process by evoking specific images. Reference to a highly appreciated social value (e.g. 'the gift of life') or a prestigious source of information (e.g. the Red Cross) may increase the receiver's tolerance to a risk,

Table 26.9 Rules for good risk communication.

Risk communication should be taken seriously.
- Failure in risk communication practices can be costly both in terms of health and money.
- Communication should be undertaken by those who are responsible and politically accountable.
- 'No risk' messages should be banished.
- Risk messages should directly address the prevalent opinion in society.
- Risk information vacuums should be avoided.
- Science should always be put in a policy context.
- Do not emphasize probability figures or risk comparisons.
- Do not lie: better to admit ignorance.

at least in the short run. By contrast, reference to detested values (e.g. 'big business', 'physicians' corporativism') decreases tolerance to risk.

Some other factors also play an important role in shaping how the public will react to a particular event. Large volumes of information and repetition by difference sources contribute to amplification independently of the accuracy and particular content of the message. Factual information on which there is not agreement among experts leads to increased anxiety if the risk was already feared by the public. Dramatization is another powerful source of risk amplification; sensational headlines magnify the risk far beyond what is supported by technical estimates, and TV images bring into our living room what otherwise would have been an exotic or never encountered hazard (Paling, 2000). Most media are private businesses run for a profit, and must compete with one another for attracting readers, listeners and viewers so they can sell advertisements. The consequence is that news is sensationalized and focused on scandals and disasters, the so-called 'infotainment'. Disagreement and conflict are overemphasized by framing most issues as though they had two – and only two – sides. Focus on individual stories of 'human interest' that are not representative of the whole spectrum contribute to distort the public perception of risk. Eventually, this leads government officers and policy-makers who are politically accountable to 'go public' to demonstrate they are in control of the situation, even before the situation has been fully appraised. Experts have identified a number of risk communication failures that often occur at this point, and which may jeopardize the whole process of risk management (Lundgren and McMakin, 1998; Morgan, 1993; Powell, 1997; Slovic, 2000). They include negating or downplaying the risk, despising public concerns as groundless, emphasizing probability estimates or risk comparisons, allowing vacuums of information that will be filled by unreliable sources, announcing measures that will not later be enforced and transferring the responsibility of public policies to scientists or others who are not politically accountable. Consequently, there is general agreement among experts on some basic principles that must guide risk communication so that it neither amplifies the public perception of danger nor poses unnecessary restrictions on the subsequent management of risk (see Table 26.9).

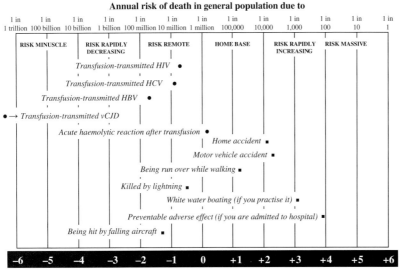

Annual risk of death in general population due to

Figure 26.4 The Paling perspective scale.

Adapted from Paling (www.johnpaling.com). The scale uses the American system of billions and trillions.

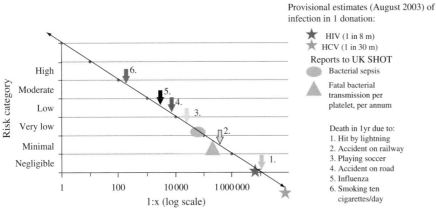

Provisional estimates (August 2003) of infection in 1 donation:

★ HIV (1 in 8 m)
★ HCV (1 in 30 m)

Reports to UK SHOT
◯ Bacterial sepsis

△ Fatal bacterial transmission per platelet, per annum

Death in 1yr due to:
1. Hit by lightning
2. Accident on railway
3. Playing soccer
4. Accident on road
5. Influenza
6. Smoking ten cigarettes/day

Figure 26.5 Are we at risk from blood that is donated?

Courtesy of Barbara, J. and Soldon, K.: Adapted from Health of the Nation, Dr K. Calman, Department of Health (DoH), UK, 1996. (http://www.dh.gov.uk/en/Publicationandstatistics/Publications/PublicationsPolicyAndGuidance/DH_4006909)

The idea of considering transfusion risks (especially microbial ones) in comparison with other health care risks and even risks in everyday life had been thought of early on, as discussed at a symposium of the European School of Transfusion Medicine (Barbara *et al.*, 2000). Graphical or pictorial representation of levels of risk and comparison of risks can help laypersons in putting transfusion risks into perspective (see Figures 26.4 and 26.5), though it has not been shown to be more effective than written materials in achieving this goal (Lee and Mehta, 2003a). Whichever way risk is illustrated, studies have proved that communication interventions changed not only what people knew about transfusion risk, but also what they felt about that risk, mainly by reducing the perceived dread and severity of risk (Lee and Mehta, 2003a). This emphasizes even more the paramount importance of good risk communication.

Some fundamentals of cost-effectiveness analysis in risk management

Cost-effectiveness (CE) analysis can be regarded as an expansion of risk assessment. The main additional scope includes identifying and measuring all resources consumed either when the risk materializes (i.e. used in the treatment of a TTI) or by the risk reduction measures (e.g. a new deferral criterion or laboratory test). Resources are very diverse and include personnel, capital (e.g. buildings, computers, auto-analysers, etc.), drugs, laboratory materials, imports of blood, and so forth. Because of the large variety of resources that are involved, a universal unit of valuation is needed, and monetary units are the most commonly used. The rationale is that any resource can be exchanged for a quantity of monetary units, which in turn can be converted into an amount of another resource. In addition to its role as a means of exchange, money has the advantage of being a store of value, so that resources valued in monetary units can be exchanged or compared over time.

A similar problem arises when one tries to value the health that is lost to an 'injury' or gained from a risk reduction intervention. Experts have devised the quality-adjusted life year (QALY) for this purpose because it permits comparison of an intervention that increases survival with another mostly aimed at ameliorating quality of life. For instance, an intervention that increases survival by ten years, which are lived with half the quality of perfect health, has the same value (10 years × 0.5 quality factor = 5 QALYs) as another resulting in five-year survival in perfect health (5 years × 1.0 quality factor = 5 QALYs).

Once cost of resources and health gains have been quantified for a particular intervention, the result can be summarized in the CE ratio.

$$\text{CE ratio} = \frac{\text{Net cost of intervention (in monetary units)}}{\text{Net health gain from intervention (in QALYs)}}$$

The net cost is the difference between the cost of introducing the intervention (e.g. new laboratory test) and the monetary value of resources that will be freed as a consequence of it (e.g. costs of treating TTI). The same applies to net health gain when the intervention implies a reduction, often temporary, of health (e.g. coronary-artery bypass graft surgery now, to decrease the risk of myocardial infarction later). When interventions vary in intensity (e.g. dosage or frequency) incremental CE ratios are calculated, so the ratio expresses the additional cost per each additional unit of outcome obtained. An intervention is said to be 'dominated' by an alternative when the latter produces more health at lower cost. Dominated interventions are automatically excluded from further analysis. The usual case, however, is that interventions producing more health are also costlier.

Two concepts employed in cost-effectiveness analysis are worth specific comment. The first is discounting. Since one Euro (or any other currency) paid in the future is worth less than one Euro paid now, the effect of time on the value of money must be taken into account for interventions where the costs or savings are spread over time. This has nothing to do with inflation. One Euro is worth more now than it will be in ten years because it can be invested in, say, Treasury Bonds at a 5 % annual interest rate, and get a return of 1.62 Euros at ten years. Likewise, psychological studies have shown that people prefer one year of life that is lived from now over one year lived from anytime in the future. By discounting costs and health gains that will be realized in the future we get a present value for both parameters, which allows comparisons to be established between interventions with rather different temporal profiles for their health and economic effects. There is no reason to choose a particular discount rate, provided that the same rate is applied to discounting health and economic effects, but consensus has been gathered to use a 3% rate after it was proposed by the Expert Panel on Cost-Effectiveness in Health and Medicine (Gold *et al.*, 1996).

The second concept deals with the perspective from which the analysis is conducted. Essentially, the perspective refers to who will meet the expenses of the new intervention and who will benefit from the health gains and cost savings that will result. For the sake of a fair analysis, gainers and losers should belong to the same financial body or institution. There are several possible perspectives: a particular hospital or health management organization, a third-party payer, a national health service, or society as a whole. Many analysts favour a societal perspective because it takes into account all the effects derived from the new intervention, but this gives rise to the problem of valuing some intangibles and indirect costs which are difficult to evaluate (e.g. leisure time, lost or impaired ability to work, pensions and other transfer

costs). Consequently, a national health service perspective, which takes into account only the health-related direct costs, is often used as a surrogate for societal perspective.

Once the CE ratio has been calculated for a set of risk reduction interventions competing for a fixed budget, rules of rational decision making establish that interventions should be ranked in a league table according to their CE ratio, and that funding must start at the most cost-effective one and work down the list until resources run out. The rationale is maximizing the benefit accrued from a fixed budget by minimizing the opportunity cost. This latter concept denotes the benefit (i.e. lives saved, health gained) that would have been accrued by the next best alternative for using the resources we have allocated to a particular intervention. The concept of opportunity cost is vital whenever we face the allocation of a limited amount of resources among competing alternatives. In health and medicine it raises an ethical issue too: how to explain away that more lives would have been saved or a higher level of health would have been attained if resources had been allocated in another way? However, it is not rare that political agendas dictate diversion of high resource for interventions of high profile, but minimal benefit, from others with more benefit, often less costly, but with less political impact.

Caution must be exercised when comparing CE ratios between preventive and therapeutic interventions, or programmes aimed at populations with quite different lives. Programmes aimed at prevention of disease may seem less cost-effective than therapeutic interventions because the benefit by the few who avoid the disease is averaged among all the people who receive the programme, most of whom incur the cost but take no benefit. Likewise, interventions aimed at people with low life expectancy (e.g. because of advanced age) will always seem less efficient than interventions aimed at populations with better baseline survival.

A clarification on two opposite meanings of 'cost-effectiveness' is necessary before ending this section: intervention A is *more cost-effective* (i.e. more efficient) than intervention B if intervention A has a *lower cost-effectiveness ratio*.

Cost-effectiveness of transfusion safety interventions

Technological change, population ageing and the higher expectations that people place on health care services have led to health care costs growing well above the average inflation rate over the past two decades. This has led policy-makers to implement cost-containment strategies and to make increasing use of cost-effectiveness analysis for deciding how to prioritize new health interventions and programmes. Blood transfusion has been affected by this new climate too, but the impact of cost-effectiveness analysis in shaping policies regarding TTI has been negligible.

Early tests that have resulted in a substantial decrease in the risk of TTI were remarkably cost-effective. HIV-antibody testing was introduced at a CE ratio of $3600 per QALY gained (AuBuchon *et al.*, 1997). Serum transaminase determination as a surrogate marker for non-A, non-B hepatitis and specific HCV-antibody assays actually reduced overall health care costs (Busch

Table 26.10 Cost-effectiveness ratio for selected interventions aimed at reducing the risk of TTI.

Intervention	Comparator	Cost per QALY gained	Reference
NAT for HIV and HCV (mini-pool).	Serologic assays[a]	$ 4.3 million	Jackson *et al.*, 2003
NAT for HIV and HCV (single-donor).	Serologic assays[a]	$ 7.3 million	Jackson *et al.*, 2003
NAT for HCV.	HCV EIA-3	$ 1.8 million	Pereira and Sanz, 2000
Enhanced HBsAg assays.	Current HBsAg assay	€ 0.8 million	Pereira, 2003
NAT for HBV (single-donor).	Current HBsAg assay	€ 5.8 million	Pereira, 2003
NAT for HBV (single-donor).	Enhanced HBsAg assay	€ 53 million	Pereira, 2003
NAT for West Nile virus (single-donor)[b].	No testing	$ 0.9 million	Custer *et al.*, 2005
NAT for West Nile virus (mini-pool)[b].	No testing	$ 0.5 million	Custer *et al.*, 2005
Virus inactivated plasma.	Fresh frozen plasma	$ 2.2 million	Pereira, 1999
Solvent/detergent treated plasma.	Fresh frozen plasma	$ 9.7 million	Jackson *et al.*, 1999
Autologous predeposit transfusion. (Only for prevention of viral diseases.)	Allogeneic transfusion	$ 3.5 million	Sonnenberg *et al.*, 1999
Post-operative cell salvage in joint arthroplasty.	Allogeneic transfusion	$ 5.7 million	Jackson *et al.*, 2000
Epoetin alone in coronary artery bypass graft surgery.	Allogeneic transfusion	$ 7 million	Marchetti and Barosi, 2000
Epoetin and autologous transfusion in coronary artery bypass graft surgery.	Allogeneic transfusion	$ 5 million	Marchetti and Barosi, 2000

[a] Assumes discontinuation of HIV p24 testing.
[b] Nationwide in the USA.

Table 26.11 Cost-effectiveness ratio for selected interventions in cancer, cardiovascular diseases, infections and accidents[a], based on USA data.

Intervention	Comparator	Cost per QALY gained
Pap smear every four years	No screening	$ 16 000
Annual foecal occult blood test for colorectal cancer	No screening	$ 18 000
Testing and mitigation of radon in homes	No programme	$ 57 000
Annual mammography	Clinical breast exam only	$ 150 000
Coronary angiography and revascularization if indicated	Medication only	$ 17 500–$ 45 000
Tissue plasminogen activator for acute myocardial infarction	Streptokinase	$ 38 000
HBV vaccination (newborns, infants and adolescents)	No vaccination	Cost saving
Behavioral intervention to decrease HIV transmission (high-risk men)	No programme	Cost saving
Behavioral intervention to decrease HIV transmission (high-risk women)	No programme	$ 2206
Compulsory helmet use (motorcyclists)	Voluntary use	Cost saving
Frontal airbag for car drivers	Safety belt only	$ 24 000
Frontal airbag for passengers	Driver-only airbag	$ 61 000

[a] Extracted from Graham *et al.*, (1998).

et al., 1995a; Pereira and Sanz, 2000). In contrast, recent safety measures have been introduced at CE ratios well above the threshold that is usually applied to new interventions in other health care areas. Table 26.10 shows the CE ratio for some recent developments in the prevention of TTI. Table 26.11, in turn, shows similar data for several medical and public health measures. By comparing data on both tables it is evident that some kind of economic exceptionality applies to TTI, because risk reduction measures aimed at TTI are introduced at a degree of inefficiency that would be unacceptable elsewhere in the health care system. Several factors related to the economic and

regulatory structure of the blood industry are behind the exceptional nature of TTI.

Regulatory agencies that oversee blood safety are not responsible for the economic effects of decisions they make, so they lack any incentive for taking into account the cost-effectiveness aspects of new regulations. In fact, both the USA FDA and the European Council explicitly disregard cost-effectiveness issues in their decision-making process about blood safety (Farrugia, 2002). Blood banks, mainly large regional blood centres, operate as a monopoly and have no economic disincentive to implement costly procedures as long as they can shift the increased cost to the blood products they sell to hospitals (Pereira, 2002). Furthermore, in a climate of concern about TTIs and their legal consequences, being the first to make available the new technology may provide a market advantage in places where there is competition between blood suppliers. If the new technology takes advantage of economics of scale and it is finally taken as a standard of industry or enforced by regulations, small competitors may be forced out of business, thus increasing the market share of the most powerful ones. In the USA, some mix of the above reasons may have been behind both the successful spreading of NAT and the attempts to implement virus-inactivated plasma and pre-storage leucoreduction of all blood components.

In countries where governments are responsible for both issuing regulations on blood safety and paying for health care costs, as in most of Western Europe, a principal-agent conflict of interest may be entertained. Policy-makers are highly influenced by the political and legal aftermath of the transfusion-transmitted AIDS epidemic, so they are strongly motivated to issue self-protective regulations, with little attention to cost. The 'rule of rescue' may also apply to this case: decision-makers show preference for financing interventions that avoid a few deaths for a small, but definite and visible group, over a larger (aggregate) benefit distributed among a less visible group (AuBuchon et al., 1997).

There is also what can be regarded as a 'domino effect'. Within the above scenario of mixed incentives, actions undertaken by a local blood centre or plasma fractionator give rise immediately to a new international standard that overcomes any sound scientific data (evidence base) or cost consideration.

Insensibility to cost-effectiveness issues seems to be greater in Europe than in the USA, perhaps because the predominant European model of government-run health care systems gives precedence to political accountability over economical responsibility. For instance, while most countries in Western Europe have implemented virus-inactivated plasma and pre-storage leucoreduction of all blood components, both measures have met a great deal of opposition in the USA.

REFERENCES

Allen, J. G. and Sayman, W. A. (1962) Serum hepatitis from transfusion of blood: epidemiologic study. *JAMA*, **180**, 1079–85.

Alvarez, M., Oyonarte, S., Rodriguez, P. M., *et al.* (2002) Estimated risk of transfusion-transmitted viral infections in Spain. *Transfusion*, **42**, 994–8.

Atance, R., Pereira, A. and Ramirez, B. (2001) Transfusing methylene blue-photoinactivated plasma instead of FFP is associated with an increased demand for plasma and cryoprecipitate. *Transfusion*, **41**, 1548–52.

AuBuchon, J. P. and Birkmeyer, J. D. (1994). Safety and cost-effectiveness of solvent-detergent-treated plasma: in search of a zero-risk blood supply. *JAMA*, **272**, 1210–14.

AuBuchon, J. P., Birkmeyer, J. D. and Busch, M. P. (1997) Safety of the blood supply in the United States: opportunities and controversies. *Ann Intern Med*, **127**, 904–9.

Ayyub, B. M. (2001) Elicitation of expert opinions for uncertainty and risk. Boca Raton, FL, USA, CRCPress.

Barbara J. A. J. and Howell D. R. (1994) Error rate for manual microbiological testing. *Transfus Med*, **4**, 24.

Barbara, J. A. J., Leikola, J. and Rossi, U. (2000) Risk perception and risk communication in Transfusion Medicine: how to achieve a sound transfusion practice based on scientific truth. Proceedings ESTM Residential Course in Brussels (Belgium). Milano, ESTM.

Barrera, J. M., Bruguera, M., Ercilla, M. G., *et al.* (1995a) Persistent hepatitis C viremia after acute self-limiting post-transfusion hepatitis C. *Hepatology*, **21**, 639–44.

Barrera, J. M., Francis, B., Ercilla, M. G., *et al.* (1995b) Improved detection of anti-HCV in post-transfusion hepatitis by a third-generation ELISA. *Vox Sang*, **68**, 15–18.

Biggerstaff, B. J. and Petersen, L. R. (2002) Estimated risk of transmission of the West Nile virus through blood transfusion in the US. *Transfusion*, **43**, 1007–17.

Bird, S. M. (2004) Recipients of blood or blood products 'at vCJD risk'. *BMJ*, **328** 118–19.

Birkmeyer, J. D., AuBuchon, J. P., Littenberg, B., *et al.* (1994) Cost-effectiveness of preoperative autologous donation in coronary-artery bypass grafting. *Ann Thorac Surg*, **57**, 161–8.

Bøgh, M., Machuca, R., Gerstof, J., *et al.* (2001) Subtype-specific problems with qualitative Amplicor HIV-1 DNA PCR test. *J Clin Virol*, **20**, 149–53.

Brennan, T. A., Leape, L. L., Laird, M. M., *et al.* (1991) Incidence of adverse events and negligence in hospitalized patients: results of the Harvard Medical Practice Study I. *N Eng J Med*, **324**. 370–6.

Busch, M. P., Glynn, S. and Schreiber, G. (1997) Potential increased risk of virus transmission due to exclusion of older donors because of concern over Creutzfeldt-Jakob disease: the National Heart, Lung and Blood Institute Retrovirus Epidemiology Donor Study. *Transfusion*, **37**, 996–1002.

Busch, M. P., Korelitz, J. J., Kleinman, S. H., *et al.* (1995a) Decaying value of alanine aminotransferase in screening of blood donors to prevent post-transfusion hepatitis B and C virus infection: the Retrovirus Epidemiology Donor Study. *Transfusion*, **35**, 903–10.

Busch, M. P., Lee, L. L., Satten, G. A., *et al.* (1995b) Time course of viral and serological markers preceding human immunodeficiency virus type 1 seroconversion: implications for screening of blood and tissue donors. *Transfusion*, **35**, 91–7.

Busch, M. P., Watanabe, K. K., Smith, J. W., *et al.* (2000) False-negative testing errors in routine viral marker screening of blood donors. *Transfusion*, **40**, 585–9.

Centers for Disease Control (1982) Epidemiologic notes and reports Pneumocystis carinii pneumonia among persons with hemophilia A. *MMWR*, **27**, 365.

Chemin, I., Jeantet, D., Kay, A., *et al.* (2001) Role of silent hepatitis B virus in chronic hepatitis B surface antigen(-) liver disease. *Antivir Res*, **52**, 117–23.

Chiavetta, J. A., Ennis, M., Gula, C. A., *et al.* (2000) Test-seeking as motivation in volunteer blood donors. *Transfus Med Rev*, **14**, 205–15.

Chiavetta, J. A., Escobar, M., Newman, A., *et al.* (2003) Incidence and estimated rates of residual risk for HIV, hepatitis C, hepatitis B and human T-cell lymphotropic viruses in blood donors in Canada, 1990–2000. *CMJ*, **169**, 767–73.

Ciaravino, V., McCullough, T. and Cimino, G. (2003) The role of toxicology assessment in transfusion medicine. *Transfusion*, **43**, 1481–92.

Custer, B., Busch, M. P., Marfin, A. A., *et al.* (2005) The cost-effectiveness of screening the US blood supply for West Nile virus. *Ann Intern Med*, **143**, 486–92.

Department of Health (2006) http://www.dh.gov.uk/en/Publicationsand statistics/Publication/PublicationsPolicyAndGuidance/DH_4006909.

Dodd, R. Y., Notari, E. P. and Stramer, S. L. (2002) Current prevalence and incidence of infectious disease markers and estimated window-period risk in the American Red Cross blood donor population. *Transfusion*, **42**, 975–9.

Dzik, W., AuBuchon, J., Jeffries, L., *et al.* (2000) Leukocyte reduction of blood components: public policy and new technology. *Transfus Med Rev*, **14**, 34–52.

Eiras, A., Sauleda, S., Planellas, D., *et al.* (2003) HCV screening in blood donations using RT-PCR in mini-pool: the experience in Spain after routine use for two years. *Transfusion*, **43**, 713–20.

Engstrand, M., Engstrand, L., Hogman, C. F., *et al.* (1995) Retrograde transmission of Proteus mirabilis during platelet transfusion and the use of arbitrarily primed polymerase chain reaction for bacteria typing in suspected cases of transfusion-transmission of infection. *Transfusion*, **35**, 871–3.

Evatt, B., Austin, H., Barnhart, E., *et al.* (1998) Surveillance for Creutzfeldt-Jakob disease among persons with hemophilia. *Transfusion*, **38**, 817–20.

Farrugia, A. (2002) The regulatory pendulum in transfusion medicine. *Transfus Med Rev*, **16**, 273–82.

Ferguson, E., Farrell, K., Lowe, K. C., *et al.* (2001) Perception of risk of blood transfusion: knowledge, group membership and perceived control. *Transfus Med*, **11**, 129–35.

Finucane, M. L., Slovic, P. and Mertz, C. K. (2000) Public perception of the risk of blood transfusion. *Transfusion*, **40**, 1017–22.

Gabel, R. A. (2002) Counting deaths due to medical errors (letter). *JAMA*, **288**, 2404.

Glynn, S. A., Kleinman, S. H., Schreiber, G. B., *et al.* (2000) Trends in incidence and prevalence of major transfusion-transmitted infections in US blood donors, 1991 to 1996. *JAMA*, **284**, 229–35.

Gold, M. R., Siegel, J. E., Russell, L. B., *et al.* (1996) *Cost-effectiveness in Health and Medicine*. NY, USA, Oxford University Press.

Graham, J. D., Corso, P. S., Morris, J. M., *et al.* (1998) Evaluating the cost-effectiveness of clinical and public health measures. *Ann Rev Public Health*, **19**, 125–52.

Hayward, R. A. and Hofer, T. P. (2001) Estimating hospital deaths due to medical errors: preventability is in the eye of the reviewer. *JAMA*, **286**, 415–20.

Heye, N., Hansen, S. and Müller, N. (1994) Creutzfeldt-Jakob disease and blood transfusion. *Lancet*, **343**, 298–9.

Holman, R. C., Khan, A. S., Belay, E. D., *et al.* (1996) Creutzfeldt-Jakob disease in the United States, 1979–1994: using national mortality data to assess the possible occurrence of variant cases. *Emerg Infect Dis*, **2**, 333–7.

Iwamoto, M., Jernigan, D. B., Guasch, A., *et al.* (2003) Transmission of West Nile virus from an organ donor to four transplant recipients. *N Eng J Med*, **348**, 2196–203.

Jackson, B. R., AuBuchon, J. P. and Birkmeyer, J. L. (1999) Update of cost-effectiveness analysis for solvent-detergent-treated plasma (letter). *JAMA*, **282**, 329.

Jackson, B. R., Busch, M. P., Stramer, S. L., *et al.* (2003) The cost-effectiveness of NAT for HIV, HCV and HBV in whole-blood donations. *Transfusion*, **43**, 721–9.

Jackson, B. R., Umlas, J. and AuBuchon, J. P. (2000) The cost-effectiveness of post-operative recovery of RBCs in preventing transfusion-associated virus transmission after joint arthroplasty. *Transfusion*, **40**, 1063–6.

Janssen, R. S., Satten, G. A., Stramer, S. L., *et al.* (1998) New testing strategy to detect early HIV-1 infection for use in incidence estimates and for clinical and prevention purposes. *JAMA*, **280**, 42–8.

Kahneman, D., Slovic, P. and Tversky, A. (1982) *Judgment under Uncertainty: Heuristics and Biases*. Cambridge, UK, Cambridge University Press.

Kitchen, A. D. and Barbara, J. A. J. (2000) Which agents threaten blood safety in the future? *Baillière's Clin Haematol*, **13**, 601–14.

Kleinman, S. (1999) New variant Creutzfeldt-Jakob disease and white cell reduction: risk assessment and decision making in the absence of data. *Transfusion*, **39**, 921–4.

Kleinman, S., Busch, M. P., Korelitz, J. J., *et al.* (1997) The incidence/window period model and its use to assess the risk of transfusion-transmitted human immunodeficiency virus and hepatitis C virus infection. *Transfus Med Rev*, **11**, 155–72.

Kleinman, S., Chan, P. and Robillard, P. (2003) Risk associated with transfusion of cellular blood components in Canada. *Transfus Med Rev*, **17**, 120–62.

Kleinman, S., Stramer, S., Mimms, L., *et al.* (2000) Comparison of preliminary observed yield of HCV and HIV minipool (MP) nucleic acid testing (NAT) with predictions from the incidence-window period (INC/WP) model [abstract]. Transfusion, **40** (Suppl.), S6–030a.

Kleinman, S. A. and Busch, M. P. (2000) The risks of transfusion-transmitted infection: direct estimations and mathematical modelling. *Ballière's Clin Haematol*, **13**, 631–49.

Korelitz, J. J., Busch, M. P. and Williams, A. E. (1996) Antigen testing for human immunodeficiency virus (HIV) and the magnet effect: will the benefit of a new test be offset by the numbers of higher risk, test-seeking donors attracted to blood centers? Retrovirus Epidemiology Donor Study. *Transfusion*, **36**, 203–8.

Lee, C. A., Ironside, J. W., Bell, J. E., *et al.* (1998) Retrospective neuropathologic review of prion disease in UK haemophilic patients. *Thromb Haemost*, **80**, 909–11.

Lee, D. H. and Mehta, M. D. (2003) Evaluation of a visual risk communication tool: effects on knowledge and perception of blood transfusion risk. *Transfusion*, **43**, 779–89.

Lee, D. H., Mehta, M. D. and James, P. D. (2003) Differences in the perception of blood transfusion risk between laypeople and physicians. *Transfusion*, **43**, 772–8.

Lee, W. M. (1997) Hepatitis B virus infection. *N Eng J Med*, **337**, 1733–45.

Lelie, P. N., Cuypers, H. T., Reesink, H. W., *et al.* (1992) Patterns of serological markers in transfusion-transmitted hepatitis C virus infection using second-generation HCV assay. *J Med Virol*, **37**, 203–9.

Lowe, K. C. and Ferguson, E. (2003) Mini-symposium: benefit and risk perception in transfusion medicine – blood and blood substitutes. *J Intern Med*, **253**, 498–507.

Lundgren, R. and McMakin, A. (1998) *Risk Communication: a Handbook For Communicating Environment, Safety and Health Risks*. Columbus, OH, USA, Battelle Press.

Lupton, D. (1999) *Risk*. New York, USA, Routledge.

Marchetti, M. and Barosi, G. (2000) Cost-effectiveness of epoetin and autologous blood donation in reducing allogeneic blood transfusions in coronary artery bypass graft surgery. *Transfusion*, **40**, 673–81.

Mimms, L. T., Mosley, J. W., Hollinger, F. B., *et al.* (1993) Effect of concurrent infection with hepatitis C virus on acute hepatitis B virus infection. *BMJ*, **307**, 1095–7.

Montagnier, L. (2002) A History of HIV discovery. *Science*, **298**, 1727–8.

Morgan, M. G. (1993). Risk analysis and management. *Scientific American*, **296**(1), 32–41.

Muder, R. R., Yee, Y. C., Rihs, J. D., *et al.* (1992) *Staphylococcus epidermidis* bacteriemia from transfusion of contaminated platelets: application of bacterial DNA analysis. *Transfusion*, **32**, 771–4.

Murthy, K. K., Henrard, D. R., Eichberg, J. W., *et al.* (1999) Redefining the HIV-infectious window period in the chimpanzee model: evidence to suggest that nucleic acid testing can prevent blood-borne transmission. *Transfusion*, **39**, 688–93.

National Academy of Sciences (NAS) (1983) *Risk Assessment in the Federal Government: Managing the Process*. Washington DC, USA, National Academy Press.

National Academy of Sciences (NAS) (1994) *Science and Judgment in Risk Analysis*. Washington DC, USA, National Academy Press.

Paling, J. (2000) Uma revisão abrangente do mundo dos riscos [A comprehensive review of the world of risk]. *ABO-Revista de Medicina Transfusional*, **4**, 50–8.

Pealer, L. N., Marfin, A. A., Petersen, L. R., *et al.* (2003) Transmission of West Nile virus through blood transfusion in the United States in 2002. *N Engl J Med*, **349**, 1236–45.

Pereira, A. (1999) Cost-effectiveness of transfusing virus-inactivated plasma instead of standard plasma. *Transfusion*, **39**, 479–87.

Pereira, A. (2002) Determinants of cost in blood services: blood transfusion from an economic perspective. *Expert Rev Pharmacoeconomics Outcomes Res*, **2**, 201–10.

Pereira, A. (2003) Health and economic impact of post-transfusion hepatitis B and cost-effectiveness analysis of expanded HBV testing protocols of blood donors: a study focused on the European Union. *Transfusion*, **43**, 192–201.

Pereira, A. (2004) Methylene-blue photoinactivated plasma (MBPIP) and its contribution to blood safety (letter). *Transfusion*, **44**, 948–50.

Pereira, A. and Sanz, C. (2000) A model of the health and economic impact of post-transfusion hepatitis C: application to cost-effectiveness analysis of further expansion of HCV screening protocols. *Transfusion*, **40**, 1182–91.

Petersen, L. R., Satten, G. A., Dodd, R., *et al.* (1994) Duration of time from onset of human immunodeficiency virus type 1 infectiousness to development of detectable antibody. The HIV Seroconversion Study Group. *Transfusion*, **34**, 283–9.

Pillonel, J., Laperche, S., Saura, C., *et al.* (2002) Trends in residual risk of transfusion-transmitted viral infections in France between 1992 and 2000. *Transfusion*, **42**, 980–8.

Popovsky, M. A. and Moore, S. B. (1985) Diagnostic and pathogenic considerations in transfusion-related acute lung injury. *Transfusion*, **25**, 573–7.

Popovsky, M. A., Whitaker, B. and Arnold, N. L. (1995) Severe outcomes of allogeneic and autologous blood donation: frequency and characterization. *Transfusion*, **35**, 734–7.

Powell, L. W. (1997) *Mad Cows and Mother's Milk: the Perils of Poor Risk Communication.* Montreal, Canada, McGill-Quen's University Press.

Prat, I., Ortiz, M., Retamero, M. D., *et al.* (2003) Detection of a healthy carrier of HCV with no evidence of antibodies for over four years. *Transfusion*, **43**, 953–7.

Roth, W. K., Weber, M., Buhr, S., *et al.* (2002) Yield of HCV and HIV-1 NAT after screening of 3.6 million blood donations in central Europe. *Transfusion*, **42**, 862–8.

Sanz, C. and Pereira, A. (2003) HCV NAT (minipool RT-PCR) and HCV core antigen ELISA – Reply (letter). *Transfusion*, **43**, 118–19.

Schreiber, G. B., Busch, M. P., Kleinman, S. H., *et al.* (1996) The risk of transfusion-transmitted viral infections. *N Eng J Med*, **334**, 1685–90.

Schreiber, G. B., Glynn, S. A., Satten, G. A., *et al.* (2002) HIV seroconverting donors delay their return: screening test implications. *Transfusion*, **42**, 414–21.

Seed, C. R., Cheng, A., Ismay, S. I., *et al.* (2002) Assessing the accuracy of three viral risk models in predicting the outcome of implementing HIV and HCV NAT donor screening in Australia and implications for future HBV NAT. *Transfusion*, **42**, 1365–72.

Slovic, P. (2000) *Perception of Risk.* London, UK, Earthscan Publications Ltd.

Soldan, K., Barbara, J. A. J., Ramsay, M. E., *et al.* (2003) Estimation of the risk of hepatitis B virus, hepatitis C virus and human immunodeficiency virus infectious donations entering the blood supply in England, 1993–2001. *Vox Sang*, **84**, 274–86.

Sonnenberg, F. A., Gregory, P., Yomtovian, R., *et al.* (1999) The cost-effectiveness of autologous transfusion revisited: implications of an increased risk of bacterial infection with allogeneic transfusion. *Transfusion*, **39**, 808–17.

Stern, P. C. and Fineberg, V. (1996) *Understanding Risk: Informing Decisions in a Democratic Society.* Washington DC, USA, National Academy Press.

Stramer, S. L., Glynn, S. A., Kleinman, S. H., *et al.* (2004) Detection of HIV-1 and HCV infections among antibody-negative blood donors by nucleic acid-amplification testing. *N Eng J Med*, **351**, 760–8.

Thomas, E. J., Studdert, D. M., Burstin, H. R., *et al.* (2000) Incidence and types of adverse events and negligent care in Utah and Colorado. *Med Care*, **38**, 247–9.

Tobler, L. H., Stramer, S. L., Lee, S. R., *et al.* (2003) Impact of HCV 3.0 EIA relative to HCV 2.0 EIA on blood-donor screening. *Transfusion*, **43**, 1452–9.

Tosti, M. E., Solinas, S., Prati, D., *et al.* (2002) An estimate of the current risk of transmitting blood-borne infections through blood transfusion in Italy. *Br J Haematol*, **117**, 215–19.

Tynell, E., Norda, R., Shanwell, A. and Bjorkman, A. (2001) Long-term survival in transfusion recipients in Sweden, 1993. *Transfusion*, **41**, 251–5.

Vamvakas, E. C. (1996) Epidemiology of red blood cell utilization. *Transfus Med Rev*, **10**, 41–61.

Vamvakas, E. C. (2003) Ten-year survival of transfusion recipients identified by hepatitis C look-back (letter). *Transfusion*, **43**, 418–19.

Vamvakas, E. C. and Taswell, H. F. (1994a) Epidemiology of blood transfusion. *Transfusion*, **34**, 464–70.

Vamvakas, E. C. and Taswell, H. F. (1994b) Long-term survival after blood transfusion. *Transfusion*, **34**, 471–7.

Van Duijn, C. M., Delasnerie-Lauprête, N., Masullo, C., *et al.* (1998) Case-control study of risk-factors of Creutzfeldt-Jakob disease in Europe during 1993–95. *Lancet*, **351**, 1081–5.

Velati, C., Romanò, L., Baraffi, L., *et al.* (2002) Residual risk of transfusion-transmitted HCV and HIV infection by antibody-screened blood in Italy. *Transfusion*, **42**, 989–93.

Ward, J. W. (1993) Transfusion-associated (T-A)-AIDS in the United States. *Dev Biol Stand*, **81**, 41–3.

Wientjens, D. P. W. M., Davanipour, Z., Hofman, A., *et al.* (1996) Risk factors for Creutzfeldt-Jakob disease: a re-analysis of case-control studies. *Neurology*, **46**, 1287–91.

Williams, A. E., Thomson, R. A., Schreiber, G. B., *et al.* (1997) Estimates of infectious disease risk factors in US blood donors: Retrovirus Epidemiology Donor Study. *JAMA*, **277**, 967–72.

Wilson, R. and Crouch, E. A. C. (2001) *Risk-benefit Analysis.* Cambridge, MA, USA, Harvard University Press.

Wu, W.-C., Rathore, S. S., Wang, Y., *et al.* (2001) Blood transfusion in elderly patients with acute myocardial infarction. *N Eng J Med*, **345**, 1230–6.

Zimmerman, R., Büscher, M., Linhardt, C., *et al.* (1997) A survey of blood component utilization in a German university hospital. *Transfusion*, **37**, 1075–83.

Zuck, T. F., Thomson, R. A., Schreiber, G. B., *et al.* (1995) The Retrovirus Epidemiology Donor Study (REDS): rationale and methods. *Transfusion*, **35**, 944–51.

27 THE REGULATORY ENVIRONMENT IN EUROPE

Virge James

Introduction

When we look at the chequered history of the blood industry, a thrilling account of which is given by Douglas Starr (Starr, 1999) it is not surprising that legislation covering blood, blood components and industrially prepared plasma derivatives is increasing throughout the world.

The regulatory environments are complex and vary in different countries, as they depend on political structures, institutions and legal systems; all such environments change with time. The legislation in force is thus both time and place dependent.

This chapter will give a general overview of the regulatory environment in Europe in 2004, dealing with the legislation in the 25 member states of the European Union (European Union Member States in 2004: Germany, United Kingdom, France, Italy, Spain, Netherlands, Greece, Belgium, Portugal, Sweden, Austria, Denmark, Finland, Ireland, Luxembourg, Poland, Czech Republic, Hungary, Slovakia, Lithuania, Latvia, Slovenia, Estonia, Cyprus, Malta (total population: approx 470 million)). Whilst this legislation applies only in EU member states, the key issues are those generally addressed by legislation in one form or another throughout the world.

European Union legislation forms part of the 'acquis communautaire' of the EU and as countries join the EU (current candidate countries are Bulgaria, Romania, Croatia and Turkey) they will need to adopt the acquis and all it involves.

A clear distinction has to be made between two very distinct approaches to achieving blood safety: guidelines and law. Guidelines, recommendations and best practice are generally written in a language which allows interpretation; they are not legally binding. The law demands observance and the wording cannot allow for ambiguity of interpretation.

In Europe, recommendations and guidelines emanate from national professional organizations and the Council of Europe, whereas legislation emanates from the European Union and is transposed into the existing legal framework of the country. Transposition is the writing of community law into national legislation. The legislation is based on existing guidelines and the same experts and professionals are generally involved in deciding which guidelines should have the force of law. The wording and emphasis may be adjusted by politicians and lawyers but the essence of what becomes law lies in the hands of national experts.

To ensure that blood transfusion and therapy with medicinal products of human origin are medical interventions which are as safe as possible, all countries need both appropriate guidelines and enforceable legislation.

Whilst guidelines are not legally binding, in many legal systems such as in the UK, abiding by professional guidelines may be regarded as best and therefore expected practice; in this sense they have a certain legal standing.

The regulatory environment in countries outside the European Union is not within the scope of this chapter.

Relevant organizations

World Health Organization (WHO)

The WHO was established in 1948 as the United Nations' specialized agency for health (information available at: www.who.int. Its aim is the attainment of the highest possible levels of health by all people. It is governed by 192 member states through the World Health Assembly.

The department of Blood Safety and Clinical Technology has a wide remit to ensure that all individuals have access to blood and blood products that are as safe as possible. To this end the WHO is active in producing recommendations, programmes and educational materials. It recognized that with increased movement of populations and also of plasma and plasma derived medicinal products, it was only through collaboration that blood safety would be improved. The Global Collaboration in Blood Safety programme started in 1995 and operates through consensus proposals and recommendations addressed to the participant countries.

The World Health Organization guidelines and recommendations reflect good practice but are not legally binding in any of the 192 countries. However, European Union legislation in this field states that the advice emanating from the WHO has to be taken into account by the member states when formulating their legislation.

Distinction between Council of Europe and the European Union

The Council of Europe (CoE) and the European Union (EU, preceded by the European Economic Community, EEC, until 1992) are two totally distinct entities although they are easily confused as they use much of the same or very similar terminology. In 2004, the Council of Europe has 45 member states and the European Union 25. The member states of the EU are all member states of the CoE and it is expected that other member states of the CoE will enter the EU over the next decade.

The recommendations emanating from the Council of Europe are not legally binding in the European Union although they have to be taken into account. The EU Directives, however, are legally binding in the member states and have to be transposed into the

Transfusion Microbiology, eds John A. J. Barbara, Fiona A. M. Regan and Marcela C. Contreras. Published by Cambridge University Press. © Cambridge University Press 2008.

existing laws of the member states within clearly defined time-frames and defined mandatory practice.

Council of Europe

The Council of Europe was founded in 1949 (CoE, 1999; further information available at: www.coe.int). One of its founding principles was to promote increasing cooperation between member states to improve the quality of life for the population of Europe. It has consistently addressed ethical issues in the field of blood transfusion and transplantation. The most important of these is the non-commercialization of human substances: blood, tissues and organs.

Cooperation among the member states in blood transfusion activities started in the 1950s. Since then, many agreements, binding on the member states that ratify them, have been reached and a programme aimed at ensuring good quality blood, blood components and blood derivatives has been established. The CoE, through its committees and working parties composed of national experts, has produced recommendations to ensure the quality of blood components and tissues. The annexes to the recommendations are published as guidelines and updated regularly to take account of advances in worldwide knowledge and technology (CoE, 2003; 2004).

Council of Europe recommendations are not legally binding but are generally regarded as constituting basic best practice and many form the basis of EU Directives.

European Pharmacopoeia (*Ph Eur*)

This is an initiative of the CoE, ratified by the EU and 30 participating member states (further information available at: www.pheur.org).

The monographs of the *Ph Eur* 2002, on individual fractionated plasma derivatives, set common compulsory standards to guarantee the quality of medicines in all member states; the organization promotes uniform analytical methods and standardizes all substances used in human and veterinary medicine.

The *Ph Eur* is mandatory in the 30 signatory member states and is also adopted by many others.

European Union

The European Union was first proposed by the French Foreign Minister Robert Schuman in 1950, following the devastation of the Second World War (see: www.europa.eu.int). It was conceived to prevent further such wars. Initially, it consisted of six countries and was concerned with trade and the economy; coal and steel had played a major role in the Second World War and cooperation over these assets was seen as a prophylactic measure to prevent further hostilities. The European Economic Community was created by the Treaty of Rome in 1957. The European Union was created in 1992 by the Treaty of Maastricht when the former EEC was renamed the European Union (EU). From this point the Directives are no longer issued as Directives of the EEC but the EU. As the EU has expanded it has also, through various treaties,

taken on more 'competencies', a term meaning a subject over which it has legislative powers. The competencies of the EU are detailed in the acquis communautaire. Competence in the field of blood and blood components was conferred on the EU by the Treaty of Amsterdam 1999 Article 152. This article also stipulates that 'Member States cannot be prevented from maintaining or introducing more stringent protective measures as regards standards of quality and safety of blood and blood components'.

In 2004, the EU does not have competence over member states' health care services nor clinical practice. This means that the laws covering blood, blood components and tissues extend to the safety of the products and *not to their clinical use*.

There are five key EU institutions, all with differing roles:
- European Parliament: elected by the peoples of the member states
- Council of the European Union: representing the governments of the member states
- European Commission: the driving force and executive body
- European Court of Justice: ensuring compliance with EU law
- European Court of Auditors: controlling sound and lawful management of the European budget.

The EU Constitution proposed in 2004, if adopted, will amend both the institutions and their roles.

The European Commission is the only body that can initiate legislation: the processes whereby legislation is proposed and finally adopted are complex and not within the scope of this chapter.

There is open consultation on any proposed legislation. The texts of the Directives and stages in the consultation process can be found on: www.europarl.eu.int.

European Union legislation relevant to blood transfusion and tissue transplantation in 2004

The wonderland of EU Directives is very difficult to explore; the 'maps' are ever changing as Directives are amended and superseded and impact on each other.

European Union Directives relevant to blood and plasma derivatives can be regarded in three separate categories:
(1) Those affecting medicinal products of human origin (industrially prepared plasma derivatives). In some European countries, blood components are regarded as medicinal products in national legislation and this may lead to confusion.
(2) Those affecting blood components and tissues.
(3) Other Directives which impact directly on blood transfusion and tissue transplantation.

Directives covering medicinal products

The essential aim of any rules governing the production, distribution and use (through pharmacovigilance systems) of medicinal products is to safeguard public health.

Directive 2001/83/EC 'on the Community code relating to medicinal products for human use' assembles all previous Directives governing medicinal products. A medicinal product is defined as any substance or combination of substances presented for treating or preventing disease in human beings. A substance is defined as 'any matter irrespective of origin which may be... human, animal, vegetable or chemical'. This Directive therefore applies to industrially prepared plasma derivatives and also blood components as starting material for the manufacture of proprietary medicinal products. The Directive states that member states 'need to take measures to prevent the transmission of infectious diseases, apply the monographs of the European Pharmacopoeia and recommendations of the Council of Europe and WHO as regards, in particular, the selection and testing of blood and plasma donors. The member states should also promote community self-sufficiency and encourage voluntary unpaid donations.' The Directive specifically excludes blood and blood components.

Directive 2003/94/EC lays down the principle and guidelines of good manufacturing practice in respect of medicinal products for human use and investigational medicinal products for human use. Two books explain the contents of the Directives in greater detail: *Good Manufacturing Practice for Medicinal Products* (1998) and *Rules and Guidance for Pharmaceutical Manufacturers and Distributors* (Medicines Control Agency, 2002).

Blood, blood components and tissues

Bearing in mind the freedom of movement of citizens within the community territory, European Community legislation should ensure that blood and its components are of comparable quality and safety throughout the transfusion chain in all member states. Blood and blood components were specifically excluded from the Directive on medicinal products, but member states were not applying the guidelines emanating from WHO, the CoE and indeed a previous recommendation for the EU with any degree of uniformity.

The European Commission therefore proposed further legislation and Directive 2002/98/EC 'setting standards of quality and safety for the collection, testing, processing, storage and distribution of human blood and blood components' was adopted, coming into force in 2003 with an implementation date of 2005.

Directives come into force on the day they are published in the *Official Journal of the European Union* (OJ) but time for transposition and implementation is allocated, so implementation dates may be set for a few years following the publication of a Directive and may vary from country to country.

Recognizing that knowledge and technology advance rapidly in this field and that laws are difficult to change, the Directive sets up a Regulatory Committee of the Commission whose task it is to ensure that detailed technical requirements are adapted to technical and scientific progress. The regulatory committee, consisting of representatives from the member states and invited by the Commission, has to take account of certain recommendations of the CoE, the monographs of the European Pharmacopoeia and recommendations of the WHO. It also takes account of member states' interests.

Commission Directive 2004/33/EC implementing Directive 2002/98/EC as regards certain technical requirements for blood and blood components becomes legally binding at the same time as Directive 2002/98/EC. Further Commission Directives dealing with detailed quality management aspects and traceability of blood components from donor to recipient and haemovigilance followed in 2005/2006.

Directive 2005/62/EC details standards and specifications related to quality systems. It came into effect in August 2006 and lays down general principles of quality systems pointing out that 'quality shall be the responsibility of all persons involved in the process... with management ensuring a systematic approach'.

Tissues

Legislation on human organs and tissues followed a similar pattern. Directive 2004/23/EC on setting standards of quality and safety for the donation, procurement, testing, processing, preservation, storage and distribution of human tissues and cells, came into force in April 2004 and is expected to be implemented in member states by April 2007. Just as for blood and blood components, a Commission Directive, dealing with more detailed technical aspects such as procurement and testing, taking account of the work of the CoE and WHO, came into effect in November 2006.

Directive 2006/17/EC implements 2004/23/EC regarding technical requirements for donation, testing and procurement of human cells and tissues The annexes detail donor selection criteria, laboratory tests and also procurement procedures and reception at tissue establishments. Some technical aspects for the testing and processing of donations are covered by two complex Directives.

In Directive 98/79/EC an in vitro diagnostic medical device is defined as any medical device which is a reagent, reagent product, calibrator, control material, kit, instrument, apparatus equipment or system whether used alone or in combination intended by the manufacturer to be used in vitro for the examination of specimens including blood and tissue donations derived from the human body solely or principally for the purpose of providing information:

- Concerning a physiological or pathological state
- Concerning a congenital abnormality
- To determine the safety and compatibility with potential recipients
- To monitor therapeutic measures.

Directive 2000/70/EC amended Directive 93/42/EEC on medical devices to include devices incorporating stable derivatives of human blood or human plasma.

A 'medical device' is defined (inter alia) as 'any instrument, apparatus, appliance, material or other article, whether used alone or in combination, including the software necessary for its proper application, intended by the manufacturer to be used for human beings for the purpose of: diagnosis, prevention, monitoring, treatment or alleviation of disease'.

These two Directives appear to cover all equipment and reagents, including software used in the transfusion services; their far reaching implications are still being unravelled. In the UK these have been transposed into the Medical Devices Regulations 2002.

Other Directives impacting on transfusion and transplantation: consumer protection; confidentiality

Directive 85/374/EEC covers 'the approximation of laws, regulations and administrative provision of the member states concerning liability for defective products'. Article 6 of the Directive states that a product is defective if it does not provide the safety that persons generally are entitled to expect. Blood/blood components and plasma derivatives are products under this Directive. In the UK this Directive was transposed into the Consumer Protection Act 1987. Hepatitis C litigation in England in 2001 was brought under this Act and resulted in far reaching judgments.

Directive 95/46/EC describes the protection of individuals with regard to processing of personal data, and free movement of such data also applies to the transfusion and transplantation services. In the UK this was transposed into the Data Protection Act 1998.

Key features of 'Blood Directives' 2002/98/EC and 2004/33/EC

The objective of the Directive 2002/98/EC is to lay down standards of quality and safety of human blood and of blood components, in order to ensure a high level of human health protection.

The Directive is wide ranging in scope. It covers:

- The collection and testing of human blood and blood components, *whatever their intended purpose* (therefore including source plasma for the manufacture of blood derivatives and donations used for further manufacture).
- The collection, testing, storage and distribution when intended for transfusion (this includes pre-deposit autologous donations).

Definitions

Member states all have different health care systems and the introduction of legally binding Directives demands that clear and agreed definitions be used to avoid misunderstandings and misinterpretations.

The Directives therefore contain many definitions, some of which will inevitably have to be further elaborated. Only the key ones are listed here.

- Blood: whole blood collected from a donor and processed either for transfusion or for further manufacturing.
- Blood component: a therapeutic constituent of blood (red cells, white cells, platelets, plasma) that can be prepared by various methods.
- Blood product: any therapeutic product derived from human blood or plasma.
- Autologous transfusion: transfusion in which the donor and the recipient are the same person and in which pre-deposited blood and blood components are used.
- Blood establishment: any structure or body that is responsible for any aspect of the collection and testing of human blood or blood components, whatever their intended purpose, and their

processing, storage and distribution when intended for transfusion. This does not include hospital blood banks.

- Hospital blood bank: a hospital unit which stores and distributes and may perform compatibility tests on blood and blood components exclusively for use within hospital facilities, including hospital based transfusion activities.
- Serious adverse event: any untoward occurrence associated with the collection, testing, processing, storage and distribution, of blood and blood components that might lead to death or life-threatening, disabling or incapacitating conditions for patients, or which results in, or prolongs, hospitalization or morbidity.
- Serious adverse reaction: an unintended response in donor or in patient associated with the collection or transfusion of blood or blood components that is fatal, life-threatening, disabling, incapacitating, or which results in, or prolongs, hospitalization or morbidity.
- Haemovigilance: a set of organized surveillance procedures relating to serious adverse or unexpected events or reactions in donors or recipients, and the epidemiological follow-up of donors

These definitions are gaining wide acceptance.

Competent authorities

Member states must designate competent authorities for implementing the requirements of the Directives. In European countries the designated competent authority is generally the Minister for Health, who then delegates this authority to an appropriate national organization.

This competent authority will authorize, accredit or license blood establishments. They will use inspection and control measures to ensure that blood establishments comply with the requirements.

Serious adverse events and reactions, as defined, must be reported to the competent authority who may take appropriate control measures

Personnel

Blood establishments must designate a responsible person whose qualifications and role are described. Personnel directly involved in collection, testing, processing, storage and distribution of human blood and blood components must be qualified to perform those tasks and be provided with timely, relevant and regularly updated training. It is left to the member states to decide what is timely, relevant or regular.

Quality management

Blood establishments must have a quality system, maintain documentation on operational procedures, guidelines, training and reference manuals and reporting forms. Details of the quality systems are expected in a further Commission Directive.

Haemovigilance

There must be full traceability from donor to recipient and vice versa and these records are to be kept for 30 years. The law does not stipulate how this is to be achieved. The 30-year time limit results from fears related to transmission of vCJD and the possible incubation period for this particular infection.

Testing of donations; annex IV: basic testing requirements

The legally required testing of donations is very basic:

- ABO group (not for source plasma for fractionation)
- RhD group (not for source plasma for fractionation)
- HBsAg
- Anti-HCV
- Anti-HIV 1/2

Additional tests may be required for specific components, or donors, or epidemiological situations (this is left to the member states).

Hospital blood banks: as defined

In order to ensure that the quality and safety of blood and blood components are maintained during the whole transfusion chain, the provisions relevant to these activities within hospital blood banks are also covered by several articles in the Directive.

Whilst inspection of hospital blood banks is not explicitly specified, it is clear that member states cannot fulfil their obligations without such inspection and accreditation. Exactly how this is dealt with is a decision of the individual member states. Without the full cooperation of blood banks, as defined, the traceability requirements of the Directive cannot be met.

Penalties

The Directives make provision for penalties: 'Member States shall lay down the rules on penalties for infringement of the national provisions adopted pursuant to this Directive and shall take all measures necessary to ensure that they are implemented. The penalties provided for must be effective, proportionate and dissuasive.'

Commission Directive 2004/33/EC

The Directive covers detailed requirements concerning donors and donations. Information to be obtained from, and given to, donors is carefully specified; eligibility criteria for blood donors, including age, body weight, haemoglobin, protein and platelet levels are listed. Permanent and temporary deferral criteria are specified. Whilst the Directive is meant to address only those issues which are relevant to the safety of the product it nevertheless introduces criteria which have some bearing on the safety of the donor.

The Directive also outlines the quality and safety requirements for blood and blood components including storage and distribution conditions.

The transposition of these Directives into national legislation requires careful use of language and definitions to avoid pitfalls. Consultation with lawyers at an early stage in the transposition process is essential. Depending on different interpretations and transposition processes, the laws applicable in the EU, whilst aiming for uniformity of standards, may nevertheless be very variable.

Implementation of Directives

Current EU member states and countries aspiring to join have to embrace the 'acquis communautaire'. The blood transfusion services in these countries need to either incorporate into their existing laws or develop laws governing blood transfusion and tissues which reflect the EU Directives.

Many countries already have transfusion laws (Mascaretti *et al.*, 2004; Rossi & Aprili 2002) but these will need to be amended accordingly. This may take longer than stipulated in the Directives.

Apart from financial concerns, the most common problems encountered are related to structure and organization of the blood transfusion/transplantation services, the concept of an independent competent authority and the expectation that all blood donors should be unpaid volunteers.

In many countries, hospitals themselves function as both blood establishments and hospital blood banks. The Directive is forcing clear thinking with regard to the organization of the services and the responsibilities of the governments towards enabling various degrees of reorganization.

The designated competent authorities must be independent of the blood transfusion services. This authority is responsible either directly, or by delegated authority, for the inspection, accreditation and licensing of the blood establishments. The independence of the competent authority from the blood establishments is crucial, but not always accepted.

The Directive states that 'Member states shall take the necessary measures to encourage voluntary unpaid donations with a view to ensuring that blood and blood components are in so far as possible provided from such donations'.

It does not demand this. Many acceding countries are dependent on paid and remunerated donors (even if only as 'replacement' donors) and many more may be so in the future. The Directive is therefore cautious in this area.

Conclusion

This chapter has outlined the regulatory environment in a large and expanding part of the world: the European Union. It has attempted to explain briefly the background for the need for legislation as distinct from guidelines and the interrelationships between professionals, relevant organizations and the EU regulatory machinery.

Some key features of the current legislation are detailed, and possible interpretation and implementation difficulties mentioned. Since the 'blood directives' did not have to be implemented until later in 2005, and the 'tissue directives' in 2007, the overall effectiveness of the legislation in maintaining and improving blood and tissue safety in the European Union will only become apparent towards the end of the decade. The author has deliberately refrained from any comment on the actual content of the legislation: that is for the reader.

REFERENCES

Council of Europe (1999) *The Conscience of Europe* ISBN 92-871-4030-8. Council of Europe Publishing Strasbourg.

Council of Europe (2003) *Guide to the Preparation, Use and Quality Assurance of Blood Components*. 10th edn. ISBN 92-871-5393-0. Council of Europe publishing, F-67075 Strasbourg, Council of Europe Publishing.

Council of Europe (2004) *Guide to the Safety and Quality Assurance for Organs, Tissues and Cells*. 2nd edn. ISBN 92-871-4891-0. Council of Europe publishing, F-67075 Strasbourg, Council of Europe Publishing.

Commission Directive 2004/33/EC implementing Directive 2002/98/EC as regards certain technical requirements for blood and blood components becomes legally binding at the same time as Directive 2002/98/EC, European Parliament.

Commission Directive 2005/62/EC *OJ* L256/41, European Parliament.

Commission Directive 2006/17/EC *OJ* L38/40, European Parliament.

Directive 85/374/ EEC On the approximation of laws, regulations and administrative provision of the member states concerning liability for defective products. *OJ* L210 7 August 85, European Parliament.

Directive 95/46/EC Protection and processing of personal data and the free movement of such data. *OJ* L 281 23 November 1995, European Parliament.

Directive 98/79/EC In vitro diagnostic Medical Devices. *OJ* L331/1 7 December 98, European Parliament.

Directive 2000/70/EC Amending Directive 93/42/EEC on Medical Devices. *OJ* L313/12 13 December 2000, European Parliament.

Directive 2001/83/EC On the Community code relating to medicinal products for human use. *OJ* L 311/67 28 November 2001, European Parliament.

Directive 2002/98/EC Setting standards of quality and safety for the collection, testing, processing and storage and distribution of human blood and blood components. *OJ* L33/30 14 October 2003, European Parliament.

Directive 2003/94/EC Laying down the principle and guidelines of good manufacturing practice in respect of medicinal products for human use and investigational medicinal products for human use. *OJ* L 262/22 14 October 2003, European Parliament.

Directive 2004/23/EC On setting standards of quality and safety for the donation, procurement, testing, processing, preservation, storage and distribution of human tissues and cells. *OJ* L102/48 7 April 2004, European Parliament.

European Pharmacopoeia (2002) 4th edn ISBN 92-871-4587-3.

United Kingdom Regulations

Blood Safety and Quality Regulations 2005 Statutory Instrument 2005 no. 50.

Medical Devices Regulations 2002 Statutory Instrument 2002 no. 618

Medicines Control Agency – Rules and Guidance for Pharmaceutical Manufactures and Distributors (Orange Guide).

Good Manufacturing Practice for Medicinal Products (1998) ISBN 92-828-2092-X Office of official publications of the EEC

Mascaretti, L. J. V., Barbara, J. Cardenas, J. M., *et al.* (2004) Comparative analysis of national regulations concerning blood safety across Europe. *Transfusion Medicine*, **14**, 105–111.

Rossi, U. and Aprili, G. (2002) *Present and Future Problems of Transfusion Medicine in South-east Europe.* Editors SIMTI edn ISBN 88-87075-21-2.

Starr, D. (1999) *Blood: an Epic History of Blood and Commerce.* Little Brown and Company, Harper Perennial.

Websites

Council of Europe: www.coe.int

Direct access to EU legislation: www.europarl.int

European Pharmacopoeia: www.pheur.org

European Union: www.eu.int

UK Regulations: www.hmso.gov.uk

World Health Organization: www.who.int

BLOOD SAFETY IN DEVELOPING COUNTRIES

Jean-Pierre Allain, Elizabeth Vinelli and Yasmin Ayob

General introduction

When compared with the standards of most developed countries, blood transfusion in developing countries is generally considered not to be as safe. This belief has led some organizations to set up a transfusion supply to Westerners travelling in developing countries. In the past decade, due to both the efforts of WHO and the political determination of some governments, blood products prepared in many countries with a medium development index have reached a level of safety meeting the highest standards.

While blood safety is considered of paramount importance, blood supply remains the priority in the developing world. In developed countries, the number of units of blood collected per 1000 inhabitants ranges between 30 and 75 units, whereas in developing countries it ranges between 1 and 15. As a result of this limited supply, indications for transfusion are limited to severe anaemia with a transfusion trigger often set at a haemoglobin of 5 g/dl. In addition, the lack of resources and technology to perform bone marrow or organ transplantation limits the demand for platelet concentrates and either whole blood or plasma-depleted red cells are the main products transfused.

Despite the fact that blood for transfusion is in limited supply, it is critical that the available blood is safe, but achieving this objective is hampered by a broad range of problems specific to the developing world, which represents 80% of the world population. The prevalence of persistent infections that are relevant to transfusion is almost always high: the prevalence of people positive for HBsAg ranges between 1 and 25%, anti-HIV and anti-HCV both range between <1 and 15%. Consequently, as the incidence of infections is higher, the frequency of 'window-period' cases is also likely to be higher. In addition, developing countries have specific infectious diseases such as malaria, dengue (and in Latin America, Chagas' disease) that are not, or at least not yet, a major cause of clinical disease in developed countries, although screening may be needed in travellers to such endemic countries. Individuals presenting themselves as blood donors are usually family members of a patient who are willing to donate blood to replace the blood transfused to their relative and therefore pay less for their care. These 'replacement' donors are usually males, 30 years or older and more at risk of having sexually transmissible infections than younger, female, donors. In many of these countries, paid, semi-professional donors who are a notoriously 'high-risk' group across the world remain part of the donor pool. In fact, in many countries a proportion of the 'family replacement' donors are often paid donors, but paid privately by the family to provide the blood required. Volunteer blood donors are relatively difficult to find and to retain as regular donors. This contrasts with the situation in developed countries where the transfusion system has been developed for over 50 years, and where being a blood donor has become part of the culture. In these countries, approximately 80% of donations are from regular volunteer blood donors.

In contrast with the trend in developed countries, where blood banking operations are concentrated in large units collecting and processing >100 000 units of blood per year, it is the norm for small, hospital-based, blood banks in developing countries to collect less than 20 units per day. The setting is often isolated, poorly funded and staffed and unable to procure the necessary materials and reagents needed to operate effectively. Equipment is too expensive for the limited resources and, if purchased, cannot be maintained. Small daily testing runs may also consume large numbers of controls, depending upon the technology used, which substantially increases the testing costs.

The large diversity of cultures and traditions in populations across the world leads to equally diversified attitudes towards giving blood. One of the challenges of blood banking in developing countries is to adapt the general principles of donor recruitment, donor selection and donor screening to the sociology, epidemiology and financial means of the local populations. For these reasons, this chapter is structured around three large areas of the world: Asia, Africa and Latin America. Problems and potential solutions for blood safety will be discussed according to these broad divisions. Despite the considerable diversity between these large areas, it is clear that they share many of the same difficulties.

Blood safety in Asia

Introduction

Asia is made up of countries of various sizes and populations with different cultures, religions, languages and economies. The development of the blood transfusion service, blood availability and accessibility, more or less reflect the socio-economic development of the country. Japan has one of the best transfusion services in the world, while there are other large and small countries in Asia where the blood programme is non-existent and, if one does exist, it is fragmented, with variable standards even within an individual country. It is not unusual to find a 'state of the art' blood service in the capital city with rather poor services provided in the remote areas, where the blood supply is not assured and is of doubtful safety.

However, the situation is changing as there are countries making tremendous efforts to provide blood to their citizens in line with the progress made in other fields within the health sector.

Transfusion Microbiology, eds John A. J. Barbara, Fiona A. M. Regan and Marcela C. Contreras. Published by Cambridge University Press. © Cambridge University Press 2008.

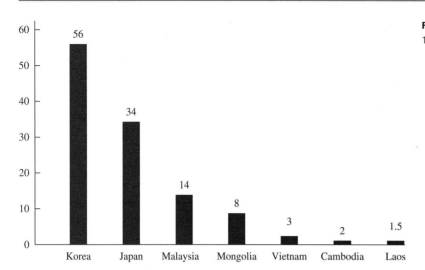

Figure 28.1 Comparison of the number of blood donations per 1000 inhabitants recorded in various Asian countries.

Government commitment in setting up an effective and reliable transfusion service is of utmost importance. The economic situation and, occasionally, political turmoil and social upheaval may prohibit the development of an efficient and effective transfusion service even though resources are available. Sometimes physical barriers, such as oceans, mountains and dense jungle make communication and transportation difficult, thus hindering the implementation of centralized services.

The transfusion service can be examined from different aspects: organization, resources, infrastructure, technical, donor issues and clinical transfusion practices. Safety of blood can be viewed from the standpoint of blood procurement, availability of tests, blood processing and transfusion practices as well as the quality system.

Collection rates in Asia are less than 20 units per 1000 population and, in the majority of countries, less than 10 per 1000 population. Figure 28.1 shows rates of collection in some Asian countries.

Blood procurement

In most Western Pacific countries, the transfusion service grew out of hospitals as part of the laboratory or pathology services. Thus, the hospitals collect blood, process, test and supply according to requests or their needs. It is natural that many hospitals depend on replacement donors. While this is convenient for the hospital, it poses many difficulties for the patients and their relatives (Shan *et al.*, 2002). They are burdened with the problem of deciding who is willing to donate blood in a very stressful situation. Sometimes the patient is from a remote area and finding a donor is difficult. A commercial donor or a paid donor may then be sought. Replacement donors are generally people who are donating for the first time and have never been tested for transfusion-transmitted infection (TTI). Paid donors usually have dubious backgrounds and, under normal circumstances, would not be allowed to donate blood (Luby *et al.*, 2001).

With the emergence of HIV in the 1980s, efforts were made in many countries to phase out replacement donors as the risk of TTI, including HIV, was higher in these individuals (Nantachit *et al.*, 2003). The recruitment of voluntary non-remunerated donors was advocated by the member states in the World

Assembly Resolution WHA 28–72 and is one of the WHO core strategies in developing a national blood transfusion service with the provison of safe blood. This principle was also promoted by the International Federation of Red Cross and Red Crescent Societies and by the International Society of Blood Transfusion.

In Malaysia, the rate of use of replacement donors was 30% in the 1970s. By 2002 the rate had fallen to just over 1%. This is because in remote areas of the country where communication is difficult due to the terrain, the small hospitals do not store enough blood. When there is a sudden need for blood, as in emergencies, donors are called in. A majority of these are relatives of the patient and because of the peculiarities of blood types in these groups of people, only their relatives can donate. However, the situation is different in other parts of Asia. While in Japan and Hong Kong, donors are entirely voluntary and non-remunerated, other countires are still largely dependent on replacement donors.

Strategies are being put in place to phase out replacement donors and to increase voluntary donors. Many countries focus on mobile collections instead of waiting for donors to come to the blood centres, making mobile collection a source of procurement accounting for up to 85% of the total blood supply. Other strategies adopted have been the recruitment of donors from colleges and institutes of higher learning (Abdul-Mujeeb *et al.*, 2000). In Cambodia, for instance, the proportion of youths amongst blood donors rose from 6% in 1998 to 26% in 2002. In Malaysia, 12% of donors were students in 1992 but this rose to 20% by 2002. Similarly, over 70% of donors in Hong Kong are 18–30 years of age.

Sometimes, blood centres have to work within cultures that view blood donation as taboo. In Malaysia, the ethnic Chinese community, which constitutes 40% of the population, only provided 17% of donated blood in 1982. In 2003, 35% of donations came from Chinese donors, reflecting a change in attitude. This is the result of public education and of targeting the young even before they reach an age at which they can donate blood.

Transfusion-transmitted infections

In Asia, it is widely accepted that blood donated for transfusion should be tested for HIV, hepatitis B and syphilis. While screening

Table 28.1 Testing and prevalence of infections in different countries.

Countries	Percentage volunteer	Serological marker prevalence (%)				Type test	National strategy
		HIV	HBsAg	HCV	Syphilis		
Cambodia 2001	21	2.2	10.2	2.1	3.1	EIA/rapid	Yes
China 2001	88	1.8	1.7	0.8	0.22	EIA	Yes
Kiribati 2001	5	2	20	ND	10	Rapid	Yes, before collection
Lavas 2001	89	0.01	7	0.8	0.0	Rapid	Yes
Malaysia 2002	99	0.03	1.5	0.3	0.3	EIA	Yes
Micronesia 2001	15	0	5	ND	3	Rapid	Yes
Mongolia 2001	100	0	10.1	13.3	7.4	EIA/rapid	Yes
Papua New Guinea 2002	30	0.02	17	ND	ND	Rapid	In process
Tonga 2001	33	0.0	10	ND	0	Rapid	Yes, before collection
Vietnam 2001	88	1.8	1.7	0.8	0.22	EIA	Yes

for these TTIs is carried out by almost 100% of countries, hepatitis C is not screened for, for a variety of reasons, but mainly due to high cost (Liu *et al.*, 1997). However, there are countries, especially remote islands, where hepatitis C infection is not prevalent in the general population. Therefore, it seems reasonable not to test for this virus in donated blood. Where the test is offered but the cost is prohibitive, countries choose to screen for hepatitis C only in blood intended for children. In a few countries blood is screened for hepatitis C when the tests are available. Some countries also screen donated blood for malaria parasites, while others screen for this infection only in endemic areas or in donors from endemic areas (Anonymous, 1998; Vu *et al.*, 1995).

Most countries in the region use classical enzyme immunoassays for screening. A few use rapid tests. The reasons for using rapid tests include the small number of units collected, inconsistent electrical and water supplies and fragmented or isolated services due to the remoteness of certain areas or islands (see Table 28.1). A few countries choose to test for hepatitis, syphilis and HIV before blood is collected ('pre-donation testing') using rapid tests. In these countries the rate of hepatitis B infection is high, ranging between 10% and 20% of donors, most of them being replacement donors. Pre-donation testing in these countries has resulted in reducing the amount of blood discarded after donation. However, the same levels of quality are required for pre- as for post-donation testing. (See 'Blood safety in Africa' section.) Sadly, there are still a few countries that have no strategy for screening donated blood for TTIs, no tests are carried out on donated blood and no data are available to determine the prevalence of infections in their population.

Little data is available on transmission of blood-borne infections through blood transfusion. Nucleic acid testing (NAT) is not performed on donated blood in developing countries of Asia, except on a research basis (Bodhiphala *et al.*, 1999; Xing *et al.*, 2002). However, Malaysia performs NAT on donated blood to confirm hepatitis C only when the blood is found anti-HCV EIA reactive and RIBA indeterminate. (Please refer back to Chapter 1.)

Table 28.1 shows epidemiological data from some countries in the region. It is clear that the prevalence of hepatitis B is high in these areas. Where voluntary donations are few, the rate of hepatitis B carriage is higher than where voluntary donations predominate. HIV prevalence in Asia is relatively low compared with developing countries in other regions of the world, except in Thailand, where HIV prevalence is high (Nantachit *et al.*, 2003; Urwijitaroon *et al.*, 1996). Even when the percentage of paid donors is high, the prevalence of HIV amongst donors (which ranges between 0 and 2.2%) is low compared with the prevalence of hepatitis B which ranges between 1.5% and 20% (Louisirirotchanakul *et al.*, 2002; Sulaiman *et al.*, 1995). The true prevalence of HCV is not known, but where HCV testing is performed, the range is between 0.3% and 13.3% (Abdul-Mujeeb *et al.*, 2000; Duraisamy *et al.*, 1993; Khattak *et al.*, 2002; Ng *et al.*, 1995; Tang, 1993; Wang *et al.*, 1994). Regular, voluntary, non-remunerated donors clearly show a much lower rate of transfusion-transmissible infections. For example, in Malaysia, the regular voluntary donors provide approximately 50% of the total annual donations. The rate of TTI in these donations is almost negligible. The donations positive for markers of infection generally come from first-time donors. In an area where the rate of replacement donors is 13%, the prevalence of hepatitis B is 3.5%, while in areas were 100% of donors are voluntary the prevalence is 0.8%. Similarly, in Cambodia the prevalence of hepatitis B and C, HIV and syphilis is much higher amongst replacement donors compared with voluntary donors (see Figure 28.2). In the National Blood Transfusion Centre in Phnom Penh, Cambodia, donors are divided into three categories: spontaneous, external and replacement. Spontaneous donors are those who come to the centre to donate, external donors are those who donate at mobile sessions, and replacement donors are those donating to replace blood that is needed by a particular patient. Where donor selection is in place, the prevalence of infection amongst donors is much lower than in the general population. For example, the prevalence of HIV in donors is 0.03% while, in the general population, it is estimated to be 3.5%. A pre-donation interview is of value, as it was found that 6.6% of deferred donors belonged to a high-risk population. This is especially helpful as

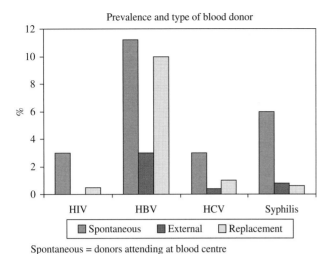

Spontaneous = donors attending at blood centre
External = donors attending at mobile sessions

Figure 28.2 Prevalence of HIV, HBV and HCV markers in volunteer donors at the hospital (spontaneous), volunteer blood collected in mobile sessions (external) and replacement donors from Cambodia. The safety advantage of mobile volunteer blood collection sessions is obvious.

some donors do not understand the donor questionnaire which must be filled out before consent is given.

Little data on disease transmission through blood transfusion in Asia is available. With a very high prevalence of hepatitis B, a considerable number of window-period donations might be expected, for example through sexual transmission to those uninfected in early life. This is difficult to prove, especially when replacement donors are involved, since they may donate but remain untraceable (Chuansumrit *et al.*, 1996; Wang *et al.*, 1994). In many instances they may never donate again. However, where donor information is not recorded centrally, an already identified infected donor may donate in another centre. The need for more effective screening strategies in Asia is apparent.

Conclusion

The blood supply in Asia is safer than it ever was. However, the prevalence of TTI, especially HBV, is high as replacement donors remain a major source of blood. The high cost of some reagents (e.g. anti-HCV) may force some countries to provide untested blood for transfusion or to test only when reagents are available. As children have the greatest potential for longevity, a country with limited resources may choose to test only blood intended for this group of patients. Some countries screen donors before donation proceeds, as the prevalence of HBV may reach 20%. In such settings, no blood is discarded, thus providing some cost-saving. Generally, national policies are evolving towards voluntary non-remunerated donation to collect safer blood. Public education and motivation are then critically needed. When funds are limited and expertise is lacking, it is easy for the policy-makers to focus more on testing rather than ensuring that only safe donors donate blood. However, this actually increases cost as a substantial amount of donated blood is discarded due to TTI.

Blood safety in Africa

In sub-Saharan Africa, blood safety is compromised by many factors. First, the prevalence of TTIs is very high. Second, the transfusion infrastructure comprises mostly small, hospital-based units without the means to implement equipment-dependent assays. Third, in several countries, there is no health expenses coverage and costs are entirely paid for by the patients' families, whose average yearly income ranges between $400 and $1000. As a result, the cost of transfusion has to remain very low to be affordable, hence the massive reliance on external aid which in turn compromises sustainability. However, in a number of countries, blood costs are supported by the governments or hospitals either entirely as in Botswana or Côte d'Ivoire, or only in part, so that the rest of the real cost is recovered from patients. Fourth, national or local strategies to achieve an acceptable level of safety are often devised from 'top-down' instead of the sustainable and more efficient 'bottom-up' approach.

Epidemiology

The epidemiological background of blood-borne viral infections is dominated by the centuries-old endemic HBV infection and the recent epidemic spread of HIV. Table 28.2 shows data collected in the past ten years, mostly from small numbers of blood donors. These figures are only indicative, but reveal a prevalence of HIV antibody positivity ranging between 0.5 and 16%. In first-time donors, it tends to remain below 5% in West Africa, below 10% in East and Central Africa and above 10% in Southern Africa. Rates of hepatitis B indicated by the presence of circulating HBsAg range between 5 and 25% of the population, including blood donors (Allain *et al.*, 2003). This is mainly due to the mode of transmission, which is in part vertical, but mostly horizontal in young children in the virtual absence of national vaccination programmes. Prevalence data in blood donors is not entirely reliable since it depends heavily on the sensitivity of the screening assays used (Allain *et al.*, 2003). HBsAg tends to be more prevalent in West Africa (10–25%) than in East or Central Africa (5–10%); the lowest prevalence is found in Southern Africa (5% or less). Antibody to HCV is not routinely screened for in many parts of Africa but the prevalence of this infection ranges between 0.5 and 3% and reaches 10–15% in Egypt or in localized areas, suggesting the important contribution of local factors such as various types of injections and past diagnostic or vaccination campaigns in the spread of infection (Frank *et al.*, 2000). Most countries do not consider screening for HTLV to be worthwhile since the prevalence is low. In addition, post-transfusion pathogenicity is more of a concern in a few immunosuppressed patients who would be very rare in Africa. Screening for syphilis is debatable, for, while the prevalence is usually high, active infections are rare and refrigeration of blood would inactivate *Treponema pallidum*.

In the few cases where it was studied, the prevalence of *Plasmodium* sp. in donor blood is very high (16–40%), particularly during the rainy season (Achidi *et al.*, 1995; Ibhanesebhor *et al.*, 1996). As a result, all African blood is considered potentially infectious for malaria and preventive treatment of transfused

Table 28.2 Prevalence of transfusion-transmissible agents in sub-Saharan African blood donors.

Country	Year collected	Prevalence (%)					
		HIV	HBV	HCV	HTLV	Syphilis	Malaria
Benin	1998	0.5–3	12	1.4–2.3	0.3–5.4	—	33.5
Botswana	2000	10	5	1	—	—	—
Cameroon	1994–1998	4.1–5.8	10–16	1.6	—	—	—
Ghana	1998–2002	1.7–3.8	15	1.7–8.4	0.5	13.5	—
Kenya	1994	6.4	—	—	—	—	—
	1995–1998	4.5–3.0	4.2–3.9	1.5–1.8	—	—	—
Malawi	2000	10.7	8.1	6.8	2.5	—	—
Nigeria	1992–1998	3.9–5.4	15–20	12.3	0.7	—	19–41
RDC	1998	6.4	9.2	4.3	—	—	—
RSA[a]	2001	4.5	5	0.5	—	—	—
Tanzania	1998	8.7	11	8–10.3	0	12.7	—
Togo	1995–2000	—	—	3.3	1.8	—	—
Uganda	2000	3.9–5.4	—	—	—	—	—
Zambia	1991–1995	8–16	6.5	—	—	—	—
Zimbabwe	1997	8.8	2.5–15.4	—	0.1	—	—

[a] Donors of African origin

RDC = Republique Democratique du Congo (formally Zaire)

RSA Republic of South Africa

young children with anti-malarial drugs is considerably more cost-effective than screening of blood (Ibhanesebhor *et al.*, 1996; Kinde-Gazard *et al.*, 2000).

Organization of transfusion services in sub-Saharan Africa

There is marked variability in the organization of transfusion services in sub-Saharan Africa. For many years, the WHO has encouraged governments to develop national blood policies and create blood centre networks. Considerable effort has gone into developing quality assurance and standard programmes to improve the quality of available blood (Dhingra *et al.*, 2003). A few countries such as Côte d'Ivoire, Benin and Kenya have invested significant resources in blood transfusion services (often with financial and advisory support from European or North American governments) and have committed to establishing centralized systems based on the blood bank model used in wealthy nations (Table 28.3). These centres typically collect over 10 000 units a year, use automated equipment and produce some components. Blood donor recruitment, screening and the processing of donated blood are carried out in specifically designed premises away from the hospitals where blood is transfused.

However, at present, most countries in sub-Saharan Africa do not operate a centralized blood transfusion service. Each hospital recruits donors for its own patients and processes the blood for local transfusion. These hospitals often handle less than 1000 units a year (Nwagbo *et al.*, 1997; Rukundo *et al.*, 1997; Sengeh *et al.*, 1997) and experience difficulties in standardization, quality assurance and maintenance of high quality reagent supply. Recruiting

voluntary donors from the community is complex and expensive and depends on regular education programs, mobile collection teams, vehicles and cold storage. Because of these difficulties, the majority of donors in poorer countries are 'replacement', not volunteer, donors. Patients in poorer countries are usually hospitalized late in the course of their disease and the delays and lack of stored blood inherent in the replacement donor system mean that patients may die before a blood transfusion can be organized. Furthermore, they are often not transfused in most of these countries; the major reasons for blood use in sub-Saharan Africa are childhood anemia (malaria), pregnancy and childbirth, and trauma. Chronic disease is simply not diagnosed, let alone treated. In many of the poorly developed countries blood is often not available and would be allocated on a 'high-priority' basis.

Improving the blood supply and safety with volunteer blood

In most parts of Africa, replacement donors are the main resource for blood donation and account for >80% of the blood supply in sub-Saharan Africa (see Table 28.3). They are typically young males at relatively high risk of HIV infection and other sexually transmitted viruses (Jacobs *et al.*, 1994; McFarland *et al.*, 1998; Sarkodie *et al.*, 2000). Cultural taboos and lack of education about donating blood, with prevailing common beliefs such as 'men will become impotent if they donate blood', or 'HIV can be caught from the blood bag needle', make relatives reluctant to donate, leading to a preference for purchasing blood from 'professional donors'.

As the availability of replacement donors is limited, the most effective way to improve the availability of blood is to recruit and

Table 28.3 Some basic facts about blood transfusion in some sub-Saharan African countries[a].

Country	Units/1000[b]	Percentage replacement donors	Viruses screened for[c]	Cost (US$) Real	Cost (US$) To patients
Cameroon	1.6	88	HIV, HBV	40	6
Rep. Congo	7		HIV, HBV	—	—
Cote d'Ivoire	4.7	<20	HIV, HBV, HCV	45	No cost
Gabon	11.3	—	HIV, HBV, HCV	45	No cost
Guinea	2.2	—	HIV, HBV	40	8
Mali	2.2	—	HIV, HBV	40	8
Rep. Dem. Congo	1.4	—	HIV 50–100%	—	—
Senegal	3.8	—	HIV, HBV, HCV	45	8
Botswana	7	0	HIV, HBV, HCV	10 (supplies)	No cost
Ghana	3	80	HIV, HBV, HCV[d]	15	10–14[e]
Kenya	1.6	60	HIV, HBV	—	—
Malawi	2.5	90	HIV, HBV	12	No cost
Nigeria	—	95	HIV, part HBV	—	—
Tanzania	3.7	>80	HIV, part HBV	12.6–25	—
Zimbabwe	—	0	HIV, HBV, HCV	20–30	Insurance

[a] Most data have been tabulated from abstracts published at the 3rd African Congress of Blood Transfusion (Tunis, 2002) or the French National Congress of Transfusion (St Etienne, France, 2003).

[b] Units of blood collected per 1000 inhabitants.

[c] Screening is performed with EIA in capital blood centres collecting 10–70 000 units/year and with rapid tests in regional or other types of health care settings.

[d] HCV screening started nationwide in 2003.

[e] For patient's families who provide a replacement donor, cost is reduced by 50%.

retain secondary school students as volunteer donors (McFarland et al., 1998; Sarkodie et al., 2000). These are younger (age range 16 to 20), generally less sexually active than older donors, include a larger proportion of females and are five to ten times less likely to be infected with HIV than replacement donors.

Several strategies have been devised to encourage repeat voluntary donors in an attempt to further reduce the risk from virus transmission (Savarit et al., 1992; Schutz et al., 1993) but these recruitment and retention programmes require dedication and funds that are not always available. In Zimbabwe, 'Pledge 25 Club', a programme using education and incentive to attract school students to give blood 25 times, has been largely successful (Mvere 2002). A less ambitious 'Club 5' could also be very effective in many areas. However, during school holidays, alternative strategies need to be devised. These include recruiting donors from faith-based organizations or collaborating with radio stations to organize and promote blood donation sessions (Opare-Sem et al., 2002).

Ultimately, the objective should be that the exclusive source of blood is regular volunteer donors, as already achieved in Botswana and Zimbabwe. However, this will take time, dedication and funds.

Blood screening for blood-transmitted infections

Human immunodeficiency virus has clearly dominated blood safety concerns during the past 15 years and major progress has been made. Some studies have attributed 5–10% of HIV infections in adults to transfusion and up to 40% in children (Beal et al., 1992; Shaffer et al., 1990). At present, on the basis of data provided by the governments of individual countries, the WHO consider that 95% of the blood transfused in sub-Saharan Africa is screened for antibody to HIV. This does not necessarily reflect the situation in the field, particularly in small, remote hospitals, where regular supply remains a major issue. Lack of quality assurance, training of operators and poor kit storage conditions considerably affect the residual risk of transfusion-related infections (Dhingra et al., 2003; Moore et al., 2001).

It is estimated that screening for HBsAg is performed in approximately 70% of the donors but no more than 20% are screened for anti-HCV. In many hospitals, HBsAg is screened with latex agglutination or other rapid tests which have a sensitivity ranging between 50 and 90% compared with EIAs (Allain et al., 2003). The WHO has undertaken some evaluations of both enzyme imunoassays and rapid tests, including test costs to guide developing countries in their choice of reagent. Many rapid tests for anti-HIV but also HBsAg and some for anti-HCV are available on the market but their performance both in terms of sensitivity and specificity, their ease of use and their cost vary greatly. Some of these tests are performed in a single step, with results obtained in 10–15 minutes using whole blood, plasma or serum samples. The best assays have a sensitivity similar to EIA for anti-HIV, detecting 1ng/ml of HBsAg and having >95% sensitivity for anti-HCV and a specificity of >98%.

This is information is based on a commentary by Clark *et al.*, (2005) on an article by Owusu-Ofori *et al.* (2005).

Pre-donation testing – advantages and disadvantages

This approach to blood testing in high endemic, low resource areas was recently described (Opare-Sem *et al.*, 2004; Owusu-Ofori *et al.*, 2005). The advantages include savings on the cost of blood collection bags, a cheaper testing method that does not require instruments, collecting only safe blood, avoiding potential confusion between tested and untested blood, avoiding to increase iron deficiency unnecessarily in unsuitable donors and offering the unique opportunity to indicate to the deferred candidate donor that there is an anomaly in his/her blood, preventing blood donation and requiring confirmation and follow-up. Genomic testing on rapid test negative blood units indicated complete efficacy for anti-HIV, 96% for HBsAg and 65% for anti-HCV. As a result, a new strategy associating front-end pre-donation rapid testing and back-end multiplex NAT was developed and implemented (Owusu-Ofori *et al.*, 2005).

Potential disadvantages of this approach to blood screening were pointed out without offering supporting data (Clark *et al.*, 2005). There are turnaround times of up to two hours to complete the full blood collection process. This may discourage volunteer donors from repeating donation, introduce errors in transcribing results, confidentiality issues and stigmata regarding HIV when blood drives are conducted in public settings. Magnet effect for test seekers and lower skill of operators affecting quality assurance (Clark *et al.*, 2005). Data provided by the group who developed this strategy clearly indicated that these assumptions were neither supported by experience nor evidence in this particular setting in West Africa (Owusu-Ofori *et al.*, 2005).

Residual risk of transfusion-transmission of blood-borne viruses

The present residual risk of viral transmission by transfusion has been assessed for HIV. In studies conducted in Kenya, Zambia and the Democratic Republic of the Congo, the risk of HIV transmission by transfusion was estimated to range between 1 and 3%, related in part to prevalence but also to test performance, storage conditions and staff training (Consten *et al.*, 1997; Mbendi-Nlombi *et al.*, 2001). The residual risk of HBV infection remains substantial in Ghana because of the large proportion of donations containing low, undetected levels of HBsAg or HBV DNA (Allain *et al.*, 2003). This risk remains high for children below age ten, but is, however, mitigated by the very high prevalence of adult recipients carrying HBV markers (60–90%). Our own studies conducted in Ghana evaluated the residual risk of HIV, HCV and HBV transmission at 1:2578, 1:1450 and 1:326, respectively, when using EIA screening (Allain *et al.*, 2003; Candotti *et al.*, 2001). These risks are essentially due to the window period for HIV and HCV and to 'occult' (low level) chronic carriage for HBV (i.e. donors who are HBsAg negative/DNA positive).

Cost of transfusion services in sub-Saharan Africa

Many countries in sub-Saharan Africa have introduced 'fee-for-service' in the health system. In these countries, costs of transfusion are entirely or partially paid for by the patients' families, who have an average income of $400–$1000 per annum. As a result, the cost of transfusion has to remain very low in order to be affordable. This leads to compromises on the quality and safety of blood or to heavy reliance on external aid, thereby threatening sustainability. The cost of a unit of blood should not be so high that patients are discouraged from using it.

Some countries, particularly in the Central and West African French speaking countries, have established government or hospital-financed systems that cover blood costs either totally, as in Côte d'Ivoire and Gabon, or partially, with families paying a fixed price of $7–10/unit that represents less than 25% of the actual cost, as in Guinea, Burkina-Faso or Senegal (see Table 28.3). This situation seems to be specific for blood transfusion, as it does not apply to other health costs.

In most English speaking countries with a 'fee-for-service' policy, blood is provided at cost (when known) or at a centrally established price. In most cases, a replacement donor system, rather than one relying on volunteer donors, reduces the processing cost by 50% to $4–8.

When a transfusion service is provided by individual hospitals, it places an enormous burden on laboratory resources. In a typical district hospital in Malawi in 1997, 39% of all tests performed by the laboratory were transfusion-related. The overall cost of the transfusion service, including consumables, proportional amounts for capital equipment and depreciation, staff time and overheads, was 36% of total laboratory costs. Extrapolating from these figures, each unit of whole blood cost the laboratory approximately $12 to collect and process (Jacobs and Mercer, 1999).

The challenge for Africa is that safe blood should be accessible to all in a continent which has limited health services and extremely limited resources. The majority of the cost of a blood unit originates from imported goods such as the blood bags and grouping and screening assays. Staff costs are a relatively small proportion of the overall costs because salaries are low and negligible resources are put into staff training, supervision and auditing mechanisms. According to published studies, a unit of blood may cost between $10 and $40 (Jacobs and Mercer, 1999), which is not affordable by most families in sub-Saharan Africa. Because blood transfusion is such an expensive service, the costs are often subsidized by the government or external agencies, making resources for transfusion services vulnerable to fickle political and non-sustainable fluctuations (Hensher and Jefferys, 2000). Developing systems that rely more on local resources means that they may be more dynamic, productive and sustainable (Nnodu *et al.*, 2003).

Theoretically, there are several possible cost-saving strategies for transfusion services in sub-Saharan Africa. For example:

(1) Using cheap but effective rapid tests that do not require equipment
(2) A reduction in prices by diagnostic companies for resource-poor countries

Table 28.4 Prevalence of infectious disease markers in blood donors in the region of the Americas during 2001.

Country	anti-HIV	HBsAg	anti-HCV	anti-syphilis	Anti-*T. cruzi*	TOTAL
Argentina	0.18	0.60	0.66	0.92	4.50	6.86
Bolivia	0.04	0.57	0.28	1.54	9.91	12.34
Brazil	0.33	0.88	0.78	1.08	0.65	3.72
Chile	0.04	0.16	0.13	0.88	0.61	1.82
Columbia	0.25	0.48	0.56	1.56	0.67	3.52
Costa Rica	0.05	0.16	0.21	0.38	0.58	1.38
Cuba	0.01	0.70	0.74	0.55	Not required	2.00
Ecuador	0.24	0.27	0.20	0.52	0.08	1.31
El Salvador	0.20	0.43	0.25	0.93	3.70	5.51
Guatemala	3.71	0.93	1.08	2.38	1.48	9.58
Honduras	0.38	0.43	0.65	0.85	1.40	3.71
Mexico	0.20	0.05	0.07	0.02	0.05	0.39
Nicaragua	0.17	0.52	0.28	1.06	0.06	2.09
Panama	0.10	1.70	0.60	0.40	0.90	3.70
Paraguay	0.20	0.52	0.59	4.42	4.46	10.19
Peru	0.10	0.82	0.50	0.89	0.29	2.60
Dominican Rep.	0.42	1.20	0.64	0.86	Not required	3.12
Uruguay 1999	0.07	0.24	0.33	0.57	0.45	1.66
Venezuela	0.25	0.94	0.56	1.40	0.67	3.82
Average	0.37	0.61	0.48	1.12	1.79	4.17

The Pan American Health Organization, Laboratory and Blood Services (2002a) is the source of data for the countries shown.

(3) The avoidance of additional costs to intermediaries

(4) Limiting blood bag waste by pre-donation screening where appropriate (Allain *et al.*, 2003; Mvere *et al.*, 1996).

Confirmatory testing is an expensive process and the WHO has advocated that confirmation of reactive samples with an alternative screening assay, rather than an expensive, highly specific, confirmatory assay is adequate in regions where prevalence is high. This approach contributes to cost reduction. It might also be argued that a test specificity >99.8% is sufficient to avoid the need for confirmation. Much more research that compares the cost-effectiveness of various strategies is needed to further improve the supply of safe blood to patients who live in resource-poor settings.

Latin America

Latin America is composed of 20 countries: Argentina, Bolivia, Brazil, Chile, Colombia, Costa Rica, Cuba, Dominican Republic, Ecuador, El Salvador, Guatemala, Honduras, Mexico, Nicaragua, Panama, Paraguay, Peru, Dominican Republic, Uruguay and Venezuela. The quality of blood banking and transfusion practices throughout these countries is highly variable. Blood banks in major cities like São Paolo and Buenos Aires are essentially comparable with those in developed countries with regard to donor services, infectious disease screening and transfusion practices. In contrast, poverty, high prevalence of infectious diseases, fragmented blood systems and an almost total reliance on replacement donors, are common factors found in most countries. Blood banks are usually less developed appendices of the clinical laboratory and are considered as diagnostic services. This has

led to an over-emphasis on serological testing and relatively little effort is concentrated on donor recruitment and retention, or on encouraging the appropriate use of blood and blood components. Many blood services lack medical direction and technical staff assume overall responsibility. This section will attempt to address the economic, social, cultural, epidemiological and technical factors affecting the quality of blood services in Latin America.

Epidemiology

The epidemiological scenario in Latin America is very complex. In 2001 alone, there were 350 000 cases of dengue fever, and over a million cases of malaria; 50–60:100 000 inhabitants have tuberculosis and close to 4 million people are living with HIV (Pan American Health Organization, 2002a). Table 28.4 shows that, on average, the prevalence of HIV antibody in donors for 2001 was 0.37%; 0.61% for HBsAg; 0.48% for antibodies to HCV and 1.79% for *Trypanosoma cruzi*. Every year, reactivity in screening tests for one or more infectious disease markers defers 4–5% of donors (Pan American Health Organization, 2002b).

Schumins *et al.* estimated that, in 1998, the risk of acquiring an infectious disease through blood transfusion was highest in Bolivia (233:10 000 transfusions) and lowest in Honduras (9:10 000 transfusions) (Schumins *et al.*, 1998). These numbers have improved considerably since this time, as the percentage of screened units has increased substantially. It is important to note, however, that the risk was estimated only on the basis of number of units not screened and that the residual risk due to the window period or testing errors was not included in the calculation.

Table 28.5 National coordination, number of blood banks per country, number of blood units collected from volunteer non-remunerated blood donors, number of blood units collected per blood bank and number of blood units collected per day in 18 countries in the Region of the Americas during 2001.

Country	National coordination	Number of blood banks	Units from VNRBD	Units collected/ blood bank	Units collected/day
Argentina	No	752	ND	1069	4.11
Bolivia	No	60	2700	412	1.59
Brazil	No	3000	0	588	2.26
Chile	No	162	0	1299	5.00
Ecuador	No	39	23 500	1679	6.46
Guatemala	No	47	563	928	3.57
Panama	No	35	514	1,225	4.71
Average		**585**	**4546**	**1029**	**4**
Columbia	Yes	161	75 044	2479	9.54
Costa Rica	Yes	35	27 311	1592	6.12
Cuba	Yes	42	575 203	13 695	52.67
El Salvador	Yes	59	7036	1230	4.73
Honduras	Yes	29	8378	1268	4.88
Mexico	Yes	529	54 499	2146	8.26
Nicaragua	Yes	24	20 207	2056	7.91
Paraguay	Yes	23	1113	2105	8.09
Peru	Yes	160	66 672	2170	8.35
Dominican Republic	Yes	81	10 153	864	3.32
Venezuela	Yes	264	19 200	1310	5.04
Average		**127.91**	**78 620**	**2810.45**	**10.81**

The Pan American Health Organization, Laboratory and Blood Services (2002a) is the source of data for the countries shown.

Trypanosoma cruzi poses by far the highest risk of TTI in the region. Poverty and lack of opportunities have forced migration from rural to urban areas and currently nearly 60% of the population live in or around the cities, increasing the risk of transfusion-transmitted Chagas' disease (Schmunis, 1999). In 2002, almost 450 000 units were not screened for *T. cruzi* (Pan American Health Organization, 2002b). Performance characteristics of certain types of *T. cruzi* screening assays are highly variable and the pressure to use lower-cost kits only increases the risk of poor diagnosis and transmission of this infectious agent.

Structure of transfusion services

In Latin America the number of blood banks ranges between 23 and 150 in the majority of countries; but in countries such as Brazil, Argentina and Mexico the number is much higher (2583, 878 and 524, respectively) (Pan American Health Organization, 2002b; 2003). Blood banks are usually hospital based, and are operated by the ministry of health, the social security system, the Red Cross, the private sector and, in some cases, the armed forces.

Over the past four years the Pan American Health Organization (PAHO) Regional Safe Blood Initiative has been supporting countries in the establishment of nationally coordinated blood programmes. Sixteen countries report having a functional national blood commission; 18 have a national policy and plan but only 12

have a designated budget (Pan American Health Organization, 2002b). Table 28.5 shows that countries with a nationally coordinated blood programme or those working towards one have, on average, fewer blood banks, collect twice as many units per blood bank and have ten times as many volunteer blood donors as countries that are not nationally coordinated.

In 2001, all the countries in Latin America reported having laws and regulations that prohibit paid blood donation and which recognize voluntary blood donation as the optimal strategy for a safe blood supply. Current legal frameworks have provisions for obligatory infectious disease screening and ensure that the ministries of health regulate blood bank operations. However, only 14 countries indicated the existence of an infrastructure regulating the quality of services (Periago, 2003).

Blood screening for transfusion-transmitted infections

Great progress has been made in the region in screening of blood units for infectious agent markers. In 1997, the percentage of blood units that remained untested were 1% for HIV; 1.3% for HBV; 5.8% for hepatitis C and nearly 50% for Chagas' disease. From the latest data available, 7.12 million units were collected in 2002 and the number of untested units has reduced dramatically. Currently, only 0.14% of units are not screened for HIV, 0.21% for HBV, 0.52

for HCV, 0.11% for syphilis and 6.8% for *T. cruzi* (Pan American Health Organization, 2002a; 2003).

The quality of results from serological testing has also greatly improved due to better laboratory practices, training efforts, infectious disease surveillance networks and external quality assessment schemes. The majority of countries in the region also have their own national quality assessment programmes.

There are still many challenges ahead in terms of improving the quality of screening of all donated blood in Latin America, but trying to reduce the number of blood banks carrying out this activity is by far the greatest challenge. In 2002, the average number of units collected per day per blood bank was 8.5 (Pan American Health Organization, 2003). Having such a low number of available units to test daily, forces blood banks either to delay testing until a suitable number of units is assembled, or to test what is available and consume large amounts of controls. Only in well organized, regional centres can resources and the necessary range of staff be concentrated for a more efficient and safer process.

Donor demographics

In order to determine the number of available donors in Latin America it is useful to examine the latest demographic data. In 2002, over half of the population of Latin America was between 17–60 years of age (the accepted upper and lower age limits for blood donation). In any given year, 2% of the population are women of childbearing age, pregnant and unable to donate blood. Women in Latin America have an average of 4.5 children, which eliminates them from the donor pool for 12–15 years. Therefore, it is not surprising that 70% of donors in Latin America are males (Pan American Health Organization, 2002a).

The economic status of the country also has clear implications for the availability of safe blood donors. The World Bank estimated that, in the year 2002, 50% of the population in Latin America lived below the poverty level, earning less than $2 per day (Pan American Health Organization, 2002a). As these individuals are themselves struggling to survive, the number of potential donors is greatly reduced.

Financial resources required to promote and retain volunteer blood donors are scarce. The collection rate for Latin America is approximately 14 units per 1000 inhabitants (Schmunis, 1999). Only Cuba reports that 100% of units transfused are obtained from voluntary blood donors (Pan American Health Organization, 2002b) but, in the majority of countries, donors are usually family or friends of patients who are asked to replace transfused blood. Information on the number of paid donations is not available since most paid donors present themselves as family members or friends. Countries such as Honduras estimate that 8–9% of donors are paid (Honduras National Blood Commission, 2003), and, in 2001, Panama reported that 47.9% of units collected were from paid donors (Pan American Health Organization, 2002b).

There are few studies that determine the risk of transfusion-transmitted infections according to the status of the donors. Salles *et al.* have shown that in a very large blood bank in São Paulo (Brazil) the number of blood units discarded because of infectious disease marker reactivity decreased from 20% to 9% over a ten-year period. This was attributed to the fact that over that period of time, the number of regular donors had increased from 10% in 1991 to 50% in 2001 (Salles *et al.*, 2003). Vinelli and Velàsquez have reported that replacement donors in Honduras are at least three times more likely to test positive for an infectious disease marker than voluntary blood donors (Vinelli, 2005).

In 2001, the PAHO Laboratory and Blood Services Unit carried out a study to determine knowledge, attitude and practices relating to voluntary blood donation in the region. Fifteen countries participated in the study. It revealed that donation venues were uncomfortable and unattractive, waiting times unacceptably long and donor selection criteria inconsistent from one blood bank to another. Donors expressed a need for more information in order to overcome fears and myths and reiterated the fact that they would like to be reminded of the need to donate blood regularly (Gutiérrez *et al.*, 2003).

Notification and counselling of donors carrying an infectious agent is an essential element in ensuring a safe blood supply. There is no official data as to how many Latin American countries actually notify donors about their serological status, but it is our opinion that the lack of availability of confirmatory tests, rudimentary record systems that limit donor traceability and the fact that only a few countries have access to treatment for infectious donors, are all factors that negatively affect the notification of donors.

Cost

The Pan American Health Organization has estimated that the cost of processing a unit of blood in Latin America ranges from US $30 to $150 (Pan American Health Organization, 2002b). This variability is due primarily to the technical and financial efficiency of the different blood banks. In the year 2000, the total allocation for health care per capita was $52 in Honduras, $53 in Guatemala and $36 in Haiti (Pan American Health Organization, 2002a). The cost of collecting, testing and storing a unit of donated blood in these countries in most instances exceeds the annual per capita budget allocation to health care (Cruz Roja Hondureña, 2003).

As mentioned earlier, almost half of all Latin American countries have no formal budget allocation to sustain blood activities, thus forcing patients and family members to support this cost themselves, which in turn greatly reduces access to safe blood products for a substantial fraction of the population. Cruz and Perez have reported that, in Latin America, the countries with the highest Gross National Product (GNP) have 8.5 times as much blood available per capita as the lowest GNP countries (1.79/0.21) (Cruz and Pérez-Rosales, 2003).

Conclusion

Despite the considerable progress made by the developing world to ensure a sufficient supply of safer blood in spite of the lack of resources, many improvements are still needed. This requires a clear strategy at central government level to organize volunteer donor recruitment, and a continuous supply of high quality reagents and quality assurance programmes. However, most of the burden remains with the blood banks themselves to find ways of improving supply and safety by astutely choosing what best meets their local needs and means. External support is critical, provided it is dispensed within the local context and has the key objective of ensuring sustainability. In the coming few years, it would be unrealistic to believe that the standards prevalent in Western countries can be met until the basic infrastructure of communication, power supply and equipment maintenance is in place and corruption within the system is reduced to a minimum.

Acknowledgements

The authors thank Dr Yu Junping, WHO Manila and Dr Chhorn Samnang, NBTC Phnom Penh, Cambodia for their contribution. They also thank Dr S. Owusu-Ofori from Komfo Anokye Teaching Hospital, Kumasi, Ghana and Dr I. Bates, Liverpool School of Tropical Medicine, Liverpool, UK.

REFERENCES

Abdul-Mujeeb, S., Aamir, K. and Mehmood, K. (2000) Seroprevalence of HBV, HCV and HIV infections among college-going first-time voluntary blood donors. *J Pak Med Assoc*, **50**, 269–70.

Achidi, E. A., Perlmann, H. and Berzins, K. (1995) Asymptomatic malaria parasitaemia and seroreactivities to *Plasmodium falciparum* antigens in blood donors from Ibadan, south-western Nigeria. *Ann Trop Med Parasitol*, **89**, 601–10.

Allain, J.-P., Candotti, D., Soldan, K., *et al.* (2003) The risk of hepatitis B virus infection by transfusion in Kumasi, Ghana. *Blood*, **101**, 2419–25.

Anonymous (1998) Malaria situation in the People's Republic of China in 1997. *Zhongguo Ji Sheng Chong Xue Yu Ji Sheng Chong Bing Za Zhi*, **16**, 161–3.

Beal, R. W., Bontick, M. and Fransen, L. (eds) (1992) Safe blood in developing countries. *Brussels: EEC AIDS Task Force*, 11–2.

Bodhiphala, P., Chaturachumroenchai, S., Chiewsilp, P., *et al.* (1999) Detection of HBV genome by gene amplification method in HBsAg negative blood donors. *J Med Assoc Thai*, **82**, 491–5.

Candotti, D., Sarkodie, F. and Allain, J.-P. (2001) Residual risk of transfusion in Ghana. *Br J Haematol*, **113**, 37–9.

Chuansumrit, A., Varavithya, W., Isarangkura, P., *et al.* (1996) Transfusion-transmitted AIDS with blood negative for anti-HIV and HIV-antigen. *Vox Sang*, **71**, 64–5.

Clark, K., Kataaha, P., Mwangi, J., *et al.* (2005) Predonation testing of potential blood donors in resource-restricted settings. *Transfusion*, **45**, 130–2.

Consten, E. C., van der Meer, J. T., de Wolf, F., *et al.* (1997) Risk of iatrogenic human immunodeficiency virus infection through transfusion of blood tested by inappropriately stored or expired rapid antibody assays in a Zambian hospital. *Transfusion*, **37**, 930–4.

Cruz, J. and Pérez-Rosales, M. (2003) Availability, safety, and quality of blood for transfusion in the Americas. *Rev Panam Salud Publica/Pan Am J Public Health*, **13**, 103–9.

Cruz Roja Hondureña (2003) Reporte Anual de Actividades 2002. Comayaguela, MDC. cenasa@honduras.cruzroja.org.

Dhingra, N., Hafner, V. and Xueref, S. (2003) Hemovigilance in countries with scarce resources – a WHO perspective. *Transf Alt Transf Med*, **5**, 277–84.

Duraisamy, G., Zuridah, H. and Ariffin, M. Y. (1993) Prevalence of hepatitis C virus antibodies in blood donors in Malaysia. *Med J Malaysia*, **48**, 313–6.

Frank, C., Mohammed, M. K., Strickland, G. T., *et al.* (2000) The role of parenteral antischistosomal therapy in the spread of hepatitis C virus in Egypt. *Lancet*, **355**, 887–91.

Gutierrez, M., Sáenz, E. and Cruz, J. (2003) Estudio de factores socioculturales relacionados con la donación voluntaria de sangre en las Américas. *Rev Panam Salud Publica/Pan Am J Public Health*, **13**, 85–90.

Hensher, M. and Jefferys, E. (2000) Financing blood transfusion services in sub-Saharan Africa: a role for user fees? *Health Policy Plan*, **15**, 287–95.

Honduras National Blood Commission (2003). Report of the Current Situation of Blood Banks and Transfusion Services. Tegucigalpa, MDC.

Ibhanesebhor, S. E., Otobo, E. S. and Ladipo, O. A. (1996) Prevalence of malaria parasitaemia in transfused donor blood in Benin City, Nigeria. *Ann Trop Paediatr*, **16**, 93–5.

Jacobs, B. and Mercer, A. (1999) Feasibility of hospital-based blood banking: a Tanzanian case study. *Health Policy Plan*, **14**, 354–62.

Jacobs, B., Berege, Z. A., Schalula, P. J. J., *et al.* (1994) Secondary school students: a safer blood donor population in an urban area with high HIV prevalence in East Africa. *East Afr Med J*, **71**, 720–3.

Khattak, M. F., Salamat, N., Bhatti, F. A., *et al.* (2002) Seroprevalence of hepatitis B, C and HIV in blood donors in northern Pakistan. *J Pak Med Assoc*, **5**, 398–402.

Kinde-Gazard, J., Oke, J., Gnahoui, I., *et al.* (2000) The risk of malaria transmission by blood transfusion at Cotonou, Benin. *Sante*, **10**, 389–92.

Liu, P., Shi, Z. X., Zhang, Y. C., *et al.* (1997) A prospective study of a serum-pooling strategy in screening blood donors for antibody to hepatitis C virus. *Transfusion*, **37**, 732–6.

Louisirirotchanakul, S., Myint, K. S., Srimee, B., *et al.* (2002) The prevalence of viral hepatitis among the Hmong people of northern Thailand. *Southeast Asian J Trop Med Public Health*, **33**, 837–44.

Luby, S. P., Niaz, Q., Siddiqui, S., *et al.* (2001) Patients' perceptions of blood transfusion risks in Karachi, Pakistan. *Int J Infect Dis*, **5**, 24–6.

Mbendi-Nlombi, C., Longo-Mbenza, B., Mbendi-Nsukini, S., *et al.* (2001) Prevalence du VIH et de l'antigene HBs chez les donneurs du sang. Risque residuel de contamination chez les receveurs de sang a Kinshasa-est, Republique Democratique du Congo. *Med Trop*, **61**, 139–42.

McFarland, W., Mvere, D., Shamu, R., *et al.* (1998) Risk factors for HIV seropositivity among first-time blood donors in Zimbabwe. *Transfusion*, **38**, 279–84.

Moore, A., Herrera, G., Nyamongo, J., *et al.* (2001) Estimated risk of HIV transmission by blood transfusion in Kenya. *Lancet*, **358**, 657–60.

Mvere, D., Constantine, N. T., Katsawde, E., *et al.* (1996) Rapid and simple hepatitis assays: encouraging results from a blood donor population in Zimbabwe. *Bull World Health Organ*, **74**, 19–24.

Mvere, D. A. (2002) Evaluation of the pledge 25 club: a youth donor recruitment programme in Zimbabwe. 27th Int Congress of the ISBT, Vancouver, abstract 684.

Nantachit, N., Robison, V., Wongthanee, A., *et al.* (2003) Temporal trends in the prevalence of HIV and other transfusion-transmissible infections among blood donors in northern Thailand, 1990 through 2001. *Transfusion*, **43**, 730–5.

Ng, K. P., Saw, T. L., Wong, N. W., *et al.* (1995) The prevalence of anti-HCV antibody in risk groups and blood donors. *Med J Malaysia*, **50**, 302–5.

Nnodu, O. E., Odunukwe, N., Odunubi, O., *et al.* (2003) Cost effectiveness of autologous blood transfusion: a developing country hospital's perspective. *West Afr J Med*, **22**, 10–2.

Nwagbo, D., Nwakoby, B. and Akpala C. (1997) Establishing a blood bank at a small hospital, Anambra State, Nigeria. The Enugu PMM Team *Int J Gynaecol Obstet*, **59** (Suppl. 2), S135–9.

Opare-Sem, O., Owusu-Ofori, S. and Allain, J.-P. (2002) A novel approach to blood safety: pre-donation screening of blood donors for viral markers. *Africa Sanguine*, **5**, 12–6.

Owusu-Ofori, S., Temple, J., Sarkodie, F., *et al.* (2005) Predonation screening of blood donors with rapid tests: implementation and efficacy of a novel approach to blood safety in resource poor settings. *Transfusion*, **45**, 133–40.

Owusu-Ofori, S., Temple, J., Sarkodie, F., *et al.* (2005) Pre-donation of blood donors in resource-poor settings. *Transfusion*, **45**, 1542–3.

Pan American Health Organization (2002a) *La Salud en las Américas.* **1**, pp. 6–8, 100, 169, 332, 335, 337–9, 344. Washington, OPS.

Pan American Health Organization. (2002b) *Medicina Transfusional en América Latina.* pp. 39–47. Washington, OPS/HSE-LAB/09.

Pan American Health Organization (2003) *Medicina Transfusional en América Latina.* pp. 55–9. Washington OPS/EV-LAB/01.

Periago, M. (2003) Promoting Quality Blood Services in the region of the Americas. *Rev Panam Salud Publica/Pan Am J Public Health*, **13**, 73–4.

Rukundo, H., Tumwesigye, N. and Wakwe, V. C. (1997) Screening for HIV I through the regional blood transfusion service in southwest Uganda: the Mbarara experience. *Health Transit Rev*, **7** (Suppl.), 101–4.

Salles, S., *et al.* (2003) Descarte de bolsas de sangue e prevalencia de doencas infecciosas em doadores de sangue da Fundacao Prò-Sangue/Hemocentro de Sao Paolo. *Rev Panam Salud Publica/Pan Am J Public Health*, **13**, 111–5.

Sarkodie, F., Adarkwa, M., Adu-Sarkodie, Y., *et al.* (2000) Screening for viral markers in volunteer and replacement blood donors in West Africa. *Vox Sang*, **80**, 142–7.

Savarit, D., De Cock, K. M., Schutz, R., *et al.* (1992) Risk of HIV infection from transfusion with blood negative for HIV antibody in a west African city. *BMJ*, **305**, 498–502.

Schmunis, G. (1999) Riesgo de la Enfermedad de Chagas a través de la Transfusión en las Américas. *Medicina (Buenos Aires)*, **59** (Suppl. II), 125–34.

Schumins, G. A., Zxicer F., Pinheiro F., *et al.* (1998) Risk for Transfusion Transmitted Infectious Diseases in Central and South America. *Jour of Emerg Infec Dis*, **4**, 5–11.

Schutz, R., Savarit, D., Kadjo, J. C., *et al.* (1993) Excluding blood donors at high risk of HIV infection in a West African city. *Brit Med J*, **307**, 1517–9.

Sengeh, P., Samai, O., Sidique, S. K., *et al.* (1997) Improving blood availability in a district hospital, Bo, Sierra Leone. *The Bo PMM Team. Int J Gynaecol Obstet*, **59** (Suppl. 2), S127–34.

Shaffer, N., Hedberg, K. and Davachi F. (1990) Trends and risk factors for HIV-1 seropositivity among outpatient children, Kinshasa, Zaire. *AIDS*, **4**, 1231–6.

Shan, H., Wang, J. X., Ren, F. R., *et al.* (2002) Blood banking in China. *Lancet*, **360**, 1770–5.

Sulaiman, H. A., Julitasari, Sie, A., *et al.* (1995) Prevalence of hepatitis B and C viruses in healthy Indonesian blood donors. *Trans R Soc Trop Med Hyg*, **89**, 167–70.

Tang, S. (1993) Seroepidemiological study on hepatitis C virus infection among blood donors from various regions in China. *Zhonghua Liu Xing Bing Xue Za Zhi*, **14**, 271–4.

Urwijitaroon, Y., Barusrux, S., Romphruk, A., *et al.* (1996) Reducing the risk of HIV transmission through blood transfusion by donor self-deferral. *Southeast-Asian J Trop Med Public Health*, **27**, 452–6.

Vinelli, E. (2005) Taking a closer look at blood donation in Latin America. *Dev Biol*, **120**, 139–44.

Vu, T. T., Tran, V. B., Phan, N. T., *et al.* (1995) Screening donor blood for malaria by polymerase chain reaction. *Trans R Soc Trop Med Hyg*, **89**, 44–7.

Wang, Y. J., Lee, S. D., Hwang, S. J., *et al.* (1994) Incidence of post-transfusion hepatitis before and after screening for hepatitis C virus antibody. *Vox Sang*, **67**, 187–90.

Xing, W., Xu, H., Ma, R., *et al.* (2002) HCV RNA assessment by PCR technique for screening post-transfusion HCV infection among blood donors. *Zhonghua Gan Zang Bing Za Zhi*, **10**, 211–2.

SUBJECT INDEX

Note: Glossary is located on pages xviii–xix